CONTENTS

SECTION 1

Principles of Patient-Focused Therapy

Section Editor: *Terry L. Schwinghammer*

SECTION 2

Cardiovascular Disorders

Section Editor: *Julia M. Koehler*

SECTION 3

Respiratory Disorders

Section Editor: *Julia M. Koehler*

SECTION 4

Gastrointestinal Disorders

Section Editor: *Jill S. Borchert*

SECTION 5

Renal Disorders

Section Editor: *Jill S. Borchert*

Schwinghammer's
Pharmacotherapy
Casebook

Schwinghammer's Pharmacotherapy Casebook

A Patient-Focused Approach

Twelfth Edition

Editors

Terry L. Schwinghammer, PharmD, FCCP, FASHP, FAPhA

Professor Emeritus
Department of Clinical Pharmacy
School of Pharmacy
West Virginia University
Morgantown, West Virginia

Julia M. Koehler, PharmD, FCCP

Professor and Associate Dean for Clinical Education and External Affiliations
College of Pharmacy and Health Sciences
Butler University
Indianapolis, Indiana

Jill S. Borchert, PharmD, BCACP, BCPS, FCCP

Professor and Vice Chair
Department of Pharmacy Practice
College of Pharmacy
Midwestern University
Downers Grove, Illinois

Douglas Slain, PharmD, BCPS, FCCP, FASHP

Professor and Chair
Department of Clinical Pharmacy
School of Pharmacy
West Virginia University
Infectious Diseases Clinical Specialist
WVU Medicine and Ruby Memorial Hospital
Morgantown, West Virginia

Sharon K. Park, PharmD, MEd, BCPS

Associate Professor and Assistant Dean for Academic Affairs
Department of Clinical and Administrative Sciences
School of Pharmacy
Notre Dame of Maryland University
Clinical Pharmacy Specialist
Drug Information and Medication Use Policy
The Johns Hopkins Hospital
Baltimore, Maryland

A companion workbook for *DiPiro's Pharmacotherapy: A Pathophysiologic Approach,* 12th ed.
DiPiro JT, Yee GC, Haines ST, Nolin TD, Ellingrod V, Posey LM, eds. New York, NY: McGraw Hill, 2023.

New York   Chicago   San Francisco   Athens   London   Madrid   Mexico City
Milan   New Delhi   Singapore   Sydney   Toronto

Schwinghammer's Pharmacotherapy Casebook: A Patient-Focused Approach, Twelfth Edition

Copyright © 2023 by McGraw Hill. All rights reserved. Printed in the United States of America. Except as permitted under the United States Copyright Act of 1976, no part of this publication may be reproduced or distributed in any form or by any means, or stored in a database or retrieval system, without the prior written permission of the publisher.

1 2 3 4 5 6 7 8 9   LWI   28 27 26 25 24 23

ISBN 978-1-264-27848-0
MHID 1-264-27848-9

This book was set in Minion by KnowledgeWorks Global Ltd.
The editors were Michael Weitz and Peter J. Boyle.
The production supervisor was Richard Ruzycka.
Project management was provided by Nitesh Sharma, KnowledgeWorks Global Ltd.
The designer was Alan Barnett.
This book was printed on acid-free paper.

Cataloging-in-publication data for this book is on file at Library of Congress.

McGraw Hill books are available at special quantity discounts to use as premiums and sales promotions, or for use in corporate training programs. To contact a representative, please visit the Contact Us pages at www.mhprofessional.com.

SECTION 10

Urologic Disorders

Section Editor: *Terry L. Schwinghammer*

SECTION 11

Immunologic Disorders

Section Editor: *Terry L. Schwinghammer*

SECTION 12

Bone and Joint Disorders

Section Editor: *Sharon K. Park*

SECTION 13

Eyes, Ears, Nose, and Throat Disorders

Section Editor: *Terry L. Schwinghammer*

SECTION 14

Dermatologic Disorders

Section Editor: *Terry L. Schwinghammer*

SECTION 15

Hematologic Disorders

Section Editor: *Terry L. Schwinghammer*

SECTION 16

Infectious Diseases

Section Editor: *Douglas Slain*

SECTION 17

Oncologic Disorders
Section Editor: Terry L. Schwinghammer

SECTION 18

Nutrition and Nutritional Disorders

Section Editor: *Terry L. Schwinghammer*

SECTION 19

Complementary and Alternative Therapies
(Level III) 423

Section Editor: *Terry L. Schwinghammer*

APPENDICES

CONTRIBUTORS

Marie A. Abate, BS, PharmD

Professor of Clinical Pharmacy, Department of Clinical Pharmacy, School of Pharmacy, West Virginia University; Assistant Dean for Assessment and Strategic Planning, West Virginia University, School of Pharmacy, Morgantown, West Virginia

Stephanie Abel, PharmD, BCPS

Opioid Stewardship Program Coordinator, University of Kentucky HealthCare, Lancaster, Kentucky

Nicole Paolini Albanese, PharmD, CDE, BCACP

Clinical Associate Professor, Department of Pharmacy Practice, School of Pharmacy and Pharmaceutical Sciences, University at Buffalo; Clinical Pharmacist in Ambulatory Care, Buffalo Medical Group, P.C., Buffalo, New York

Kwadwo Amankwa, PharmD, BCPS

Clinical Pharmacy Specialist, Advanced Heart Failure and Recovery Program, Norton Audubon Hospital, Louisville, Kentucky

Jarrett R. Amsden, PharmD, BCPS

Associate Professor, Department of Pharmacy Practice, Butler University College of Pharmacy & Health Sciences; Infectious Diseases Clinical Pharmacist, Community Health Network, Indianapolis, Indiana

Sarah L. Anderson, PharmD, FASHP, FCCP, BCACP, BCPS

Scientific Director, Clinical Care Options, Denver, Colorado

Lori T. Armistead, MA, PharmD

Senior Research Associate, Division of Practice Advancement and Clinical Education, UNC Eshelman School of Pharmacy, Chapel Hill, North Carolina

Albert Bach, PharmD, APh

Assistant Professor of Pharmacy Practice, Chapman University School of Pharmacy, Irvine, California

Elizabeth Bald, PharmD, BCACP

Assistant Professor (Clinical), Department of Pharmacotherapy, University of Utah College of Pharmacy; Clinical Pharmacist, Madsen Family Health Clinic, Salt Lake City, Utah

Aimee M. Banks, PharmD, BCPS, MSCS

Pharmacy Clinical Team Lead, Specialty Pharmacy Services, Multiple Sclerosis and Neuroimmunology Clinic, Vanderbilt University Medical Center, Nashville, Tennessee

Kimberly M. Beck, PhD, RPh

Associate Professor and Pharmacy Program Director, Pharmaceutical Sciences, College of Pharmacy and Health Sciences, Butler University, Indianapolis, Indiana

Morgan Belling, PharmD, BCOP

Clinical Pharmacy Specialist – Stem Cell Transplant and Cellular Therapy, The University of Texas MD Anderson Cancer Center, Houston, Texas

Erin L. Berry, PharmD, BCPS

Clinical Assistant Professor, Department of Pharmacy Practice, College of Pharmacy, Idaho State University, Pocatello; Clinical Pharmacist in Adult Medicine, Eastern Idaho Regional Medical Center, Idaho Falls, Idaho

Michael A. Biddle, Jr., PharmD, BCPS

Ambulatory Care Pharmacist, Saint Luke's Health System, Boise, Idaho

Amie Taggart Blaszczyk, PharmD, BCPS, BCGP, FASCP

Professor & Division Head – Geriatrics, Department of Pharmacy Practice, Texas Tech University HSC School of Pharmacy – Dallas/Fort Worth, Dallas, Texas

Meghan M. Bodenberg, PharmD, BCPS

Professor of Pharmacy Practice and Director of Advanced Experiential Education and Preceptor Development, Butler University College of Pharmacy & Health Sciences, Indianapolis, Indiana

Scott Bolesta, PharmD, BCPS, FCCM, FCCP

Associate Professor, Department of Pharmacy Practice, Nesbitt School of Pharmacy, Wilkes University; Clinical Pharmacist in Critical Care, Wilkes-Barre General Hospital, Wilkes-Barre, Pennsylvania

Kevin M. Bozymski, PharmD, BCPS, BCPP

Assistant Professor, Department of Clinical Sciences, Medical College of Wisconsin School of Pharmacy, Milwaukee, Wisconsin

Jessica H. Brady, PharmD, BCPS

Clinical Professor and Associate School Director, School of Clinical Sciences, College of Pharmacy, University of Louisiana Monroe; Clinical Pharmacist in Internal Medicine, Ochsner-LSU Health Monroe Medical Center, Monroe, Louisiana

Trisha N. Branan, PharmD, BCCCP

Clinical Associate Professor and Assistant Department Head – Professional Education, Department of Clinical and Administrative Pharmacy, University of Georgia College of Pharmacy, Athens, Georgia

Jamal Brown, PharmD, BCGP

Associate Professor of Pharmacy Practice, Florida A&M University, Tampa; Clinical Pharmacist in Ambulatory Care, Tampa General Medical Group, Tampa, Florida

Rodrigo M. Burgos, PharmD, MPH

Clinical Assistant Professor, College of Pharmacy, Department of Pharmacy Practice, University of Illinois at Chicago, Infectious Diseases Pharmacotherapy Section, Chicago, Illinois

Elizabeth A. Cady, PharmD, BCPS

Clinical Assistant Professor, Department of Pharmacy Practice, Southern Illinois University at Edwardsville School of Pharmacy, Edwardsville; Clinical Infectious Diseases Pharmacist, HSHS St. John's Hospital, Springfield, Illinois

Lauren Camaione, BS, PharmD, BCPPS

Pediatric Infectious Diseases Clinical Specialist, University of Rochester Medical Center, Rochester, New York

Matthew A. Cantrell, PharmD, BCPS

Clinical Associate Professor, Department of Pharmacy Practice & Science, University of Iowa College of Pharmacy; Clinical Pharmacy Specialist, Iowa City VA Health Care System, Iowa City, Iowa

Krista D. Capehart, PharmD, MS, BCACP, FAPhA, AE-C

Clinical Associate Professor, Department of Clinical Pharmacy, School of Pharmacy, West Virginia University, Morgantown; Director of Professional and Regulatory Affairs at the West Virginia Board of Pharmacy, Charleston, West Virginia

Katie E. Cardone, PharmD, BCACP, FNKF, FASN, FCCP

Associate Professor and Doctor of Pharmacy Program Director, Department of Pharmacy Practice, Albany College of Pharmacy and Health Sciences, Albany, New York

Juliana Chan, PharmD, FCCP, BCACP

Clinical Associate Professor, College of Pharmacy, Deparment of Pharmacy Practice, College of Medicine, Division of Gastroenterology and Hepatology, University of Illinois at Chicago; Clinical Pharmacist, Gastroenterology/Hepatology, Illinois Department of Corrections Hepatology Telemedicine, University of Illinois Hospital and Health Sciences System, Chicago, Illinois

Stephanie Chase, PharmD, BCOP

Clinical Pharmacist Specialist – Malignant Hematology/Bone Marrow Transplantation & Cellular Therapy, University of Colorado Hospital, Aurora, Colorado

Jennifer Y. Chen, MD

Assistant Professor, Department of Neurology, Robert Wood Johnson School of Medicine, Rutgers University, New Brunswick, New Jersey

Amber Chiplinski, PharmD, BCPS

Clinical Pharmacy Specialist, Antithrombotic Stewardship, WVU Medicine J.W. Ruby Memorial Hospital, Morgantown, West Virginia

Christo L. Cimino, PharmD, BCPS, BCIDP

Clinical Pharmacist Specialist, Infectious Diseases, PGY2 Infectious Diseases Pharmacy Residency Program Director, Nashville, Tennessee

Amber B. Cipriani, PharmD, BCOP

Precision Medicine Pharmacy Coordinator, UNC Health Medical Center; Clinical Assistant Professor, Division of Pharmacotherapy and Experimental Therapeutics, UNC Eshelman School of Pharmacy, Chapel Hill, North Carolina

Rebecca Clawson, MAT, PA-C

Clinical Assistant Professor, PA Program, School of Allied Health Professions, Louisiana State University Health Sciences Center – Shreveport, Shreveport, Louisiana

Tracy J. Costello, PharmD, BCPS

Associate Professor of Pharmacy Practice, Butler University College of Pharmacy and Health Sciences, Indianapolis, Indiana; Clinical Pharmacy Specialist, Family Medicine, Community Health Network, Indianapolis, Indiana

Elizabeth A. Coyle, PharmD, FCCM, BCPS

Associate Dean for Academic Affairs, Clinical Professor, Department of Pharmacy Practice and Translational Research, University of Houston College of Pharmacy, Houston, Texas

Brian L. Crabtree, PharmD

Dean and Professor of Pharmacy Practice, Mercer University College of Pharmacy, Atlanta, Georgia

Daniel J. Crona, PharmD, PhD, CPP

Assistant Professor, Division of Pharmacotherapy and Experimental Therapeutics, UNC Eshelman School of Pharmacy, University of North Carolina; Clinical Pharmacist Practitioner, Genitourinary Malignancies, Department of Pharmacy, University of North Carolina Health Care and the North Carolina Cancer Hospital, Chapel Hill, North Carolina

Aaron Cumpston, PharmD, BCOP

Pharmacy Clinical Specialist – BMT/Hematological Malignancy, West Virginia University Medicine, Morgantown, West Virginia

Kendra M. Damer, PharmD

Associate Professor of Pharmacy Practice, Butler University College of Pharmacy and Health Sciences, Indianapolis, Indiana

Jessica Michaud Davis, PharmD, BCOP, CPP

Clinical Pharmacist Coordinator, Adult Hematology/Oncology, Levine Cancer Institute, Charlotte, North Carolina

Lisa E. Davis, PharmD, FCCP, BCPS, BCOP

Clinical Professor, Department of Pharmacy Practice & Science, R. Ken Coit College of Pharmacy, The University of Arizona; Clinical Pharmacist, Hematology-Oncology, Banner University Medical Center Tucson/The University of Arizona Cancer Center, Tucson, Arizona

Christopher M. Degenkolb, PharmD, BCPS

Clinical Pharmacy Specialist, Internal Medicine, Richard L. Roudebush Veterans Affairs Medical Center, Indianapolis, Indiana

Paulina Deming, PharmD, PhC

Clinical Associate Professor, Department of Pharmacy Practice, College of Pharmacy, University of New Mexico Health Sciences Center; Clinical Pharmacist, Center for Digestive Diseases HCV Clinic, University of New Mexico, Albuquerque; Assistant Director – Viral Hepatitis Programs, Project ECHO, University of New Mexico Health Sciences Center, Albuquerque, New Mexico

Brandon Dionne, PharmD, BCPS-AQ ID, BCIDP, AAHIVP

Associate Clinical Professor, Department of Pharmacy and Health Systems Sciences, School of Pharmacy and Pharmaceutical Sciences, Northeastern University; Clinical Pharmacist – Infectious Diseases, Brigham and Women's Hospital, Boston, Massachusetts

Holly S. Divine, PharmD, BCACP, BCGP, CDCES, FAPhA

Clinical Professor, Department of Pharmacy Practice and Science, University of Kentucky College of Pharmacy, Lexington, Kentucky

Gabriella Douglass, PharmD, BCACP, AAHIVP, BC-ADM, TTS

Clinical Pharmacist and Residency Program Director, ARcare, Searcy, Arkansas

Emily Drwiega, PharmD, BCIDP, BCPS, AAHIVP

Infectious Diseases Pharmacy Fellow, University of Illinois Chicago, College of Pharmacy, Chicago, Illinois.

David P. Elliott, PharmD, FASCP, FCCP, AGSF, BCGP

Professor and Associate Chair, Department of Clinical Pharmacy, School of Pharmacy, West Virginia University Health Sciences Charleston Campus; Internal Medicine Clinic Pharmacist, Charleston Area Medical Center, Charleston, West Virginia

Kathy Eroschenko, PharmD

Pharmacy Program Manager, Federal Employee Program, Eagle, Idaho

Brian L. Erstad, PharmD, FCCP, MCCM, FASHP

Professor and Head, Department of Pharmacy Practice and Science, The University of Arizona College of Pharmacy, Tucson, Arizona

Alisa K. Escano, PharmD, BCPS

Assistant Professor, Virginia Commonwealth University School of Pharmacy, Inova Campus, Falls Church, Virginia

Jeffery D. Evans, PharmD

Director and Associate Professor, School of Clinical Sciences, College of Pharmacy, University of Louisiana Monroe, Monroe, Louisiana

Virginia H. Fleming, PharmD, BCPS

Clinical Associate Professor, Department of Clinical and Administrative Pharmacy, University of Georgia, College of Pharmacy, Athens, Georgia

Rachel W. Flurie, PharmD, BCPS

Assistant Professor, Department of Pharmacotherapy & Outcomes Science, School of Pharmacy, Virginia Commonwealth University, Richmond; Clinical Pharmacist in Internal Medicine, Virginia Commonwealth University Health System, Richmond, Virginia

Ryan Flynn, PharmD

PGY 2 Infectious Diseases Pharmacy Resident, HSHS St. John's Hospital, Hartley, Iowa

Michelle Fravel, PharmD, BCPS

Clinical Associate Professor, Department of Pharmacy Practice and Science, University of Iowa College of Pharmacy, Iowa City, Iowa

Mary E. Fredrickson, PharmD, BCPS

Assistant Professor of Pharmacy Practice, Director of Instructional Labs, Director of Alumni Relations, Northeast Ohio Medical University, College of Pharmacy, Rootstown, Ohio

Sharon Gatewood, PharmD, BCACP, FAPhA

Associate Professor, Department of Pharmacotherapy & Outcomes Science, Virginia Commonwealth University, School of Pharmacy, Richmond, Virginia

Jane M. Gervasio, PharmD, FCCP, BCNSP

Professor of Pharmacy Practice, College of Pharmacy and Health Sciences, Butler University, Indianapolis, Indiana

Brett E. Glasheen, PharmD

Clinical Pharmacist, Rheumatology and Gastroenterology, University of Utah Health, Salt Lake City, Utah

Michael J. Gonyeau, BS, MEd, PharmD, FNAP, FCCP, BCPS

Clinical Professor, Department of Pharmacy and Health Systems Sciences, School of Pharmacy and Pharmaceutical Sciences, Northeastern University; Clinical Pharmacist in Internal Medicine, Brigham and Women's Hospital, Boston, Massachusetts

Jean-Venable "Kelly" R. Goode, PharmD, BCPS, FAPhA, FCCP

Professor and Director, PGY-1 Community-Based Pharmacy Residency Program, School of Pharmacy, Virginia Commonwealth University, Richmond, Virginia

Jaime L. Gray, PharmD, BCCCP, FCCM

System Directory Medication Safety & Policy, Temple University Health System, Philadelphia, Pennsylvania

Anthony J. Guarascio, PharmD, BCPS

Associate Professor and Division Head, Division of Pharmacy Practice, Duquesne University School of Pharmacy, Pittsburgh, Pennsylvania

Wayne P. Gulliver, MD, FRCPC

Professor of Medicine and Dermatology, Faculty of Medicine, Memorial University of Newfoundland, Newfoundland, Canada

John G. Gums, PharmD, FCCP

Associate Dean for Clinical and Administrative Affairs, College of Pharmacy, University of Florida; Professor of Pharmacy and Medicine, Colleges of Pharmacy and Medicine, University of Florida, Gainesville, Florida

Jennifer R. Guthrie, MPAS, PA-C

Associate Professor and Director of Experiential Education for the Physician Assistant Program, Butler University College of Pharmacy & Health Sciences, Indianapolis, Indiana

Sasha Haarberg, PharmD, BCOP

Clinical Oncology Pharmacist, Siteman Cancer Center, Washington University School of Medicine, St. Louis, Missouri

Deanne Hall, PharmD, CDCES, BCACP

Associate Professor of Pharmacy and Therapeutics, University of Pittsburgh School of Pharmacy, Ambulatory Care Clinical Specialist, UPMC Heart and Vascular Institute; Director PGY2 Ambulatory Care Residency, UPMC Presbyterian Shadyside, Pittsburgh, Pennsylvania

Suzanne C. Harris, PharmD, BCPP, CPP

Assistant Professor, Clinical Pharmacist Practitioner – Psychiatry, Director of Well-Being and Resilience, UNC Eshelman School of Pharmacy, UNC Hospitals and Clinics, Chapel Hill, North Carolina

Deborah A. Hass, PharmD, BCOP, BCPS

Associate Professor of Pharmacy Practice, West Coast University School of Pharmacy, Los Angeles, California

Jason J. Heavner, MD, FCCP

Chair for Department of Pulmonary and Critical Care Medicine and Associate Chair of Medicine, University of Maryland Baltimore Washington Medical Center, Glen Burnie, Maryland

Mojdeh S. Heavner, PharmD, BCPS, BCCCP, FCCM

Associate Professor and Vice Chair for Clinical Services, Department of Pharmacy Practice and Science, University of Maryland School of Pharmacy, Baltimore, Maryland

Keith A. Hecht, PharmD, BCOP

Associate Professor Pharmacy Practice, Southern Illinois University Edwardsville, School of Pharmacy, Edwardsville, Illinois

Brian A. Hemstreet, PharmD, FCCP, BCPS

Associate Dean for Student Affairs and Professor, Department of Clinical Pharmacy, University of Colorado, Skaggs School of Pharmacy and Pharmaceutical Sciences, Aurora, Colorado

Karl Hess, PharmD, APh, CTH, CMWA, FCPhA, FAPhA

Associate Professor of Pharmacy Practice, Director of Community Pharmacy Practice Innovations, Chapman University School of Pharmacy, Irvine, California

Sarah Hittle, PharmD, BCCCP

Medical ICU Clinical Pharmacy Specialist, Ascension St. Vincent Indianapolis Hospital, Indianapolis, Indiana

Brittany Hoffmann-Eubanks, PharmD, MBA

Founder & CEO, Banner Medical LLC, Frankfort, Illinois

Jennifer Hoffmann, MS, CRNP-BC, MPH

Nurse Practitioner, University of Maryland Baltimore School of Medicine, Baltimore, Maryland

Lisa M. Holle, BS Pharm, PharmD, BCOP, FHOPA, FISOPP

Clinical Professor, University of Connecticut School of Pharmacy, Department of Pharmacy Practice and Clinical Professor, University of Connecticut School of Medicine, Carole & Ray Neag Comprehensive Cancer Center, Storrs, Connecticut

Vanthida Huang, PharmD, FCCP

Professor, Department of Pharmacy Practice, College of Pharmacy-Glendale Campus, Midwestern University, Glendale; Clinical Pharmacist in Infectious Disease, HonorHealth John C. Lincoln Medical Center, Phoenix, Arizona

Yvonne C. Huckleberry, PharmD, BCPS, FCCM

Critical Care Pharmacist, Medical Intensive Care Unit, Banner University Medical Center Tucson; Clinical Associate Professor, Department of Pharmacy Practice and Science, University of Arizona College of Pharmacy, Tucson, Arizona

Franklin Huggins, PharmD, BCPPS, BCCCP

Clinical Associate Professor, Department of Clinical Pharmacy, West Virginia University School of Pharmacy; Pediatric Clinical Specialist, CAMC Women & Children's Hospital, Charleston, West Virginia

Carrie L. Isaacs, PharmD, CDCES, MLDE

Clinical Pharmacy Specialist in Primary Care, Lexington VA Medical Center, Lexington, Kentucky

Timothy J. Ives, PharmD, MPH, FCCP, CPP

Professor of Pharmacy and Medicine, UNC Eshelman School of Pharmacy, Chapel Hill, North Carolina

Haley N. Johnson, PharmD, BCPS

Assistant Professor, Pharmacy Practice, St. Louis College of Pharmacy at University of Health Sciences and Pharmacy in St. Louis; Clinical Pharmacy Specialist, Internal Medicine, Barnes-Jewish Hospital, St. Louis, Missouri

Alexis R. Jones, PharmD, BCOP, CPP

Clinical Pharmacist, Gynecologic Oncology, UNC Health Medical Center; Adjunct Assistant Professor of Clinical Education, UNC Eshelman School of Pharmacy, Chapel Hill, North Carolina

Laura L. Jung, BS Pharm, PharmD

Senior Medical Writer, PRECISIONscientia, Yardley, Pennsylvania

Marina Kanos, MSN, FNP-C, RN, BSBA

Advanced Practice Provider, Adult Medical Oncology, Levine Cancer Institute, Charlotte, North Carolina

Michael D. Katz, PharmD

Professor, Dept. of Pharmacy Practice & Science; Director of Residency Programs; Director of International Programs, R. Ken Coit College of Pharmacy, University of Arizona, Tucson, Arizona

David M. Kaylor, PharmD

PGY2 Internal Medicine Pharmacy Resident, Department of Pharmacy, UofL Health – UofL Hospital, Louisville, Kentucky

Michael B. Kays, PharmD, FCCP, BCIDP

Associate Professor, Department of Pharmacy Practice, Purdue University College of Pharmacy, West Lafayette and Indianapolis, Indiana; Adjunct Associate Professor, Department of Medicine, Indiana University School of Medicine; Clinical Specialist, Infectious Diseases, Eskenazi Health, Indianapolis, Indiana

S. Travis King, PharmD

Clinical Pharmacy Specialist, Department of Pharmacy, Ochsner Medical Center – New Orleans, New Orleans, Louisiana

Cynthia K. Kirkwood, PharmD, BCPP

Professor and Executive Associate Dean for Academic Affairs, School of Pharmacy, Virginia Commonwealth University, Richmond, Virginia

Erika L. Kleppinger, PharmD, BCPS

Associate Clinical Professor, Department of Pharmacy Practice, Harrison School of Pharmacy, Auburn University, Auburn, Alabama

Jonathan M. Kline, PharmD, BCPS, CDE

Director of Pharmacy, Jefferson Medical Center; Adjunct Clinical Professor of Pharmacy, West Virginia University School of Pharmacy, Morgantown, West Virginia

Vanessa T. Kline, PharmD, BCPS

Pharmacist, Winchester Medical Center, Winchester, Virginia

Julia M. Koehler, PharmD, FCCP

Associate Dean for External Affiliations; Professor, Department of Pharmacy Practice, College of Pharmacy & Health Sciences, Butler University, Indianapolis, Indiana

Denise M. Kolanczyk, PharmD, BCPS

Associate Professor, Department of Pharmacy Practice, Midwestern University College of Pharmacy Downers Grove Campus, Downers Grove; Clinical Pharmacist in Internal Medicine, Loyola University Medical Center, Maywood, Illinois

Brian J. Kopp, PharmD, BCCCP, BCPS, FCCM

Clinical Pharmacist, Surgical Trauma ICU, Banner – University Medical Center Tucson; Clinical Associate Professor, Department of Pharmacy Practice and Science, The University of Arizona College of Pharmacy, Tucson, Arizona

Michael D. Kraft, PharmD, BCNSP

Clinical Professor, Department of Clinical Pharmacy, College of Pharmacy, University of Michigan; Assistant Director–Education & Research, Department of Pharmacy Services, Michigan Medicine, Ann Arbor, Michigan

Margaret Landis, PharmD

Pharmacist, Kroger Pharmacy, Blacksburg, Virginia

Kena J. Lanham, PharmD, BCPS, BCGP, BCCP

Clinical Pharmacist Specialist, Cardiothoracic Vascular Transplant Unit, Ascension Saint Vincent Indianapolis, Indianapolis, Indiana

Lisa LaVallee, MD

Family Medicine Residency Program Director, MAHEC, Asheville; Clinical Associate Professor, UNC School of Medicine Division of Family Medicine, Chapel Hill, North Carolina

Rebecca M. Law, BScPharm, PharmD

Associate Professor, School of Pharmacy and Faculty of Medicine, Memorial University of Newfoundland, St. John's, Newfoundland

Mary Lee, PharmD, BCPS, FCCP

Professor of Pharmacy Practice, Midwestern University College of Pharmacy – Downers Grove; Vice President and Special Assistant to the President, Midwestern University, Downers Grove, Illinois

Cara Liday, PharmD, CDCES

Associate Professor & Co-Chair, Department of Pharmacy Practice, College of Pharmacy, Idaho State University; Clinical Pharmacist, InterMountain Medical Clinic, Pocatello, Idaho

Kristen L. Longstreth, PharmD, BCPS

Associate Professor of Pharmacy Practice, Director of Workforce Development Office of Student Success, Northeast Ohio Medical University, College of Pharmacy, Rootstown, Ohio

Cheen Lum, PharmD, BCPP

Clinical Specialist in Behavioral Care, Community Hospital North; Ambulatory Care Pharmacist, Behavioral Care, Community Health Network, Indianapolis, Indiana

Cole D. Luty, PharmD, BCPS

Assistant Professor of Pharmacy Practice, Manchester University College of Pharmacy, Natural and Health Sciences; Clinical Pharmacy Specialist, Internal Medicine, Parkview Health, Fort Wayne, Indiana

Mark Lutz, MPAS, PA-C

Assistant Professor, Department of PA Studies, College of Pharmacy & Health Sciences, Butler University, Indianapolis, Indiana

Robert MacLaren, BSc (Pharm), PharmD, MPH, FCCM, FCCP

Professor, University of Colorado Skaggs School of Pharmacy and Pharmaceutical Sciences, Aurora, Colorado

Rebecca J. Mahan, PharmD, BCGP, BCACP, FASCP

Assistant Professor – Geriatrics, Department of Pharmacy Practice – Abilene, Texas Tech University HSC School of Pharmacy, Abilene, Texas

Howard I. Maibach, MD

Professor, Department of Dermatology, School of Medicine, University of California San Francisco, San Francisco, California

Erik D. Maki, PharmD, BCPS

Associate Professor and Chair, Clinical Sciences Department, College of Pharmacy and Health Sciences, Drake University, Des Moines, Iowa

Jonathan W. Malara, PharmD, BCOP

Clinical Pharmacy Specialist, Breast Medical Oncology, Division of Pharmacy, The University of Texas MD Anderson Cancer Center, Houston, Texas

Joel C. Marrs, PharmD, MPH, FAHA, FASHP, FCCP, FNLA, BCACP, BCCP, BCPS, CLS

Professor and Coordinator of Clinical Outreach, Department of Clinical Pharmacy & Translational Science, College of Pharmacy, the University of Tennessee Health Science Center, Nashville, Tennessee

Jay L. Martello, PharmD, BCPS

Clinical Associate Professor, Department of Clinical Pharmacy, School of Pharmacy, West Virginia University; Clinical Pharmacist in Internal Medicine, West Virginia University Medicine, Morgantown, West Virginia

Craig Martin, PharmD, MBA

Professor and Associate Dean (Chief Operating Officer), University of Kentucky College of Pharmacy, Lexington, Kentucky

Michelle T. Martin, PharmD, FCCP, BCPS, BCACP

Clinical Associate Professor, Department of Pharmacy Practice, College of Pharmacy, University of Illinois at Chicago; Clinical Pharmacist, University of Illinois Hospital and Health Sciences System, Chicago, Illinois

Katelynn Mayberry, PharmD

Clinical Assistant Professor, Department of Pharmacy Practice, Atlanta, Georgia

Lena Maynor, PharmD, BCPS

Professor, Department of Clinical Pharmacy, School of Pharmacy, West Virginia University; Director of Student Affairs and Academic Initiatives, West Virginia University Health Sciences Centre, Morgantown, West Virginia

Ziemowit Mazur, PhD, EdM, MS, PA-C

Associate Program Director, Rosalind Franklin University of Medicine and Science, College of Health Professions, Physician Assistant Program, North Chicago, Illinois

James W. McAuley, RPh, PhD, FAPhA

Professor of Pharmacy Education & Innovation and Neurology; Associate Dean for Academic Affairs, The Ohio State University College of Pharmacy, Columbus, Ohio

Sea-Oh McConville, DO

Associate Director and Women's Health Director, Heritage Valley Family Medicine Center, Beaver Falls, Pennsylvania

William McGhee, PharmD

Clinical Pharmacist, UPMC Children's Hospital of Pittsburgh, Pittsburgh, Pennsylvania

Ashlee McMillan, PharmD, BCACP

Clinical Associate Professor, Department of Clinical Pharmacy, School of Pharmacy, West Virginia University, Morgantown, West Virginia

Brian McMillan, MD

Clinical Associate Professor, Department of Ophthalmology, West Virginia University School of Medicine, Morgantown, West Virginia

Sarah T. Melton, PharmD, BCPP, BCACP, FASCP

Professor of Pharmacy Practice, Gatton College of Pharmacy at East Tennessee State University, Johnson City, Tennessee

Renee-Claude Mercier, PharmD, PhC, BCPS-AQID, FCCP

Professor of Pharmacy and Medicine, University of New Mexico Health Sciences Center; Associate Medical Director, Truman Health Services, UNM Medical Group, Albuquerque, New Mexico

Lindsey Miller, PharmD, BCPP

Associate Professor, Pharmacy Practice, Lipscomb University College of Pharmacy; Clinical Pharmacist, Vanderbilt Psychiatric Hospital, Nashville, Tennessee

Ronni Miller, PharmD, BCOP

Clinical Pharmacist, Thoracic Oncology, University of Colorado Hospital; Clinical Course Instructor, University of Colorado, Skaggs School of Pharmacy and Pharmaceutical Sciences, Aurora, Colorado

Rachel C. Minrath, PharmD

PGY1 Pharmacy Resident, Lexington VA Medical Center, Lexington, Kentucky

Benjamin Miskle, PharmD

Clinical Assistant Professor, University of Iowa College of Pharmacy; Clinical Pharmacy Specialist – Psychiatry, University of Iowa Health Care, Iowa City, Iowa

Marta A. Miyares, PharmD, BCPS, BCCP, CACP

Clinical Pharmacy Specialist, Internal Medicine & Anticoagulation, Jackson Memorial Hospital
Director, PGY1 Residency Program, Miami, Florida

Christie R. Monahan, PharmD

Pharmacy Postdoctoral Fellow, Departments of Pharmacotherapy & Translational Research and Community Health & Family Medicine, Colleges of Pharmacy and Medicine, University of Florida, Gainesville, Florida

Cynthia Moreau, PharmD, BCACP

Clinical Ambulatory Pharmacy Specialist
Baptist Health South Florida, Boca Raton, Florida

Allison L. Morse, PharmD, BCOP

Pharmacist, Clinical Coordinator, Department of Hematologic Oncology and Blood Disorders, Levine Cancer Institute, Charlotte, North Carolina

Scott W. Mueller, PharmD, FCCM, FCCP, BCCCP

Clinical Associate Professor, University of Colorado Skaggs School of Pharmacy and Pharmaceutical Sciences; Burn Service Pharmacy Clinical Specialist, University of Colorado Health, Aurora, Colorado

Ryan P. Mynatt, PharmD, BCPS

Clinical Pharmacist, Infectious Diseases and Outpatient Parenteral Antimicrobial Therapy (OPAT), University of Kentucky HealthCare, Lexington, Kentucky

James J. Nawarskas, PharmD, BCPS

Associate Professor, Department of Pharmacy Practice and Administrative Sciences, College of Pharmacy, University of New Mexico, Albuquerque, New Mexico

Leigh Anne Nelson, PharmD, BCPP

Professor, Pharmacy Practice and Administration, University of Missouri-Kansas City School of Pharmacy, Kansas City, Missouri

Branden D. Nemecek, PharmD, BCPS

Associate Professor, Division of Pharmacy Practice, Duquesne University School of Pharmacy; Clinical Pharmacist, University of Pittsburgh Medical Center – Mercy Hospital, Pittsburgh, Pennsylvania

Jenna Nikolaides, MD

Assistant Professor of Emergency Medicine, Medical Toxicology and Addiction Medicine, Departments of Emergency Medicine and Psychiatry; Medical Director, Substance Use Intervention Team, Department of Psychiatry, Rush University Medical Center, Chicago, Illinois

Jason Noel, PharmD, BCPP

Associate Professor, University of Maryland School of Pharmacy, Baltimore, Maryland

Kimberly J. Novak, PharmD, BCPS, BCPPS, FPPA

Advanced Patient Care Pharmacist, Pediatric and Adult Cystic Fibrosis, Nationwide Children's Hospital; Clinical Assistant Professor (adjunct), The Ohio State University, College of Pharmacy, Columbus, Ohio

Cindy L. O'Bryant, PharmD, BCOP

Professor, Department of Clinical Pharmacy, Skaggs School of Pharmacy and Pharmaceutical Sciences; Clinical Pharmacist Specialist – Gastrointestinal Cancer and Phase 1 Clinical Trials, University of Colorado Cancer Center, Aurora, Colorado

Dannielle C. O'Donnell, BS, PharmD

Adjunct Clinical Assistant Professor, College of Pharmacy, The University of Texas, Austin, Texas

Vishal Ooka, PharmD, BCCCP

Trauma Neuro Critical Care Clinical Pharmacy Specialist, Ascension St. Vincent Indianapolis Hospital, Indianapolis, Indiana

Linda B. Ou, BScPharm, PharmD, MSc

Clinical Pharmacist, Department of Pharmacy, Sunnybrook Health Sciences Centre, Toronto, Ontario, Canada

Manjunath (Amit) P. Pai, PharmD, FCP

Professor and Chair, Department of Clinical Pharmacy, Deputy Director of the PK Core, College of Pharmacy, University of Michigan, Ann Arbor, Michigan

Neha Sheth Pandit, PharmD, AAHIVP, BCPS

Associate Professor, Department of Pharmacy Practice and Science, University of Maryland School of Pharmacy, Baltimore, Maryland

Laura Panko, MD, FAAP

Assistant Professor of Pediatrics, University of Pittsburgh School of Medicine, Pediatric Hospitalist, Paul C. Gaffney Division of Pediatric Hospital Medicine, UPMC Children's Hospital of Pittsburgh, Pittsburgh, Pennsylvania

Dennis Parker, Jr., PharmD, FCCM

Associate Professor Pharmacy Practice, Eugene Applebaum College of Pharmacy and Health Sciences, Wayne State University, Detroit, Michigan

Robert B. Parker, PharmD, FCCP

Professor, University of Tennessee Health Science Center, Department of Clinical Pharmacy and Translational Science, Memphis, Tennessee

Chris Paxos, PharmD, BCPP, BCPS, BCGP

Professor, Pharmacy Practice; Director, Pharmacotherapy, Northeast Ohio Medical University, Rootstown, Ohio

Jacob R. Peters, PharmD, BCPP, BCPS

Assistant Professor of Pharmacy Practice, College of Pharmacy and Health Sciences, Butler University; Psychiatric Clinical Pharmacy Specialist, Indiana University Health, Indianapolis, Indiana

Rebecca S. Pettit, PharmD, MBA, BCPS, BCPPS, FCCP

Pediatric Pulmonary Ambulatory Pharmacy Specialist; PGY2 Pediatric Residency Program Director, Riley Hospital for Children at Indiana University Health, Indianapolis, Indiana

Nicole C. Pezzino, PharmD, BCACP, CDCES

Director of Community Outreach & Innovation, Wilkes University, Nesbitt School of Pharmacy, Associate Professor of Pharmacy Practice, Wilkes University, Nesbitt School of Pharmacy; Director of PGY-1 Community-based Residency Program, Weis Markets/Wilkes University, Wilkes-Barre, Pennsylvania

Beth Bryles Phillips, PharmD, FCCP, FASHP, BCPS, BCACP

Rite Aid Professor and Assistant Department Head for Residency Programs, University of Georgia College of Pharmacy, Athens, Georgia

Melissa R. Pleva, PharmD, BCNPS, BCCCP

Pharmacy Manager – CVC, Surgery and Cardiovascular Services, Michigan Medicine; Adjunct Clinical Assistant Professor, University of Michigan College of Pharmacy, Ann Arbor, Michigan

Charles D. Ponte, BS, PharmD, BC-ADM, BCPS, CDES, FADCES, FAPhA, FASHP, FCCP, FNAP

Professor Emeritus of Clinical Pharmacy and Medicine, School of Pharmacy and School of Medicine, West Virginia University, Morgantown, West Virginia

Brecon C. Powell, PharmD

Clinical Associate Professor, Idaho State University College of Pharmacy, Idaho Falls, Idaho

Caroline Quinn, PharmD, BCOP

Clinical Pharmacy Specialist, Breast Medical Oncology, Division of Pharmacy, The University of Texas MD Anderson Cancer Center, Houston, Texas

Erin C. Raney, PharmD, FCCP, BCPS, BC-ADM

Professor of Pharmacy Practice, Midwestern University College of Pharmacy, Glendale Campus, Glendale, Arizona

Paul M. Reynolds, PharmD, BCCCP

Assistant Professor, University of Colorado Skaggs School of Pharmacy and Pharmaceutical Sciences, Aurora, Colorado

Denise H. Rhoney, PharmD, FCCP, FCCM, FNCS

Ron and Nancy McFarlane Distinguished Professor, UNC Eshelman School of Pharmacy, Chapel Hill, North Carolina

Tamara Richards, PharmD, BCPS

Assistant Professor of Pharmacy Practice, Florida A&M University, Tampa; Clinical Pharmacist in Internal Medicine, Tampa General Hospital, Tampa, Florida

Natalie I. Rine, PharmD, BCPS, BCCCP

Clinical Assistant Professor of Pharmacy Practice, Northeast Ohio Medical University College of Pharmacy, Rootstown; Clinical Toxicology Fellow, Central Ohio Poison Center – Nationwide Children's Hospital, Columbus, Ohio

Kami Roake, PharmD

Clinical Pharmacist, Rheumatology and Gastroenterology, University of Utah Health and Clinics, Salt Lake City, Utah

Kelly C. Rogers, PharmD, BCCP, FCCP, FACC

Professor, Department of Clinical Pharmacy and Translational Science, University of Tennessee Health Science Center, Memphis, Tennessee

Carol J. Rollins, MS, RD, PharmD, BCNSP, FASPEN, FASHP

Clinical Professor, Department of Pharmacy Practice and Science, College of Pharmacy, The University of Arizona, Tucson, Arizona

Rochelle Rubin, PharmD, BCPS, CDCES

Assistant Director, Ambulatory Pharmacy Services, Lahey Hospital and Medical Center, Acton, Massachusetts

Laura Ruekert, PharmD, BCPP, BCGP

Clinical Specialist in Behavioral Care, Community Hospital North; Associate Professor of Pharmacy Practice, Butler University, Indianapolis, Indiana

Rachel Marie E. Salas, MD, MEd, FAAN, FANA, FAASM

Professor, Neurology and Nursing at Johns Hopkins Medicine; Director, Interprofessional Education and Interprofessional Collaborative Practice; Director, Neurology Clerkship, Baltimore, Maryland

Laurel Sampognaro, PharmD

Director of Student Success, Clinical Professor, School of Clinical Pharmacy, College of Pharmacy, University of Louisiana Monroe, Monroe, Louisiana

Elizabeth J. Scharman, PharmD, DABAT, BCPS, FAACT

Professor, Department of Clinical Pharmacy, School of Pharmacy, West Virginia University Health Sciences Center Charleston Division; Clinical Toxicologist and Director, West Virginia Poison Center, Charleston, West Virginia

Justin M. Schmidt, PharmD, BCPS

Clinical Pharmacist in Home-Based Primary Care, Edward Hines Jr. VA Hospital, Hines, Illinois

Kristine S. Schonder, PharmD

Associate Professor, Department of Pharmacy and Therapeutics, University of Pittsburgh School of Pharmacy, Pittsburgh, Pennsylvania

Christie Schumacher, PharmD, BCPS, BCACP, BCCP, BC-ADM, CDCES, FCCP

Professor, Pharmacy Practice, Director, PGY2 Ambulatory Care Residency Program, Midwestern University College of Pharmacy, Downers Grove; Clinical Pharmacist, Advocate Medical Group, Chicago, Illinois

Terry L. Schwinghammer, PharmD, FCCP, FASHP, FAPhA

Professor Emeritus, Department of Clinical Pharmacy, School of Pharmacy, West Virginia University, Morgantown, West Virginia

Mollie Ashe Scott, PharmD, BCACP, CPP, FASHP

Regional Associate Dean and Clinical Associate Professor, UNC Eshelman School of Pharmacy, Asheville, North Carolina

Roohollah Sharifi, MD, FACS

Professor of Surgery and Urology, University of Illinois at Chicago College of Medicine; Section Head of Urology, Jesse Brown Veterans Administration Medical Center, Chicago, Illinois

Amy Heck Sheehan, PharmD

Professor, Department of Pharmacy Practice, Purdue University College of Pharmacy; Drug Information Specialist, Indiana University Health Center for Medication Management, Indianapolis, Indiana

Kelly M. Shields, PharmD

Associate Dean and Professor of Pharmacy Practice, College of Pharmacy, Ohio Northern University, Ada Ohio

Carrie A. Sincak, PharmD, BCPS, FASHP

Associate Dean of Clinical Affairs, Professor of Pharmacy Practice, Midwestern University College of Pharmacy, Downers Grove, Illinois

Douglas Slain, PharmD, BCPS, FCCP, FASHP

Professor & Chair, Department of Clinical Pharmacy; Infectious Diseases Clinical Specialist, West Virginia University, Morgantown, West Virginia

Carmen B. Smith, PharmD, BCPS

Associate Professor, Pharmacy Practice, St. Louis College of Pharmacy at University of Health Sciences and Pharmacy in St. Louis; Clinical Pharmacy Specialist, Internal Medicine, SSM Health Saint Louis University Hospital, St. Louis, Missouri

Steven M. Smith, PharmD, MPH, FCCP

Assistant Professor of Pharmacy, Department of Pharmacotherapy & Translational Research, College of Pharmacy, University of Florida; Associate Director, Center for Integrative Cardiovascular and Metabolic Disease, University of Florida, Gainesville, Florida

Susan E. Smith, PharmD, BCCCP, BCPS

Clinical Associate Professor, Department of Clinical and Administrative Pharmacy, University of Georgia College of Pharmacy, Athens, Georgia

Mikayla L. Spangler, PharmD, BCPS

Associate Professor of Pharmacy Practice and Family Medicine, Creighton University School of Pharmacy and Health Professions and School of Medicine, Omaha, Nebraska

Tracy L. Sprunger, PharmD, BCPS

Professor of Pharmacy Practice, Butler University College of Pharmacy and Health Sciences, Indianapolis, Indiana

Sneha Baxi Srivastava, PharmD, BCACP, CDCES, DipACLM, CDE

Associate Professor and Associate Director of Skills Education, Rosalind Franklin University College of Pharmacy; Clinical Pharmacist, Lake County Health Department, North Chicago, Illinois

Mary K. Stamatakis, PharmD

Professor, Department of Clinical Pharmacy, Senior Associate Dean of Academic Affairs and Educational Innovation, School of Pharmacy, West Virginia University, Morgantown, West Virginia

Autumn Stewart-Lynch, PharmD, BCACP, BC-ADM, CTTS

Associate Professor, Department of Pharmacy Practice, Duquesne University School of Pharmacy, Pittsburgh; Clinical Pharmacist, Heritage Valley Family Medicine, Beaver Falls, Pennsylvania

Rebecca H. Stone, PharmD, BCPS, BCACP, FCCP

Clinical Associate Professor, Department of Clinical and Administrative Pharmacy, College of Pharmacy, University of Georgia, Athens, Georgia

Siddharth F. Swamy, PharmD, BCPS, BCIDP

Clinical Assistant Professor, Department of Pharmacy Practice and Administration, Ernest Mario School of Pharmacy, Rutgers University, Piscataway; Clinical Pharmacy Specialist, Infectious Diseases, Hackensack University Medical Center, Hackensack, New Jersey

Jennifer L. Swank, PharmD, BCOP

Clinical Pharmacy Specialist Medical Oncology, Moffitt Cancer Center, Tampa, Florida

Gregory B. Tallman, PharmD, MS, BCPS, BCIDP

Assistant Professor, Department of Pharmacy Practice, School of Pharmacy, Pacific University, Hillsboro, Oregon

Heather M. Teufel, PharmD, BCCCP

Associate Director of Pharmacy, Penn Medicine Chester County Hospital, West Chester, Pennsylvania

Teresa C. Thakrar, PharmD, BCOP

Clinical Pharmacist in Hematology/Stem Cell Transplant/Cellular Therapies, Indiana University Health, Indianapolis, Indiana

Sterling C. Torian, PharmD

PGY2 Critical Care Pharmacy Resident & Instructor, University of Colorado, Skaggs School of Pharmacy and Pharmaceutical Sciences, Aurora, Colorado

Trent G. Towne, PharmD, BCPS, BCIDP

Professor and Vice Chair of Pharmacy Practice, Manchester University College of Pharmacy, Natural and Health Sciences; Clinical Pharmacy Specialist, Infectious Diseases, Parkview Health, Fort Wayne, Indiana

Tran H. Tran, PharmD, BCPS

Associate Professor, Department of Pharmacy Practice, Midwestern University, Downers Grove; Clinical Pharmacist, Substance Use Intervention Team, Department of Psychiatry, Rush University Medical Center, Chicago, Illinois

Natalie Tucker, PharmD, BCPS, BCIDP

Clinical Pharmacy Specialist, Antimicrobial Stewardship; PGY2 Infectious Diseases Residency Program Director, HSHS St. John's Hospital, Springfield, Illinois

Kevin M. Tuohy, PharmD, BCPS

Associate Professor of Pharmacy Practice, Butler University College of Pharmacy and Health Sciences; Clinical Pharmacy Specialist – Internal Medicine, IU Health Methodist Hospital, Indianapolis, Indiana

R. Brigg Turner, PharmD

Associate Professor, Department of Pharmacy Practice, School of Pharmacy, Pacific University, Hillsboro, Oregon

Veronica P. Vernon, PharmD, BCPS, BCACP, NCMP

Assistant Professor of Pharmacy Practice, Butler University College of Pharmacy and Health Sciences, Indianapolis, Indiana

Carol G. Vetterly, PharmD, BCPPS

Clinical Coordinator, Pharmacy Services; Clinical Pharmacist, UPMC Children's Hospital of Pittsburgh, University of Pittsburgh School of Pharmacy, Pittsburgh, Pennsylvania

Regan M. Wade, PharmD, BCPS

Clinical Pharmacist, Internal Medicine, Department of Pharmacy, UofL Health – UofL Hospital, Louisville, Kentucky

Mary L. Wagner, PharmD, MS

Associate Professor, Department of Pharmacy and Administration. Ernest Mario School of Pharmacy, Rutgers, The State University of New Jersey, Piscataway, New Jersey

Alison Walton, PharmD, BCPS

Associate Professor, Department of Pharmacy Practice, College of Pharmacy & Health Sciences, Butler University, Indianapolis, Indiana

Sheila K. Wang, PharmD, BCPS, BCIDP

Associate Professor, Department of Pharmacy Practice, Midwestern University College of Pharmacy, Downers Grove; Clinical Pharmacist in Infectious Diseases, Northwestern Memorial Hospital, Chicago, Illinois

Kyle A. Weant, PharmD, BCPS, BCCCP, FCCP

Clinical Assistant Professor, Department of Clinical Pharmacy and Outcome Sciences, College of Pharmacy, University of South Carolina; Emergency Medicine Clinical Pharmacy Specialist, Prisma Health Richland Hospital, Columbia, South Carolina

Zachary A. Weber, PharmD, BCPS, BCACP, CDCES, FASHP

Director of Interprofessional Education, Clinical Professor of Pharmacy Practice, Purdue College of Pharmacy; Assistant Dean for Education, Indiana University Interprofessional Practice and Education Center, Indianapolis, Indiana

Jeff T. Wieczorkiewicz, PharmD, BCPS

Associate Professor of Pharmacy Practice, Midwestern University College of Pharmacy, Downers Grove; Clinical Pharmacy Specialist, Internal Medicine, Edward Hines, Jr. Veterans Affairs Hospital, Hines, Illinois

Jon P. Wietholter, PharmD, BCPS, FCCP

Clinical Associate Professor, Department of Clinical Pharmacy, School of Pharmacy, West Virginia University; Internal Medicine Clinical Pharmacist, WVU Medicine J.W. Ruby Memorial Hospital, Morgantown, West Virginia

Susan R. Winkler, PharmD, BCPS, FCCP

Professor and Chair, Department of Pharmacy Practice, Midwestern University College of Pharmacy, Downers Grove, Illinois

Nancy S. Yunker, PharmD, FCCP, BCPS

Professor Emeritus, Department of Pharmacotherapy and Outcomes Science, Virginia Commonwealth University School of Pharmacy, Richmond, Virginia

Erin H. Zacholski, PharmD, BCOP

Assistant Professor, Department of Pharmacotherapy & Outcomes Science, School of Pharmacy, Virginia Commonwealth University; Clinical Pharmacist in Oncology, Virginia Commonwealth University Health System, Richmond, Virginia

PREFACE

The purpose of this 12th edition of the *Pharmacotherapy Casebook* is to help students in the health professions and practicing clinicians develop and refine the skills required to identify and resolve medication therapy problems by using realistic patient cases. Case studies can actively involve students in the learning process, foster self-confidence, and promote the development of skills in independent self-study, problem analysis, decision making, oral communication, and teamwork. Patient case studies can also be used as the focal point of discussions about pathophysiology, medicinal chemistry, pharmacology, and the pharmacotherapy of individual diseases. By integrating the biomedical and pharmaceutical sciences with pharmacotherapeutics, case studies can help students appreciate the relevance and importance of a sound scientific foundation in preparation for practice.

The patient cases in this book are intended to complement the scientific and clinical information in the 12th edition of *DiPiro's Phamacotherapy: A Pathophysiologic Approach*. This casebook edition contains 160 unique patient cases, with case chapters organized into organ system sections corresponding to the *Pharmacotherapy* textbook. Learners should read the relevant textbook chapter to become thoroughly familiar with the pathophysiology and pharmacotherapy of each disease state before attempting to identify and address the drug therapy problems of the patients described in this casebook. *Pharmacotherapy* textbook, casebook, and other useful learning resources are also available on *AccessPharmacy.com* (subscription required). By using these realistic cases to practice creating, defending, and implementing pharmacotherapeutic care plans, students can begin to build the skills and confidence that will be necessary to make the real decisions required in professional practice.

The knowledge and clinical experience required to answer the questions associated with each patient presentation vary from case to case. Some cases deal with a single disease state, whereas others have multiple diseases and drug therapy problems. As a guide for instructors, each case is identified as being one of three complexity levels; this classification system is described in more detail in Chapter 1.

Casebook Section 1: Principles of Patient-Focused Therapy includes five chapters that provide guidance on use of the casebook and six patient cases related to managing special patient populations (pediatrics, geriatrics, palliative care) and toxicology situations.

Chapter 1 describes the format of case presentations and how users can maximize usefulness of the casebook. The case questions and answers use the Joint Commission of Pharmacy Practitioners (JCPP) Pharmacists' Patient Care Process (PPCP; https://jcpp.net/patient-care-process/). The disease state chapters in *DiPiro's Pharmacotherapy* textbook also include an outline of the PPCP for the disorders. Clinicians should use a consistent process in delivering care so patients and other healthcare providers know what to expect from them. In addition, the PPCP is similar to the patient care process used by other healthcare professionals, and the Accreditation Council for Pharmacy Education (ACPE) requires schools/colleges of pharmacy to teach the PPCP in the curriculum.

Chapter 2 presents the philosophy and implementation of active learning strategies. This chapter sets the tone for the casebook by describing how these approaches can enhance student learning. The chapter provides useful active learning strategies for instructors and provides advice to students on how to maximize their learning opportunities in active learning environments.

Chapter 3 discusses the importance of patient communication and offers strategies to get the most out of the time that the clinician shares with the patient during each encounter. The information can be used as the basis for simulated counseling sessions related to the patient cases.

Chapter 4 describes in detail the steps involved in the PPCP: (1) Collect, (2) Assess, (3) Plan, (4) Implement, and (5) Follow-up: Monitor and Evaluate. The chapter includes example of patient case vignettes to demonstrate implementation of the PPCP. Implementing the PPCP provides a common terminology patient care services and focuses on quality improvement, provider collaboration, improved patient outcomes, and cost savings regardless of practice setting.

Chapter 5 describes the process of documenting patient encounters and interventions to serve as a record of patient care services provided and to communicate effectively with other healthcare providers. The authors discuss documentation of medication therapy management (MTM) and comprehensive medication management (CMM) encounters, as well as use of the traditional SOAP note for documenting the identification and resolution of drug therapy problems. A sample case presentation is provided to illustrate construction of a SOAP note with appropriate documentation of drug therapy problems.

Casebook Sections 2 through 18 contain patient cases organized by organ systems that correspond to those of the *Pharmacotherapy* textbook. Section 19 (Complementary and Alternative Therapies) contains patient vignettes that are directly related to patient cases that were presented earlier in this casebook. Each scenario involves the potential use of one or more dietary supplements. Additional follow-up questions are then asked to help the reader gain the scientific and clinical knowledge required to provide evidence-based recommendations about use of the supplement in that particular patient. Sixteen different dietary supplements are discussed: garlic, fish oil (omega-3 fatty acids), ginger, butterbur, feverfew, St. John's wort, kava, melatonin, cinnamon, α-lipoic acid, black cohosh, soy, *Pygeum africanum*, glucosamine, chondroitin, and elderberry.

We are grateful for the broad acceptance that previous editions of the casebook have received. It has been adopted by many schools of pharmacy and advanced practice provider programs. It has also been used in institutional staff development efforts and by individual pharmacists striving to upgrade their pharmacotherapy skills. It is our hope that this new edition will be even more valuable in assisting healthcare practitioners to meet society's need for safe and effective drug therapy.

ACKNOWLEDGMENTS

The editors would like to thank the 223 case and chapter authors from more than 100 schools of pharmacy, healthcare systems, and other institutions in the United States and Canada who contributed their scholarly efforts to this casebook. We especially appreciate their diligence in meeting deadlines, adhering to the PPCP casebook format, and providing up-to-date pharmacotherapy information. The next generation of healthcare practitioners will benefit from their willingness to share their expertise.

We also thank the individuals at McGraw Hill whose cooperation, guidance, and commitment were instrumental in maintaining the high standards of this publication, especially Michael Weitz, Melinda Avelar, and Peter Boyle. We appreciate the meticulous attention to composition provided by Nitesh Sharma, Senior Project Manager at KnowledgeWorks Global Ltd. Finally, we are grateful to our spouses for their understanding, support, and encouragement during the preparation of this new edition.

Terry L. Schwinghammer, PharmD, FCCP, FASHP, FAPhA
Julia M. Koehler, PharmD, FCCP
Jill S. Borchert, PharmD, BCACP, BCPS, FCCP
Douglas Slain, PharmD, BCPS, FCCP, FASHP
Sharon K. Park, PharmD, BCPS

Schwinghammer's
Pharmacotherapy
Casebook

SECTION 1
PRINCIPLES OF PATIENT-FOCUSED THERAPY

CHAPTER

1

Introduction: How to Use This Casebook

TERRY L. SCHWINGHAMMER, PharmD, FCCP, FASHP, FAPhA

USING PATIENT CASES TO ENHANCE STUDENT LEARNING

Case-based learning (CBL) is based on the principle that learning is more effective when realistic, relevant examples are used that create memorable mental images for learners that trigger knowledge recall later during actual clinical practice. CBL helps develop the skills of self-learning, critical thinking, problem identification, and decision making. When patient cases from this *Casebook* are used in the curricula of the healthcare professions or for independent study by practitioners, the focus should be on learning the *process* of identifying and resolving drug therapy problems rather than simply finding answers to the individual case questions. Students do learn scientific and clinical facts as they resolve case study problems, but they can also learn as much or more from their own independent study and discussions with their peers as they do from instructors. Educational programs that rely heavily on traditional lectures tend to concentrate on dissemination of scientific and clinical content with rote memorization of facts rather than developing higher-order thinking and problem-solving skills.

CBL in the health professions provides the personal history of a patient and information about one or more healthcare problems that require resolution. The learner's job is to collect the relevant patient information, assess that clinical data, develop hypotheses about the underlying cause of problems, consider possible solutions to problems identified, decide on and implement optimal solutions, perform follow-up to identify the consequences of one's decisions, and then make adjustments in the plan as needed.[1] The role of the teacher is to serve as coach and facilitator rather than as the source of "the answer." In fact, in many situations, there is more than one acceptable answer to a given case question. Students become self-directed learners through independent self-study, and instructors and students learn from each other during thoughtful discussion of the case.

PREPARATION FOR LEARNING WITH PATIENT CASES

The patient cases in this *Casebook* can be used for independent self-learning by individual students and for in-class problem-solving discussions by student groups and their instructors. If meaningful learning and discussion are to occur, students must come to class sessions prepared to discuss the case material rationally, to make informed recommendations, and to defend their patient care plans. This requires a strong commitment to independent self-study prior to the session. The cases in this book were designed to correspond with the scientific and clinical information contained in the 12th edition of *DiPiro's Pharmacotherapy: A Pathophysiologic Approach.*[2] For this reason, thorough understanding of the corresponding textbook chapter is recommended as the principal method of student preparation. The McGraw Hill online learning center *AccessPharmacy* (www.AccessPharmacy.com, subscription required) contains *DiPiro's Pharmacotherapy* textbook, this *Pharmacotherapy Casebook*, and many other educational resources that can be beneficial in answering case questions. The patient cases in the *Casebook* can also be used with the textbook *Pharmacotherapy Principles & Practice*, 6th edition[3] or other therapeutics textbooks. Primary literature should also be consulted as necessary to supplement textbook readings.

Most of the cases in the *Casebook* represent common diseases likely to be encountered by generalist practitioners. As a result, not all of the medical disorders discussed in the *DiPiro's Pharmacotherapy* textbook have an associated patient case in the *Casebook*. On the other hand, textbook chapters that discuss multiple diseases may have several corresponding cases in the *Casebook*.

LEVELS OF CASE COMPLEXITY

Each case is identified at the top of the first page as being one of the three levels of complexity. Instructors may use this classification system to select cases for discussion that correspond to the experience level of the student learners. These levels are defined as follows:

Level I—An uncomplicated case; only a single textbook chapter is required to complete the case questions. Little prior knowledge of the disease state or clinical experience is needed.

Level II—An intermediate-level case; several textbook chapters or other reference sources may be required to complete the case. Prior clinical experience may be helpful in resolving all of the issues presented.

Level III—A complicated case; multiple textbook chapters, additional readings, and substantial clinical experience may be required to solve all of the patient's drug therapy problems.

USING LEARNING OBJECTIVES TO FOCUS LEARNING

Learning objectives are included at the beginning of each case for student reflection. The focus of these outcomes is on eventually achieving clinical competence rather than simply learning isolated clinical and scientific facts. These objectives reflect some of the knowledge, skills, and abilities that students should possess after reading the relevant textbook chapter(s), studying the case, preparing a patient care plan, and defending their recommendations. Of course, true clinical competence can only be gained by direct interaction with real patients in various healthcare environments.

The learning objectives provided are meant to serve as a starting point to stimulate student thinking, but they are not intended to be all-inclusive. In fact, students should also generate their own personal ability outcome statements and learning objectives for each case. By so doing, students take greater control of their own learning, which serves to improve personal motivation and the desire to learn.

FORMAT OF THE CASEBOOK

PATIENT PRESENTATION

The format and organization of cases reflect those usually seen in actual clinical settings. The patient's medical history, physical examination findings, and laboratory results are provided in the following standardized outline format.

Chief Complaint

The chief complaint (CC) is a brief statement from the patient describing the symptom, problem, condition, or other reason for a medical encounter. The CC is stated in the patient's own words and forms the basis for the healthcare provider's initial differential diagnosis. Medical terms and diagnoses are generally not used in the CC, so the patient's symptoms are documented accurately. The appropriate medical terminology is used only after an appropriate evaluation (ie, medical history, physical examination, laboratory and other testing) leads to a medical diagnosis.

In the United Kingdom, the term "presenting complaint" (PC) may be used. Other synonyms include reason for encounter (RFE), presenting problem, problem on admission, or reason for presenting.

History of Present Illness

The history of present illness (HPI) (called the history of presenting complaint or HPC in the United Kingdom) is a more complete description of the patient's symptom(s). Items usually included in the HPI are:

- Date of onset
- Precise location
- Nature of onset, severity, and duration
- Presence of exacerbations and remissions
- Effect of any treatment given
- Relationship to other symptoms, bodily functions, or activities (eg, activity, meals)
- Degree of interference with daily activities

Past Medical History

The past medical history (PMH) includes serious illnesses, surgical procedures, and injuries the patient has experienced previously. Minor complaints (eg, influenza, colds) are usually omitted unless they might have a bearing on the current medical situation.

Family History

The family history (FH) includes the age and health of parents, siblings, and children. For deceased relatives, the age and cause of death are recorded. In particular, heritable diseases and those with a hereditary tendency are noted (eg, diabetes mellitus, cardiovascular disease, malignancy, rheumatoid arthritis, obesity).

Social History

The social history (SH) includes the social characteristics of the patient as well as environmental factors and behaviors that may contribute to development of disease. Items that may be documented are the patient's marital status, number of children, educational background, occupation, physical activity, hobbies, dietary habits, and use of tobacco, alcohol, or other drugs.

Medication History

The medication history (Meds) should include an accurate record of the patient's current use of prescription medications, nonprescription products, dietary supplements, and home remedies. Because there are thousands of prescription and nonprescription products available, it is important to obtain a complete medication history that includes the names, doses, routes of administration, schedules, and duration of therapy for all medications, including dietary supplements and other alternative therapies.

Allergies

Allergies (All) to drugs, food, pets, and environmental factors (eg, grass, dust, pollen) are recorded. An accurate description of the reaction that occurred should also be included. Care should be taken to distinguish adverse drug effects ("upset stomach") from true allergies ("hives").

Review of Systems

In the review of systems (ROS), the examiner questions the patient about the presence of symptoms related to each body system. In a brief ROS, only the pertinent positive and negative findings are recorded. In a complete ROS, body systems are generally listed starting from the head and working toward the feet and may include symptoms related to the skin, head, eyes, ears, nose, mouth and throat, neck, cardiovascular, respiratory, gastrointestinal, genitourinary, endocrine, musculoskeletal, and neuropsychiatric systems. The purpose of the ROS is to identify patient complaints related to each body system and prevent omission of pertinent information. Findings that were included in the HPI are generally not repeated in the ROS.

Physical Examination

The exact procedures performed during the physical examination (PE) vary depending on the CC, medical history, and type of encounter. A complete physical examination may be performed for annual screening, employment, or insurance purposes. In most clinical situations, only a limited physical examination is performed that is focused on the reason for the encounter. In psychiatric practice, greater emphasis is usually placed on the type and severity of the patient's symptoms than on physical findings. Most of the cases in this *Casebook* include comprehensive physical examination data, so students become familiar with common procedures and learn which findings are relevant to the CC and which are routine, normal findings. A suitable physical assessment textbook should be consulted for the specific procedures that may be conducted for each body system. The general sections for the PE are outlined as follows:

- **General Appearance (Gen)**—This brief statement represents a subjective impression of the patient's general state of being. An astute clinician observer may identify diagnostic clues about underlying disease; severity of illness; and the patient's values, social status, and personality.
- **Vital Signs (VS)**—Blood pressure, pulse, respiratory rate, and temperature. In hospital settings in particular, the presence of acute and chronic pain should be assessed when appropriate, but pain is no longer referred to as "the fifth vital sign."[4] For ease of use and consistency in this *Casebook*, weight and height are included in the vital signs section, but they are not actually considered to be vital signs.
- **Skin** (or Integumentary)
- **Head, Eyes, Ears, Nose, and Throat (HEENT)**
- **Neck/Lymph Nodes**
- **Lungs/Thorax** (or Pulmonary)
- **Breasts** (if female)
- **Cardiovascular (Cor** or **CV)**
- **Abdomen (Abd)**
- **Genitalia/Rectal (Genit/Rect)**
- **Musculoskeletal and Extremities (MS/Ext)**
- **Neurologic (Neuro)**

Laboratory Data

The results of laboratory tests are included with most cases in this *Casebook*. **Appendix A: Conversion Factors and Anthropometrics** contains common conversion factors and anthropometric information that will be helpful in solving many case answers. Normal (reference) ranges for the laboratory tests used throughout the *Casebook* are included in **Appendix B: Common Laboratory Tests.** Values in the appendix are provided in both traditional units and SI units (*le système International d'Unités*). The reference range for a given laboratory test is determined from a representative sample of the general population. The upper and lower limits of the range usually encompass two standard deviations from the population mean, which includes a range within which about 95% of healthy persons would fall. The term *normal range* may therefore be misleading, because a test result may be abnormal for a given individual even if it falls within the so-called normal range. Furthermore, given the statistical methods used to calculate the range, about 1 in 20 normal, healthy individuals will have a value for a test that lies outside the range. For these reasons, the term *reference range* is preferred over *normal range*. Reference ranges differ among laboratories, so the values given in Appendix B should be considered only as a general guide. Institution-specific reference ranges should be used in actual clinical settings.

All of the cases include some physical examination and laboratory findings that are within normal limits. For example, a description of the cardiovascular examination may include a statement that the point of maximal impulse is at the fifth intercostal space; laboratory evaluation may include a serum sodium level of 140 mEq/L (140 mmol/L). The presentation of actual findings (rather than simple statements that the heart examination and the serum sodium were normal) reflects what will be seen in actual clinical practice. More importantly, listing both normal and abnormal findings requires students to carefully assess the complete database and identify the pertinent positive and negative findings for themselves. A valuable portion of the learning process is lost if students are only provided with findings that are abnormal and are known to be associated with the disease that is the focus of the patient case.

HUMANISTIC CONSIDERATIONS

CBL provides an opportunity to employ inclusive practices using social justice principles, and issues of race, ethnicity, and gender deserve thoughtful consideration. Social identities are described carefully in the *Casebook* to avoid common stereotypes that reinforce bias.[5]

Race is defined as a category of humankind that shares certain distinctive physical traits. *Ethnicity* relates to groups of people classed according to common racial, national, tribal, religious, linguistic, or cultural origin or background. Race and ethnicity are cultural constructs, but they can have biological implications. In this edition, the patient's race is not identified if it has no bearing on the clinical situation. Adult patients in this *Casebook* are usually referred to as men or women, rather than males or females, to promote sensitivity to human dignity.

In contrast to previous *Casebook* editions, case patients have not been assigned fictitious names because they could inadvertently suggest a particular race or ethnicity, thereby introducing social bias. For example, instead of stating, "Robert Jackson is a 38-year-old man with a history of alcoholic cirrhosis who is admitted to the hospital…" that case in this edition would begin with the statement, "A 38-year-old man with a history of alcoholic cirrhosis is admitted to the hospital…" Avoidance of patient names is also consistent with actual clinical practice, where patient privacy and confidentiality are of utmost importance. Real patient names should not be used during group discussions in patient care areas unless absolutely necessary.

The patient cases in this *Casebook* include medical abbreviations and both generic and proprietary drug names, just as medical records do in actual practice. Although abbreviations and brand names are sometimes the source of clinical problems, the intent of their inclusion is to make the cases as realistic as possible. **Appendix C** lists the medical abbreviations used in the *Casebook*. This list is limited to commonly accepted abbreviations; thousands more exist, which can make it difficult for novice practitioners to efficiently assess patient databases. An accreditation standard of the Joint Commission International (JCI) mandates that healthcare institutions ensure the standardized use of approved symbols and medical abbreviations across the hospital.[6] Clinicians must be aware of this institutional document and use only approved symbols and abbreviations in the medical record system. Appendix C of this *Casebook* also lists abbreviations and designations that should be avoided. Given the immense human toll resulting from medical errors, this section should be considered "must" reading for all student learners. Medical abbreviations were ubiquitous throughout the paper medical charts used in physician offices, clinics, and hospitals prior to the advent of electronic health records. Fortunately, abbreviations are used less frequently now with the widespread adoption of electronic health records that have click boxes for sections of the medical history, PE, and other areas, along with physician dictation of progress notes.

The *Casebook* also contains some photographs of commercial drug products. These illustrations are provided as examples only and are not intended to imply endorsement of those particular products.

SOCIETAL NEED FOR COMPREHENSIVE MEDICATION MANAGEMENT SERVICES

Medication therapy plays a crucial role in improving human health by enhancing quality of life and extending life expectancy. The advent of biotechnology has led to the introduction of unique compounds for the prevention and treatment of disease that were unimagined just a decade or two ago. Each year the US Food and Drug Administration (FDA) approves a wide range of new drug products.

In 2021, the FDA approved 50 new molecular entities and therapeutic biological products.[7] Although the cost of new therapeutic agents often receives intense scrutiny, appropriate drug therapy can be cost-effective and reduce total healthcare expenditures by decreasing the need for surgery, avoiding adverse drug reactions, preventing hospital admissions and readmissions, shortening hospital stays, and preventing emergency department and physician visits.[8]

Unfortunately, use of medication regimens that have not been optimized for individual patients has been estimated to cost the United States $528 billion (2016 data), resulting in more than 275,000 deaths annually.[9] Various types of drug therapy problems frequently interfere with the ability of healthcare providers and patients to achieve the desired health outcomes. One analysis concluded that more than 250,000 Americans die each year from medical errors, and that if medical error were a disease, it would rank as the third-leading cause of death in the United States.[10] Medical errors include not only drug therapy problems but also any unintended act (either of omission or commission) or an act that does not achieve its intended outcome, failure of a planned action to be completed as intended, use of a wrong plan to achieve a goal, or deviation from the process of care that may or may not cause harm to the patient. Considering the magnitude of this problem, there is a clear societal need for better medication use.

Comprehensive medication management (CMM) is the standard of care that ensures that each patient's medications (prescription, nonprescription, nutritional supplements, and other types) are assessed to determine that each one is appropriate for the patient, effective for the medical condition, safe given patient comorbidities and other medications being taken, and able to be taken by the patient as intended.[11] When drug therapy problems are identified, pharmacists and other healthcare providers collaborate in a team-based approach to develop and implement an individualized care plan with specific therapeutic goals, drug therapy interventions, patient education, and follow-up evaluation to determine the actual patient outcomes achieved. Throughout this process, it is imperative that the patient understand, agree with, and participate actively in the treatment plan to optimize the medication experience and clinical outcomes. Widespread implementation of CMM in patient-centered medical homes (PCMHs) and other clinical settings has the potential to optimize medication use and improve healthcare for society.

CATEGORIES OF DRUG THERAPY PROBLEMS

A drug therapy problem has been defined as "any undesirable event experienced by a patient that involves, or is suspected to involve, drug therapy and that interferes with achieving the desired goals of therapy and requires professional judgment to resolve."[12] Seven distinct types of drug therapy problems have been identified that may potentially lead to an undesirable event that has physiologic, psychological, social, or economic ramifications.[12] These seven problem types relate to the assessment of medication appropriateness, effectiveness, safety, or adherence:

Appropriate indication for the medication:

1. The medication is unnecessary because the patient does not have a clinical indication at this time.

2. Additional drug therapy is required to treat or prevent a medical condition.

Effectiveness of the medication:

3. The medication being used is not effective at producing the desired patient response.

4. The dosage is too low to produce the desired patient response.

Safety of the medication:

5. The medication is causing an adverse reaction.

6. The dose is too high, resulting in actual or potential undesirable effects.

Adherence to the medication:

7. The patient is not able or willing to take the drug therapy as intended.

These drug therapy problems are discussed in more detail in **Chapter 4**. Because this *Casebook* is intended to be used as a companion for *DiPiro's Pharmacotherapy* textbook, one of its purposes is to serve as a tool for learning about the pharmacotherapy of disease states. For this reason, the primary drug therapy problem requiring identification and resolution for many patients in the *Casebook* is the need for additional drug treatment for a specific medical indication (problem 2 above). Other actual or potential drug therapy problems may coexist during the initial presentation or may develop during the clinical course of the disease.

APPLYING A CONSISTENT PATIENT CARE PROCESS TO CASE PROBLEMS

In this *Casebook*, each patient presentation is followed by a set of questions that are similar for each case. These questions are applied consistently to each case to demonstrate that clinicians should use a systematic patient care process for identifying, preventing, and resolving drug therapy problems regardless of the disease state being addressed. The *Casebook* has adopted the Joint Commission of Pharmacy Practitioners (JCPP) *Pharmacists' Patient Care Process* (PPCP)[13] as the framework for this purpose. The PPCP is the standard patient care process taught in schools and colleges of pharmacy in the United States. The 2016 Accreditation Council for Pharmacy Education (ACPE) Standard 10.8 states that "the curriculum prepares students to provide patient-centered collaborative care as described in the Pharmacists' Patient Care Process model endorsed by the Joint Commission of Pharmacy Practitioners."[14] Although the PPCP includes the word "pharmacists," the process mirrors the patient care process used by other healthcare providers. Thus, teaching pharmacy students to employ this process in clinical practice will help ensure that they "speak the same language" as other healthcare providers when they become healthcare providers.

Prior to embarking upon the patient care process for a given individual, the clinician must establish an appropriate professional relationship with the patient, family, and caregivers that will support active engagement and effective communication. Throughout the process, the medication management expert must continually collaborate, document, and communicate with physicians, pharmacists, and other healthcare professionals to provide safe, effective, and coordinated care. See **Chapter 4, Fig. 4-1** for an illustration of how the PPCP is implemented in clinical practice. A description of how the case questions in this *Casebook* employ the steps of the PPCP is included in the following paragraphs.

1. COLLECT INFORMATION

1.a. What subjective and objective information indicates the presence of (the primary problem or disease)?

The first step is to collect the necessary subjective and objective information to understand the patient's medical and medication history and his/her clinical status. Therefore, the first case question in the *Casebook* asks the learner to identify the subjective and objective information that indicates the presence of the patient's primary disease state that is associated with the reason for the patient encounter.

Subjective information is obtained by communicating with the patient and cannot usually be verified by the clinician. As examples, a patient may report having chest pain, palpitations, shortness of breath, dizziness, or feelings of depression. Subjective information usually begins with the CC, which includes one or more symptoms. Subjective information is also obtained from the ROS, as discussed previously.

Objective information can be measured and verified by the clinician using the physical examination procedures of inspection, auscultation, palpation, and percussion as well as vital signs (heart rate, blood pressure, respiratory rate, temperature). Laboratory data and other diagnostic test results also provide objective information.

For purposes of CMM in real patient situations, it is critically important to obtain accurate and complete information about all of the patient's medications, including prescription, nonprescription, alternative therapies, vitamins, nutritional supplements, and products used from family or friends, regardless of who prescribed them. It is also important to identify where the products were dispensed, purchased, or otherwise obtained. Even though not all of this information will be provided or known for the patient cases in the *Casebook*, it is important for students to realize the importance of collecting this information.

1.b. What additional information is needed to fully assess this patient's primary problem?

In many *Casebook* cases (just as in real life), some important pertinent information is missing from the patient presentation. A separate case question will ask the student to list other additional information that would be needed to fully assess the patient's main problem. Providing precise recommendations for obtaining the additional information needed to satisfactorily assess the patient's problems can be a valuable contribution to the patient's care. Therefore, it is important for students to have an in-depth understanding of the patient's medical conditions and medication therapy and be able to recognize the subjective and objective information that is available, as well as the pertinent information that may be missing from the case presentation.

2. ASSESS THE INFORMATION

2.a. Assess the severity of the primary problem or disease based on the subjective and objective information available.

The next step is to review the information collected to assess the severity of the patient's clinical condition and determine whether drug therapy problems exist. Each medication should be assessed for its appropriateness, effectiveness, safety, and patient adherence. It is important to differentiate the process of identifying drug therapy problems from making a disease-related medical diagnosis. In fact, the primary medical diagnosis is often known for patients seen by pharmacists. However, pharmacists must be able to assess the patient's database to determine whether drug therapy problems exist that warrant a change in drug therapy. In the case of preexisting chronic diseases, such as asthma or rheumatoid arthritis, one must be able to assess information that may indicate a change in severity of the disease.

2.b. Create a list of the patient's drug therapy problems and prioritize them. Include assessment of medication appropriateness, effectiveness, safety, and patient adherence.

Novice student learners often struggle with writing statements of drug therapy problems. Simply put, a drug therapy problem statement must include a medical condition (disease) or health-related issue and a problem related to drug therapy. These statements should be clear, concise, and easily understood by other healthcare

professionals. They must also contain sufficient detail so others can understand the magnitude of the problem. Provided here are several examples of well-written drug therapy problem statements:

- Established rheumatoid arthritis (>6 months duration) with high disease activity (DAS28 score >5.1) inadequately treated with the current regimen of methotrexate monotherapy.

- Newly diagnosed stage IIIB classic Hodgkin lymphoma requiring treatment with pharmacotherapy that offers the best chance for cure.

- Dyslipidemia with need for change in statin therapy due to drug interaction (simvastatin and verapamil) and dose too low (inappropriate statin intensity).

- Allergic rhinitis treated with a medication (diphenhydramine) that is inappropriate for the patient and is likely causing an adverse reaction (excessive sedation).

- Recurrent falls, possibly related to medication use (diphenhydramine, metoprolol succinate, donepezil) and other factors.

The clinician should create a prioritized list of all of the drug therapy problems that were identified. Problems of the highest priority should be addressed first (immediately during the current encounter), whereas those of lower priority may be addressed later (eg, later in the course of a hospital stay or at subsequent follow-up visits). For many cases in the *Casebook*, the major drug therapy problem (highest priority) will be an untreated or inadequately treated indication. Other problems related to the primary or secondary diseases might be improper drug selection leading to ineffectiveness, subtherapeutic dosage, overdosage, failure to receive or take the drug(s) prescribed, adverse drug reactions, drug interactions, or drug use without indication.

2.c. *Optional Question*: What economic, psychosocial, cultural, racial, and ethical considerations are applicable to this patient?

Some patient cases will include a question related to these unique considerations that must be identified and addressed. For example, the patient may not have medical insurance or be able to afford high-cost biologic drug products for diseases such as inflammatory bowel disease, plaque psoriasis, or rheumatoid arthritis. Other patients may have family, social, or cultural issues that could interfere with effective drug therapy. Addressing these issues is an important part of developing an effective and comprehensive patient care plan.

3. DEVELOP A CARE PLAN

After all relevant patient information has been collected and assessed and the patient's drug therapy problems have been identified and prioritized, the pharmacist or other medication management expert develops an individualized patient-centered medication management plan in collaboration with other healthcare professionals and the patient (or caregiver). The plan must be evidence-based, cost-effective, and likely to be adhered to by the patient.

3.a. What are the goals of pharmacotherapy for the primary problem in this case?

The first step in designing a care plan is to establish treatment goals for each medical condition. The primary therapeutic outcomes include:

- Cure of disease (eg, bacterial infection)

- Reduction or elimination of symptoms (eg, pain from cancer)

- Arresting or slowing of the progression of disease (eg, rheumatoid arthritis, HIV infection)

- Preventing a disease or symptom (eg, coronary heart disease)

Other important outcomes of pharmacotherapy include:

- Not complicating or aggravating other existing disease states
- Avoiding or minimizing adverse effects of treatment
- Providing cost-effective therapy
- Maintaining the patient's quality of life

Sources of information for this step may include the patient or caregiver, the patient's physician or other healthcare professionals, medical records, and *DiPiro's Pharmacotherapy* textbook or other literature references. Importantly, although national guidelines may stipulate population-level goals (eg, A1C <7% for type 2 diabetes), goals must be individualized for each patient based on potential risk, comorbidities, concomitant drug therapy, patient preference, and physician intentions.[13]

3.b. What nondrug therapies might be useful for this patient's primary problem?

After the intended outcomes have been defined, attention can be directed toward identifying the types of treatments that might be beneficial in achieving those outcomes. The clinician should consider all feasible nondrug and pharmacotherapeutic alternatives available for achieving the predefined therapeutic outcomes before designing a regimen. Nondrug therapies that might be useful such as lifestyle measures (eg, diet, weight loss, and exercise), physical therapy, relaxation techniques, and surgical procedures should be included in the list of therapeutic alternatives.

3.c. What feasible pharmacotherapeutic options are available for treating the primary disease or drug therapy problem?

All feasible drug therapy options should be considered while assessing the potential benefits and limitations of each one in light of the patient's particular situation. Some first-line agents may need to be avoided due to inadequate efficacy, potential for adverse effects, concomitant comorbidities or drugs, or high cost. For example, an asthma patient who requires new drug therapy for hypertension might better tolerate treatment with a thiazide diuretic rather than a β-blocker. On the other hand, a hypertensive patient with gout may be better served by use of a β-blocker rather than a thiazide diuretic. Useful sources of information on therapeutic options include *DiPiro's Pharmacotherapy* textbook and other references, as well as the clinical experience of the healthcare provider and other healthcare professionals on the patient care team.

There has been a resurgence of interest in dietary supplements and other alternative therapies in recent years. The public spends billions of dollars each year on supplements for which there is little scientific evidence of efficacy, that are not standardized for potency and purity, and that are not regulated by the FDA as drug products. Furthermore, some products are hazardous, and others may interact with a patient's prescription medications or aggravate concurrent disease states. On the other hand, scientific evidence of efficacy does exist for some dietary supplements, and the National Institutes of Health Office of Dietary Supplements maintains fact sheets that give an overview of individual vitamins, minerals, and other dietary supplements.[15] Healthcare providers must be knowledgeable about these products and prepared to answer patient questions regarding their efficacy and safety.

The *Casebook* contains a separate section devoted to dietary supplements (see **Section 19**). This portion of the *Casebook* contains a number of fictitious patient vignettes that relate to patient cases that were presented earlier in the *Casebook*. Each scenario involves the potential use of one or more dietary supplements by the patient. Additional follow-up questions are then asked to help the reader gain the scientific and clinical knowledge required to provide an evidence-based recommendation about use of the supplement in that particular patient. The use of 16 different dietary supplements

for 12 different disorders is included in this section: α-lipoic acid (type 2 diabetes), black cohosh (menopausal symptoms), butterbur (migraine prevention, allergic rhinitis), cinnamon (diabetes), elderberry (influenza), feverfew (migraine prevention), fish oil (diabetes, dyslipidemia), garlic (dyslipidemia), ginger (nausea/vomiting), glucosamine and/or chondroitin (osteoarthritis), kava (anxiety), melatonin (insomnia), *Pygeum africanum* (benign prostatic hypertrophy), soy (menopausal symptoms), and St. John's wort (depression). Current reference sources are provided for all of the supplements.

3.d. Create an individualized, patient-centered, team-based care plan to optimize medication therapy for this patient's primary disease and other drug therapy problems. Include specific drugs, dosage forms, doses, schedules, and durations of therapy.

The purpose of this step is to determine the specific drugs, dosage forms, doses, routes of administration, schedules, and durations of therapy that are best suited to resolve each drug therapy problem that has been identified. Each pharmacotherapy regimen should be evidence-based and individualized for the specific patient. Thus, the learner should be prepared to defend the rationale for the regimens selected and provide logical reasons for avoiding specific regimens in the care plan. Some potential reasons for drug avoidance include drug allergy, drug–drug or drug–disease interactions, patient age, renal or hepatic impairment, adverse effects, inconvenient dosage schedule, likelihood of poor adherence, pregnancy, and high treatment cost.

The specific dose selected may depend on the severity of the medical condition. For example, the initial oral dose of the loop diuretic furosemide for edema ranges from 20 to 80 mg per day and may be titrated up to 600 mg per day for severe edematous states.[16] Appropriate dosage also may vary depending on the indication for the drug; for example, the analgesic effect of the nonsteroidal anti-inflammatory drug ibuprofen may be achieved at lower doses than those required for anti-inflammatory activity.[17] The likelihood of adherence with the regimen and patient tolerance come into play in the selection of dosage forms. For example, some patients receiving the tumor necrosis factor inhibitor golimumab for rheumatoid arthritis may prefer to self-administer the medication subcutaneously at home; others may require golimumab intravenous infusions because they are either unwilling or unable to use subcutaneous injections. The economic, psychosocial, and ethical factors that are applicable to the patient should also be given due consideration in designing the pharmacotherapeutic regimen.

In many clinical situations, there is more than one acceptable drug regimen, so it is important for the healthcare team to agree on all drug therapy regimens selected for a given patient.

3.e. *Optional question*: What alternatives would be appropriate if the initial care plan fails or cannot be used?

This optional question is included only for select patients in the *Casebook*. However, it is a good idea to always have an appropriate backup plan in place if the initial therapy fails or cannot be used.

4. IMPLEMENT THE CARE PLAN

In real-life clinical situations, the care plan that was agreed upon by the healthcare team and patient then requires thoughtful, collaborative implementation. Steps to be taken during the implementation process include[13]:

- Addressing medication- and health-related problems that exist or may arise
- Performing preventive care strategies, including administering vaccines

- Initiating, modifying, discontinuing, and administering medication therapy as authorized
- Providing education and self-management training to the patient or caregiver
- Contributing to coordination of care, including patient referral or transition to another healthcare professional
- Scheduling follow-up care as needed to achieve goals of therapy

4.a. What information should be provided to the patient to enhance adherence, ensure successful therapy, and minimize adverse effects?

As described previously, CMM requires that healthcare providers establish a professional and personal relationship with the patient. Patients are our partners in healthcare, and our efforts may be for naught without their informed participation in the process. For chronic diseases such as diabetes mellitus, hypertension, and asthma, patients may have a greater role in managing their diseases than do healthcare professionals. Self-care is becoming widespread as increasing numbers of prescription medications receive over-the-counter status. For these reasons, patients must be provided with sufficient information to enhance compliance, ensure successful therapy, and minimize adverse effects. **Chapter 3** describes patient interview techniques that can be used efficiently to determine the patient's level of knowledge. Additional information can then be provided as necessary to fill in knowledge gaps.

In the questions posed with individual cases, students are asked to provide the kind of information that should be given to the patient who has limited knowledge of his or her disease. The information should be provided with the intent of improving adherence, ensuring successful therapy, and minimizing adverse effects. Under the Omnibus Budget Reconciliation Act (OBRA) of 1990, for patients who accept the offer of counseling, pharmacists should consider including the following items[18]:

- Name and description of the medication (which may include the indication)
- Dosage, dosage form, route of administration, and duration of therapy
- Special directions and precautions for preparation, administration, and use
- Common and severe adverse effects, interactions, and contraindications (with the action required should they occur)
- Techniques for self-monitoring
- Proper storage
- Prescription refill information
- Action to be taken in the event of missed doses

Instructors may wish to have simulated patient-interviewing sessions for new and refill prescriptions during case discussions to practice medication education skills. Factual information should be provided as concisely as possible to enhance memory retention. Various online and print resources are available for consumer information about individual drug products. MedlinePlus is the National Institute of Health's free website for consumers that contains information on prescription and nonprescription drugs, dietary supplements, medical conditions, wellness, diagnostic tests, and other medical information.[19]

4.b. Describe how care should be coordinated with other healthcare providers.

As part of the team-based approach, patient care must be coordinated among healthcare providers and the patient, family, and caregivers.

Learner responses to this *Casebook* question should include more than simple descriptions of the roles of other healthcare professionals. More importantly, learners should be able to thoughtfully express how each unique professional role is integrated with others in providing collaborative, team-based care.

For pharmacists and some other providers, their roles include (in part) initiating, modifying, discontinuing, and administering medication therapy as authorized. Others involved in team-based care might include primary care physicians, specialist physicians, surgeons, nurses, physical therapists, occupational therapists, social workers, dentists, dietitians, psychologists, and others. Consider which of them should be involved in the patient's care and how their efforts serve to coordinate and optimize care. For example:

- Who will educate the patient about their primary disease(s), and the impending changes in care?
- Who will discuss the disease prognosis with the patient?
- Who will counsel the patient about new medications, nondrug therapies, and lifestyle changes?
- Who will provide an updated medication list to the patient?
- Who will discuss options for surgical intervention or discharge to an assisted-care facility?
- If referrals to specialists or other transitions of care are needed, how will this be accomplished? For example, should the patient be referred to a diabetes or anticoagulation management expert for chronic care? Does the patient need dental care? Is a social worker needed to manage the patient's social/home situation?
- Who will be involved in follow-up visits, and who will communicate with the patient about them?
- How will team members communicate with each other during this patient encounter and in planning and conducting future visits?
- Who will document treatment plans in the record?

Documenting the medication therapy plan in the medical record is necessary to ensure accurate communication among practitioners. Oral communication alone can be misinterpreted or transferred inaccurately to others. This is especially true because there are many drugs that sound alike when spoken but have far different therapeutic uses.

The SOAP (Subjective, Objective, Assessment, and Plan) format has been used by clinicians for many years to assess patient problems and to communicate findings and plans in the medical record. Writing SOAP notes may not be the optimal process for learning to solve drug therapy problems because several important steps taken by experienced clinicians are not always apparent and may be overlooked. For example, the precise therapeutic outcome desired is often unstated in SOAP notes, leaving others to presume what the desired treatment goals are. Healthcare professionals using the SOAP format also commonly move directly from an assessment of the patient (diagnosis) to outlining a diagnostic or therapeutic plan, without conveying whether careful consideration has been given to all available feasible diagnostic or therapeutic alternatives. The plan itself as outlined in SOAP notes may also give short shrift to the monitoring parameters required to ensure successful therapy and to detect and prevent adverse drug effects. Finally, SOAP notes often do not include the treatment information that should be conveyed to the most important individual involved: the patient. If SOAP notes are used for documenting drug therapy problems, consideration should be given to including each of these components.

In **Chapter 5**, the SOAP note is presented as the traditional method for documenting care plans in the patient's health record.

Although preparation of written communication notes is not included in written form with each set of case questions in the *Casebook*, instructors are encouraged to include the composition of a SOAP note as one of the requirements for successfully completing each case study assignment. A well-written SOAP note focusing on drug therapy problems should provide a clear statement of the drug therapy problem, the clinician's findings relevant to the problem, assessment of the findings, an actual or proposed plan for resolving the problem, and the clinical and laboratory parameters required for follow-up and monitoring.

Clinicians responsible for the outcomes of drug therapy should create and maintain a record of each patient's drug therapy problem list, the plans for resolving each problem, the interventions actually made, and the subsequent therapeutic outcomes achieved.

5. FOLLOW-UP: MONITOR AND EVALUATE

5.a. Explain how to monitor and evaluate the care plan for medication appropriateness, effectiveness, safety and patient adherence by using clinical and laboratory data, patient feedback and other information.

Monitoring the care plan and modifying it in collaboration with other healthcare professionals and the patient (or caregiver) is performed to assess[13]:

- Medication appropriateness, effectiveness, and safety
- Patient adherence
- Clinical endpoints that contribute to the patient's overall health
- Outcomes of care achieved

The outcome parameters are evaluated against the predetermined goals of therapy to determine the progress made toward achieving the therapeutic goals and to determine if any new drug therapy problems have developed that could interfere with safe and effective medication use.[8]

Clinicians must identify the clinical and laboratory parameters necessary to assess the therapy for achievement of the therapeutic goals and to detect and prevent adverse effects. Each outcome parameter selected should be specific, measurable, achievable, directly related to the therapeutic goals, and have a defined endpoint. As a means of remembering these points, the acronym SMART has been used (*S*pecific, *M*easurable, *A*chievable, *R*elated, and *T*ime bound). If the goal is to cure bacterial pneumonia, learners should outline the subjective and objective clinical parameters (eg, relief of chest discomfort, cough, and fever), laboratory tests (eg, normalization of white blood cell count and differential), and other procedures (eg, resolution of infiltrate on chest X-ray) that provide evidence of bacterial eradication and clinical cure of the disease. The intervals at which data should be collected are dependent on the outcome parameters selected and should be established prospectively. Some expensive or invasive procedures may not be repeated after the initial diagnosis is made.

Adverse effect parameters must also be well-defined and measurable. For example, it is insufficient to state that one will monitor for potential drug-induced "blood dyscrasias." Rather, one should identify the likely specific hematologic abnormality (eg, anemia, leukopenia, or thrombocytopenia) and outline a prospective schedule for obtaining the appropriate parameters (eg, obtain monthly hemoglobin/hematocrit, white blood cell count, or platelet count).

Monitoring for adverse events should be directed toward preventing or identifying serious adverse effects that have a reasonable likelihood of occurrence. For example, it is not cost-effective to obtain periodic liver function tests in all patients taking a drug that causes mild abnormalities in liver injury tests only rarely, such

as omeprazole. On the other hand, the antipsychotic drug clozapine requires therapy-long periodic monitoring of white blood cell counts and absolute neutrophil counts to enable early detection of drug-induced leukopenia and agranulocytosis.

Patient follow-up should occur at intervals that are appropriate for the patient's clinical situation, the medical conditions being treated, and the drug therapy being used. Follow-up should be carefully coordinated with members of the healthcare team and the patient to avoid interfering with other ongoing patient care activities.[8] The return time may be short when there is a patient safety concern when a new potent medication is started that may have serious adverse effects. Longer intervals may be needed to allow a suitable time frame for new medications to exert either partial or full therapeutic effect, such as medications for dyslipidemia or depression.

CLINICAL COURSE

The patient care process requires assessment of the patient's progress to ensure movement toward achieving the desired therapeutic outcomes. A description of the patient's clinical course is included with many cases in this *Casebook* to reflect this process. Some cases follow the progression of the patient's disease over months to years and include both inpatient and outpatient treatment. Follow-up questions directed toward ongoing evaluation and problem-solving are included after the presentation of the clinical course.

SELF-STUDY ASSIGNMENTS

Each case concludes with several study assignments related to the patient case or the disease state that may be used as independent study projects for students to complete outside class. These assignments may require students to obtain additional information that is not contained in the corresponding *Pharmacotherapy* textbook chapter.

LITERATURE REFERENCES AND INTERNET SITES

Literature references relevant to the patient case are included at the end of each presentation. References selected for inclusion will be useful to students for answering the questions posed. Most of the citations relate to major clinical trials or meta-analyses, authoritative review articles, and clinical practice guidelines. The *Pharmacotherapy* textbook contains a more comprehensive list of references pertinent to each disease state.

Some cases list internet sites as sources of drug therapy information. The sites listed are recognized as authoritative sources of information, such as the FDA (*www.fda.gov*) and the Centers for Disease Control and Prevention (*www.cdc.gov*). Students should be advised to be wary of information posted on the internet that is not from highly regarded healthcare organizations or publications. The uniform resource locators (URLs) for internet sites sometimes change, and it is possible that not all sites listed in the *Casebook* will remain available for viewing.

DEVELOPING ANSWERS TO CASE QUESTIONS

The use of case studies for independent learning and in-class discussion may be unfamiliar to many learners. For this reason, students may find it difficult at first to devise complete answers to the case questions. **Appendix D** contains the answers to two cases in order to demonstrate how case responses might be prepared and presented. The authors of the cases contributed the recommended answers provided in the appendix, but they should not be considered the sole "right" answer. Thoughtful students who have prepared well for the discussion sessions may arrive at additional or alternative answers that are also appropriate.

With diligent self-study, practice, and the guidance of instructors, students will gradually acquire the knowledge, skills, and self-confidence to develop and implement patient care plans for their own future patients in collaboration with other members of the healthcare team. The goal of the *Casebook* is to help students progress along this path of lifelong learning.

REFERENCES

1. Herreid CF. Case studies in science: a novel method of science education. J Coll Sci Teach. 1994;23:221–229.

2. DiPiro JT, Yee GC, Posey LM, Haines, ST, Nolin TD, Ellingrod VL, eds. DiPiro's Pharmacotherapy: A Pathophysiologic Approach. 12th ed. New York, NY: McGraw Hill, 2023.

3. Chisholm-Burns MA, Schwinghammer TL, Malone PM, Kolesar JM, Bookstaver PB, Lee KC, eds. Pharmacotherapy Principles & Practice. 6th ed. New York, NY: McGraw Hill, 2022.

4. Baker DW. The Joint Commission's pain standards: origins and evolution. Oakbrook Terrace, IL: The Joint Commission; 2017.

5. Okoro ON, Arya V, Gaither CA, Tarfa A. Examining the inclusion of race and ethnicity in patient cases. Am J Pharm Educ 2021;83(9): Article 8583.

6. Joint Commission International. Use of codes, symbols, and abbreviations. Oak Brook, IL; 2018. *https://store.jointcommissioninternational.org/assets/3/7/April_JCInsight_2018.pdf*. Accessed April 9, 2022.

7. United States Food and Drug Administration. Novel drug approvals for 2021. *https://www.fda.gov/drugs/new-drugs-fda-cders-new-molecular-entities-and-new-therapeutic-biological-products/novel-drug-approvals-2021*. Accessed April 9, 2022.

8. Dalton K, Byrne S. Role of the pharmacist in reducing healthcare costs: current insights. Integr Pharm Res Pract. 2017;6:37–36. *https://www.ncbi.nlm.nih.gov/pmc/articles/PMC5774321/*. Accessed April 9, 2022.

9. Watanabe JH, McInnis T, Hirsch JD. Cost of prescription drug–related morbidity and mortality. Ann Pharmacother. 2018;52:829–837.

10. Makary MA, Daniel M. Medical error—the third leading cause of death in the US. BMJ. 2016;353:i2139. doi: 10.1136/bmj.i2139.

11. McFarland MS, Finks SW, Smith L, et al. Medication optimization: integration of comprehensive medication management into practice. Am Health Drug Benefits. 2021;14(3):111–114.

12. Cipolle RJ, Strand LM, Morley PC. Drug therapy problems. In: Cipolle RJ, Strand LM, Morley PC, eds. Pharmaceutical Care Practice: The Patient-Centered Approach to Medication Management Services. 3rd ed. New York, NY: McGraw-Hill, 2012:chap 5. *https://accesspharmacy.mhmedical.com/book.aspx?bookid=491*. Accessed April 9, 2022.

13. Joint Commission of Pharmacy Practitioners. Pharmacists' Patient Care Process. May 29, 2014. *https://jcpp.net/patient-care-process/*. Accessed April 9, 2022.

14. Accreditation Council for Pharmacy Education. Professional program in pharmacy leading to the doctor of pharmacy degree standards. *https://www.acpe-accredit.org/pdf/Standards2016FINAL.pdf*. Accessed April 9, 2022.

15. National Institutes of Health Office of Dietary Supplements. Dietary Supplement Fact Sheets. *https://ods.od.nih.gov/factsheets/list-all/*. Accessed April 9, 2022.

16. Drug monographs: furosemide. *www.accesspharmacy.com*. Accessed April 9, 2022.

17. Drug monographs: ibuprofen. *www.accesspharmacy.com*. Accessed April 9, 2022.

18. Martin S. What you need to know about OBRA '90. J Am Pharm Assoc. 1993;NS33(1):26–28.

19. MedlinePlus: Trusted Health Information for You. National Library of Medicine, U.S. Department of Health and Human Services, National Institutes of Health; Bethesda, MD: 2022. *https://medlineplus.gov/*. Accessed April 9, 2022.

RACHEL W. FLURIE, PharmD, BCPS
ERIN H. ZACHOLSKI, PharmD, BCOP
CYNTHIA K. KIRKWOOD, PharmD, BCPP

CHAPTER 2

Active Learning Strategies

Healthcare practitioners face situations that require the use of effective problem solving, critical thinking, and communication skills on a daily basis. Therefore, providing students with knowledge alone is insufficient to equip them with the tools needed to be valuable contributors to patient care. Students must understand that it is imperative to provide more than just drug information, which is readily obtained in today's world from internet sites, smartphone applications, and online reference texts. They must be able to evaluate, analyze, and synthesize information, and apply their knowledge to prevent and resolve drug-related problems. As clinicians, they will be required to contribute their expertise to team discussions about patient care, ask appropriate questions, integrate information, and develop action plans.

Professional students must also recognize that learning is a lifelong process. Scores of new drugs are approved every year, drug use practices change, and innovative research alters the way that diseases are treated. Students must be prepared to proactively expand their knowledge base and clinical skills to adapt to the changing profession.

Warren identified several traits that prepare students for future careers: analytic thinking, polite assertiveness, tolerance, communication skills, understanding of one's own physical well-being, and the ability to continue to teach oneself after graduation.[1] To prepare students to become healthcare professionals who are essential members of the healthcare team, many healthcare educators are using active learning strategies in the classroom.[2,3]

ACTIVE LEARNING VERSUS TRADITIONAL TEACHING

Active learning has numerous definitions, and various methods are described in the educational literature. Simply put, *active learning is the process of having students engage in activities that require reflection on ideas and how students use them.*[3] Active learning is learner-focused and helps students take responsibility for their own learning.[2] Most proponents of active learning strategies agree that compared with passively receiving lectures, active engagement of students promotes deeper learning, enhances critical thinking skills, provides feedback to students and instructors, and promotes social development. Learning is reinforced when students are actively engaged and apply their knowledge to new situations.[3]

In contrast, traditional teaching involves a teacher-centered approach. At the beginning of the course, students are given a course syllabus packet that contains "everything they need to know" for the semester. In class, the teacher lectures on a predetermined topic that does not require student preparation and allows students to be passive recipients of information. The testing method is usually a written examination that employs a multiple-choice or short-answer format, which focuses on the student's ability to recall isolated facts that the teacher has identified as being important. They do not

learn to apply their knowledge to situations that they will ultimately encounter in practice. The reward is an external one (ie, exam or course grade) that may or may not reflect a student's actual ability to use the knowledge they have to improve patient care.

To teach students to be lifelong learners, it is essential to stimulate them to be inquisitive and actively involved with the learning that takes place in the classroom. This requires that teachers move away from more comfortable teaching methods and learn new techniques that will help students "learn to learn." In classes with active learning formats, students are involved in much more than listening. The transmission of information is deemphasized and replaced with the development of skills and application of knowledge. Active learning shifts the control of learning from the teacher to the students; this provides an opportunity for students to become active participants in their own learning.[2]

ACTIVE LEARNING STRATEGIES

Teachers implement active learning exercises into classes in a variety of ways. While some strategies engage individual students with the material, such as giving students the opportunity to pause and recall information, other active learning strategies involve the use of student groups, such as problem-based learning (PBL), team-based learning (TBL), or cooperative or collaborative learning whereby students work together to perform specific tasks in a small group (ie, solve problems, discuss case studies).[2,4] A flipped classroom approach, whereby the typical lecture and application elements of a course are switched, naturally pivots the focus of in-class time to active learning.[5] Technology is increasingly used in active learning in numerous ways to maximize the use of class time for higher-order thinking tasks such as analysis, synthesis, and evaluation.[6,7] The following are the examples of active learning strategies that involve students in the learning process.

EXERCISES FOR INDIVIDUAL STUDENTS

These exercises can complement lectures and are easily implemented. Quick writing tasks can assess student understanding of (or reaction to) material. Writing helps students to identify knowledge deficits, clarify understanding of the material, and organize thoughts in a logical manner. The "minute paper" or "half-sheet response" has students provide written responses to a question asked in class.[8] Example questions might be, "What was the main point of today's class session?" or "What was the muddiest point of today's class session?" In-class quizzes can be strategically placed to break up lecture time and engage students. Quizzes given at the beginning of class on pre-class readings help stimulate students to review information they did not know and listen for clarification during class. Quizzes can also be given throughout class (eg, using electronic audience response systems [ARS]) and may or may not be graded. ARS can help instructors engage students in lecture content, promote interactivity, identify misconceptions, and stimulate discussion.[6] ARS questions posed immediately after the presentation of the content will more likely test immediate recall than substantive knowledge. Quizzes at the end of class allow students to use their problem-solving skills by applying what they have just learned to a patient case or problem.

DISCUSSION-BASED LEARNING

Discussion-based learning emphasizes the use of communication among learners and can include several types of active learning strategies. One such strategy involves questions and answers that can increase student involvement and comprehension. "Wait time" is a method whereby the instructor poses a question and asks students to think about it.[9] After a brief pause, the instructor can ask for volunteers or randomly call on a student to answer the question. This wait time forces every student to think about the question rather than relying on those students who immediately raise their hands to answer questions. With the "fish bowl" method, students are asked to write questions related to the course material for discussion at the end of class or at the beginning of the next class session.[9] Instructors then draw several questions out of the "fish bowl" to discuss or ask the class to answer. Questions can also be submitted electronically, using a learning management system or programs such as Google Forms or Poll Everywhere. In classes that use active learning, much of the learning will come from class discussion. However, many students may not pay attention to their classmates, but rather wait for instructors to either repeat or clarify what one of their classmates has said. To promote active listening, after one student has volunteered to answer a question, instructors could ask another student if they agree with the previous response and why.

The "think–pair–share" exercise involves providing students with a question or problem to solve.[2] After working on the assignment individually (think) for 2–5 minutes, they discuss their ideas for 3–5 minutes with the student sitting next to them (pair). Finally, student pairs are chosen to share their ideas with the whole class (share). By sharing ideas with a partner first, students are kept on task and can have a more intimate discussion to work out problems before sharing with others. This method provides immediate feedback and can lead to productive class discussion. Another type of sharing involves small-group discussions. Preassigned small groups of three to four students work together throughout the course to complete activities. Groups may have 20–30 minutes for discussion and apply a topic presented in class to a new situation. To create heterogeneity for discussion, one example is to group students with different experiences (eg, community vs hospital IPPE).[10] Assigning functional roles and role-playing can create multiple perspectives.

Cooperative or collaborative learning strategies involve students in the generation of knowledge.[11] Students are randomly assigned to groups of four to six at the beginning of the school term. Several times during the term, each group is given a patient case and a group leader is selected. Each student in the group volunteers to work on a certain portion of the case. The case is discussed in class, and each member receives the same grade. After students have finished working in their small groups or during large-group sessions, the teacher serves as a facilitator of the discussion rather than as a lecturer. Students actively participate in the identification and resolution of the problem(s). The integration of this technique helps with development of skills in teamwork, interdependency, and communication.[10] Group discussions help students formulate opinions and recommendations, clarify ideas, and develop new strategies for clinical problem solving. These skills are essential for lifelong learning and will be used by the students throughout their careers.

CONCEPT MAPPING

Concept maps are diagrams used to visually connect concepts. This strategy can be used to link new information to previously learned material, critically think through a process, or simply describe ideas in a pictorial form. Concept mapping can reveal how students organize their knowledge, understand relationships between various concepts, and display their creativity in incorporating new information.[12] This may be particularly useful in clinical therapeutics courses where foundational theories are connected with pharmacotherapy. The activity can help students organize information about a disease state and focus on relevant information for clinical decision making.[13] There are several free web-based programs available to build concept maps, but paper or any computer-based drawing tool is equally acceptable. Many different topics can be visualized using a concept map; therefore, detailed instructions and clear expectations are necessary for successful implementation of the activity. In the classroom, concept maps work best when used during group activities to facilitate collaborative and cooperative learning.[14]

PROBLEM-BASED/CASE-BASED LEARNING

Problem-solving skills can be developed during a class period by applying knowledge of pharmacotherapy to a patient case. This is commonly referred to as problem-based learning (PBL) or case-based learning (CBL). Application reinforces the previously learned material and helps students understand the relevance of the topic in a real-life situation. PBL is a teaching and learning method in which a complex problem is used as the stimulus for developing critical thinking and problem-solving skills, group skills, and investigative techniques. The process of PBL starts with the student identifying the problem in a patient case. The student spends time either alone or in a group exploring and analyzing the case and identifying learning resources needed to solve the problem. After acquiring the knowledge, the student applies it to solve the problem.[15] Interactive PBL computer tools and the use of real patient cases also stimulate learning both outside and inside the classroom.[16] Computer-assisted PBL can provide instant feedback throughout the process and incorporate other methods of active learning such as quizzes.[17] Programs that create virtual patients can be used creatively in PBL cases to simulate actual patient outcomes based on student recommendations.[18]

CBL is used by many professional schools to teach pharmacotherapy.[2,16] CBL involves a written description of a real-world problem or clinical situation. Only the facts are provided, usually in chronological sequence, similar to what would be encountered in a patient care setting. Many times, as in real life, the information given is incomplete, or important details are not available. When working through a case, the student must distinguish between relevant and irrelevant facts and realize that there is no single "correct" answer. CBL promotes self-directed learning because the student is actively involved in the analysis of the facts and details of the case, selection of a solution to the problem, and defense of his or her solution through discussion of the case.[19] During class, active participation is essential for the maximum learning benefit to be achieved. Because of their various backgrounds, students learn different perspectives when dealing with patient problems. Both PBL and CBL may support knowledge construction and elicit higher-order learning competencies such as critical thinking and decision making that bridge the gap between classroom and pharmacy practice.[20]

TEAM-BASED LEARNING

Team-based learning (TBL) is a learner-centered, instructor-directed, small-group learning strategy that can be implemented in large-group educational settings. The course is structured around the activity of teams of five to seven students who work together over an entire semester. TBL focuses on deepening student learning and enhancing team development. This is accomplished by the TBL structure, which involves: (1) pre-class preparation, (2) assurance of readiness to apply learned concepts, and (3) application of content to real-world scenarios through team problem-solving activities in class. A peer-review process provides important feedback to help team members develop the attitudes, behaviors, and skills that contribute positively to individual learning and effective teamwork.[4,21,22] A growing number of schools are adopting this strategy, resulting in various combinations and permutations of TBL. Guidance documents describing the core elements of TBL that should be incorporated to maximize student engagement and learning within teams have been published.[22,23]

TECHNOLOGY IN ACTIVE LEARNING

Educational technology use has become widespread among colleges and schools of pharmacy.[24] Technology can be used to enrich active learning when applied to the techniques above. In addition to the examples provided, a range of instructional technologies is available.[6,16] Learning management systems, like Blackboard™ and Canvas™ provide platforms for electronic teacher-student communication, assessment, and real-time feedback. Web conferencing and interactive video conferencing not only allow for distance learning but may include ARS, text chat, and small-group conference functionality. This technology, as well as proprietary and open-access document collaboration software (eg, Google Docs), provides platforms that can support student PBL, CBL, and TBL. Some teachers may choose to utilize social media platforms and blogging or microblogging technologies like Twitter™ to promote student engagement with the material, or model lifelong learning.[24] Particularly in health science education, the use of technology to conduct "serious gaming" has emerged. These interactive games used to practice and learn skills have been recognized as motivating, low-stakes, collaborative active learning experiences.[25] Finally, electronic simulations and virtual reality (VR) platforms can provide opportunities to bring real-life learning experiences into the classroom.[24,26]

ADVICE ON ACTIVE LEARNING FOR STUDENTS AND INSTRUCTORS

The use of active learning strategies provides students with opportunities to take a dynamic role in the learning process. Willing students, innovative teachers, and administrative support within the school are required for active learning to take place and be successful.[27]

ADVICE FOR STUDENTS

Students may have concerns about active learning. Some students may be accustomed to passively receiving information and feel uncomfortable participating in the learning process. Taking initiative is the key to deriving the benefits of active learning.

Prepare for class. Assigned readings, pre-recorded lectures, and homework must be completed before class in order to use class time efficiently for questions and discussion. Time management is important.[28] When reading assignments, take notes and summarize the information using tables or charts. Alternatively, make lists of questions from class or readings to discuss with your colleagues or faculty or try to answer them on your own.[28]

Seek to understand versus memorize. To develop appropriate therapeutic recommendations or answers to a question, you may have to look beyond the required reading materials. You may need to review notes from previous courses or perform literature searches and use the library or the internet to retrieve additional information. It is important that you understand "why" and "how" and not just memorize "what." Memorizing results in short-term retention of knowledge, whereas understanding results in long-term retention and will enable you to better justify your clinical recommendations. In active learning, much of what you learn you will learn on your own. You will probably find that you read more, but you will gain understanding from reading. At the same time, you are developing a critical lifelong learning skill.

During class, take an active role in the learning process. Be an active participant in class or group discussions; lively debates about pharmacotherapy issues allow more therapeutic options to be discussed. Discussing material helps you to apply your knowledge, verbalize the medical and pharmacologic terminology, engage in active listening, think critically, and develop interpersonal skills. When working in groups, all members should participate in problem solving because teaching others is an excellent way to learn the subject matter. Listen carefully to and be respectful of the thoughts and opinions of classmates. Writing about a topic develops critical thinking, communication, and organization skills. Stopping to write allows you to reflect on the information you have just heard and reinforces learning. Although many options for digital note-taking are available, it is not known whether these enhance or deter learning.[29] Taking an active role through team discussions, note-taking, identifying connections between patient cases, and applying what you have learned to the current cases will promote development of self-directed and autonomous learning skills.

ADVICE FOR INSTRUCTORS

Instructors may also have concerns about incorporating active learning strategies. They may feel that their class is too large to accommodate active learning, have concerns that they will not be able to cover all the content or that it will take too much time to change their course, or even fear that students may be resistant to active learning strategies.[27] Some of the hesitation may lie in the belief that active learning is an alternative to lecture. Rather, active learning strategies can be incorporated into didactic lectures to enhance learning sessions. Educators can move some course content online by assigning pre-class mini-lectures or quizzes.[2] Several strategies can be used to increase the successful implementation of active learning.

Discuss course expectations. Take time to describe teaching, learning, and assessment methods and how students can be successful in the course. Help students to understand the benefits of active learning.[27]

Consider slowly implementing a change in the classroom. To implement active learning strategies, teachers must overcome the anxiety that change often creates. Experiment with simple active learning methods (ie, the pause technique) and slowly implement other active learning approaches.

Consider techniques to maximize student discussion. Allowing students to discuss content in pairs or small groups before asking them to share their ideas with the entire class can help minimize student anxiety about engaging in classroom discussions. Consider moving around the room during discussions, if possible, and make an effort to learn student names.

Take a stepwise approach. Learners become self-directed in stages, not in one single moment of transformation. Sequence activities and assignments that gradually develop all three stages: learning, intellectual development, and interpersonal skills.[30]

Prepare students for group learning. Group learning is not intuitive. Instructors who use group learning should create a workable environment, ensure that expectations of students are understood, and structure the learning sessions to maximize student engagement and learning within teams.[27]

Have a preconceived plan for how the learning session will go and stick to it. Determine what learning objectives you would like to achieve during the session. Consider developing an outline for the learning session, estimating the time that will be spent on each active learning activity.[2]

USING THE CASEBOOK

The *Casebook* was prepared to assist in the development of each student's understanding of a disease and its management as well as problem-solving skills. It is important for students to realize that learning and understanding the material is guided through problem solving. Students are encouraged to solve each of the cases individually or with others in a study group before discussion of the case and topic in class. These cases can be used as an active learning strategy by allowing time for students to work on the cases during class as an application exercise for TBL.[21] Teams or individuals can then report verbally on the questions and debate various treatment options.

SUMMARY

The use of case studies and other active learning strategies will enhance the development of essential skills necessary to practice in any setting. The role of the healthcare professional is constantly changing; thus, it is important for students to acquire the knowledge, skills, behaviors, and attitudes to develop the lifetime skills required for continued learning. Teachers who incorporate active learning strategies into the classroom are facilitating the development of lifelong learners who will be able to adapt to change that occurs in their profession.

REFERENCES

1. Warren RG. Carpe Diem: A Student Guide to Active Learning. Landover, MD: University Press of America; 1996.
2. Gleason BL, Peeters MJ, Resman-Targoff BH, et al. An active learning strategies primer for achieving ability-based educational outcomes. Am J Pharm Educ. 2011;75(9):186. doi:10.5688/ajpe759186.
3. Michael J. Where's the evidence that active learning works? Adv Physiol Educ. 2006;30(4):159–167. doi:10.1152/advan.00053.2006.
4. Ofstad W, Brunner LJ. Team-based learning in pharmacy education. Am J Pharm Educ. 2013;77(4):70. doi:10.5688/ajpe77470.
5. Rotellar C, Cain J. Research, perspectives, and recommendations on implementing the flipped classroom. Am J Pharm Educ. 2016;80(2):34. doi:10.5688/ajpe80234.
6. Cain J, Robinson E. A primer on audience response systems: current applications and future considerations. Am J Pharm Educ. 2008;72(4):77.
7. DiVall MV, Hayney MS, Marsh W, et al. Perceptions of pharmacy students, faculty members, and administrators on the use of technology in the classroom. Am J Pharm Educ. 2013;77(4):75. doi:10.5688/ajpe77475.
8. Stead DR. A review of the one-minute paper. Act Learn High Educ. 2005;6(2):118–131. doi:10.1177/1469787405054237.
9. Paulson DR, Faust JL. Active Learning for the College Classroom. Cal State LA. October 22, 2013. Available at: *https://www.calstatela.edu/dept/chem/chem2/Active/main.htm*. Accessed November 11, 2021.
10. Sylvia LM, Barr JT. Pharmacy Education: What Matters in Learning and Teaching. Sudbury, MA: Jones & Bartlett, 2011.
11. Sawyer J, Obeid R. Cooperative and collaborative learning: getting the best of both worlds. In: Obied R, et al., eds. How We Teach Now: The GSTA Guide to Student-Centered Teaching. 2017. Available at: *https://teachpsych.org/ebooks/howweteachnow#:~:text=How%20We%20Teach%20Now%20provides,teamwork)%20in%20addition%20to%20discipline%2D*. Accessed November 11, 2021.
12. Hill LH. Concept mapping in a pharmacy communications course to encourage meaningful student learning. Am J Pharm Educ. 2004;68(5):109. doi:10.5688/aj6805109.
13. Carr-Lopez SM, Galal SM, Vyas D, Patel RA, Gnesa EH. The utility of concept maps to facilitate higher-level learning in a large classroom setting. Am J Pharm Educ. 2014;78(9):170. doi:10.5688/ajpe789170.
14. Schwendimann B. Concept maps as versatile tools to integrate complex ideas: from kindergarten to higher and professional education. Knowl Manag E-Learn Int J. 2015;7(1):73–99. doi:10.34105/j.kmel.2015.07.006.
15. Strohfeldt K, Grant DT. A model for self-directed problem-based learning for renal therapeutics. Am J Pharm Educ. 2010;74(9):173.
16. Raman-Wilms L. Innovative enabling strategies in self-directed, problem-based therapeutics: enhancing student preparedness for pharmaceutical care. Am J Pharm Educ. 2001;65:56–64.
17. McFalls M. Integration of problem-based learning and innovative technology into a self-care course. Am J Pharm Educ. 2013;77(6):127. doi:10.5688/ajpe776127.
18. Benedict N. Virtual patients and problem-based learning in advanced therapeutics. Am J Pharm Educ. 2010;74(8):143.
19. Thistlethwaite JE, Davies D, Ekeocha S, et al. The effectiveness of case-based learning in health professional education. A BEME systematic review: BEME Guide No. 23. Med Teach. 2012;34(6):e421–e444. doi:10.3109/0142159X.2012.680939.
20. Tawfik AA, Fowlin J, Kelley K, Anderson M, Vann SW. Supporting case-based reasoning in pharmacy through case sequencing. J Form Des Learn. 2019;3(2):111–122. doi:10.1007/s41686-019-00035-0.
21. Conway SE, Johnson JL, Ripley TL. Integration of team-based learning strategies into a cardiovascular module. Am J Pharm Educ. 2010;74(2):35.
22. Haidet P, Levine RE, Parmelee DX, et al. Perspective: guidelines for reporting team-based learning activities in the medical and health sciences education literature. Acad Med 2012;87(3):292–299. doi:10.1097/ACM.0b013e318244759e.
23. Parmelee D, Michaelsen LK, Cook S, Hudes PD. Team-based learning: a practical guide: AMEE Guide No. 65. Med Teach. 2012;34(5):e275–e287. doi:10.3109/0142159X.2012.651179.
24. Monaghan MS, Cain JJ, Malone PM, et al. Educational technology use among US colleges and schools of pharmacy. Am J Pharm Educ. 2011;75(5):87. doi:10.5688/ajpe75587.
25. Cain J, Piascik P. Are serious games a good strategy for pharmacy education? Am J Pharm Educ. 2015;79(4):47. doi:10.5688/ajpe79447.
26. Coyne L, Merritt TA, Parmentier BL, Sharpton RA, Takemoto JK. The past, present, and future of virtual reality in pharmacy education. Am J Pharm Educ. 2019;83(3):7456. doi:10.5688/ajpe7456.
27. Whitley HP, Bell E, Eng M, et al. Practical team-based learning from planning to implementation. Am J Pharm Educ. 2015;79(10):149. doi:10.5688/ajpe7910149.
28. McKeirnan KC, Colorafi K, Kim AP, et al. Study behaviors associated with student pharmacists' academic success in an active classroom pharmacy curriculum. Am J Pharm Educ. 2020;84(7):ajpe7695. doi:10.5688/ajpe7695.
29. Stacy EM, Cain J. Note-taking and handouts in the digital age. Am J Pharm Educ. 2015;79(7):107. doi:10.5688/ajpe797107.
30. Weimer M. Learner-Centered Teaching: Five Key Changes to Practice. 2nd ed. San Francisco, CA: Jossey-Bass; 2013.

CHAPTER

3

Patient Communication: Getting the Most Out of That One-on-One Time

KRISTA D. CAPEHART, PharmD, MS, BCACP, FAPHA, AE-C

Talking with patients is a crucial component of the medication use process. Regardless of practice area, healthcare providers have the opportunity to teach and learn from people they interact with each day. In addition to having a wealth of scientific knowledge and clinical skills, providers must also possess excellent communication skills. This chapter focuses on key elements of communication in various practice settings. The intricacies of interpersonal communication can be found in other resources.[1-3]

PATIENT-CENTERED CARE AND THE ROLE OF COMMUNICATION

With the movement toward value-based, accessible, high-quality care, provision of interprofessional, team-based care is vital. The Patient Protection and Affordable Care Act of 2010 fostered development of accountable care organizations (ACOs) and patient-centered medical homes (PCMHs). The National Center for Quality Assurance defines a PCMH as "a way of organizing primary care that emphasizes care coordination and communication to transform primary care into 'what patients want it to be.'"[4] A team-based approach that includes pharmacists with medication expertise and good communication skills can optimize the medication use process and ensure that the patient truly is at the center of care.

In patient-centered care, the patient participates in his/her own health care through shared decision making with healthcare providers. Shared decision making involves decision aids or a process to facilitate patient understanding when multiple treatment options could be used.[5] Shared decision making increases knowledge and improves patient understanding of the risks of their care and makes patients more likely to receive care that is consistent with their values and beliefs.[6]

Consequently, the patient–clinician interaction must involve more than simply collecting information during a medication history interview or conveying verbal or written information about a prescription. Active listening skills must be employed to understand the patient's concerns about medication therapy, engage the patient in his/her care, and develop the trust required for a positive long-standing relationship. Establishing a trusting relationship is necessary for effective communication, but trust does not come quickly or easily. In the community pharmacy, it may result from a caring pharmacist always taking the time to ask how a patient's medications are working. In an ambulatory clinic, it could come from a nurse practitioner or pharmacist teaching about diabetes care and improving A1C levels. Pathways to a trusting relationship may vary, but the ultimate goal is for patients to feel that they can confide in and rely on their healthcare providers about medication-related needs.

Patient interactions vary depending on the practice setting, clinician training, the purpose of the interaction, and other factors.

In 2015, the Joint Commission of Pharmacy Practitioners (JCPP) published the Pharmacist's Patient Care Process, which is similar to the patient care process used daily by other healthcare providers and is intended to standardize the patient's experiences in each encounter with the pharmacist.[7] The steps of the Pharmacists' Patient Care Process include: (1) Collect, (2) Assess, (3) Plan, (4) Implement, and (5) Follow-up: Monitor and Evaluate (see **Chapter 4, Fig. 4–1**).

Optimal communication is necessary in the *Collect, Implement,* and *Follow-up* parts of the process. During the *Collect* portion, the pharmacist gathers information about the patient and the present medical situation. The information available may vary by practice site, but the process remains the same. During the *Implement* stage, the pharmacist has the opportunity to educate the patient about the care plan. This may include new medications, lifestyle modifications, changes in therapy, or referrals to other healthcare providers. *Monitor* and *Evaluate* can involve gathering information from the patient regarding how the medication is working, whether any adverse events have occurred, and vital adherence data. The key to successful use of the patient care process is collaboration with the patient and other healthcare team members.

IMPROVING THE PATIENT ENCOUNTER

Talking with a patient and collecting information require patience, empathy, and the ability to direct the conversation. The clinician should use open-ended questions, which start with *who, what, when, where, why,* or *how.* Close-ended questions are those that permit the patient to respond with a simple *yes* or *no* and tend to leave much unsaid. With a close-ended question, the patient may not provide complete information. For example, if a provider asks, "Have you been taking your warfarin as the doctor prescribed?" the patient may simply respond, "Yes." However, it could be that the patient understood and adhered to the one-tablet-daily directions that were initially prescribed but did not realize that the directions were recently changed to one tablet Monday, Wednesday, Friday, and Saturday, and one-half tablet the other days of the week. An open-ended question such as, "How are you taking your warfarin each day?" requires more explanation from the patient, allowing the clinician to collect more accurate information to assess the patient's medication/medical history and status. There is a place for close-ended questions; after most of the information has been collected, close-ended questions can be used to narrow down the details about the patient's situation.

Healthcare providers must be exceptional listeners, open to what the patient is sharing and not sharing. Becoming an active listener is not always easy in busy patient care environments. It includes removing distractions, empathizing with the patient, acknowledging the patient's individuality, and recognizing nonverbal signals from the patient.

TABLE 3-1	Nonverbal Cues to Demonstrate Good Listening
Letter	Meaning
S	Squarely face the patient (do not have your body angled in another direction)
O	Open posture (do not cross your legs and arms)
L	Lean toward the patient (not encroaching on personal space) to show interest
E	Eye contact
R	Relax

Regardless of practice setting, distractions should be minimized to ensure that the patient is the primary focus of the provider's attention. In community pharmacies, separate counseling rooms may be used, if available. Attempts to maintain privacy help demonstrate the pharmacist's focus on the patient.

Empathy and sympathy are often confused. Empathy is the ability to understand the patient's feelings and share them, whereas sympathy is feeling sorry for the patient. Acknowledging emotions, reassuring the patient, and providing answers to questions helps to improve the interaction and outcomes. Each patient enters the medical encounter with a set of experiences, beliefs, and expectations; understanding them through active listening facilitates creation and implementation of the therapeutic plan.

Nonverbal communication can be as important as what the patient relates verbally, and clinicians must recognize these as well. Nonverbal cues may include body language, use of time, tone of voice, touch, distance, and physical environments. Body language clues include crossing the arms (a sign the patient is closing themselves off) or nodding the head (an indication the listener is paying attention or agreeing). Time can be used to delay (as with dramatic pauses) or to rush through situations that may be uncomfortable. Tone of voice is revealing because it includes pitch and intonation and can relate anger, fascination, confusion, and a variety of other emotions. Touch, distance, and physical environment are specific to the individual. Some patients are comfortable with a touch on the arm for reassurance or to show concern, whereas others require much greater personal space and shy away from physical contact. Generally, people prefer approximately 2 feet of personal space when having a one-on-one encounter. Maintaining an appropriate distance that makes the patient comfortable may take time to master, and it's important to maintain awareness of the patient's reaction to your proximity to them. The physical environment the clinician creates for the encounter serves as a nonverbal cue. For example, an open room with chairs arranged in a circle creates a welcoming space for individuals to gather for conversation. A lecture-style setup creates a more formal setting where the focus is on the presenter with less individual sharing. The clinician must be aware of the nonverbal cues he or she is giving as well. Egan developed a mnemonic to assist in demonstrating nonverbal cues for good listening (SOLER), which can help build a trusting patient relationship (Table 3-1).[8]

EXAMPLES OF COMMUNICATION WITHIN THE PHARMACIST–PATIENT RELATIONSHIP

Although the principles discussed in this section are directed toward pharmacy practice, many of them can also be used by other healthcare providers in any environment in which medication counseling and education occur. The opportunities to talk with patients vary with practice settings and expectations. For example, hospital pharmacists or nurses may perform counseling on all discharge medications or discuss injectable medications being started with the patient. The community pharmacist may counsel on new or refill medications or help select an over-the-counter (OTC) medication for a particular problem. Pharmacists communicate with patients to undertake medication therapy management, participate in collaborative drug therapy management, and perform medication reconciliation.

THE MEDICATION AND MEDICAL HISTORY

It is important to collect comprehensive information when conducting a patient medication interview. Using the tips presented previously, information can be gathered from the patient to improve patient care and safety.

Initially, collect demographic information about the patient, including name, address, and date of birth, unless this information is already available. Use an open-ended question to inquire about the patient's allergies (medication, environmental, and food), such as, "What medication allergies have you experienced in the past?" Be sure to document what happened when the patient experienced the reaction. It may be necessary at some point in the future to evaluate risk versus benefit and determine if a true allergy exists. Query the patient regarding social history related to drug and substance use, including tobacco use, alcohol consumption, recreation and medical marijuana use, illicit drug use, and caffeine intake. Asking about social history can sometimes make both the clinician and the patient uncomfortable. One method to ease tension is to advise the patient that some medications interact with alcohol or tobacco, and that it is important for information to be complete to evaluate drug–drug interactions. Remember to identify the type of substance, quantity, and frequency of use as well.

When verifying the patient's current prescription medications, it is helpful to start by asking whether the patient has either brought their medications or a written list to the visit. This is a good practice in the emergency department and many other clinical settings. Regardless of whether the patient has a list, ask, "What prescription medications do you take?" For each medication, specifically document the name, strength, route of administration, prescriber, and how he or she takes the medication. The way the patient actually takes each medication can be compared to the label directions to assess patient adherence. Remember that nonadherence could be due to misunderstanding the correct directions, attempting to save money, or any of a number of reasons other than simply choosing **not** to take the medication as directed. Also, be sure to ask the patient why each medication was prescribed. Remind each patient about nonoral routes of administration also. This could be a close-ended question followed up by an open-ended one, such as, "Do you use any medications that you apply to your skin? What other medications do you use that you don't swallow by mouth?" This may prompt the patient to remember some medications they may have forgotten.[9]

Patients should be asked about nonprescription items used, including OTC medications, herbals, vitamins, and dietary supplements. Patients may have the misconception that OTC or "natural" substances do not interact with prescription medications or medical conditions. This is an opportunity to educate the patient about the potential dangers of incorrect use of these products.

Pharmacists and other providers conducting medication interviews must also have or collect information on diagnosed medical conditions, but there is flexibility in when this occurs. One option is to address medical conditions after asking about allergies and before beginning questions on medications. This gives the interviewer an idea of the therapeutic categories of medications the patient may be taking. The other option is to cover diagnosed medical conditions after collecting the list of prescription and nonprescription medications. Using this order of questioning enables the interviewer to ask the patient "What are you taking X medication for?" if the patient fails to list an indication for a medication named earlier.

The comprehensive medication interview is optimal for the provision of medication reconciliation, medication therapy management, and collaborative drug therapy management. However, it is not always feasible to perform an interview directly with the patient. Sometimes, the information may need to be collected from the pharmacy dispensing record, a family member, or another source. Information not obtained personally from the patient may need to be reconfirmed later.

COUNSELING ON A NEW PRESCRIPTION

The Omnibus Budget Reconciliation Act of 1990 (OBRA 90) was passed, in part, to help ensure safe medication use for Medicaid patients. While OBRA 90 is often considered to be the law that mandated the offer to counsel on medications, it also gave rise to new record-keeping requirements and mandated that pharmacists complete a prospective drug utilization review for all Medicaid patients. Requirements vary by state regarding what must be done for drug counseling, but OBRA 90 required making an offer to counsel, not that counseling must actually be performed.[10] Since 1990, some states have passed various additional requirements for patient counseling and education from merely complying with OBRA 90 to not permitting a patient to decline the offer of counseling. It is important to be familiar with your state's patient counseling requirements.

Counseling on medications increases the patient's knowledge and comfort level in using their medication correctly.[11] Part of the patient's comfort can derive from the process as well as from the information. The counseling should occur in a private area, if possible. If a separate room is not available, use a divider or area that makes the counseling space relatively easy to maintain patient confidentiality and privacy. A patient may be uncomfortable receiving counseling on certain types of medication, such as a medication for a vaginal infection; speaking in a confidential tone in a private area will improve patient satisfaction with the encounter.

Educating the patient on new medications should start by assessing what the patient already knows about the medication that has been prescribed. The Indian Health Service (IHS) began providing patient medication counseling services in the 1970s and 1980s.[12] The IHS would go on to develop a commonly used method for counseling on new and refill prescriptions. The method is referred to as the Three Prime Questions technique (Fig. 3-1).[13]

Asking "What did your doctor tell you the medicine was for?" is an excellent way to begin the session. After determining the patient's knowledge about the medication, state the medication name (including whether it is generic) and strength. Then ask, "How did the doctor tell you to take the medicine?" Next, provide information about the route of administration, dosing schedule, duration of treatment, storage, and administration. Inquire about the patient's daily activities and attempt to incorporate the schedule into routine daily activities to increase adherence. Finally, the third question enables the pharmacist to provide information regarding adverse effects and how to monitor effectiveness. Explain the medication in terms of what condition it is intended to treat, what the expected action is, and how the patient can self-monitor for efficacy. The patient should realize if and when he/she should "feel different." For example, with medications for hypertension and dyslipidemia, the patient may not notice a difference in how they feel and should be counseled about the importance of laboratory testing or other monitoring. Potential adverse effects can be discussed by dividing them into two categories: (1) those that are more likely to occur but are not serious, and (2) those that are rare but serious. Provide guidance on how the patient can avoid some of the most common adverse effects, if possible, and what should be done if a serious one occurs. Also inform the patient about other drugs or conditions that interact with the medication and how to manage the interaction. In finishing this portion of the session, discuss storage information, what to do if a dose is missed, and any pertinent refill information.

As the counseling session is concluding, verify the patient's understanding of the information covered during the session. One of the best methods for this is the "teach-back method," which is used to determine what the patient understands and to correct any misunderstandings.[14] To avoid the impression that you are testing the patient, a good approach is to say, "I have covered quite a bit of information about your new medication. Just to make sure that I did not forget anything, how are you going to take the medication when you get home?" This places the appearance of responsibility for remembering everything on the healthcare provider and reduces stress for the patient. Studies have compared lecture-based counseling and interactive counseling similar to the Three Prime Questions style for preference and retention of information. Approximately two-thirds of standardized patients who experienced both types preferred interactive counseling over lecture-based counseling.[13] Another study examined retention among actual patients and found them to be four times more likely to correctly answer how to take their medication than those who received traditional lecture-based counseling.[15] The style of counseling may need to be individualized to a particular patient by picking up on nonverbal cues and the patient interaction.

COUNSELING ON A REFILL

Counseling on a medication refill is an abbreviated process of counseling for a new medication. The IHS has an additional three prime questions for refills (see Fig. 3-1). The purpose of the medication and how to take it is reviewed, but the focus changes from how to take the medication to monitoring the patient with queries such as, "What kinds of problems are you having?" Counseling on refills is especially important when the use of a device is involved. For example, metered-dose inhalers are difficult to use correctly. Correct inhaler use decreases over time, even in as little as 2–3 months, and studies show that pharmacist counseling improves correct inhaler technique and adherence.[16] Additionally, it is important to follow up with the patient to answer any questions that have arisen since the last fill and to provide contact information for any future questions that arise.

New Prescriptions	• What did the doctor tell you the medicine was for? • How did the doctor tell you to take the medicine? • What did the doctor tell you to expect?
Refills Prescriptions	• What do you take the medicine for? • How do you take it? • What kind of problems are you having?

FIGURE 3-1. Indian Health Service Three Prime Question counseling method. (Reproduced with permission from Lam N, Muravez SN, Boyce RW. A comparison of the Indian Health Service counseling technique with traditional, lecture-style counseling. *J Am Pharm Assoc* (2003). 2015;55(5):503-510.)

OVER-THE-COUNTER MEDICATION SELECTION

Assisting a patient with selection of self-care products also requires effective communication skills. The first steps are to assess the patient's complaints and evaluate whether self-management with OTC medications is appropriate or whether referral is needed. There are a variety of mnemonics to assist clinicians in asking all necessary questions before recommending a product. These include: (1) CHAPS-FRAPS (Chief complaint, History of present illness, Allergies, Past medical history, Social history, Family history, Review of Systems, Assessments, Plans, and SOAP); (2) The Basic Seven (location, quality, severity, timing, context, modifying factors, and associated symptoms); and (3) PQRST (Palliation and provocation, Quality and quantity, Region and radiation, Signs and symptoms, Temporal relationship).[17-19] The most comprehensive mnemonic is the QuEST/SCHOLAR approach.[20] This method enables the clinician to evaluate the patient and most accurately select the best non-prescription product. The QuEST/SCHOLAR process includes:

1. **Qu**ickly and accurately assess the patient.
   Ask about the current complaint (SCHOLAR), other medications, and allergies:
   - ✓ **S**ymptoms
   - ✓ **C**haracteristics
   - ✓ **H**istory
   - ✓ **O**nset
   - ✓ **L**ocation
   - ✓ **A**ggravating factors
   - ✓ **R**emitting factors
2. **E**stablish that the patient is a self-care candidate.
   - ✓ No severe symptoms, symptoms do not persist or return, patient is not using self-care to avoid medical care
3. **S**uggest appropriate self-care strategies.
   - ✓ Recommend the medication and nonpharmacologic therapy
4. **T**alk with the patient.
   - ✓ How the drug is going to work, when it should be taken, expected adverse events

For example, Joe comes into your pharmacy requesting assistance in selecting an OTC product for heartburn. Utilizing the QuEST/SCHOLAR process, you could:

1. **Qu**ickly and accurately assess the patient: "Let's talk a little about the type of problems you have been having."
   Ask about the current complaint (SCHOLAR), other medications, allergies:
   - ✓ **S**ymptoms: "What symptoms are you having?"
   - ✓ **C**haracteristics: "How would you describe the pain…burning, sharp, shooting?"
   - ✓ **H**istory: "Have you experienced this before? What have you tried already? Did it work?"
   - ✓ **O**nset: "When did the symptoms start?"
   - ✓ **L**ocation: "Where is the pain you are describing as heartburn?"
   - ✓ **A**ggravating factors: "What makes it worse?"
   - ✓ **R**emitting factors: "What makes it better?"
2. **E**stablish that the patient is a self-care candidate:
   - ✓ "Based on this information, I think it would (or would not) be appropriate for you to use OTC treatment."
3. **S**uggest appropriate self-care strategies:
   - ✓ "I would recommend _____ and some non-medication strategies, too."
4. **T**alk with the patient:
   - ✓ "You can take ___ tablet(s) every ___ hours to help with symptoms. This medication will work by _____. You should start to notice improvement in _____ minutes. Also, try lifestyle changes like avoiding spicy foods and raising the head of the bed. If your symptoms persist for more than 2 weeks or do not improve, see your doctor. The OTC medications can cover up symptoms that need to be checked out further by your doctor."

The QuEST/SCHOLAR method provides a technique for systematically assessing patients in the pharmacy and providing a thorough but efficient evaluation. It is vital to maintain the patient's privacy (using a private area, if possible) and be cognizant of topics that make patients uncomfortable. These occur with OTC items, too; recognizing this and being prepared will help put the patient at ease. Try to employ the teach-back method with OTCs, herbals, and dietary supplements to ensure patient understanding of the information discussed.

BARRIERS TO COMMUNICATION

Patient communication does not always happen the way we plan. There are common barriers to communication, and knowing them can help you to be prepared. Communication barriers can be divided into three common categories: (1) patient barriers, (2) clinician barriers, and (3) healthcare setting barriers. Patient barriers may include the patient literacy level, misconceptions regarding the purpose of the visit, aging, or visual/hearing difficulties. A clinician may lack training with certain types of patient encounters or have a negative attitude about patient counseling. A patient and clinician combined barrier can include misconceptions regarding cultural beliefs and household influence on healthcare decisions. Healthcare setting barriers posing communication issues can include lack of privacy, space, or resources to serve their specific patient population.

Because the patient is ultimately in charge of his/her health care, patient barriers can be some of the most difficult to overcome. Lack of education and poor health literacy can be substantial barriers. The aging patient brings unique challenges to communication, such as changes in physical health, depression, cognitive decline, and changes in hearing, vision, voice, and speech processes.[21] Also, you may be communicating with the caregiver and not the patient, and he/she may be in a rush or may not have all of the patient information needed.

HEALTH LITERACY

Health literacy is defined as the degree to which individuals have the capacity to obtain, process, and understand basic health information and services needed to make appropriate health decisions. It is not enough for patients to simply "understand" information about their health. They must be able to make decisions about what to do—to be able to navigate the healthcare system and be somewhat confident about it. Health literacy may or may not be tied to the level of education completed. For example, a patient with an MBA degree who is highly educated and very successful in the corporate world may not realize that it is unsafe to take OTC acetaminophen and an OTC cough and cold product also containing acetaminophen. On the other hand, a woman who only completed the 10th grade and has a young child with a pediatric cancer may be well versed in the healthcare system and able to tell you more about her child's medications and medical needs than some members of the healthcare team. Simply put, clinicians cannot determine the level of health literacy by looking at a patient and making assumptions about his/her education or social status.

A sense of shame often accompanies a patient's low health literacy. Because patients do not typically volunteer their lack of knowledge, identifying low health literacy is important, especially in light of its association with medication nonadherence.[22] Some indicators that health literacy may be a problem with a given patient are leaving forms partially filled out, referring to medications by their color (instead of by name), opening the bottle to look at the medication rather than the label, making excuses like "I forgot my glasses," postponing appointments, chronic nonadherence, failing to look at written materials, or bringing someone with them.

Once you recognize that a patient presents health literacy concerns, it is vital to remain respectful, considerate, and maintain privacy. Failure to be sensitive to the needs of these patients can result in loss of the relationship that was forming and loss of an opportunity to impact the patient's health outcomes. Recognizing that time is a limitation, there are some tips to help with patient understanding. First, limit the number of main counseling points to two or three. Covering too many topics can be overwhelming. Second, demonstrate the procedure or technique. One example of this is to show the patient how to use an inhaler and spacer device. Then ensure that understanding is complete with the teach-back method discussed previously. Pictures can also be used to convey information about medication instructions and safety. Standard pictograms created by the United States Pharmacopeia are available for download at *http://www.usp.org/usp-healthcare-professionals/related-topics-resources/usp-pictograms/download-pictograms*. Finally, summarize the information and be positive, communicating in an open manner while maintaining eye contact.

Using plain language is one of the most important tenets for working with patients with low health literacy. This involves using common words instead of medical jargon to improve understanding of complex situations. An example is to use "water pill" instead of "diuretic", "a medication that helps open the airways" instead of "bronchodilator," and "sore" instead of "abscess." Additional examples can be found at *http://www.plainlanguage.gov./populartopics/health_literacy/index.cfm* under the Plain Language Thesaurus.

AGING

The aging patient may experience many physiologic changes such as cognitive decline and dementia that can make communication more difficult. Sensory loss, including both hearing and vision, may also occur with aging.[21] Because these are challenging in their own right, living with them while navigating the healthcare system can be frustrating for patients.

Some general techniques can make the encounter with these patients more effective. Know the patient's strengths and weaknesses and cater to them. Select educational materials that are most appropriate for that patient. Be prepared to take some extra time with the patient to ensure full understanding and buy-in of the information. Use an environment that is conducive to the conversation—a place with minimal distractions. If the patient has difficulty hearing, speaking louder will not help; it will only distort the sound. Speak slowly and simplify your sentences. Use plain language when speaking, making sure to avoid medical jargon that can be confusing and overwhelming. Finally, if the patient has visual difficulties, ensure that they have their glasses and be prepared to provide the materials in a larger font. You may also want to determine whether your prescription filling software can print prescription label information in a larger font for easier reading.

CULTURAL COMPETENCE AND PATIENT BELIEFS

Patients come to healthcare visits with a set of personal beliefs and strongly held cultural backgrounds. Clinicians should be prepared with training on cultural competence and cultural humility to understand that a patient's ultimate healthcare decision will not be based solely on what the clinician says. Successful communication strategies involve not only being aware of the patient's beliefs but endeavoring to honor their beliefs and values.[23] Studies show that when both the clinician and the healthcare organization take steps including education about the cultures in the patient population, hiring a diverse population, and having culture-specific programs that both patient outcomes and satisfaction can be improved.[24,25]

TEAM-BASED CARE AND PATIENT COMMUNICATION IN THE FUTURE

With the widespread implementation of electronic health records, more patients requiring chronic care management, and a value-based reimbursement system, a clinician's ability to develop masterful patient communication skills is becoming essential. Employing a collaborative, team-based approach to patient care and the tips for patient communication can help to ensure optimal health outcomes. Maximizing use of technology such as the electronic health record for referral to and communication with other clinicians who provide necessary services can meet needs that may seem impossible in a single clinic or pharmacy. Each healthcare team member brings special skills and communicates with the patient to obtain additional information. The best care is provided when providers come together at the same location (or virtually) to collaborate and meet the overall needs of each patient. In some settings, this may be collaborative drug therapy management working with the healthcare team to optimize medication therapy and overall health outcomes. In other settings, it may include clinicians working to coordinate with health educators in the community to provide services such as diabetes self-management classes.

CONCLUSION

Effective patient communication is a mandatory skill for all healthcare providers. Good communication involves developing a positive clinician–patient relationship, demonstrating a real interest in the patient's health, listening carefully to the patient's complaints, involving the patient in the decision-making process, and providing education in a way that the patient can understand. The ultimate goal is to improve the patient's health, and effective communication is the key to making this happen.

REFERENCES

1. Patterson K, Grenny J, McMillan R, Switzler A. Crucial Conversations. 2nd ed. New York, NY: McGraw Hill; 2012.

2. Rantucci M. Pharmacists Talking with Patients: A Guide to Patient Counseling. 2nd ed. Philadelphia, PA: Lippincott, Williams, & Wilkins; 2007.

3. Berger B. Communication Skills for Pharmacists: Building Relationships, Improving Patient Care. 3rd ed. Washington, DC: American Pharmacists Association; 2009.

4. Ncqa.org. Patient-Centered Medical Home (PCMH). 2018. Available at: *http://www.ncqa.org/Programs/Recognition/Practices/PatientCentered MedicalHomePCMH.aspx*. Accessed August 30, 2021.

5. Shafir A, Rosenthal J. Shared-Decision Making: Advancing Patient-Centered Care through State and Federal Implementation. 1st ed. Washington, DC: National Academy for State Health Policy; 2012. Available at: *http://www.nashp.org/sites/default/files/shared.decision.making.report.pdf*. Accessed October 28, 2021.

6. Stacey D, Bennett C, Barry M. Decision aids for people facing health treatment or screening decisions. Cochrane Database Syst Rev. 2011;10:CD001431.

7. Bennett M, Kliethermes M. How to Implement the Pharmacists' Patient Care Process. Washington, DC: American Pharmacist Association; 2015.

8. Egan G. The Skilled Helper. Belmont, CA: Brooks Cole, Cengage Learning; 2010.

9. Ahrq.gov. Figure 9: Tips for Conducting a Patient Medication Interview. Agency for Healthcare Research & Quality. 2012. Available at: *http://www.ahrq.gov/professionals/quality-patient-safety/patient-safety-resources/resources/match/matchfig9.html*. Accessed October 28, 2021.

10. Drug Diversion Toolkit. Controlled Substance Integrity-Documentation from Drop-off to Pickup, 1st ed. Baltimore, MD: Center for Medicare and Medicaid Services; 2016. Available at: *https://www.homestatehealth.com/content/dam/centene/home-state-health/pdfs/drugdiversion-controlledsubstancedoc-booklet.pdf*. Accessed October 28, 2021.

11. Erickson S, Kirking D, Sandusky M. Michigan Medicaid recipients perceptions of medication counseling as required by OBRA 90. J Am Pharm Assoc. 1998;38(3):333–338.

12. Fisher R, Brands A, Herrier R. History of the Indian Health Service Model of Pharmacy Practice: Innovations in Pharmaceutical Care. Pharmacy in History. 1995;37(3):107–122.

13. Lam N, Muravez S, Boyce RW. A comparison of the Indian Health Service counseling technique with traditional, lecture-style counseling. J Am Pharm Assoc. 2015;55(5):503–510.

14. Schillinger D, Piette J, Grumbach K, et al. Closing the loop: physician communication with diabetic patients who have low health literacy. Arch Intern Med. 2003;163(1):83–90.

15. Guirguis LM, Nusair MB. Standardized patients' preferences for pharmacist interactive counseling style: a mixed method approach. J Am Pharm Assoc. 2016;56(2):123–128.

16. Mehuys E, Van Bortel L, De Bolle L, et al. Effectiveness of pharmacist intervention for asthma control improvement. Eur Respir J. 2008;31(4):790–799.

17. McCallian DJ, Cheigh NH. The pharmacist's role in self-care. J Am Pharm Assoc. 2002;42(5 Suppl 1):S40–S41.

18. Boyce R, Herrier R. Obtaining and using patient data. Am Pharm. 1991;31:65–71.

19. Bates B, Bates B, Northway D. PQRST: a mnemonic to communicate a change in condition. J Am Med Direct Assoc. 2002;3(1):23–25.

20. Leibowitz K, Ginsburg D. Counseling self-treating patients quickly and effectively. In: APhA Inaugural Self-Care Institute. Washington, DC: American Pharmacist Association; 2002.

21. Yorkston K, Bourgeois M, Baylor C. Communication and aging. Phys Med Rehab Clin North Am. 2010;21(2):309–319.

22. Ngoh L. Health literacy: a barrier to pharmacist–patient communication and medication adherence. J Am Pharm Assoc. 2009;49(5):e132–e149.

23. Stubbe D. Practicing cultural competence and cultural humility in the care of diverse patients. Focus. 2020;18(1):49–51. Available at *focus.psychiatryonline.org*.

24. Clifford A, McCalman J, Bainbridge R, Tsey K. Interventions to improve cultural competence in healthcare for indigenous peoples of Australia, New Zealand, Canada, and the USA: a systematic review. Int J Quality in Health Care. 2015;27(2):89–98.

25. Handtke O, Schilgen B, Mosko M. Culturally competent healthcare—a scoping review of strategies implemented in healthcare organizations and a model of cultural competent healthcare provision. PLoS ONE. 2019;14(7):e0219971.

CHAPTER 4

Implementing the Pharmacists' Patient Care Process

ERIKA L. KLEPPINGER, PharmD, BCPS

INTRODUCTION

Historically, the profession of pharmacy has referred to patient care services by a variety of titles, such as pharmaceutical care, medication therapy management (MTM), comprehensive medication management (CMM), and individualized medication assessment and planning. While a pharmacist's activities generally focus on (1) identifying, resolving, and preventing drug therapy problems, (2) improving medication use, and (3) optimizing a patient's pharmacotherapeutic outcomes,[1] terminology tends to be inconsistent among practice settings, making it difficult to communicate the role of a pharmacist clearly with other healthcare professionals. Without a clear, consistent patient care process, pharmacists cannot demonstrate to patients, caregivers, or other healthcare professionals their contributions to improved medication-related outcomes. The Pharmacists' Patient Care Process (PPCP), as published by the Joint Commission of Pharmacy Practitioners (JCPP), provides a standardized process applicable to a wide variety of patient care services and highlights a pharmacist's medication expertise.[2] While a consistent process of care applied to every patient is a foundational principle of most healthcare professions, the PPCP differs from processes in other professions because of a pharmacist's unique approach to assessing a patient's medication regimen to ensure that medications are appropriately indicated, effective, safe, and able to be taken by the patient as intended. The JCPP states that the goals of the PPCP are to (1) promote consistency across the profession, (2) provide a framework for delivering patient care in any practice setting, (3) be a contemporary and comprehensive approach to patient-centered care delivered in collaboration with other members of the healthcare team, and (4) be applicable to a variety of patient care services delivered by pharmacists, including medication management.[3] Pharmacists in different practice settings have varying levels of intensity in implementing the PPCP. In some situations, pharmacists may not be responsible for all steps in the process or share responsibility with other pharmacists, yet all pharmacists will follow these basic steps to some degree. This chapter summarizes the steps in the PPCP and applies the steps to various patient care situations.

DRUG THERAPY PROBLEMS

The primary role of pharmacists when participating in the patient care process is to identify, resolve, and prevent drug therapy problems.[4] A drug therapy problem is defined as "any undesirable event experienced by a patient which involves, or is suspected to involve, drug therapy and that interferes with achieving the desired goals of therapy and requires professional judgment to resolve."[4] Pharmacists must assess patient factors, drug therapy, and information on the patient's medical conditions to thoroughly assess the appropriateness of medication regimens and identify potential drug therapy problems. This process involves a logical sequence of steps. It begins with evaluating each medication regimen for appropriateness of indication, then optimizing the drug and dosage regimen to ensure maximum effectiveness, and finally, individualizing drug therapy to make it as safe as possible for the patient. After completing these three steps, the practitioner considers other issues such as cost, adherence, and convenience.

As described in **Chapter 1**, drug therapy problems can be separated into seven distinct categories related to medication appropriateness, effectiveness, safety, or adherence:

Appropriate indication for the medication:

1. The medication is unnecessary because the patient does not have a clinical indication at this time.
2. Additional drug therapy is required to treat or prevent a medical condition.

Effectiveness of the medication:

3. The medication being used is not effective at producing the desired patient response.
4. The dosage is too low to produce the desired patient response.

Safety of the medication:

5. The medication is causing an adverse reaction.
6. The dose is too high, resulting in actual or potential undesirable effects.

Adherence to the medication:

7. The patient is not able or willing to take the drug therapy as intended.

To resolve or prevent a drug therapy problem, the underlying cause of the problem must be clearly understood. Table 4-1 provides a list of potential causes of drug therapy problems based on each of the seven categories.[4] This list of causes provides factors to consider when identifying drug therapy problems.

STEPS IN THE PHARMACISTS' PATIENT CARE PROCESS

The core of the PPCP is patient-centered care and establishing a relationship with the patient.[2] Including the patient, his/her family, and caregivers in the process allows for open communication and engagement in managing their own health problems. Communication, collaboration, and documentation are also key components incorporated into many, if not all, of the steps in the process. Collaboration among patients, pharmacists, physicians, and other healthcare providers is essential in providing optimal patient care. These topics are covered in more detail in **Chapters 3** and **5**.

TABLE 4-1	Causes of Drug Therapy Problems
Drug Therapy Problem Category	**Possible Causes of Drug Therapy Problems**
Unnecessary drug therapy	No valid medication indication for the drug at this time
	Multiple drug products are used when only single-drug therapy is required
	The condition is better treated with nondrug therapy
	Drug therapy is used to treat an avoidable adverse drug reaction associated with another medication
	The medical problem is caused by drug abuse, alcohol use, or smoking
Need for additional drug therapy	A medical condition exists that requires initiation of new drug therapy
	Preventive therapy is needed to reduce the risk of developing a new condition
	A medical condition requires combination therapy to achieve synergistic or additive effects
Ineffective drug	The drug is not the most effective one for the medical problem
	The drug product is not effective for the medical condition (drug not indicated)
	The condition is refractory to the drug product being used
	The dosage form is inappropriate
	The drug is contraindicated because of patient risk factors
Dosage too low	The dose is too low to produce the desired outcome
	Clinical or laboratory monitoring parameters are needed to determine if the dosage is too low
	The dosage interval is too infrequent
	A drug interaction reduced the amount of active drug available
	The duration of therapy is too short
	The drug was administered by an inappropriate route or method
	The drug was stored incorrectly resulting in lost potency
Adverse drug reaction	The drug product causes an undesirable reaction that is not dose related
	A safer drug is needed because of patient risk factors
	A drug interaction causes an undesirable reaction that is not dose related
	The drug was administered by an incorrect route or method
	The drug dosage was administered or escalated too rapidly
	The product caused an allergic reaction
Dosage too high	The dose is too high for the patient
	Clinical or laboratory monitoring parameters are needed to determine if the dosage is too high
	The dosing frequency is too short
	The duration of therapy is too long
	A drug interaction caused a toxic reaction to the drug product
Adherence	The patient does not understand the instructions
	The patient cannot afford the drug therapy or monitoring recommendations
	The patient prefers not to take the medication
	The patient forgets to take the medication
	The patient cannot swallow or self-administer the medication properly
	The drug product is not available to the patient

Reproduced with permission from Cipolle RJ, Strand LM, Morley PC. *Pharmaceutical Care Practice: The Patient-Centered Approach to Medication Management Services*, 3rd ed. New York, NY: McGraw-Hill, 2021.

The steps of the PPCP include *Collect, Assess, Plan, Implement,* and *Follow-up: Monitor and Evaluate*, and are illustrated as a circle to indicate the cyclical nature of the process, with *Follow-up* leading back to *Collect* at a future patient encounter (Fig. 4-1).[2] Each of the steps is summarized below followed by a short patient case vignette example.

COLLECT

Collection of subjective and objective information provides the basis for identifying drug therapy problems. This information can be obtained directly from the patient or caregiver through review of existing health records or by communicating with other healthcare professionals. In all practice settings, a primary function of pharmacists is to conduct a medication history as the initial step in identifying drug therapy problems. This is especially important during patient transitions of care. A complete medication history includes the prescription and nonprescription medications the patient is currently taking; dietary supplements, herbal products, and complementary medicine approaches; and recent previous medications the patient has taken. Other relevant health data such as a medical history, health and wellness information, biometric test results, and physical assessment findings may also be collected. Beyond conducting medication and health histories, other important factors to gather include lifestyle habits, a patient's preferences and/or beliefs, health and functional goals, and socioeconomic factors. This additional information can help to provide a holistic approach to patient care. A sample of specific types of information to collect is provided as follows:[2,4]

Patient Information

- Name, address, and phone number (for future contact and follow-up evaluation)
- Primary care physician
- Demographic and background information: age (date of birth), gender, sexual orientation, gender identity, race, ethnicity, height, weight (important for weight-based dosing)
- Social history (SH): living arrangements, occupation, tobacco, alcohol, substance use (include name of substance, amount, and frequency when possible)
- Family history (FH): relevant health histories of parents and siblings
- Insurance information: name of health plan and policy number (important for accurate billing of services)

Disease Information

- Past medical history (PMH)
- Current medical problems
- History of present illness (HPI)
- Pertinent information from the review of systems (ROS), physical examination, laboratory results, and X-ray/imaging results
- Immunization history

Drug Information

- Allergies and adverse medication effects (include the name of the medication and the reaction that occurred)
- Current prescription medications; for each medication include start date, indication for use, drug name, strength, dosage regimen, and how the patient is actually taking it. The *actual* regimen may differ from the *prescribed* regimen because patients do not always take medications as directed. Also ask about effectiveness, adverse effects, and patient questions or concerns about current medications for a complete medication history.
- Current nonprescription medications, vitamins, dietary supplements, and alternative/complementary therapies
- Recent past prescription and nonprescription medications (include the stop date)

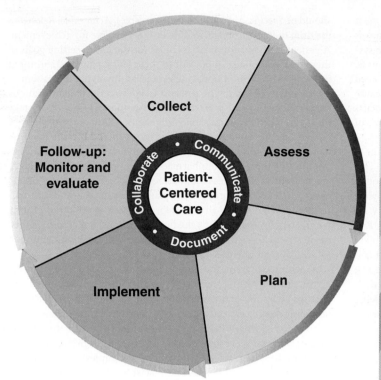

Pharmacists' patient care process
Pharmacists use a patient-centered approach in collaboration with other providers on the health care team to optimize patient health and medication outcomes.

Using principles of evidence-based practice, pharmacists:

Collect
The pharmacist ensures the collection of the necessary subjective and objective information about the patient in order to understand the relevant medical/medication history and clinical status of the patient.

Assess
The pharmacist assesses the information collected and analyzes the clinical effects of the patient's therapy in the context of the patient's overall health goals in order to identify and prioritize problems and achieve optimal care.

Plan
The pharmacist develops an individualized patient-centered care plan, in collaboration with other healthcare professionals and the patient or caregiver that is evidence-based and cost-effective.

Implement
The pharmacist implements the care plan in collaboration with other healthcare professionals and the patient or caregiver.

Follow-up: Monitor and evaluate
The pharmacist monitors and evaluates the effectiveness of the care plan and modifies the plan in collaboration with other healthcare professionals and the patient or caregiver as needed.

FIGURE 4-1. The pharmacists' patient care process. (Reproduced with permission from Joint Commission of Pharmacy Practitioners Pharmacists' Patient Care Process, May 29, 2014. https://jcpp.net/patient-care-process/. Accessed November 11, 2021.)

The amount and type of information collected by pharmacists will vary based on the patient care service or practice setting. For example, in a community pharmacy, there will be excellent data on a patient's refill history, but laboratory tests are not as readily available. The pharmacist will rely mostly on communicating with the patient to obtain information but may also conduct point-of-care testing, blood pressure measurement, or other screening tests when available. In hospital and clinic settings, pharmacists have access to laboratory and test results, physician physical exam information, and other objective data; however, they still rely on interviewing the patient to obtain subjective data to fully describe the problem.

Example Case Vignette

A 32-year-old man presents to the pharmacy today for a refill of his lorazepam. He states that he only has a few tablets left and doesn't want to run out. He was recently diagnosed with generalized anxiety disorder and started on sertraline and lorazepam. A review of the patient profile in the computer system reveals the following:

- *Sertraline (Zoloft) 50 mg, take one tablet daily, quantity #30, 1 refill (started 2 weeks ago)*
- *Lorazepam (Ativan) 0.5 mg, take one tablet up to 3 times per day as needed for severe anxiety, quantity #20, no refills (started 2 weeks ago)*
- *Acetaminophen (Tylenol) 500 mg, take one to two tablets as needed for headaches (OTC medication)*

What additional information is needed to identify potential drug therapy problems in this patient?

First, it is important to ask the patient about his medications, specifically what he takes his medications for, how he takes his medications, and any problems he may be experiencing with them. A brief

medication history can also be obtained. These questions reveal the following information: *He takes lorazepam twice a day on most days because his doctor told him he could take it whenever he needed it for anxiety. He admits to taking it even when his anxiety is not severe. He has only three tablets remaining. He takes sertraline as prescribed and is not experiencing any adverse effects; however, he doesn't think it is working very well. He does not use any other prescription or nonprescription medications and uses acetaminophen twice a day about four to five times per month.*

After learning about his medications, it is important to determine what the patient knows about his generalized anxiety disorder, especially since it is a recent diagnosis. *He is seeing a therapist to help him with nonpharmacologic strategies for dealing with anxiety, particularly when he has to travel for work. He wasn't told a lot about the medications when he started them 2 weeks ago and he wonders why he was prescribed two different medications.*

ASSESS

A great deal of time is spent analyzing the drug therapy in the context of the patient's overall health goals. Assessment of a patient's health and medications helps to identify and prioritize drug therapy problems. To identify potential drug therapy problems, pharmacists can ask five questions when assessing a patient's drug therapy:

1. Is there an appropriate indication for each medication?
2. Is the drug therapy effective?
3. Is the drug therapy safe for this patient?
4. Can the patient comply with the drug therapy and other aspects of their care plan?
5. Is there an untreated indication that needs drug therapy?

Asking these questions will allow the pharmacist to determine if the patient's drug therapy is appropriate, effective, safe, and convenient for the patient. When asked in this order, pharmacists can systematically assess for potential drug-related problems. For example, if a medication is not appropriate for the patient, one does not need to ask about its effectiveness, safety, or patient adherence because these questions would not be applicable. Additionally, pharmacists can identify drug therapy problems that may interfere with goals of therapy or other potential problems that could be prevented.

After a drug therapy problem is identified, it is also important to determine the severity of the medical condition or problem. This will help in prioritizing the problem list, which is the final portion of the *Assess* step. The most urgent or severe problem should be listed first, with the remaining problems listed in order of severity. In addition to assessing drug therapy problems, pharmacists may also assess a patient's health literacy, the patient's willingness and ability to make changes, barriers to follow-up (eg, transportation difficulties, insurance limitations), vaccination status, and other preventive care needs. The *Collect* and *Assess* steps are often conducted simultaneously because pharmacists evaluate information as it is being collected. The assessment process is similar across practice settings, but the type and quantity of information available may vary.

Example Case Vignette (continued)

Prioritized problem list:

1. *Generalized anxiety disorder: no refills for lorazepam (medication indication problem–either medication is unnecessary or additional drug therapy is required). Benzodiazepine therapy for generalized anxiety disorder should be reserved for short-term use for acute management of symptoms.[5] The patient is taking lorazepam regularly even though it is only prescribed for severe symptoms, which has led to running out of his supply of medication in 2 weeks. In taking 0.5 mg twice per day most days of the week, he is below the maximum daily dose of 10 mg, but it is unclear if he requires continued therapy. A new prescription will be needed if he continues to require lorazepam for anxiety symptoms.*

2. *Generalized anxiety disorder: lack of understanding of sertraline effects (adherence problem). The patient does not seem to know that sertraline may take some time to be fully effective.*

3. *Headaches: potential for acetaminophen overuse (possible safety problem–dose too high): The patient is currently taking less than the maximum daily dose of acetaminophen (4000 mg/day). However, he should be educated on the maximum daily dose and reminded of other acetaminophen-containing products to avoid duplication of therapy and potential adverse events.*

PLAN

Once a problem list has been identified and prioritized, pharmacists must then develop an individualized, patient-centered care plan specific to the patient's needs. Collaboration with other healthcare providers may be necessary if the plan goes beyond the pharmacist's scope of practice. When formulating a care plan, it is important to include the medical condition for which the patient has drug-related needs, the specific drug therapy problems identified, clear goals of therapy, proposed interventions (nonpharmacologic and pharmacologic), and a follow-up plan. A plan should be created for all problems identified in the assessment step.

Goals of therapy for each medical condition should indicate one of the primary therapeutic outcomes as described in **Chapter 1**: cure of disease, reduction or elimination of symptoms, arresting or slowing of the progression of disease, or preventing a disease or symptom. To create clear goals, the SMART acronym can be used. Each goal

should be *Specific, Measurable* (or observable), *Achievable, Related* to the drug therapy problem, and include a *Timeline* for achievement. A patient-centered approach includes the patient in setting goals of therapy that are most important to them and seeking patient input in the prioritization of nonacute problems. Involving the patient in the care plan allows the pharmacist to address the patient's unique concerns, needs, and preferences, and empowers patients to take more responsibility in implementing their portion of the plan.

Specific drug therapy recommendations should include the drug name, dosage form, dose, route of administration, schedule, and duration of therapy. Nonpharmacologic approaches to treatment and preventive strategies (such as screenings or vaccinations) should also be included as appropriate. A plan for monitoring and care continuity is also essential in this step, including specific monitoring parameters for the patient's medical conditions and recommended medications, a specific timeframe for follow-up appointments, and information on referrals if needed.

As with *Assessment*, the process of creating a care plan is similar across practice settings and varies based on the information available for collection and assessment. Hospital and insurance formularies must be considered when developing patient care plans. In the community setting, pharmacists can recommend nonprescription products and self-care strategies but must contact a prescriber if prescription drug therapy needs to be changed, unless a collaborative practice agreement is in place. Pharmacists in all settings can address many drug therapy problems related to patient adherence issues.

Example Case Vignette (continued)

Plan:

1. *Generalized anxiety disorder: no refills for lorazepam. Goal of therapy is to alleviate acute anxiety symptoms. Contact the prescribing physician for clarification of indication for lorazepam and request a new prescription if needed.*

2. *Generalized anxiety disorder: lack of understanding of sertraline effects. Goal of therapy is to reduce anxiety symptoms. Educate the patient about sertraline, specifically its onset of action and the time needed to experience maximal effectiveness.*

3. *Headaches: potential for acetaminophen overuse. Goal is to prevent acetaminophen overdose. Educate the patient about the maximum dose of acetaminophen. Provide examples of other products that contain acetaminophen, such as over-the-counter cold medications and sleep aids.*

IMPLEMENT

A pharmacist's ability to implement care plans depends on the scope of activities allowed by state laws and regulations or through a collaborative practice agreement. Collaborative practice agreements can be broad or limited to a specific condition, such as anticoagulation. In clinical settings, pharmacists may also be a part of a healthcare team conducting collaborative patient visits or rounding. When a plan requires expertise outside a pharmacist's scope of practice, it is important to provide a referral to the appropriate healthcare provider (eg, physician, podiatrist, dietician) and explain to the patient the importance of follow-up. A main component of implementation is providing education and self-management training for the patient and/or caregiver. When counseling patients, a pharmacist can discuss reasons for drug therapy, medication actions, administration, adverse effects, what to expect from treatment (eg, when the medication will begin working, if it provides a cure or just relieves symptoms, if it relieves symptoms completely or just improves them), and appropriate follow-up (eg, proper duration of therapy, when to see a physician if the problem continues).

If authorized, implementation may include initiating, modifying, discontinuing, or administering medication therapy. Under a collaborative practice agreement, pharmacists may be able to implement these changes directly with the patient. Preventive care strategies are also important, such as vaccinations, diabetic foot exams, diet and exercise counseling, and various screenings (eg, blood pressure, cholesterol, depression, blood glucose, HIV, osteoporosis). Many of these strategies could be implemented and patients referred to appropriate providers if abnormal results are found. Communication and documentation of the plan are also important to ensure that care is coordinated with other healthcare providers.

Example Case Vignette (continued)

You call and speak with the prescribing physician about the patient's management of his anxiety. The physician confirms that the patient was instructed to take the lorazepam only when experiencing severe anxiety, and it was primarily intended for anxiety while traveling for business. The physician provides you with a verbal prescription for lorazepam 0.5 mg, with instructions to take one tablet up to three times per day as needed for severe anxiety while traveling, quantity #10, no refills. The physician states that this should be an adequate supply until the patient's next appointment in 4 weeks and that the patient will need to schedule an appointment if more lorazepam is needed prior to this appointment. The physician also asks that you talk with the patient about when he should take the lorazepam.

You speak with the patient and summarize your conversation with his physician. He admits that he probably does not need the lorazepam as much as he is taking it and agrees to take it only if his anxiety is severe or if he is traveling for business. You also inform him that it may take up to 4–6 weeks to see the full effects of sertraline, and that he should notice some effects soon. You counsel him on the importance of taking his medications as prescribed and contacting his physician if he needs more lorazepam than prescribed. You also discuss his acetaminophen use and educate him that the maximum daily dose is 4000 mg. While he is well under this dose currently, he should be aware of other medications that contain acetaminophen, including over-the-counter cold medications and sleep aids. He agrees to talk with you if he is unsure if a medication contains acetaminophen. You document your conversation with the patient in his profile in the computer system.

FOLLOW-UP: MONITOR AND EVALUATE

The final step in the PPCP clearly delineates a continual process because at some future time subjective and objective data will again need to be collected and assessed. During follow-up, the pharmacist evaluates the positive and negative impact of the care plan on the patient, identifies new drug therapy problems, and takes action to address new problems or adjust therapy. It is also important to determine an appropriate follow-up time frame to ensure that efficacy and safety parameters can be evaluated appropriately. In some settings, patients may have scheduled visits at predetermined intervals while others may be conducted primarily as a walk-in. In these situations, patient no-shows for visits can make follow-up problematic. With follow-up, various outcomes can also be tracked and reported such as:

- *Clinical outcomes:* blood pressure, A1C, medication problem resolution, adverse drug events, adherence
- *Humanistic outcomes:* patient medication knowledge, patient functioning, self-management capability, satisfaction, patient concerns about the treatment
- *Economic outcomes:* hospitalizations, emergency department visits, medication costs

When evaluating the care plan, a pharmacist should compare the goals of therapy with the patient's current status. Cipolle et al.

developed terminology to describe the patient's status, the medical condition, and the comparative evaluation of that status with the previously determined therapeutic goals.[4] These terms also describe the actions taken as a result of the follow-up evaluation:

Status	Definition
Resolved	Therapeutic goals achieved for the acute condition; discontinue therapy
Stable	Therapeutic goals achieved; continue the same therapy for chronic disease management
Improved	Progress is being made in achieving goals; continue the same therapy because more time is required to assess the full benefit of therapy
Partial improvement	Progress is being made, but minor adjustments in therapy are required to fully achieve the therapeutic goals before the next assessment
Unimproved	Little or no progress has been made, but continue the same therapy to allow additional time for benefit to be observed
Worsened	A decline in health is observed despite an adequate duration using the optimal drug; modify drug therapy (eg, increase the dose of the current medication, add a second agent with additive or synergistic effects)
Failure	Therapeutic goals have not been achieved despite an adequate dose and duration of therapy; discontinue current medication(s) and start new therapy
Expired	The patient died while receiving drug therapy; document possible contributing factors, especially if they may be drug related

Example Case Vignette (continued)

The patient returns to the pharmacy in 2 weeks to pick up his sertraline prescription. You ask him how he is doing, and he reports that he is feeling better and his anxiety has improved. He expresses appreciation for the help you provided during his last visit to the pharmacy. He reports taking lorazepam only once in the past two weeks and feels like the sertraline is starting to have some positive effects. He has an appointment with his physician in 2 weeks for follow-up. You evaluate your care plan as follows:

1. *Generalized anxiety disorder: no refills for lorazepam. Goal of therapy is to alleviate acute anxiety symptoms. Symptoms are improving and patient has a better understanding of when to take lorazepam as needed.*

2. *Generalized anxiety disorder: lack of understanding of sertraline effects. Goal of therapy is to reduce anxiety symptoms. Symptoms are improving, and the patient understands the current therapy.*

3. *Headaches: potential for acetaminophen overuse. The goal is to prevent acetaminophen overdose. The patient understands the need to avoid other acetaminophen-containing drug products; thus, this potential drug therapy problem was prevented at this time, but ongoing monitoring is advised.*

EXAMPLES OF PATIENT CARE PROCESS IMPLEMENTATION

The PPCP can be applied in a variety of patient care situations such as CMM, IV-to-oral dosing in the hospital setting, medication reconciliation during a care transition, disease state management, and provision of immunization services, to name a few. To assist pharmacists with implementing the PPCP, the Centers for Disease Control and Prevention (CDC) published a resource guide for managing patients with high blood pressure.[6] In more general terms, many pharmacists use the PPCP in providing MTM, assisting patients with self-care needs, and chronic disease state monitoring.

MEDICATION THERAPY MANAGEMENT

The American Pharmacists Association (APhA) and the National Association of Chain Drug Stores (NACDS) published core elements of MTM to assist pharmacists in providing these services consistently for patients, regardless of the setting.[7] MTM focuses on the identification and resolution of drug therapy problems, similar to the main purpose of the PPCP. Therefore, the steps of the PPCP can be easily seen in MTM's five core elements[7]:

1. *Medication therapy review (MTR):* Involves discussing the full list of the patient's medications (*Collect*), identifying and prioritizing potential drug therapy problems (*Assess*), and creating a plan to resolve the identified drug therapy problems (*Plan*). This could be conducted in person or via the telephone.

2. *Personalized medication record (PMR):* A complete record of the patient's medications including dosages and directions for use is provided for the patient (*Implement*). All prescription and nonprescription medications should appear on this list in addition to dietary supplements and herbal products. This record may also include demographic information, a complete list of allergies, the name of pharmacy, emergency contact information, and the date it was last updated.

3. *Medication-related action plan (MAP):* A document provided to the patient that includes any action items derived from the full medication therapy review (*Plan, Implement*). This plan is used by the patient to track their progress for self-management (*Follow-up*).

4. *Intervention and/or referral:* Completing any needed action steps (eg, calling a physician, making written instructions to the patient, counseling on proper inhaler use). The pharmacist either addresses the drug therapy problems directly or refers the patient to a physician or other healthcare provider (*Implement*).

5. *Documentation and follow-up:* All interventions should be documented; however, the format may vary depending on the specific area of practice. Documentation may include a full SOAP note or something as simple as documenting a brief note in the pharmacy patient profile (*Implement*). Follow-up appointments are scheduled based on the patient's needs (*Follow-up*).

SELF-CARE MANAGEMENT

Pharmacists in many settings assist patients with various self-care needs. In this capacity, pharmacists perform functions similar to a primary care provider, specifically gathering and evaluating information about the patient's problems, differentiating between self-treatable conditions and conditions requiring medical intervention, and advising and counseling the patient about the proposed course of action. To assist pharmacists with these types of encounters, the QuEST/SCHOLAR tool was developed.[8] In addition to patients presenting with a self-care complaint, the SCHOLAR-MAC questions could also be helpful to organize a patient interview for any patient presenting with a particular symptom complaint. The steps of the PPCP are clearly evident in QuEST, as described below[8]:

- *Qu*ickly and accurately assess the patient using SCHOLAR-MAC questions (*Collect*)
  - ✓ Symptoms: the main and associated symptoms
  - ✓ Characteristics: a description of the situation and evolution of the symptoms
  - ✓ History: previous experience with the problem; what has been tried so far
  - ✓ Onset: when the problem began

- ✓ Location: where the problem is located
- ✓ Aggravating factors: aspects that make the problem worse
- ✓ Remitting factors: aspects that make the problem better
- ✓ Medications: prescription and nonprescription medications, dietary supplements, herbal products, complementary therapies
- ✓ Allergies: to medications and other substances
- ✓ Conditions: all current medical conditions

- *E*stablish that the patient is an appropriate self-care candidate (*Assess*)

- *S*uggest appropriate self-care strategies (*Plan*)

- *T*alk with the patient about the suggested self-care strategies and follow-up recommendations (*Implement, Follow-up*)

CHRONIC DISEASE STATE MONITORING

In ambulatory settings, pharmacists often participate in chronic disease state monitoring in collaboration with other healthcare professionals. For example, a community pharmacist may have a collaborative practice agreement with a physician to manage their patients on chronic anticoagulation therapy. After starting anticoagulation, the physician may refer patients to the pharmacist for follow-up appointments. At these appointments, the pharmacist interviews the patient, conducts point-of-care INR testing, makes adjustments in anticoagulant therapy, and communicates those changes to the patient's physician. Pharmacists also participate in chronic disease state monitoring in clinic settings, where they would have full access to the patient's medical record. While a patient may be referred to pharmacy services for a particular indication, such as diabetes management, it is important for the pharmacist to explore all potential drug-related problems that may arise, even if they go beyond the original intent of the consult. An illustration of how the PPCP may be implemented during a chronic disease state monitoring situation is provided below:

Example case vignette

As part of a diabetes care clinic, pharmacists manage patients under a collaborative practice agreement and are an integral part of the healthcare team. A 62-year-old woman with diabetes, hypertension, and dyslipidemia presents to the pharmacy clinic today for follow-up of her diabetes management.

Collect: Because this patient has been seen previously in clinic, her medical record contains a wealth of information for the pharmacist to identify and assess the patient's medical and drug therapy problems. The encounter begins by interviewing the patient with a focus on what has changed since the last visit. It is important to assess the patient holistically and not focus exclusively on her diabetes management. Collect relevant patient information, disease information, and medication information as described previously. This information is organized in a manner appropriate for documentation in a medical record:

- *Chief complaint (CC):* "*I don't think this new medication for my diabetes is working any better than the last one.*"

  Asking the CC up front allows the pharmacist to elicit factors that are most important to the patient and may give the clinician an idea of potential drug therapy problems.

- *HPI: Last month, the physician started the patient on exenatide because her blood glucose readings were not controlled on metformin monotherapy. Exenatide is an injectable drug, so she thought that it worked like insulin and she no longer needed to take the metformin. She checks her fasting blood glucose every morning. Her daily log indicates fasting blood glucose readings* of 145–155 mg/dL, which is about the same as when she was taking metformin monotherapy.

The HPI provides more information about the CC and is a summary of the patient interview. It provides a story describing the situation from the patient's perspective. When patients present with specific symptom complaints, SCHOLAR questions can be asked as part of the HPI.

- *PMH:* type 2 diabetes (diagnosed 2 years ago), HTN (diagnosed 5 years ago), dyslipidemia (diagnosed 2 years ago).

- *FH:* mother has type 2 diabetes and dyslipidemia; father has hypertension and history of an MI at age 68.

- *SH:* (–) tobacco; (+) alcohol—one glass of wine or beer 2–3 times per week.

A complete list of the patient's medical conditions (including when they were diagnosed), relevant family history, and relevant social history are helpful in identifying and assessing drug therapy problems.

- *Medications:* The patient takes all medications as prescribed except she stopped taking metformin 1 month ago when the exenatide was started. She does not use any nonprescription medications, dietary supplements, or herbal products. At this time, she is not experiencing any adverse effects with her medication.

  ✓ Metformin 1000 mg, take one tablet twice daily with meals (started 2 years ago and titrated up to the current dose, patient has not been taking for the past month)

  ✓ Exenatide 5 mcg, inject subcutaneously twice daily 60 minutes before meals (started 1 month ago)

  ✓ Lisinopril 10 mg, take one tablet daily (started 5 years ago)

  ✓ Chlorthalidone 25 mg, take one tablet daily (started 3 years ago)

  ✓ Atorvastatin 40 mg daily, take one tablet daily (started 2 years ago)

  Documenting all of the medications the patient is currently taking, how the patient is taking them, adverse effects experienced, and adherence information is important to assist in identifying actual or potential drug therapy problems.

- *Allergies:* none

- *ROS:* No complaints of hypoglycemic symptoms, shortness of breath, or chest pain. No recent reports of polyuria, polyphagia, or polydipsia. Reports good sensation in lower extremities.

  Pertinent positive and pertinent negative information related to the patient's medical conditions and drug therapy problems should be collected and documented.

- *Vital signs:* BP 142/74 mm Hg, HR 68 bpm, weight 85 kg

  A targeted physical examination could also be conducted and included if pertinent to the situation. Review of the physician's previous physical exam information could also be included.

- *Laboratory results:*

  ✓ Fasting blood glucose 152 mg/dL (today)

  ✓ A1C 7.9% (1 month ago)

  ✓ Lipid panel: TC 164 mg/dL, LDL 98 mg/dL, HDL 42 mg/dL, TG 120 mg/dL (1 month ago)

  ✓ Electrolytes and liver function tests WNL (1 month ago)

  Document all laboratory results relevant to the patient's medical conditions and drug therapy, including the date the test was conducted. This information is helpful in assessing the patient's drug therapy problems.

- *Preventive care:* eye exam 6 months ago, foot exam last month in clinic, urine albumin screening 6 months ago (negative results).

- *Immunizations:* All childhood vaccines completed, flu vaccine annually, Tdap 5 years ago, hepatitis B vaccine 2 years ago, 2 doses of Pfizer COVID-19 vaccine received in 2021.

  Relevant preventive care tests and a complete list of vaccinations allow the pharmacist to fully assess the patient to identify additional drug therapy problems that would otherwise have been missed.

Assess: Evaluate each of the patient's medical conditions and medications to identify and prioritize all drug therapy problems. An assessment of the patient's problems is provided below. Diabetes is the problem with highest priority not only because it is the reason for the patient's clinic visit, but also because it was the patient's primary concern. Any medical condition that is currently under control (such as dyslipidemia) is prioritized at the end of the list.

1. *Type 2 diabetes:* A1C above goal of <7.0% and fasting glucose above target range 80–130 mg/dL.[9] No improvement since previous appointment. No reported episodes of hypoglycemia. Exenatide 5 mcg twice daily is an appropriate dose for this patient, and she is tolerating it well. However, she stopped taking metformin when she began using exenatide. Patient is up to date with preventive care measures for diabetes.

2. *Hypertension:* BP elevated above goal of <130/80 on lisinopril and chlorthalidone therapy.[10] Patient reports adherence with medications and good tolerability. Lisinopril is not at the maximum dose and could be increased.

3. *Vaccination status:* The recombinant zoster vaccine (RZV) is recommended for all patients 50 years of age and older.[11] The vaccine is given as a two-dose series 2–6 months apart. One dose of the pneumococcal polysaccharide vaccine (PPSV23) is recommended for all patients age 19–64 with chronic medical conditions, including diabetes.[11] According to the CDC at the time of this writing (late 2021), a COVID-19 booster dose is recommended for all people age 50 years or older who have completed the primary vaccination series at least 6 months prior.[12] This patient should receive a booster shot if she has not yet received one. The patient is up to date on all other vaccinations.

4. *Dyslipidemia:* Stable. Lipid panel is controlled on atorvastatin monotherapy (high-intensity statin therapy).[13]

Plan and implement: When documenting the plan, the problem list should appear in the same order as the assessment. All problems identified in the assessment should be provided with a plan. In addition to specific medication changes, goals of therapy and needed referrals can be included. Implementation often occurs simultaneously with the plan, and all counseling provided should be documented in the medical record. Medication therapy can be adjusted if a collaborative practice agreement is in place and it is within the pharmacist's scope of practice. Any referrals should be clearly specified and communicated with the patient.

1. *Type 2 diabetes:* Goal of therapy—HbA1c <7.0% without episodes of hypoglycemia[9] and improved medication adherence. Restart metformin 500 mg twice daily and titrate up to 1000 mg twice daily after 2 weeks if tolerated (new prescription called in to pharmacy for patient). Continue exenatide 5 mcg twice daily. Counsel patient on mechanism of action and adverse effects of medications for diabetes. Emphasized importance of checking with the clinic before stopping any medication.

2. *Hypertension:* Goal of therapy—BP <130/80.[10] Increase lisinopril to 20 mg daily for improved BP control (new prescription called in to pharmacy for patient). Continue chlorthalidone 25 mg daily. Counsel patient on new dose and adverse effects of lisinopril.

3. *Vaccination status:* Goal of therapy—up to date on all recommended vaccinations.[11,12] Have clinic nurse give one dose (0.5 mL)

RZV intramuscularly and one dose (0.5 mL) PPSV23 intramuscularly today. A second dose of RZV is needed in 2–6 months. If patient is agreeable, administer one booster dose (0.3 mL) Pfizer COVID-19 vaccine if it is at least 6 months after completion of the primary series. Counseled patient on importance of receiving the influenza vaccine annually.

4. *Dyslipidemia: Continue atorvastatin 40 mg daily. Patient does not need refills at this time.*

Follow-up: Plans for follow-up are often included when documenting plans for the identified drug therapy problems but could also be specified separately. It is important to be clear and specific not only with the monitoring parameters, but with a timeline for follow-up.

1. *Type 2 diabetes: Continue checking daily fasting glucose and recommended checking 2-hour postprandial glucose every other day. Schedule follow-up appointment with the pharmacist in 1 month. Call patient in 2 weeks to check on metformin tolerability and remind patient to increase the dose. Check A1C in 3 months.*

2. *Hypertension: Recheck BP at next clinic visit in 1 month. Encourage patient to check BP at home using an automatic monitor. Check kidney function (serum creatinine) and electrolytes in 1 month.*

3. *Vaccination status: Monitor for any soreness in the arm post-injection. Schedule an appointment for a second dose of RZV in 2 months.*

4. *Dyslipidemia—Recheck lipid panel in 1 year. Monitor for adverse effects of statin therapy, particularly myalgia.*

CONCLUSION

Implementing the PPCP throughout the profession of pharmacy provides a common terminology for pharmacist patient care services and allows the focus of the profession to shift to quality improvement, provider collaboration, improved patient outcomes, and cost savings. This process should be incorporated into the thought process for all pharmacists providing direct patient care, regardless of the practice setting, and used as a format for communication with other health professionals.

REFERENCES

1. Harris IM, Phillips B, Boyce E, et al. Clinical pharmacy should adopt a consistent process of direct patient care. Pharmacotherapy. 2014;34(8):e133–e148.

2. Joint Commission of Pharmacy Practitioners. Pharmacists' Patient Care Process. May 29, 2014. Available at: *https://jcpp.net/wp-content/uploads/2016/03/PatientCareProcess-with-supporting-organizations.pdf*. Accessed November 11, 2021.

3. Joint Commission of Pharmacy Practitioners. Pharmacists' Patient Care Process Presentation. Available at: *https://jcpp.net/wp-content/uploads/2015/09/Patient_Care_Process_Template_Presentation-Final.pdf*. Accessed November 11, 2021.

4. Cipolle RJ, Strand LM, Morley PC, eds. Pharmaceutical Care Practice: The Patient-Centered Approach to Medication Management Services. 3rd ed. New York, NY: McGraw-Hill; 2012.

5. Stein MB, Sareen J. Generalized anxiety disorder. N Engl J Med. 2015;373(21):2059–2068.

6. Centers for Disease Control and Prevention. Using the Pharmacists' Patient care Process to Manage High Blood Pressure: A Resource Guide for Pharmacists. Atlanta, GA: Centers for Disease Control and Prevention, U.S. Department of Health and Human Services, 2016. Available at: *https://www.cdc.gov/dhdsp/pubs/docs/pharmacist-resource-guide.pdf*. Accessed November 11, 2021.

7. American Pharmacists Association, National Association of Chain Drug Stores Foundation. Medication therapy management in pharmacy practice: core elements of an MTM service model (version 2.0). J Am Pharm Assoc. 2008;48(3):341–353.

8. Divine H, McIntosh T. Pharmacists' patient care process in self-care. In: Krinsky DL, Ferreri SP, Hemstreet BA, Hume AL, Rollins CJ, Teitze KJ, eds. Handbook of Nonprescription Drugs: An Interactive Approach to Self-Care. 20th ed. Washington, DC: American Pharmacists Association; 2021:27–28.

9. American Diabetes Association. Glycemic targets: standards of medical care in diabetes—2021. Diabetes Care. 2021;44(Suppl 1):S73–S84.

10. Whelton PK, Carey RM, Aronow WS, et al. 2017 ACC/AHA/AAPA/ABC/ACPM/AGS/APhA/ASH/ASPC/NMA/PCNA guideline for the prevention, detection, evaluation, and management of high blood pressure in adults: a report of the American College of Cardiology/American Heart Association Task Force on Clinical Practice Guidelines. J Am Coll Cardiol. 2018;71:e127–e248.

11. Centers for Disease Control and Prevention. Recommended Adult Immunization Schedule, United States, 2021. Available at: *https://www.cdc.gov/vaccines/schedules/downloads/adult/adult-combined-schedule.pdf*. Accessed November 11, 2021.

12. Centers for Disease Control and Prevention. Interim Clinical Considerations for Use of COVID-19 Vaccines Currently Approved or Authorized in the United States. Available at: *https://www.cdc.gov/vaccines/covid-19/clinical-considerations/covid-19-vaccines-us.html#considerations-covid19-vax-booster*. Accessed November 23, 2021.

13. Grundy SM, Stone NJ, Bailey AL, et al. 2018 AHA/ACC/AACVPR/AAPA/ABC/ACPM/ADA/AGS/APhA/ASPC/NLA/PCNA guideline on the management of blood cholesterol: executive summary: a report of the American College of Cardiology/American Heart Association Task Force on Clinical Practice Guidelines. J Am Coll Cardiol. 2018. doi:10.1016/j.jacc.2018.11.002.

5

Documentation of Patient Encounters and Interventions

LORI T. ARMISTEAD, MA, PharmD

TIMOTHY J. IVES, PharmD, MPH, FCCP, CPP

LEARNING OBJECTIVES

After reviewing this chapter, the reader should be able to:

- Describe the purposes of documenting patient encounters and interventions.
- Incorporate key components of documentation when recording patient encounters and interventions.
- Describe the benefits and disadvantages of documenting patient encounters in an electronic health record (EHR).
- Document patients' drug therapy and medical problems in a clear and concise manner, ensuring that all aspects of the Pharmacist Patient Care Process (PPCP) are included.

To ensure high-quality patient care, especially in the current environment of increasingly complex care, all healthcare providers must generate and maintain clear and concise records of each patient's health and medical conditions.[1,2] Documentation is also required for providers to receive accurate and timely payment for services. Documentation outlines the care the patient received in a chronological and organized manner and serves as a form of communication among providers, which is an important element that contributes to the quality of care provided. Each provider involved knows what evaluation has occurred, what the patient's treatment plan is, and who will provide it. Furthermore, third-party payers may require documentation from providers that ensures that the services provided are consistent with the insurance coverage.[1-3] General components of documentation include:

- A complete and legible record
- Date of service, site of service, and identity of the provider
- Documentation for each encounter with a rationale for the encounter, relevant history, physical findings, prior test results, and identified health risk factors
- An easily inferred rationale for ordering diagnostic tests or ancillary services, assessment, clinical impression (or diagnosis), and plan for care
- Patient progress, response to and changes in treatment, and revision of the original diagnosis/assessment
- Applicable diagnostic and treatment codes

Documentation should include all pertinent facts, findings, and observations about a patient's health history, including past and present illnesses, examinations, tests, treatments, medication use, and outcomes.

DOCUMENTATION IN ELECTRONIC HEALTH RECORDS

Historically, clinical documentation was paper-based; however, such records were often inaccessible at the point of care, not easily transferable or transportable, illegible, poorly organized, and missing key information. Due to these limitations, most healthcare systems have implemented electronic health records (EHRs), which have greatly enhanced workflow, usability, patient safety, and access to updated, real-time information.[2,4] Further, the 2001 Institute of Medicine report *Crossing the Quality Chasm* identified the EHR as a key component in improving provider access to medical information, facilitating decision support and data collection, and reducing medical errors and associated costs.[5] The EHR may also improve documentation with reduced clinical variation, better provision of quality care, and increased security of confidential patient information.[1,6,7] Furthermore, EHRs are associated with higher performance on certain quality measures.[1,7,8]

With the growth and evolution of EHRs, new features have been added or enhanced to facilitate ease of use and improved patient outcomes (Table 5-1). Additional benefits of EHRs include:[3,4,6,7,9–11]

- Enhanced ability of providers across the continuum of care to evaluate care, plan immediate treatment, and monitor care over time
- Easier communication and continuity of care among providers involved in the patient's care
- New modes of communicating with patients and providing them information about their care
- Increased time efficiency
- Greater adherence to practice guidelines and access to reference information
- Fewer medication errors and adverse drug events
- Improved ability to measure and track clinical, financial, humanistic, and process of care outcomes
- More accurate and timely claims review and payment
- Improved efficiency with other administrative tasks, such as patient scheduling and population management
- Greater clarity of coding (ie, Current Procedural Terminology [CPT] and International Statistical Classification of Diseases and Related Health Problems, Tenth Revision, Clinical Modification [ICD-10-CM], from the World Health Organization [WHO]) on health insurance claim forms, which must be supported by documentation in the patient record.

TABLE 5-1	Key Features of EHRs That Facilitate Ease of Use and Improved Patient Care[4,9–13]

- Health information exchange (HIE) technologies
- Clinical decision support tools (eg, evidence-based guidelines, predictive models)
- Automated clinical alerts (eg, allergy or dose alerts, drug interaction)
- Computerized provider order entry (CPOE)
- Electronic delivery of orders (eg, medication orders, lab orders) and results (eg, lab results, radiology reports)
- Medication order sets
- Documentation "smart phrases," templates, and dictation capabilities
- E-prescribing technologies
- Telehealth technologies (eg, patient-provider video visits, remote patient monitoring)
- Patient portals (for communication and sharing of information with individual patients)
- Embedded patient education materials
- Customizable EHR workflows
- Administrative tools (eg, appointment scheduling, assessing insurance eligibility)
- Data analytics capabilities for care management and research purposes
- Storage of EHR data on cloud servers versus physical servers
- Mobile app versions of the EHR

EHRs also have a number of potential disadvantages and limitations:[4,9–11,14]

- Computerized provider order entry (CPOE) may introduce errors such as selection of the wrong medication or wrong patient, even though it reduces other errors such as transcription and legibility issues.

- Community pharmacies and other external stakeholders often have limited access to patient EHR data, potentially impacting the quality of care a patient receives.

- Complex technology may generate barriers to care and communication for less tech-savvy patients.

- Too many clinical reminder alerts may cause alert fatigue in providers.

- Overuse of documentation "smart phrases" may facilitate errors in documentation or misrepresentation of services provided.

- EHRs are expensive to implement and maintain, and training for use requires a significant time investment.

Many proprietary EHR platforms are available. Some of the top systems include Epic, Cerner, Meditech, AllScripts, and Athenahealth.[15] These systems differ in a number of ways, including, but not limited to: cost, availability of training and support, interoperability with other healthcare information technology (IT) systems (operational, clinical, and financial), intuitiveness of interface, customization capabilities, and population health management features.[4,12,13,15]

DOCUMENTING A CLINICAL PROGRESS NOTE

Much of the documentation in health care is derived from a systematic patient care process. More than 50 years ago, the use of a Problem-Oriented Medical Record was proposed,[16] leading many healthcare providers to write progress notes using the Subjective, Objective, Assessment, Plan (SOAP) format. The elements of SOAP are as follows:

S = **Subjective**: Chief complaint; history of present illness; why the patient is being seen

O = **Objective**: Physical findings and measurable data such as laboratory values, drug levels, and imaging studies

A = **Assessment**: Analysis or conclusion about the patient's current health status, evidence of progress, response to intervention or medication, and change in functional status

P = **Plan**: Interventions or actions taken in response to assessment, collaboration with others, plan for follow-up, change in diagnosis, and documentation that the patient was informed of changes in interventions and/or medications.

Institutional consultant notes often use an abbreviated version of the SOAP format, often organized by pertinent disease states. This abbreviated version includes key subjective and objective information, assessments, and recommendations. In most cases, the EHR has embraced many of the key components of the above formats. EHR documentation is tailored to documenting medical encounters and history, and also to maximizing billing by meeting requirements established by the US Centers for Medicare & Medicaid Services (CMS). Historically, this documentation was performed by dictation and transcription. Today, most EHRs use predetermined templates to accept automated insertion of clinical data to facilitate the documentation process.

DOCUMENTING MEDICATION MANAGEMENT SERVICES

Pharmacists are increasingly serving as accountable and integral members of healthcare teams. As highlighted in **Chapter 4**, pharmacists provide patient-centered care through a variety of medication management services, such as medication therapy management (MTM), comprehensive medication management (CMM), chronic disease state management, and transitions of care (TOC) services. The most comprehensive of these services has been termed comprehensive medication management (CMM). CMM is a patient-centered approach to optimizing medication use and improving patient health outcomes, is delivered by a pharmacist or other clinician working in collaboration with the patient and other healthcare providers, and assesses all of a patient's medications comprehensively and holistically, not in a targeted manner.[17] CMM also requires use of a patient's medical record for collecting patient information and documenting the findings, assessments, and interventions of each patient encounter.[10,17] Where pharmacists are recognized as partners in care and have access to patients' full medical records, they have been shown to identify drug therapy problems (DTPs) with greater confidence and are better able to offer efficient CMM services.[18]

As described in **Chapters 1** and **4**, the Pharmacist Patient Care Process (PPCP) is used in this *Casebook* as the framework for identifying and resolving patient-specific DTPs and documenting patient encounters. The patient information collected (Step 1 of the PPCP) can be summarized in the S and O sections of a SOAP note, while Assess and Plan (Steps 2 and 3 of the PPCP) can be captured in the A and P sections of a SOAP note. However, Steps 4 and 5 of the PPCP (Implement the Care Plan and Follow up: Monitor and Evaluate) should not be forgotten. Clinicians must document the actual or potential drug therapy and medical problems identified and also the associated interventions they desire to implement or have implemented as well as the follow-up and monitoring required to evaluate a patient's progress effectively.

Regardless of each clinician's role on the team, collaboration, communication, and documentation are key components for the provision of high-quality care. The need for interoperable IT systems to facilitate efficient documentation and effective communication among all healthcare providers is key for optimal communication and continuity of patient care.[6] Additionally, each clinician is responsible for documenting services in a manner appropriate for evaluating patient progress and sufficient for billing purposes. The use of core documentation elements helps create consistency in documentation and information sharing among members of the healthcare team, while facilitating clinician, organization, and regional variations.

Documentation of medication management services should include the following information categories, regardless of note format:

- Patient demographics
- Known allergies, diseases (eg, heart failure), or conditions (eg, pregnancy)
- A record of all medications, including prescription, nonprescription, herbal, and other dietary supplement products
- Assessment of drug therapy problems and plans for resolution or prevention
- Therapeutic monitoring performed or needed
- Interventions or referrals made
- Education provided to the patient
- Feedback provided to providers and patients
- Schedule and plan for follow-up appointment(s)
- Amount of time spent with the patient
- Appropriate billing codes

Similarly, the American Society of Health-System Pharmacists (ASHP) has suggested the following categories of information that may need to be documented in the patient medical record, depending on the clinical context[19]:

- A summary of the patient's medication history on admission, including medication allergies and their manifestations
- Oral and written consultations provided to other healthcare professionals regarding the patient's medication therapy selection and management
- Prescribers' oral orders received directly by the pharmacist
- Clarification of medication orders
- Adjustments made to medication dosage, dosage frequency, dosage form, or route of administration
- Medications, including investigational drugs, administered
- Actual and potential drug therapy problems that warrant surveillance
- Pharmacotherapy monitoring findings, including:
  - ✓ Therapeutic appropriateness of the patient's medication regimen, including the route and method of administration
  - ✓ Therapeutic duplication in the patient's medication regimen
  - ✓ The degree of patient adherence to the prescribed medication regimen
  - ✓ Actual and potential drug–drug, drug–food, drug–laboratory test, and drug–disease interactions
  - ✓ Clinical and pharmacokinetic laboratory data pertinent to the medication regimen
  - ✓ Actual and potential medication toxicity and adverse effects
  - ✓ Physical signs and clinical symptoms relevant to the patient's pharmacotherapy
- Medication-related patient education and counseling provided

USING THE SOAP NOTE FORMAT FOR DOCUMENTATION

As discussed previously, in the SOAP note format subjective (S) and objective (O) data are recorded and then assessed (A) to formulate a plan (P). *Subjective* (S) data include patient symptoms (eg, pain), clinician observations (eg, agitation), or information obtained about the patient (eg, history of cigarette smoking). By its nature, subjective information is descriptive and generally cannot be confirmed by diagnostic tests or procedures. Much of the subjective information is obtained by speaking with the patient or their caregiver while obtaining the medical history, as described in **Chapter 1** (ie, chief complaint, history of present illness, past medical history, family history, social history, medications, allergies, and review of systems). Important subjective information may also be obtained by direct interview with the patient after the initial medical history has been performed (eg, a description of an adverse drug effect, rating of pain severity using standard scales).

A primary source of *objective* (O) information is the physical examination. Other relevant objective information includes laboratory values, serum drug concentrations (along with the target therapeutic range for each level), and the results of other diagnostic tests (eg, electrocardiogram [ECG], X-rays, culture and sensitivity tests). Risk factors that may predispose the patient to a particular problem should also be considered for inclusion. The progress note should include only the pertinent positive and negative findings. Pertinent negative findings are signs and symptoms of the disease or problem that are not present in the particular patient being evaluated.

The *assessment* (A) section outlines what the clinician thinks the patient's problem is, based on the subjective and objective information collected. This assessment often takes the form of a diagnosis or differential diagnosis. This portion of the SOAP note should include all of the reasons for the clinician's assessment. This helps other healthcare providers reading the note to understand how the clinician arrived at his or her particular assessment of the problem.

Since the primary role of the pharmacist is to identify, prevent, and resolve DTPs, this section is where pharmacists should document the patient-specific DTPs they have identified. The first step in documenting DTPs is to clearly state the nature of the medication-related problem(s), including the medication and associated medical condition to which the DTP applies. Each DTP should be addressed separately and prioritized by level of urgency. Understanding the types of pharmacotherapeutic problems that may occur facilitates identification of DTPs. As described in **Chapter 4**, seven distinct types of problems with associated causes have been identified that relate to assessment of medication appropriateness, effectiveness, safety, and adherence.[20]

The *plan* (P) may include ordering additional diagnostic tests or initiating, revising, or discontinuing treatment. If the plan includes changes in pharmacotherapy, the rationale for the specific changes recommended should be described. The drug, dose, dosage form, schedule, route of administration, and duration of therapy should be included. The plan should be directed toward achieving specific, measurable goals or endpoints, which should be clearly stated in the note. Desired therapeutic endpoints and outcomes may include both short-term goals (eg, lower blood pressure [BP] to <130/80 mm Hg in a patient with primary hypertension [HTN] [therapeutic endpoint]) and long-term goals (eg, prevent cardiovascular complications in that patient [therapeutic outcome]). The plan should also outline the efficacy and toxicity parameters that will be used to determine whether the desired therapeutic outcome is being achieved and to detect or prevent drug-related adverse events. Ideally, information about the therapy that should be communicated to the patient should also be included in the plan.

MONITORING FOR ENDPOINTS AND OUTCOMES

It is not enough to only provide a clear, concise record of the nature of a problem, the assessment that led to the conclusion that a problem exists, and the selection of a plan for resolution of the problem. To truly "close the loop" of patient care, follow-up on the plan must occur to ensure that the intended outcome was achieved. A plan for follow-up monitoring of the patient must be documented and adequately implemented. This process should include questioning the patient, gathering laboratory data, and performing the ongoing physical assessments necessary to determine the effect of the plan that was implemented to ensure that it results in an optimal outcome for the patient.

Monitoring parameters to assess efficacy generally include improvement in or resolution of the signs, symptoms, and laboratory abnormalities that were initially assessed. The monitoring parameters used to detect or prevent adverse reactions are determined by the most common and most serious events known to be associated with the therapeutic intervention. Potential adverse reactions should be precisely described along with the method of monitoring. For example, rather than stating "monitor for gastrointestinal (GI) complaints," the recommendation may be to "question the patient about the presence of dyspepsia, diarrhea, or constipation." The frequency, duration, and target endpoint for each monitoring parameter should be identified. The points at which changes in the plan may be warranted should be included. For example, in the case of a patient with type 2 diabetes mellitus (T2DM), one may recommend to "return to clinic (RTC) in 2 weeks to check blood glucose (BG) levels; recheck lipids in 4–6 weeks and A1C in 3 months. If the goal A1C of <7% is not achieved with good adherence at 3 months, increase metformin from 500 mg PO BID to metformin 1000 mg PO BID. If the A1C goal is achieved, maintain metformin 500 mg PO BID and repeat A1C in 6 months."

SUMMARY

A progress note constructed in the manner described states the clinician's subjective and objective findings, an assessment of the findings, the actual or proposed interventions for resolving the drug therapy and medical problems identified, and the parameters for follow-up and monitoring. Whether the note follows a strict SOAP format or not, it should provide a clear, logical, concise record of process, activity, and projected follow-up, clearly stating the problems identified and interventions needed

Based on recommendations from organizations such as the Institute of Medicine, CMS, and researchers involved in the provision of quality of care, EHRs will continue to proliferate and change the way pharmacists and other healthcare providers document patient care encounters. Although the format of the documentation may not strictly follow the SOAP format, the common principles of documentation will remain.

SAMPLE CASE PRESENTATION

The following case presentation illustrates how such a system can be used in practice.

CHIEF COMPLAINT (CC)

"I get a little short of breath working around the house sometimes, and my feet have really been bothering me recently."

HISTORY OF PRESENT ILLNESS (HPI)

A 71-year-old woman is seen in clinic for her first visit. She has a history of mild heart failure and had an MI 4 years ago. She lives alone and has maintained a good level of activity and self-care over the years. However, she reports watching more television recently and being more sedentary than previously. She complains that she experiences some fatigue and SOB (shortness of breath) while cleaning her house or climbing stairs. She also reports occasional pain and tingling in her feet, which has become more bothersome over the past few months.

PAST MEDICAL HISTORY (PMH)

Heart failure (HF)

Myocardial infarction (MI) 4 years ago

Atrial fibrillation (AF)

Type 2 diabetes mellitus (T2DM)

Hypertension (HTN)

FAMILY HISTORY (FH)

Father died after MVA at age 52; mother died of an MI at age 76; a son died by suicide 8 years ago

SOCIAL HISTORY (SH)

Moved to the area recently after her husband's unexpected death; has one son living in the area. Denies illicit drug use. Quit smoking 15 years ago; has a 35 pack-year history of cigarette smoking. Drinks alcohol rarely on social occasions; denies excessive use. Insured under her state's Medicare Advantage health plan; drug coverage is included. Uses a pill box to organize her medications; reports missing her morning doses rarely and her evening doses no more than once weekly.

MEDICATIONS (Meds)

Metformin 500 mg PO BID

Omeprazole 20 mg PO daily

Digoxin 0.125 mg PO Q AM

Warfarin 5 mg PO Q AM

EC aspirin 81 mg PO Q AM

Furosemide 40 mg PO Q AM

Metoprolol XL 100 mg PO Q AM

ALLERGIES (ALL)

Penicillins (rash)

REVIEW OF SYSTEMS (ROS)

Complains of occasional fatigue and DOE. Denies diarrhea, constipation, melena, hematochezia, or change in stool caliber. Also denies bruising and polyuria/polydipsia. Complains of pain/tingling in feet but has no leg pain with walking. She had a difficult time adjusting to her husband's untimely death but now feels she is doing fine. She denies symptoms of anxiety or depression. No recent changes in diet.

PHYSICAL EXAMINATION

Gen

71-year-old woman whose appearance is consistent with her stated age. Appears well developed, well nourished, and in no acute distress.

VS

BP 169/88 mm Hg, HR 62 bpm, RR 13/min, T 99°F; weight 184 lb, height 5′4″.

Skin

Unremarkable.

HEENT

Slight arteriovenous (AV) nicking, otherwise unremarkable.

Neck/Lymph Nodes

Neck supple, thyroid normal with no mass, nodules, or tenderness; jugular venous pressure (JVP) 6 cm; normal carotid pulsations; no carotid bruits.

Chest/Lungs

Slight crackles at the right and left bases; no rales, e-to-a changes, or tactile fremitus.

Breasts

Normal breasts without pain, swelling, discharge, or masses.

CV

RRR. (+) S_3 gallop; (+) hepatojugular reflux. Mild neck vein distention at 45°.

Abd

Soft, nontender, nondistended, bowel sounds normal. No hepatosplenomegaly.

Genit/Rect

Unremarkable.

MS/Ext

1–2+ pedal edema bilaterally. Ankle-brachial index (ABI) 1.02 (negative). Strength 5/5.

Neuro

Unremarkable.

Labs

Laboratory values are unremarkable except:

INR 3.5

FBG 198 mg/dL

A1C 9.5% = eAG 226 mg/dL

SCr 1.3 mg/dL

TC 183 mg/dL, LDL 128 mg/dL, HDL 38 mg/dL, TG 150 mg/dL

Digoxin level 1.0 ng/mL

Imaging

Chest X-ray (CXR): diffuse patchiness at the bases. Enlarged cardiac silhouette.

Echo: no valvular abnormalities; EF = 40%.

Electrocardiogram

Normal sinus rhythm (NSR). Changes are consistent with left ventricular hypertrophy (LVH).

Medical Assessment

1. Mild, class II–III HF with pedal edema and mild pulmonary congestion; taking digoxin, furosemide, and metoprolol.
2. AF, currently rate-controlled on digoxin and metoprolol. Warfarin anticoagulation per guidelines above target of INR 2–3.
3. T2DM, not optimally controlled with metformin.
4. Peripheral neuropathy symptoms, currently untreated.
5. HTN not optimally managed with metoprolol.
6. Clinical atherosclerotic cardiovascular disease (ASCVD; s/p MI); taking aspirin and metoprolol; no statin therapy.
7. Moderate renal insufficiency stage 3: SCr 1.3, estimated ClCr 29 mL/min, glomerular filtration rate (GFR by MDRD)[21] 43 mL/min.
8. Obesity: body mass index (BMI) 31.6 kg/m².
9. Medication with no indication: omeprazole.
10. Inconsistent patient adherence with medication use, patient unaware of medication indications.

PLAN

1. HF: Increase furosemide to 40 mg PO BID.
2. AF: Decrease warfarin dose per clinic algorithm. Continue digoxin and metoprolol at current doses.
3. T2DM: Continue metformin 500 mg PO BID. Initiate a GLP-1 receptor agonist for improved A1C control and the potential for weight loss. Provide education and review of injection technique for GLP-1 receptor agonist. Goal A1C <7%.
4. Peripheral neuropathy: Initiate gabapentin therapy at 100 mg PO Q HS, titrate as needed to manage symptoms.
5. HTN: Add an ACE inhibitor or ARB for BP reduction and renal protection. Continue metoprolol.
6. Clinical ASCVD (s/p MI): Continue metoprolol and aspirin; add a high-intensity statin.
7. Renal insufficiency: add an ACE inhibitor or ARB.
8. Obesity: Counsel on lifestyle modifications for weight reduction, add GLP-1 receptor agonist as discussed above.
9. Discontinue omeprazole.
10. Clinic appointment for follow-up in 2 weeks. Will recheck INR and basic chemistry panel and reassess medication adherence at that time.

CONSTRUCTION OF A SOAP NOTE WITH DRUG THERAPY PROBLEM DOCUMENTATION

Subjective

71-year-old woman with CC of DOE and increasing pain and tingling in feet. History of AF, T2DM, mild–moderate HF, and MI 4 years ago. She is taking her medications as prescribed, missing doses no more than once weekly. Uses a pill box to organize medications but doesn't know the indication for each.

Objective

VS: BP 169/88, HR 62, RR 13, T 99.0°F; weight 184 lb, height 5′4″

Extremities: 1–2+ BLE edema

HEENT: Slight AV nicking

CV: RRR

Meds:

  Metformin 500 mg PO BID

  Omeprazole 20 mg PO daily

  Digoxin 0.125 mg PO Q AM

  Warfarin 5 mg PO Q AM

  EC ASA 81 mg PO Q AM

  Furosemide 40 mg PO Q AM

  Metoprolol XL 100 mg PO Q AM

Labs:

  INR 3.5

  FBG 198 mg/dL

  A1C 9.5%

  SCr 1.3 mg/dL

  TC 183 mg/dL, LDL 128 mg/dL, HDL 38 mg/dL, TG 150 mg/dL

  Serum digoxin 1.0 ng/mL

Chest X-ray: Diffuse patchiness at the bases. Enlarged cardiac silhouette.

ECHO: EF = 40%

ECG: NSR, LVH

Assessment

1. Mild HF, class II (BLE edema, DOE, cardiomegaly on CXR, LVH on ECG, and diminished EF). Maintained with a β-blocker and digoxin (level within target range); no ACE inhibitor.

2. AF: Rate controlled with metoprolol and digoxin. No digoxin dose adjustment indicated. Anticoagulation: INR > target range of 2–3, no clinical complications, no identifiable cause.

3. T2DM, not well controlled. A1C above goal of <7%. Taking max metformin dose for current renal function. No ACEI or ARB for renal protective effects.

4. Untreated peripheral neuropathy in feet.

5. HTN, not optimally controlled with metoprolol (increased BP, elevated SCr, and AV nicking). Renal findings suggest significant, sustained HTN.

6. Clinical ASCVD (s/p MI): Taking low-dose ASA and metoprolol; no statin therapy.

7. Possible moderate renal insufficiency (CrCl = 29 mL/min; GFR = 43 mL/min). No renal dose adjustments necessary at this time.

8. Obesity: Classified as obese; BMI 31.6 kg/m².

9. Medication without indication (omeprazole 20 mg): No complaints related to GERD or PUD; omeprazole not needed.

10. Nonoptimal medication adherence; lack of knowledge about medication indications.

Plan

1. Mild HF:

   – Continue metoprolol and digoxin at current doses.

   – Add lisinopril 10 mg daily, titrating to 40 mg daily as tolerated.

   – Increase furosemide to 40 mg PO BID.

   – No added dietary salt.

   – Reassess status and repeat basic chemistry panel in 2 weeks.

2. AF:

   – Rate control: Continue metoprolol and digoxin at current doses.

   – Anticoagulation: Recommend warfarin 2.5 mg today and then resume 5 mg PO daily Mon–Sat and 2.5 mg on Sun (decrease in total weekly dose [TWD] by 7.1%). Recheck INR in 2 weeks.

3. T2DM:

   – Start lisinopril 10 mg daily as above per current ADA guidelines.

   – Maintain metformin at 500 mg PO BID due to renal insufficiency.

– Add Victoza 0.6 mg SC once daily for 1 week, then increase to 1.2 mg once daily. Provide patient education on proper injection technique.

– Diet: Encourage three meals and bedtime snack, with no concentrated CHO choices. Limit CHO intake per meal to 60 g; snacks 15–20 g. No added salt. Check BG daily. Refer to dietitian for nutrition review.

– Provide patient education printouts from the EHR on T2DM

4. Peripheral neuropathy: Start gabapentin 100 mg PO Q HS. Titrate dose over several weeks to 300 mg PO BID for better symptom control, as tolerated.

5. HTN (Goal BP: <130/80 [per ADA 2022 Standards of Medical Care]): Start lisinopril 10 mg PO daily as recommended above. Titrate dose to maintain BP control (and improve HF Sx); target dose = 40 mg daily. Continue metoprolol at current dose.

6. Clinical ASCVD (s/p MI):

– Continue EC ASA 81 mg PO Q AM.

– Add lisinopril 10 mg PO daily as noted above.

– Add high-intensity statin (atorvastatin 40 mg PO daily).

– Continue metoprolol XL 100 mg Q AM.

7. Renal insufficiency: Repeat SCr in 2 weeks. Initiate lisinopril 10 mg PO daily as above for renal protective effects.

8. Obesity: Counsel on lifestyle modifications for weight reduction. Adding GLP-1 receptor agonist (Victoza, as noted above) for potential for weight loss in addition to improved A1C control.

9. Medication without indication: Discontinue omeprazole 20 mg.

10. Suboptimal medication adherence: Assess and reinforce adherence to recommended therapy. Educate on purpose of each medication. Recommend use of an alarm or mobile app to improve adherence.

11. Send all updated prescriptions to Main Street Pharmacy.

Monitoring

1. Lab tests (orders entered):

– Baseline basic chemistry panel today

– INR in 2 weeks

2. Patient was counseled to monitor BG once daily, before breakfast, and to bring information on RTC.

Follow-Up

1. RTC in 2 weeks to recheck INR and basic chemistries and to assess medication changes.

2. Dietary consultation: Appointment made with the clinic's registered dietician (RD).

3. Prescribed medications after this visit:

– Digoxin 0.125 mg PO Q AM for HF symptoms and rate control (maintain dose)

– Furosemide 40 mg PO BID for HF (dose increase)

– Warfarin 5 mg PO Q AM Mon–Sat, 2.5 mg on Sun for CVA prevention (dose decrease)

– EC ASA 81 mg PO daily for secondary ASCVD prevention (maintain dose)

– Metoprolol XL 100 mg PO Q AM for s/p MI and rate control (maintain dose)

– Lisinopril 10 mg PO daily for HF, HTN, and T2DM (new medication)

– Atorvastatin 40 mg PO daily for secondary ASCVD prevention (new medication)

– Metformin 500 mg PO BID for T2DM (maintain dose)

– Victoza 0.6 mg SC daily for 1 week, then increase to 1.2 mg SC daily for T2DM and potential weight loss (new medication)

– Gabapentin 100 mg PO Q HS for peripheral neuropathy, with a 2-week titration to 300 mg PO BID (new medication)

– Discontinue omeprazole 20 mg

REFERENCES

1. McNally ME. The importance of detailed documentation in ICD-10. Bull Am Coll Surg. 2015;100(8):63–64.

2. Patterson ES, Lowry SZ, Ramaiah M, et al. Improving clinical workflow in ambulatory care: implemented recommendations in an innovation prototype for the Veteran's Health Administration. EGEMS (Washington, DC). 2015;3(2):1149.

3. Evaluation and Management Services Guide. Washington, DC: Centers for Medicare & Medicaid Services; August 2017. Available at: *www.cms.gov/Outreach-and-Education/Medicare-Learning-Network-MLN/MLNProducts/Downloads/eval-mgmt-serv-guide-ICN006764.pdf*. Accessed February 1, 2022.

4. Practice Fusion blog. EHR (electronic health record) vs. EMR (electronic medical record). May 21, 2021. Available at: *https://www.practice-fusion.com/blog/ehr-vs-emr/*. Accessed February 1, 2022.

5. Institute of Medicine. Crossing the Quality Chasm: A New Health System for the 21st Century. Washington, DC: National Academy Press; 2001.

6. Bates DW, Gawande AA. Improving safety with information technology. N Engl J Med. 2003;348:2526–2534.

7. Campanella P, Lovato E, Marone L, et al. The impact of electronic health records on healthcare quality: a systematic review and meta-analysis. Eur J Public Health. 2016;26(1):60–64.

8. Poon EG, Wright A, Simon SR, et al. Relationship between use of electronic health record features and health care quality: results of a statewide survey. Med Care. 2010;48:203–209.

9. Mills S. Electronic health records and use of clinical decision support. Crit Care Nurs Clin North Am. 2019;31(2):125–131.

10. Nelson SD, Poikonen J, Reese T, El Halta D, Weir C. The pharmacist and the EHR. J Am Med Inform Assoc. 2017;24(1):193–197.

11. Yan L, Reese T, Nelson SD. A narrative review of clinical decision support for inpatient clinical pharmacists. Appl Clin Inform. 2021;12(2):199–207.

12. Epic website. Available at: *https://www.epic.com/*. Accessed February 1, 2022.

13. Athenahealth website. Electronic health records: an EHR that lets you focus on delivering care. Available at: *https://www.athenahealth.com/solutions/electronic-health-records*. Accessed February 1, 2022.

14. Faiella A, Casper KA, Bible L, Seifert J. Implementation and use of an electronic health record in a charitable community pharmacy. J Am Pharm Assoc. 2019;59(2S):S110–S117.

15. Newman D. Top EHR vendors 2022—Epic, Cerner, Meditech, Allscripts, Athenahealth. HealthCare Skills website. January 3, 2022. Available at: *https://healthcareitskills.com/top-ehr-vendors-allscripts-athenahealth-cerner-epic-meditech/*. Accessed February 1, 2022.

16. Weed LL. Medical records that guide and teach. N Engl J Med. 1968;278:593–600, 652–657.

17. American College of Clinical Pharmacy. 2018. The Patient Care Process for Delivering Comprehensive Medication Management (CMM): Optimizing Medication Use in Patient-Centered, Team-Based Care Settings. CMM in Primary Care Research Team. Available at: *http://www.accp.com/cmm_care_process*. Accessed February 1, 2022.

18. van Lint JA, Sorge LA, Sorensen TD. Access to patients' health records for drug therapy problem determination by pharmacists. J Am Pharm Assoc. 2015;55:278–281.

19. American Society of Health-System Pharmacists. ASHP guidelines on documenting pharmaceutical care in patient medical records. Am J Health Syst Pharm. 2003;60:705–707.

20. Cipolle RJ, Strand LM, Morley PC. Pharmaceutical Care Practice: The Clinician's Guide. 3rd ed. New York, NY: McGraw-Hill; 2012.

21. Levey AS, Bosch JP, Lewis JB, Greene T, Rogers N, Roth D. A more accurate method to estimate glomerular filtration rate from serum creatinine: a new prediction equation. Modification of Diet in Renal Disease Study Group. Ann Intern Med. 1999;130:461–470.

Bilateral undescended testes
Neonatal abstinence syndrome requiring a 12-day morphine taper
Colostomy reversal and gastrostomy tube placement 5 days PTA
Failure to thrive
Immunizations: hepatitis B immune globulin and hepatitis B vaccine administered at birth; DTaP, IPV, HepB, Hib, PCV13 administered 2 months PTA

■ **FH**

Unavailable

■ **SH**

Placed with foster family 2 months prior to admission due to neglect. Foster mother at bedside and appropriately concerned.

■ **Current Meds**

Omeprazole suspension 10 mg GT daily
Pediatric multivitamin with iron 1 mL GT daily

■ **All**

NKDA

■ **ROS (As Reported By Foster Mother)**

Constitutional

Foster mother affirms that the child, although normally nonverbal, is more lethargic and unresponsive than normal. The patient has not walked but rolls himself.

HEENT

Oral secretions well controlled. Denies history of rhinitis, allergies, or ear infections. The patient ordinarily tracks visually and responds to verbal cues.

Respiratory

Denies SOB, coughing

Cardiovascular

Echocardiogram and ECG normal at birth

Gastrointestinal

G-tube feeding dependent. Prior to G-tube placement, oral feeds attempted with very limited success, usually less than an ounce per feeding, leading to failure to thrive. The patient tolerated continuous G-tube feeds of 30 kcal/oz formula at 25 mL/hr in the hospital on the day prior to discharge but vomited repeatedly at home leading to current admission. Stooled during previous admission but not at home.

Genitourinary

No wet diapers since yesterday. Follows with nephrology for single kidney. Evaluated by pediatric endocrinology for undescended testes and small penis who proposed a trial of β-hCG. If fails, will require orchiopexy.

■ **Physical Examination**

Gen

Ill appearing, mottled child who is floppy, lethargic, and barely responsive to painful stimuli

6

PEDIATRICS

The Case of Baby's Busted Belly . . . . Level III

Franklin Huggins, PharmD, BCPPS, BCCCP

LEARNING OBJECTIVES

After completing this case study, the reader should be able to:

- Recognize septic shock in a pediatric patient using age-appropriate assessment parameters.
- Design an evidence-based pharmacotherapy plan for the child in septic shock, including medications, dosing, and monitoring.
- Determine the pediatric patient's fluid and electrolyte requirements and make therapeutically sound recommendations for repletion.
- Monitor the progress of the sick child and adjust therapy as indicated using appropriate metrics.
- Employ specific techniques to ensure that medications are deployed safely for pediatric patients.
- Recommend age-appropriate vaccinations for children.

PATIENT PRESENTATION

■ **Chief Complaint**

Mother reports vomiting, poor feeding, and fever in her 15-month-old son.

■ **HPI**

A 15-month-old boy presents today with his foster mother, who reports that the child has had poor oral intake, vomiting, and fever for 1 day. A colostomy had been performed at birth due to the presence of an imperforate anus. He was subsequently lost to follow-up until 2 months prior to the current admission when he presented to the PCP for the first time since birth with severe failure to thrive (weight and weight-for-height below 1% of expected) and oral feeding intolerance. Five days prior to admission, the patient underwent reversal of a colostomy with repair of the imperforate anus and placement of a gastrostomy tube for the feeding intolerance and was discharged home 2 days ago. Yesterday, he had four episodes of vomiting and was unable to retain any of the G-tube feedings. The mother took him to the PCP where he was found to be lethargic, ill appearing, and febrile, which prompted his admission directly to the pediatric intensive care unit.

■ **PMH**

Vaginal delivery at 35 weeks gestation
No prenatal care
Intrauterine growth restriction
Birth hypoxia
Imperforate anus requiring colostomy on second day of life
Single kidney

VS

BP 114/66, HR 148, RR 36, current temperature 40.2°C, O_2 saturation 95%, height 69 cm, weight 5.6 kg

Skin

Cool, pale, mottled, and dry

HEENT

Eyes sunken, PERRLA, tympanic membranes normal, mucous membranes dry

Neck/Lymph Nodes

Supple, nontender, no masses, no lymphadenopathy, no bruit, no JVD

Chest

Tachypneic, clear to auscultation and percussion

CV

Tachycardic, monitor shows NSR, no murmur, gallop or edema, absent peripheral pulses, central pulses weak, capillary refill 6 seconds

Abd

Soft, nondistended, no masses, (+) rebound tenderness globally, no bowel sounds appreciated. G-tube in place with no erythema or drainage. Surgical scar in LLQ.

Genit/Rect

Tanner stage I, bilateral undescended testes

Ext

Flaccid, pale, cold extremities

Neuro

Lethargic, responds to painful stimuli, cranial nerves intact, reflexes intact

Laboratory Values

Na 135 mEq/L	Total protein 5.9 g/dL	WBC 1.6×10^3/mm³
K 4.7 mEq/L	Albumin 2.1 g/dL	Neutrophils 8%
Cl 101 mEq/L	Total bilirubin 0.7 mg/dL	Immature neutrophils 36%
CO_2 20 mEq/L	Alk phos 365 U/L	Lymphocytes 51%
BUN 39 mg/dL	ALT 192 U/L	Monocytes 5%
SCr 0.3 mg/dL	AST 521 U/L	Hgb 10.5 g/dL
Glu 53 mg/dL		Hct 30%
Calcium 7.6 mg/dL		Plt 62×10^3/mm³

Imaging

- Radiograph abdomen two view: Nonspecific gaseous distention of stomach and loops of bowel in the lower abdomen and right upper quadrant. No discernible evidence of free air. No acute osseous abnormalities. G-tube.
- Ultrasound abdomen limited: Focused ultrasound of the left hemiabdomen identifies complicated extraluminal fluid in the upper abdomen, particularly the left upper quadrant. It is seen adjacent to the spleen and likely insinuating itself around the stomach. Internal debris and septations are noted. Stool-filled portions of the colon are seen in the left hemiabdomen.

While there is no definite fluid collection or sonographic abnormality in the right hemiabdomen, the patient was very tender in the right hemiabdomen during real-time imaging.

■ Assessment

Critically ill child with sepsis and septic shock secondary to presumptive peritonitis

Failure to thrive secondary to malnutrition

Underimmunization

QUESTIONS

Collect Information

1.a. What subjective and objective information indicates the presence of septic shock?

1.b. What additional information is needed to fully assess this patient?

Assess the Information

2.a. Assess the severity of septic shock based on the subjective and objective information available.

2.b. Create a list of the patient's drug therapy problems and prioritize them. Include assessment of medication appropriateness, effectiveness, safety, and patient adherence.

2.c. How does the evidence supporting a diagnosis of septic shock in this patient differ from an adult patient?

Develop a Care Plan

3.a. What are the goals of pharmacotherapy for septic shock in this case?

3.b. What nondrug therapies might be useful for this patient's septic shock?

3.c. What feasible therapeutic options are available for treating pediatric septic shock?

3.d. Create an individualized, patient-centered, team-based care plan to optimize medication therapy for septic shock and the patient's other drug therapy problems. Include specific medications, dosage forms, doses, schedules, and durations of therapy.

Implement the Care Plan

4.a. What information should be provided to the patient to enhance adherence, ensure successful therapy, and minimize adverse effects?

4.b. Describe how care should be coordinated with other healthcare providers.

4.c. What pediatric-specific medication practices should be applied in this case to prevent adverse outcomes of medication therapy?

Follow-Up: Monitor and Evaluate

5. Explain how to monitor and evaluate the care plan for medication appropriateness, effectiveness, safety and patient adherence by using clinical and laboratory data, patient feedback and other information.

■ CLINICAL COURSE

After initial stabilization, the patient was taken to the operating room for an exploratory laparotomy that revealed failure of the colostomy repair from 5 days ago. The abdomen was found to be filled with fluid, stool, and pus. The abdomen was extensively irrigated and cultures sent. The colostomy was recreated, and the patient returned to the ICU with the abdomen open to facilitate further surgical intervention.

Current medications:

Famotidine 2.8 mg IV Q 12 H (1 mg/kg/day)
Piperacillin-tazobactam 560 mg IV Q 8 H (300 mg/kg/day)
Acetaminophen 80 mg IV Q 6 H (14 mg/kg/dose)
Morphine 0.6 mg IV Q 4 H PRN pain score 7–10 (0.1 mg/kg/dose)
TPN 10% dextrose + 2 g/kg/day amino acid IV
Lipid emulsion 1 g/kg/day IV

On hospital day 2, the following laboratory results were obtained:

Na 141 mEq/L	Total protein 5.1 g/dL	WBC $1.4 \times 10^3/mm^3$
K 3.1 mEq/L	Albumin 1.7 g/dL	Neutrophils 17%
Cl 108 mEq/L	Total bilirubin	Immature neutrophils 23%
CO_2 21 mEq/L	0.8 mg/dL	Lymphocytes 53%
BUN 31 mg/dL	Alk phos 304 U/L	Monocytes 7%
SCr 0.6 mg/dL	ALT 239 U/L	Hgb 7.4 g/dL
Glu 140 mg/dL	AST 600 U/L	Hct 22%
Calcium 8.0 mg/dL		Plt $37 \times 10^3/mm^3$

Anaerobic Culture—Final

Source: Peritoneal cavity
Gram stain: Many WBC, many gram-negative rods, few gram-positive rods
Light growth *Klebsiella pneumoniae*
Light growth *Proteus mirabilis*
Light growth *Bacteroides fragilis*

Antimicrobial Susceptibility (mcg/mL)

	Klebsiella Pneumoniae		Proteus Mirabilis	
Amikacin	S	≤16	S	≤16
Ampicillin	R	>16	S	≤8
Ampicillin/Sulbactam	S	8/4	S	N/A
Aztreonam	S	≤4	S	≤4
Cefazolin	S	≤4	S	4
Cefepime	S	≤2	S	≤2
Cefotaxime	S	≤2	S	≤2
Ceftazidime	S	≤1	S	≤1
Ceftriaxone	S	≤1	S	≤1
Cefuroxime	S	≤4	S	≤4
Ciprofloxacin	S	≤1	S	≤1
Ertapenem	S	≤0.5	S	≤0.5
Gentamicin	S	≤1	S	≤1
Imipenem	S	≤0.5	N/A	N/A
Levofloxacin	S	≤0.25	S	≤0.25
Meropenem	S	≤1	S	≤1
Piperacillin/Tazobactam	S	≤4	S	≤4
Tetracycline	S	≤4	R	>8
Tigecycline	S	≤2	N/A	N/A
Tobramycin	S	≤1	S	≤1
Trimethoprim/Sulfa	S	≤2/38	R	>2/38

■ FOLLOW-UP QUESTIONS

1. What is the likely cause of the elevated liver enzymes, increasing creatinine, and cytopenia in this patient?

2. Now that the patient is fully fluid resuscitated and hemodynamically stable, calculate the appropriate maintenance fluid rate.

3. What changes should be made to the patient's medication therapy based on the most recent results?

■ SELF-STUDY ASSIGNMENTS

1. Describe the challenges involved in managing parenteral nutrition in this patient.

2. Write an evidence-based paper outlining the role of corticosteroid therapy in pediatric septic shock.

CLINICAL PEARL

Children remain normotensive until very late in shock making blood pressure an unreliable indicator of perfusion status. Clinicians should carefully evaluate children for other signs of shock, such as tachycardia, decreased or weak pulses, altered mental status, oliguria, pale mottled skin, and slow capillary refill. If clinical signs of poor perfusion are present, appropriate fluid resuscitation and inotropic therapy should be initiated immediately. Hypotension in a septic child is a sign of impending cardiovascular collapse and must be addressed emergently.

REFERENCES

1. Weiss SL, Peters MJ, Alhazzani W, et al. Surviving sepsis campaign international guidelines for the management of septic shock and sepsis-associated organ dysfunction in children. Pediatr Crit Care Med. 2020;21(2):e52–e106.

2. Sterling SA, Miller WR, Pryor J, Puskarich MA, Jones AE. The impact of timing of antibiotics on outcomes in severe sepsis and septic shock: a systematic review and meta-analysis. Crit Care Med. 2015;43(9):1907–1915.

3. Solomkin JS, Mazuski JE, Bradley JS, et al. Diagnosis and management of complicated intra-abdominal infection in adults and children: guidelines by the Surgical Infection Society and the Infectious Diseases Society of America. Clin Infect Dis. 2010;50(2):133–164.

4. Tables of antibacterial drug dosages. In: Kimberlin DW, et al., eds. Red Book: 2021–2024 Report of the Committee on Infectious Diseases. Am Acad Pediatr. 2021:876–897.

5. Ventura AM, Shieh HH, Bousso A, et al. Double-blind prospective randomized controlled trial of dopamine versus epinephrine as first-line vasoactive drugs in pediatric septic shock. Crit Care Med. 2015;43(11):2292–2302.

6. Centers for Disease Control and Prevention. Recommended immunization schedule for children and adolescents aged 18 years or younger, United States, 2021. Available at: https://www.cdc.gov/vaccines/schedules/hcp/imz/child-adolescent.html. Accessed November 11, 2021.

7. Levine SR, Cohen MR, Blanchard NR, et al. Guidelines for preventing medication errors in pediatrics. J Pediatr Pharmacol Ther. 2001;6:426–442.

8. Meyers RS. Pediatric fluid and electrolyte therapy. J Pediatr Pharmacol Ther. 2009;14(4):204–211.

9. Schwartz GJ, Work DF. Measurement and estimation of GFR in children and adolescents. Clin J Am Soc Nephrol. 2009;4(11):1832–1843.

10. Lexicomp Online, Pediatric and Neonatal Lexi-Drugs Online. Waltham, MA: UpToDate, Inc.; July 30, 2021. Available at: https://online.lexi.com. Accessed November 11, 2021.

7

GERIATRICS

Forgetting and Falling .... Level II

David P. Elliott, PharmD, FASCP, FCCP, AGSF, BCGP

LEARNING OBJECTIVES

After completing this case study, the reader should be able to:

- Identify medications an older adult is taking that may not be suitable for that person and determine if a change in therapy should be considered.

- Recognize common geriatric syndromes, including falls, urinary incontinence, cognitive impairment, and frailty and identify medications that may precipitate or worsen these conditions.

- Evaluate a patient's medication use system and recommend changes for reasons related to medication regimen effectiveness, safety, adherence, and caregiver stress or burden.

- Describe the screening, assessment, and prevention of falls in older adults.

- Recommend changes in pharmacotherapy for an older adult with multiple chronic conditions based on person-centered considerations such as patient preferences, remaining life expectancy, applicability of published evidence, and treatment complexity and feasibility.

PATIENT PRESENTATION

■ Chief Complaint

"My mother has been having dizzy spells."

■ HPI

An 87-year-old woman was referred by her PCP for a pharmacotherapy consult and adverse drug event review. Patient presents with her daughter, who reports that her mother often complains of feeling dizzy and had a fall last night after getting out of bed to use the bathroom. Patient states that her hip hurts where she fell on it.

The daughter reports administering *Ginkgo biloba* to help with her mother's memory but isn't sure it has made a difference. The daughter also says that her mother has been requesting Tylenol frequently since her fall and suspects that her mother has been taking additional doses when the daughter is away from the home. The patient does not remember the other medications she is taking and says that her daughter helps her.

■ PMH

Osteoporosis, diagnosed 7 years ago
Nonvalvular atrial fibrillation, no h/o VTE
Allergic rhinitis
Major neurocognitive disorder due to Alzheimer disease, diagnosed 2 years ago

■ PSH

Cesarean section

■ FH

Noncontributory

■ SH

Patient denies using any tobacco or alcohol. She moved in with her daughter 6 months ago after the death of her husband, and her daughter assists with her daily needs. Her daughter works full-time outside the home, so the patient is alone in the house between about 8 AM and 5:30 PM each day.

■ Meds

Warfarin 2 mg Mon-Wed-Fri-Sun and 4 mg Tue-Thu-Sat
Alendronate 70 mg PO once weekly for the last 3 years
Diphenhydramine 25 mg PO TID PRN allergy symptoms
Acetaminophen OTC Extra Strength 1–2 PO PRN pain
Metoprolol succinate 50 mg PO every morning
Donepezil 5 mg PO every evening started 2 years ago
Multiple vitamin every morning
Ginkgo biloba PO every morning started a few weeks ago

■ All

Donepezil: Developed nausea and diarrhea with donepezil 10 mg daily. Patient's family declines further attempts at dosage increases or adding other drugs to enhance cognitive function.

■ ROS

Patient complains of hip pain where she fell as well as a runny nose from allergies; denies heartburn, chest pain, or shortness of breath.

■ Physical Examination

Gen

WDWN woman who appears her stated age; NAD

VS

BP 118/72 mm Hg sitting, 100/60 mm Hg standing; HR 58 bpm (irregularly irregular), RR 18/min, T 98.4°F (36.8°C), Ht 5′4″ (163 cm), Wt 55 kg

HEENT

Mildly inflamed nasal mucosa, watery nasal discharge consistent with allergic rhinitis

Heart

Rhythm is irregularly irregular; no murmurs or bruits.

Ext

Bruising and swelling over right hip. Patient reports some tenderness with palpation. Some limitations of range of motion, probably due to age-related osteoarthritis. Do not suspect a fracture.

Neuro

Motor, sensory, CNs, cerebellar, and gait normal. SLUMS score 17/30 (normal ≥27), compared with a score of 17/30 and 19/30 last year and at the initial diagnosis, respectively. Disoriented to month, date, and day of week. Good registration but impaired attention and very poor short-term memory. Able to follow commands. Displayed irritability during administration of the SLUMS (Fig. 7-1).

VAMC
SLUMS Examination
Questions about this assessment tool? E-mail aging@slu.edu

Name_____ Age___**87**_____

Is the patient alert?_____**Yes**_____ Level of education___**High School Grad**_____

1/1	**1**	1. What day of the week is it?
1/1	**1**	2. What is the year?
1/1	**1**	3. What state are we in?

4. Please remember these five objects. I will ask you what they are later.

Apple   Pen   Tie   House   Car

5. You have $100 and you go to the store and buy a dozen apples for $3 and a tricycle for $20.
- **1** How much did you spend? **23**
- **1**/3 **2** How much do you have left? **couldn't answer**

6. Please name as many animals as you can in one minute. **11**
- **2**/3
  - **0** 0–4 animals **1** 5–9 animals **2** 10–14 animals **3** 15+ animals

7. What were the five objects I asked you to remember? 1 point for each one correct. **Apple,**
- **2**/5

8. I am going to give you a series of numbers and I would like you to give them to me **House**
backwards. For example, if I say 42, you would say 24.
- **1**/2
  - **0** 87 **ok**   **1** 648 **ok**   **1** 8537 **wrong**

9. This is a clock face. Please put in the hour markers and the time at
ten minutes to eleven o'clock. **see attached**
- **2** Hour markers okay **yes**
- **2**/4 **2** Time correct **no**

1 10. Please place an **X** in the triangle.

X

- **2**/2 **1** Which of the above figures is largest? **square**

11. I am going to tell you a story. Please listen carefully because afterwards, I'm going to ask
you some questions about it.

Jill was a very successful stockbroker. She made a lot of money on the stock market. She then
met Jack, a devastatingly handsome man. She married him and had three children. They lived
in Chicago. She then stopped work and stayed at home to bring up her children. When they were
teenagers, she went back to work. She and Jack lived happily ever after.

- **2** What was the female's name? **Jill**   **2** What work did she do? **not sure**
- **4**/8 **2** When did she go back to work? **don't know**   **2** What state did she live in? **Illinois**

___**17**___ **TOTAL SCORE**

SCORING		
HIGH SCHOOL EDUCATION		**LESS THAN HIGH SCHOOL EDUCATION**
27–30	NORMAL	25–30
21–26	MILD NEUROCOGNITIVE DISORDER	20–24
1–20	DEMENTIA	1–19

_____   _____   _____
CLINICIAN'S SIGNATURE   DATE   TIME

FIGURE 7-1. Completed SLUMS form including scoring. (Reproduced with permission from Tariq SH, Tumosa N, Chibnall JT, Perry MH 3rd, Morley JE. Comparison of the Saint Louis University mental status examination and the mini-mental state examination for detecting dementia and mild neurocognitive disorder—a pilot study. *Am J Geriatr Psychiatry.* 2006;14(11):900-910.)

Clock Drawing Test

Patient's Name: _____   Date: _____

FIGURE 7-1. (Continued)

Labs

Na 139 mEq/L	Hgb 13.5 g/dL	T. bili 0.9 mg/dL	Ca 9.7 mg/dL
K 3.7 mEq/L	Hct 39.0%	D. bili 0.3 mg/dL	Phos 4.5 mg/dL
Cl 108 mEq/L	AST 25 IU/L	T. prot 7.5 g/dL	TSH 3.8 mIU/L
CO_2 25.5 mEq/L	ALT 24 IU/L	Alb 4.5 g/dL	Free T4 1.2 ng/dL
BUN 16 mg/dL	Alk phos 81 IU/L	Chol 212 mg/dL	Uric acid 6.8 mg/dL
SCr 1.1 mg/dL	GGT 22 IU/L	INR 3.1	25-OH vitamin D
Glu 78 mg/dL	LDH 85 IU/L	A1C 5.8%	21 ng/mL

Radiology

CT scan (head, 2 years ago): Mild to moderate generalized cerebral atrophy.

DXA scan results (last year): T scores in the spine and hip were −1.8 and −2.2, respectively.

ECG

Atrial fibrillation

Assessment

1. Falls, secondary to multiple factors including medications
2. Atrial fibrillation, rate controlled
3. Allergic rhinitis
4. Osteopenia

QUESTIONS

Collect Information

1.a. What additional information is needed to assess whether the patient's medications are being administered in a safe and consistent manner?

1.b. What additional details about the patient's medication list are needed to evaluate current therapy?

1.c. What additional information would be helpful to evaluate the patient's drug therapy with respect to her fall history and treatment for atrial fibrillation and osteoporosis?

Assess the Information

2.a. Which one of the patient's chronic medical problems has the greatest impact on her independent function and life expectancy?

2.b. Which of the patient's medications is/are included in the AGS Beers Criteria® as being potentially inappropriate based on her age or underlying conditions?

2.c. What are the patient's known risk factors for falls?

2.d. Create a list of the patient's drug therapy problems and prioritize them. Include assessment of medication appropriateness, effectiveness, safety, and patient adherence.

Develop a Care Plan

3.a. What are the goals of treatment for this patient?

3.b. What nondrug therapies should be implemented to prevent falls, and fractures?

3.c. Create an individualized, patient-centered, team-based care plan to optimize medication therapy for this patient. Include specific drugs, dosage forms, doses, schedules, and durations of therapy.

Implement the Care Plan

4.a. What strategies should be implemented with the patient and caregiver to reduce the medication-related burden, ensure successful therapy, and minimize adverse effects?

4.b. Describe how care should be coordinated with other healthcare providers.

Follow-Up: Monitor and Evaluate

5. Explain how to monitor and evaluate the care plan for medication appropriateness, effectiveness, safety and patient adherence by using clinical and laboratory data, patient feedback and other information.

■ SELF-STUDY ASSIGNMENTS

1. Review the 2019 AGS Beers criteria for potentially inappropriate use of medications in older adults, and consider your first-line recommendations for optimal treatment of depression, insomnia, and diabetes in the older adult.

2. Outline the changes that you would make to the pharmacotherapeutic regimen for this patient if she had each of the following comorbidities or characteristics:

   • Creatinine clearance <30 mL/min

   • Severe Alzheimer disease

3. For atrial fibrillation in this patient:

   • Based on the CHA_2DS_2-VASc, what is the patient's risk of stroke due to atrial fibrillation?

   • What tools may be used to assess the patient's risk of bleeding from anticoagulation?

   • What therapy should be offered to reduce the patient's risk of stroke? Provide a rationale for the decision. How should the different options be discussed with the patient and her daughter?

CLINICAL PEARLS

When managing drug therapy in older persons, make as few changes to the regimen at one time as possible due to the unpredictability of outcomes in older adults with multiple chronic conditions.

For older people with multiple chronic conditions taking many medications, first consider what medications could be reduced, tapered, or stopped before recommending new therapies.

REFERENCES

1. Boyd C, Smith CD, Masoudi FA, et al. Decision making for older adults with multiple chronic conditions: executive summary for the American Geriatrics Society Guiding Principles on the Care of Older Adults with Multimorbidity. J Am Geriatr Soc. 2019;67(4):665–673.

2. Ashburner JM, Go AS, Chang Y, et al. Influence of competing risks on estimating the expected benefit of warfarin in individuals with atrial fibrillation not currently taking anticoagulants: the Anticoagulation and Risk Factors in Atrial Fibrillation Study. J Am Geriatr Soc. 2017;65(1):35–41.

3. Camacho PM, Petak SM, Binkley N, et al. American Association of Clinical Endocrinologists/American College of Endocrinology clinical practice guidelines for the diagnosis and treatment of postmenopausal osteoporosis—2020 update. Endocr Pract 2020;26(Suppl 1):1–46. Available at: *https://pro.aace.com/disease-state-resources/bone-and-parathyroid/clinical-practice-guidelines/clinical-practice*. Accessed September 9, 2021.

4. Fazio S, Pace D, Maslow K, Zimmerman S, Kallmyer B. Alzheimer's Association Dementia Care Practice Recommendations. Gerontologist 2018;58(Suppl 1):S1–S9. Available at: *https://www.alz.org/professionals/professional-providers/dementia_care_practice_recommendations*. Accessed September 9, 2021.

5. The 2019 American Geriatrics Society Beers Criteria® Update Expert Panel. American Geriatrics Society 2019 Updated AGS Beers Criteria® for Potentially Inappropriate Medication Use in Older Adults. J Am Geriatr Soc. 2019;67(4):674–694.

6. Make STEADI part of your medical practice. STEADI (Stopping Elderly Accidents, Deaths & Injuries)—Older Adult Fall Prevention; CDC Injury Center. Available at: *https://www.cdc.gov/steadi/index.html*. Accessed September 9, 2021.

7. Health in Aging Tip Sheet: Aducanumab: What You Should Know. Available at: *https://www.healthinaging.org/tools-and-tips/tip-sheet-aducanumab-what-you-should-know*. Accessed November 16, 2021.

8. Lip GYH, Banerjee A, Boriani G, et al. Antithrombotic therapy for atrial fibrillation: CHEST Guideline and Expert Panel Report. Chest 2018;154(5):1121–1201.

9. Ginkgo Biloba–Warfarin. Lexicomp Online. Waltham, MA: UpToDate, Inc.; July 30, 2021. Available at: *https://online.lexi.com*. Accessed September 9, 2021.

10. Centers for Disease Control and Prevention. Table 1. Recommended Adult Immunization Schedule for ages 19 years or older, United States, 2021. Available at: *https://www.cdc.gov/vaccines/schedules/hcp/imz/adult.html*. Accessed September 9, 2021.

11. Tariq SH, Tumosa N, Chibnall JT, Perry III HM, Morley JE. Comparison of the Saint Louis University mental status examination and the mini-mental state examination for detecting dementia and mild neurocognitive disorder—a pilot study. Am J Geriatr Psych. 2006;14(11):900–910. *Available at*: https://www.slu.edu/medicine/internal-medicine/geriatric-medicine/aging-successfully/pdfs/slums_form.pdf. Accessed November 21, 2021.

8

PALLIATIVE CARE

Helpful Hospice .... Level III

Jennifer L. Swank, PharmD, BCOP

LEARNING OBJECTIVES

After completing this case study, the reader should be able to:

• Define the goals for pain management in a patient with chronic malignant pain with hospice services.

• Prepare a pharmacotherapeutic pain management plan.

• Differentiate between palliative care and hospice care.

• Recommend medication options for managing nausea in a hospice setting.

• Discuss the roles of continued nutritional support and antibiotic therapy in a hospice setting.

PATIENT PRESENTATION

■ Chief Complaint

"I have been having fevers up to 102°F and chills for 2 days. I have also noticed that my skin is orange."

■ HPI

This is a 48-year-old woman with a history of metastatic gastric adenocarcinoma diagnosed 3 years ago. Her treatment course consisted of: (1) subtotal gastrectomy and adjuvant chemoradiation with 5-FU, (2) disease progression treated with 5-FU and cisplatin,

(3) disease progression again with small bowel obstruction requiring multiple surgeries, and (4) now has a chronic gastric outlet obstruction. The patient now requires chronic parenteral nutrition and also has a percutaneous biliary drain placement for biliary obstruction due to tumor. She was recently enrolled in supportive hospice services but continues on TPN for treatment of chronic small bowel obstruction.

The patient presents to her primary oncologist office with a 2-day history of fevers and chills, abdominal pain, and recurrent jaundice. She is directly admitted from the oncologist clinics to the hospital. She had been using Tylenol suppositories for the fevers at home without relief. Her abdominal pain has worsened over the past 2 days, and she currently rates the pain as 8 out of 10. This pain is not relieved by the use of as-needed oxycodone liquid.

■ PMH

Cholangitis
Gastric outlet obstruction and small bowel obstruction
Subtotal gastrectomy 5 years ago
Sigmoid colectomy 2 years ago

■ FH

Mother—Living, with cervical cancer
Maternal aunt—Deceased from laryngeal cancer
Maternal uncle—Deceased from liver cancer

■ SH

Patient is married and has two children. She is on medical leave from her position as a grade school teacher. Denies use of alcohol or tobacco.

■ Meds

Total parental nutrition
Fentanyl 200-mcg patch, change every 72 hours
Oxycodone concentrated liquid 20 mg/mL, 1 mL PO every 3 hours PRN pain
Ondansetron 8 mg ODT, one tablet PO every 8 hours PRN nausea or vomiting
Acetaminophen suppository 650 mg, one rectally every 6 hours PRN fever

■ All

NKDA

■ ROS

Ten organ systems were reviewed. The patient reports fever, chills, nausea, vomiting, headache, and abdominal pain rated 8 out of 10. She denies chest pain, sore throat, cough, increased urinary frequency, rash, hematuria, hemoptysis, hematemesis, or black stool.

■ Physical Examination

Gen

The patient is a 48-year-old woman in acute distress holding her abdomen.

VS

BP 77/50, P 90, RR 16, T 100.9°F (38.3°C); Wt 101 lb (45.8 kg), Ht 5'2" (157.5 cm); pain
8/10 sharp, and stabbing in nature

Skin

Warm; dry; jaundice is appreciated.

HEENT

PERRLA; EOMI; sclerae jaundiced, TMs intact; moist mucous membranes

Neck

No JVD; full range of motion; no masses

Resp

CTA; no crackles, rhonchi, or wheezes

CV

Normal S_1, S_2; RRR; no murmurs

Abd

Soft and distended; (+) BS; moderate RUQ pain with deep palpation and mild guarding; biliary drain is in place and noted to be draining appropriately but with a foul-smelling, greenish liquid.

MS/Ext

Negative lower extremity edema; palpable pedal and radial pulsations

Neuro

CN II–XII intact, A&O × 3; no sensory or focal deficits apparent

■ Labs

Na 147 mEq/L	WBC 27.71 × 10³/mm³	T. prot 8 g/dL
K 4.5 mEq/L	Neutros 65%	Alb 2.4 g/dL
Cl 115 mEq/L	Bands 12%	T. bili 13.5 mg/dL
CO₂ 19 mEq/L	Lymphs 22%	D. bili 11.2 mg/dL
BUN 50 mg/dL	Eos 0%	AST 402 IU/L
SCr 1.7 mg/dL	Monos 1%	ALT 400 IU/L
Glu 101 mg/dL	Hgb 10 g/dL	Alk phos 321 IU/L
Ca 8.8 mg/dL	Hct 31.1%	Cortisol 39.8 mcg/dL
Phos 3.9 mg/dL	Plt 158 × 10³/mm³	Lactic acid 0.7 mmol/L
Mg 3.0 mg/dL		

■ Chest X-Ray

Mild increased interstitial lung markings; bilateral nonspecific changes that can be seen with pulmonary edema; no consolidation to suggest pneumonia.

■ RUQ Ultrasound

Sonographically abnormal appearance of the gallbladder, which is ill defined on this examination; no intrahepatic or extrahepatic biliary ductal dilatation; however, cholangitis cannot be excluded based on these findings.

■ Blood Cultures × 2 Sets

Pending

■ Urine Culture

Pending

■ Biliary Drainage Culture

Pending

■ Assessment

1. Acute-on-chronic abdominal pain due to peritoneal metastases from gastric cancer
2. Hypotension and probable cholangitis due to biliary obstruction
3. Chronic bowel obstruction requiring TPN for nutrition
4. Nausea due to pain medications and chronic small bowel obstruction

QUESTIONS

Collect Information

1.a. What subjective and objective information indicates the presence of an acute-on-chronic pain syndrome?

1.b. What subjective and objective data support the diagnosis of cholangitis in this patient?

1.c. What additional information is needed to fully assess this patient's pain?

Assess the Information

2.a. Assess the severity of the patient's pain using an appropriate patient assessment tool.

2.b. Create a list of the patient's drug therapy problems and prioritize them. Include assessment of medication appropriateness, effectiveness, safety, and patient adherence.

2.c. How does the role of hospice services affect the treatment plan for this patient's care?

Develop a Care Plan

3.a. What are the goals of pharmacotherapy for each of the patient's problems?

3.b. What nondrug therapies might be useful for supportive care for this patient?

3.c. Compare the pharmacotherapeutic alternatives available for treating this patient's pain.

3.d. Create an individualized, patient-centered, team-based care plan to treat this patient's pain. Include specific drugs, dosage forms, doses, schedules, and durations of therapy.

3.e. What alternatives would be appropriate if the initial therapy fails or cannot be used?

3.f. Compare the pharmacotherapeutic alternatives available for treatment of this patient's nausea and vomiting.

3.g. Create an individualized, patient-centered, team-based care plan to treat the patient's nausea.

Implement the Care Plan

4.a. What information should be provided to the patient to enhance adherence, ensure successful therapy, and minimize adverse effects?

4.b. Describe how care should be coordinated with other healthcare providers.

Follow-Up: Monitor and Evaluate

5. Explain how to monitor and evaluate the care plan for medication appropriateness, effectiveness, safety and patient adherence by using clinical and laboratory data, patient feedback, and other information.

■ CLINICAL COURSE

The patient was given IV fluids and started on empiric antibiotic therapy with meropenem 1 g IV Q 12 H, vancomycin 750 mg IV daily, and fluconazole 100 mg IV daily with improvement in blood pressure and serum creatinine. The blood and urine cultures were negative, but the biliary drainage cultures were positive for *Enterococcus faecalis* sensitive to vancomycin and *Pseudomonas stutzeri* sensitive to cefepime, ciprofloxacin, piperacillin/tazobactam, and tigecycline. The empiric antibiotic therapy was continued due to appropriate sensitivities to the antibiotics.

Interventional radiology was consulted to evaluate the biliary drain for possible obstruction due to poor output. The drain was exchanged with only mild improvement in total bilirubin to 8–10 mg/dL.

A fentanyl PCA pump was started at a basal rate of 35 mcg/hr with on-demand dosing of 10 mcg every 8 minutes with an hourly lockout of 100 mcg/hr, which resulted in adequate pain control rated 2 out of 10.

The patient's overall prognosis is poor due to chronic jaundice from biliary obstruction, worsening renal function, and infection. She has metastatic gastric adenocarcinoma of the colon and small bowel and is not a candidate for further chemotherapy or surgery. The patient and her husband discussed her overall prognosis and made the choice to transition to full hospice services. The patient chose to continue the 14-day course of IV antibiotic therapy. She was discharged home with home health services on IV meropenem 1 g IV Q 12 H, vancomycin 750 mg IV daily, and fluconazole 100 mg IV daily × 14 days, fentanyl PCA basal rate 35 mcg/hr on demand 10 mcg Q 8 minutes, and TPN. After the patient completes the IV antibiotics, she will choose to stop the TPN and continue with comfort measures only and enroll in full hospice services.

■ FOLLOW-UP QUESTIONS

1. Based on this new information of the patient discontinuing TPN and being discharged to hospice, are there any other supportive medications that may benefit the patient?

2. If the patient reports her pain to be 7 out of 10 at the time of discharge, how would you alter your treatment plan?

■ SELF-STUDY ASSIGNMENTS

1. Prepare a list of opioids and their corresponding equianalgesic dosing.

2. Prepare a set of guidelines for managing chronic malignant cancer pain reflecting the recommendations in the NCCN guidelines.

3. Prepare a list of antiemetics and dosing regimens useful in palliative care.

CLINICAL PEARL

Hospice is a specific type of palliative care team dedicated to managing patients with advanced illness who have a life expectancy of less than 6 months. Hospice has various levels of service and covers different therapies/services depending on the area in which the patient lives. Some hospice services will allow palliative therapy (ie, chemotherapy), IV antibiotics, and IV nutrition, whereas other hospice agencies require the patient to stop all such therapies prior to enrolling in their services.

REFERENCES

1. Adult Cancer Pain. NCCN Clinical Practice Guidelines in Oncology. Available at: *https://www.nccn.org/professionals/physician_gls/pdf/pain.pdf*. Accessed November 1, 2021.

2. Williamson A, Hoggart B. Pain: a review of three commonly used pain rating scales. J Clin Nurs. 2005;14:798–804.

3. Cassileth B. Psychiatric benefits of integrative therapies in patients with cancer. Int Rev Psychiatry. 2014;26:114–127.

4. World Health Organization. WHO definition of palliative care. Available at: *http://www.who.int/cancer/palliative/definition/en/*. Accessed November 1, 2018.

5. Hui D, Mori M, Parsons HA, et al. The lack of standard definitions in supportive and palliative oncology literature. J Pain Symptom Manage. 2012,43:582–592.

6. McCarberg BH, Barkin RL. Long-acting opioids for chronic pain: pharmacotherapeutic opportunities to enhance compliance, quality of life, and analgesia. Am J Ther. 2001;8:181–186.

7. Trescot AM, Datta S, Lee M, Hansen H. Opioid pharmacology. Pain Physician. 2008;11(2 Suppl):S133–S153.

8. Kress H, Von der Laage D, Hoerauf K, et al. A randomized, open, parallel group, multicenter trial to investigate analgesic efficacy and safety of a new transdermal fentanyl patch compared to standard opioid treatment in cancer pain. J Pain Symptom Manage. 2008;36:268–279.

9. Palliative Care NCCN Clinical Practice Guideline in Oncology. Available at: *https://www.nccn.org/professionals/physician_gls/pdf/palliative.pdf*. Accessed November 12, 2021.

9

CLINICAL TOXICOLOGY: ACETAMINOPHEN TOXICITY

If One Is Good, More Is Better.................... Level II

Elizabeth J. Scharman, PharmD, DABAT, BCPS, FAACT

LEARNING OBJECTIVES

After completing this case study, the reader should be able to:

- Determine when a potentially toxic acetaminophen exposure exists.

- Monitor a patient for signs and symptoms associated with acetaminophen toxicity.

- Recommend appropriate antidotal therapy for acetaminophen poisoning, and monitor its use for effectiveness and adverse effects.

- Describe the appropriate management of adverse drug reactions related to *N*-acetylcysteine.

PATIENT PRESENTATION

■ Chief Complaint

The patient is uncooperative and states that he just wants to be left alone.

■ HPI

The poison center receives a telephone call at 1:40 AM from a physician in a local ED regarding a 54-year-old man who was brought to the ED via ambulance accompanied by police because he had been belligerent and was refusing referral. According to his wife, he took a handful of pills following a heated argument she had with him earlier that evening. She estimates the time of the fight was about 6:00 PM. She left the house and came back 2 hours later. When she returned, she found him lying on the bed and saw two empty bottles in the bathroom wastepaper basket that were not there before. The wife thinks he was trying to kill himself. He states that he took a few extra pills because he had a backache and did not think one or two pills would work. The ambulance crew brings in the two empty bottles of medicine. The wife cannot remember how many pills, if any, were remaining in the bottles prior to today. According to the wife, all other medications in the house are accounted for. One of the bottles originally contained sixty 500-mg acetaminophen tablets, and the other bottle originally contained thirty 300-mg acetaminophen/ 5-mg hydrocodone tablets. The physician reports that the patient vomited twice in the ambulance and an additional four times since his arrival in the ED. He has not received any antiemetics.

■ PMH

Patient states that he is healthy. He has not seen a physician "in years" according to his wife.

■ FH

Father died of a heart attack when the patient was 12 years old. Mother is living. He has no sisters. He has one younger brother with "a bad heart."

■ SH

Smokes two packs of cigarettes a day. Drinks "about as much as anybody else" according to his wife.

■ Meds

No prescription medications.
Often takes nonprescription diphenhydramine because of insomnia.

All

None

■ Physical Examination

Gen

The patient appears drowsy. There are no external signs of trauma. The patient has vomited a total of six times. The vomitus has not been bloody. His estimated height is 5'10".

VS

BP 142/98, HR 72, RR 14, O_2 sat 98% on room air, T 37°C; Wt 98 kg

Skin

Mucous membranes are moist.

HEENT

Pupil size is normal; pupils are equal and reactive to light; retinal exam is unremarkable.

Lungs/Thorax

Occasional cough is noted.

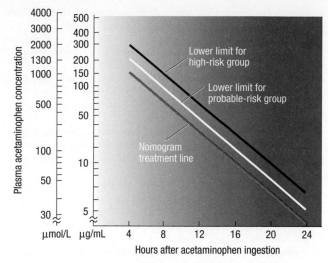

FIGURE 9-1. Nomogram for assessing hepatotoxic risk following acute ingestion of acetaminophen. (Reproduced with permission from DiPiro JT, Talbert RL, Yee GC, et al, eds. *Pharmacotherapy: A Pathophysiologic Approach.* 9th ed. New York, NY: McGraw-Hill; 2014.)

CV

No murmurs or gallops heard.

Abd

Bowel sounds are present. No guarding or tenderness.

Neuro

The patient is noticeably drowsy and uncooperative but is oriented to time and place; no tremors noted. The patient states that his headache has resolved.

■ Labs (Drawn at 01:00)

Na 142 mEq/L	Glucose 225 mg/dL	T. bili 0.8 mg/dL
K 3.1 mEq/L	Urine (+) PCP	INR 1.2
Cl 96 mEq/L	Hgb 15.7 g/dL	Salicylates (−)
CO₂ 23 mEq/L	Hct 48.2%	Acetaminophen 124 mcg/mL
BUN 24 mg/dL	AST 38 IU/L	Ethanol (EtOH) 138 mg/dL
SCr 1.1 mg/dL	ALT 42 IU/L	

■ ECG

Normal sinus rhythm

■ Assessment

The physician asks the poison center if acetaminophen toxicity is present (Fig. 9-1).

QUESTIONS

Collect Information

1.a. Is determining the amount of acetaminophen the patient ingested an important factor in determining whether acetaminophen toxicity is present? Why or why not?

1.b. What subjective and objective information indicates that acetaminophen toxicity is present?

1.c. What additional information is needed to fully assess this patient's acute overdose?

Assess the Information

2.a. What are the possible causes of vomiting in this patient?

2.b. Does toxicity from any other drug(s)/toxin(s) need to be considered in this patient? If so, which one(s) and why?

2.c. Create a list of the patient's drug therapy problems and prioritize them. Include assessment of medication appropriateness, effectiveness, safety, and patient adherence. For the secondary problems, describe the rationale behind whether they need to be managed immediately or whether they can be addressed prior to discharge.

Develop a Care Plan

3.a. What are the goals for managing acetaminophen toxicity in this case?

3.b. What feasible pharmacotherapeutic options are available for treating acetaminophen toxicity in this patient?

3.c. Create an individualized, patient-centered, team-based care plan to treat acetaminophen toxicity for this patient. Include specific drugs, dosage forms, doses, schedules, and durations of therapy.

3.d. If the physician asks the pharmacy to make an IV containing the exact dose of IV *N*-acetylcysteine for this patient, instead of rounding to the nearest dose designated in the prescribing information dosing table, how many milliliters of *N*-acetylcysteine should this patient receive? Show all calculations, including how the total dose needed was obtained and how the amount of *N*-acetylcysteine in each milliliter was calculated.

3.e. Will administration of *N*-acetylcysteine have any influence on the pharmacologic management of the patient's other problems as identified in his problem list? Why or why not?

3.f. If this patient had been a female who was human chorionic gonadotropin (β-hCG) (+), would recommendations for *N*-acetylcysteine therapy change? Why or why not?

Implement the Care Plan

4.a. What should the patient be told about the effectiveness of *N*-acetylcysteine therapy?

4.b. Describe how care should be coordinated with other healthcare providers.

Follow-Up: Monitor and Evaluate

5. Explain how to monitor and evaluate the care plan for medication appropriateness, effectiveness, safety and patient adherence by using clinical and laboratory data, patient feedback, and other information.

■ CLINICAL COURSE

At 02:20 the same day, the poison center gets a call from the patient's treating physician. He states that the patient developed flushing and urticaria at the end of the loading dose; some faint wheezes were heard, and the baseline cough is unchanged. The physician thinks the patient may be having an anaphylactic reaction and has stopped the IV *N*-acetylcysteine. He wants poison center recommendations for an alternative antidote. The poison specialist determines that the correct mg/kg dosage was administered, although the loading dose was administered over 15 minutes. Vital signs are BP 138/99, HR 68, RR 14, and nonlabored. Blood chemistries are scheduled to be repeated at 08:00. Administration of ondansetron has controlled the vomiting.

■ FOLLOW-UP QUESTIONS

1. Do you agree that this is an anaphylactic reaction? If not, what type of reaction is this and how is it different from an anaphylactic reaction?

2. What are the appropriate management options for this reaction and for continued management of acetaminophen toxicity in this patient?

3. The prescribing information for IV *N*-acetylcysteine lists one contraindication. Do you agree with this contraindication? Why or why not?

4. If this patient is discharged from the hospital on medications to treat other medical problems, how will his history of an overdose affect the healthcare provider's decision on which medication(s) to select?

■ SELF-STUDY ASSIGNMENTS

1. Defend the argument that all patients with an intentional drug overdose, no matter what their stated history, should have an acetaminophen level drawn to rule out acetaminophen toxicity.

2. If this patient had been 104 kg instead of 98 kg, the dose given would have been the same as that of a person weighing 100 kg. Why do patients weighing over 100 kg not receive an IV *N*-acetylcysteine dose calculated on an mg/kg basis, and what is the rationale for this maximum dose being clinically effective?

3. For a patient whose initial acetaminophen level is substantially elevated (defined as >300 mcg/mL) at the 4 hour post-ingestion mark, should any alternatives to standard dose IV *N*-acetylcysteine, or alternative treatment options, be considered?

CLINICAL PEARL

It is difficult to determine the best evidence-based practice for managing overdoses. It is unethical to withhold treatment or an antidote from a control group who has been poisoned. Therefore, there will never be a randomized control trial to determine an antidote's ideal dose or administration regimen. Use of historical cohort data from poisoning cases prior to antidote availability is the best available data; however, as with all retrospective studies, missing data are a limitation. For this reason, it is difficult to determine whether simplifying the FDA-approved three-bag IV *N*-acetylcysteine dosing regimen to a one- or two-bag total dose regimen has equal efficacy. Published case series using simplified regimens have only included acute acetaminophen exposures with early presentations in patients with unconfirmed exposure histories. Because the number of patients expected to progress to fulminant hepatotoxicity is so small (approximately 0.1–0.2%) if treatment is given within 10 and 16 hours, all published case series using simplified regimen have been underpowered to determine equal efficacy. Thousands of patients would be required to make a statistically valid conclusion. The use of more sensitive biomarkers of APAP hepatotoxicity (eg, microRNA rather than AST or ALT) may enable practitioners to better determine hepatotoxicity risk in the future and increase the ability to statistically compare dosing regimens.

REFERENCES

1. Dart RC, Erdman AR, Olson KR, et al. Acetaminophen poisoning: an evidence-based consensus guideline for out-of-hospital management. Clin Toxicol. (Phila) 2006;44:1–18.

2. Rumack BH, Bateman NS. Acetaminophen and acetylcysteine dose and duration: past, present and future. Clin Toxicol. 2012;50:91–98.

3. Lewis JC, Lim M, Mendoza E, Albertson TE, Chenoweth JA. Evaluation of N-acetylcysteine dose for the treatment of massive acetaminophen ingestion. Clin Toxicol. (Phila) 2021;59:932–936.

4. Dribben WH, Porto SM, Jeffords BK. Stability and microbiology of inhalant *N*-acetylcysteine used as an intravenous solution for the treatment of acetaminophen poisoning. Ann Emerg Med. 2003;42:9–13.

5. Gosselin S, Juurlink DN, Kielstein JT, Ghannoum M, Lavergne V, Nolin TD, Hoffman RS. Extracorporeal treatment for acetaminophen poisoning: recommendations from the EXTRIP workgroup. Clin Toxicol. (Phila) 2014;52:856–867.

6. Mullins ME, Yeager LH, Freeman WE. Metabolic and mitochondrial treatments for severe paracetamol poisoning: a systematic review. Clin Toxicol. (Phila) 2020;58:1284–1296.

7. Acetadote Package Insert. Nashville, TN, Cumberland Pharmaceuticals Inc., December 2016.

8. Waring WS. Novel acetylcysteine regimens for treatment of paracetamol overdose. Ther Adv Drug Saf. 2012;3:305–315.

9. Curtis RM, Sivilotti ML. A descriptive analysis of aspartate and alanine aminotransferase rise and fall following acetaminophen overdose. Clin Toxicol. (Phila) 2015;53:849–855.

10. Bateman DN, Dear JW, Thomas SH. New regimens for intravenous acetylcysteine, where are we now? Clin Toxicol. (Phila) 2016;54(s):75–78.

10

CYANIDE EXPOSURE

Expect the Unexpected .... Level II

Elizabeth J. Scharman, PharmD, DABAT, BCPS, FAACT

LEARNING OBJECTIVES

After completing this case study, the reader should be able to:

- Identify which signs, symptoms, and laboratory data indicate a possible cyanide exposure.
- Compare and contrast the two different antidotes for cyanide exposure.
- Recommend specific dosing regimens for antidotes and supportive care for children and adults.
- State monitoring parameters and management of antidote adverse effects.
- Explain the factors involved in determining the amount of cyanide antidote a hospital should stock for immediate availability.

PRESENTATION OF PATIENTS

A 60-year-old laboratory worker with a history of major depressive disorder has stayed after normal laboratory hours on the pretense of completing a project. Once his coworkers have left, he ingests a bottle containing a toxic chemical. His biochemistry laboratory is on the fifth (top) floor of a university building containing eight other offices occupying the four floors below, all of which are faculty and staff offices for the biochemistry department. He loses consciousness. Meanwhile, the heating unit in the basement of the office building catches fire that quickly spreads through the first three floors of the building. At least 10 other individuals were in the other building's offices working late. They were not able to evacuate before being overcome by smoke.

■ HPI

Firefighters and emergency medical services (EMS) personnel are at the scene. Ambulances are bringing the 11 victims from the fire to your hospital's ED; some are comatose, and others present with a variety of signs/symptoms including confusion, coughing, wheezing, and minor burns. One of the victims brought in is a man who appears to be in his sixties. He has profound cyanosis and seizure activity. Unlike the other victims, he has no soot on his clothing. The ambulance worker reports that he was found on a floor receiving very little smoke damage and no fire damage. This victim has been tagged Male Victim #1 (MV#1).

■ PMH, PSH, FH, and SH

Not available. The hospital was initially overwhelmed because the ED was nearly full before the arrival of these patients.

■ ROS

Patients are presenting with a variety of symptoms and illness severity. ED nurses and doctors are only able to do brief physical exams. Ages and weights are being estimated as needed. MV#1 is the most critically ill patient.

■ Physical Examination (Victims Excluding JD)

Gen

Four of the ten patients appear weak and are breathing rapidly. Two additional victims are unconscious and required intubation to support breathing. All six of these patients have soot in their nares and around their mouths. The remaining four patients have mild coughing, wheezing, and burning eyes; soot is not present in their nares or inside their mouths, and systemic signs and symptoms are absent. Facial burns are not evident on any of these 10 individuals.

VS

BP: The six sickest patients are hypotensive.
HR: The six sickest patients have rates between 110 and 120 bpm.
RR: The six sickest patients have rates between 22 and 26.
T: All have normal temperatures.
Pain: Patients not intubated are anxious but are not in obvious pain.
O_2 sat: Normal for all.

Skin

No notable contusions, abrasions; second- and third-degree burns are absent. Two of the ten have some mild blistering on their hands.

HEENT

Mydriasis observed in some patients.

Neck/Lymph Nodes

No lymphadenopathy

Lungs/Thorax

Rapid respiratory rate; patients complain of some chest tightness and dyspnea.

CV

Bradycardia for the six sickest patients, too noisy in ED to listen for heart sounds.

Abd

Bowel sounds present in all; the six sickest patients have nausea and some vomiting.

Genital/Rect

Deferred

MS/Ext

No abnormal movements noted.

Neuro

Two of the six sickest victims are ventilated. No convulsions are observed. The six sickest patients are confused. The remaining four fire victims are neurologically intact.

■ Pertinent Physical Findings for JD

Gen

Unresponsive; generalized convulsions are present. Oxygen saturation via pulse oximetry was 98%. An almond smell was noted by one of the medical care providers after the patient vomited; this odor was not detected by others on the healthcare team. JD has been intubated.

VS: HR 22 bpm, RR 6, BP 60/35 mm Hg, T 37.0°C.

■ Lab

Ranges for the Six Sickest Fire Victims: HCO_3^- 13–15 mEq/L from the metabolic panel; CBC within normal limits; lactate 14 mmol/L; carboxyhemoglobin 12–15%.
Reported for MV#1: HCO_3^- 8 mEq/L from the metabolic panel; CBC normal; lactate 22 mmol/L; carboxyhemoglobin 1%.
Four Remaining Fire Victims: Labs are within normal limits.

■ Other

Example initial blood gas for an intubated patient: pH 7.2, $PaCO_2$ 40 mm Hg, PaO_2 110 mm Hg, HCO_3^- 13 mEq/L.
Blood gas for JD: pH 7.1, $PaCO_2$ 40 mm Hg, PaO_2 240 mm Hg, HCO_3^- 9 mEq/L.
Blood gases were not obtained for the four fire victims without systemic symptoms.
Chest X-rays for MV#1 and the six sickest fire victims are pending.

■ Follow-Up

The ED clinical pharmacist contacts the Poison Center after overhearing one of the EMS workers mention that MV#1 was found in his laboratory next to an opened and empty chemical bottle. The poison center will check with the on-scene Incident Commander (IC) and follow up with the clinical pharmacist as quickly as possible. Based on the presenting toxidrome, the most likely chemical ingested by MV#1 is cyanide. There is agreement that products of combustion and toxic gases from smoke inhalation are causing toxicity in the six sickest patients.

QUESTIONS

Collect Information

1.a. MV#1 and the six sickest fire victims share a similar toxidrome pattern. How is this possible when only MV#1 ingested chemical from the bottle? Compare the signs and symptoms of severe cyanide poisoning with less severe intoxication.

1.b. List the laboratory tests that may be abnormal in patients exposed to cyanide. Explain the pathophysiology underlying these abnormalities.

Assess the Information

2. What are the potential short- and long-term sequelae from these cyanide exposures?

Develop a Care Plan

3.a. What are the goals of pharmacotherapy in these cases?

3.b. What nondrug measures are available to treat cyanide poisoning in these victims?

3.c. What feasible pharmacotherapeutic options are available for treating cyanide poisoning (Fig. 10-1)? Include dose(s), route(s), and repeat dosing information (if any) for both adult and pediatric patients. Also describe use of administration devices or ancillary supplies.

3.d. Create an individualized, patient-centered, team-based care plan to treat cyanide poisoning in these patients. Include

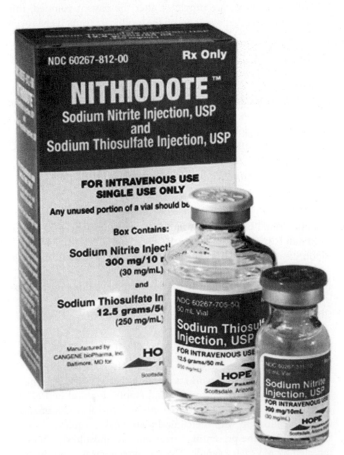

FIGURE 10-1. Nithiodote® (sodium nitrite injection and sodium thiosulfate injection for intravenous infusion). (Photo courtesy of Hope Pharmaceuticals.)

specific drugs, dosage forms, doses, schedules, and durations of therapy.

3.e. What supportive care measures may be necessary for optimal management in these patients?

Implement the Care Plan

4.a. For patients who are alert and oriented, what information would you share with them about the possible immediate adverse effects of each of the antidotes?

4.b. Describe how care should be coordinated with other healthcare providers.

4.c. How long might it take for the patients to recover from potential long-term effects of acute cyanide exposure?

Follow-Up: Monitor and Evaluate

5. Explain how to monitor and evaluate the care plan for medication appropriateness, effectiveness, and safety by using clinical and laboratory data.

■ CLINICAL COURSE

The bottle from the laboratory is confirmed to have contained cyanide. MV#1 went into cardiac arrest shortly after being intubated. He was given the cyanide antidote during the resuscitation efforts. Catastrophic hypoxic brain injury became evident, and his family requested that life-support be withdrawn. Five of the six sickest patients survived; the sixth victim died of complications from cardiac arrest and acute respiratory distress syndrome. The four ambulatory patients were discharged to home from the ED. Legal charges were brought against the building's landlord because of the faulty heating unit and the fact that over one-quarter of the emergency exits were blocked.

■ FOLLOW-UP QUESTIONS

1. For how many patients should a hospital stock the cyanide antidotes? Consider the cost of the antidotes in your answer.

2. Suppose there are 100 patients in your hospital's ED requiring a cyanide antidote and you only have enough antidote to treat 4 patients. Who may be involved in making these ethical treatment decisions, and how would these decisions be made?

■ SELF-STUDY ASSIGNMENTS

1. Cyanide is usually obtained for suicidal exposures by persons who have access to it in a workplace setting. Other exposures to pure cyanide are the result of unintentional, occupational exposures in industrial settings. The public might be exposed after a cyanide transportation accident that spills cyanide into sources of drinking water, leads to direct physical contact with the spilled cyanide, or results in the inhalation of cyanide fumes emanating from the spill. There is also the possibility that terrorists might obtain cyanide from manufacturing locations or transportation vehicles (chemical trucks, train cars). Describe which specific occupational settings utilize cyanide on a regular basis.

2. Describe why amyl nitrite is not required for the management of cyanide toxicity.

3. Describe how the toxicokinetics and toxicodynamics differ between ingestion and inhalational exposure to cyanide.

CLINICAL PEARL

Cyanide has an odor that has been described as that of "bitter almonds." Unfortunately, only a small percentage of patients with cyanide poisoning present with this finding, and it is estimated that only 10% of the population is genetically able to detect cyanide's smell. Another classically reported finding is "cherry red skin" from increased venous oxygen saturation; however, this finding also occurs in only a small percentage of cyanide poisonings and is not a reliable indicator of cyanide toxicity.

REFERENCES

1. Thompson JP, Marrs TC. Hydroxocobalamin in cyanide poisoning. Clin Toxicol. (Phila) 2012;50:875–885.
2. Hendry-Hofer TB, Ng PC, Witeof AE, et al. A review on ingested cyanide: risks, clinical presentation, diagnostics, and treatment challenges. J Med Toxicol. 2019;15(2):128–133.
3. Centers for Disease Control (CDC) Emergency Preparedness and Response [Internet]. Atlanta, GA. Facts about cyanide. Available at: *https://emergency.cdc.gov/agent/cyanide/basics/facts.asp*. Accessed November 4, 2021.
4. Baud FJ. Cyanide: critical issues in diagnosis and treatment. Hum Exp Toxicol. 2007;26():191–201.
5. Borron SW, Baud FJ. Antidotes for acute cyanide poisoning. Curr Pharm Biotechnol. 2012;13:1940–1948.
6. Baud FJ, Borron SW, Mégarbane B, et al. Value of lactic acidosis in the assessment of the severity of acute cyanide poisoning. Crit Care Med. 2002;30:2044–2050.
7. Parker-Cote JL, Rizer J, Vakkalanka JP, Rege SV, Holstege CP. Challenges in the diagnosis of acute cyanide poisoning. Clin Toxicol. 2018;56:609–617.
8. Dalkiran T, Kandur Y, Ozaslan M, Acipayam C, Olgar S. Role of hemodialysis in the management of cyanide intoxication from apricot kernels in a 3-year-old child. Pediatr Emerg Care. 2020;36(10):e582–e584.
9. Nithiodote Package Insert. Scottsdale, AZ: Hope Pharmaceuticals, November 2017.
10. Cyanokit Package Insert. Columbia, MD: Meridian Medical Technologies™, Inc., December 2018.

11

CHEMICAL THREAT AGENT EXPOSURE

Name That Poison . . . . Level II

Elizabeth J. Scharman, PharmD, BCPS, DABAT, FAACT

LEARNING OBJECTIVES

After completing this case study, the reader should be able to:

- Identify one of the toxidromes associated with a chemical threat agent attack.

- Determine the indications for antidotes and supportive care options based on patient signs and symptoms.

- State the difference between the utilization of a medical model and a mass care model during a public health emergency.

- Identify antidote and drug treatment stockpile sources and when state or national stockpile options may be utilized.

PATIENT PRESENTATION

■ Patient Scenario

Via the disaster response radio in the emergency department (ED), hospital staff learn that attendees at an outdoor concert have suddenly become ill. A series of four loud popping sounds had been heard immediately prior. EMS personnel are on scene donning personal protective equipment (PPE) and setting up decontamination stations. Some concert attendees have been fleeing the scene despite orders from law enforcement to stay on site for decontamination. At least four backpacks have been observed in the area via binoculars but have not yet been examined. They are suspicious because backpacks were not allowed at the concert venue and attendees were checked for large bags prior to entry. Due to the large number of attendees, it is suspected that security measures were imperfect.

■ HPI

The on-scene incident commander ensures that the communication chief notifies all local EDs (total of four) to stand up their emergency operation centers (EOC). The concert venue held 1000, and seats had been sold out. Hospital 1 is the largest of the four and is also a Level I trauma center. Within 20 minutes of the notification, patients begin arriving at that hospital's outdoor staging and decontamination areas via car, by foot, and via ambulance. Hospital security personnel have donned full PPE and are working to ensure that those not arriving via ambulance (and therefore lacking prior decontamination) do not enter the ED until they have been through the hospital's decontamination stations, which are in the final stages of being set up. Security personnel are also directing friends and family members of the victims to a waiting area across the street so those needing care are not lost in the crowd.

An emergency triage center is established just outside ED entrance of Hospital 1. It is staffed by a lead physician, three nurses, two nursing aides, two medical residents, and the ED clinical pharmacist. Dozens of victims are in the staging area awaiting decontamination, and they appear to be in various states of illness and anxiety levels. Victims arriving in the triage area via ambulance are unconscious.

In the triage area, the large number of victims and mass panic are creating chaos, making thorough individual assessment impossible. After ensuring that triage staff are properly gowned and double gloved, the ED lead physician at Hospital 1 instructs the nursing aides to obtain patient vital signs on those arriving via ambulance. Nurses are directed to establish an IV line in each comatose patient. The medical residents are assigned to triage patients into four groups based on need for immediate threats to life, focusing on prominent findings observed with a brief physical exam. The clinical pharmacist is instructed to call the poison center for information on what the chemical threat agent is likely to be based on the cluster of symptoms being observed and to obtain antidote information.

■ PMH, PSH, FH, AND SH

Not obtained

■ ROS

At Hospital 1, at least 300 victims are waiting for care. In the triage area, patients are tagged with color-coded bracelets into one of four groups:

- *Red*—Unconscious and having immediate life-threatening symptoms.
- *Yellow*—Severe but not immediately life-threatening symptoms; awake but not ambulatory and not conversing well.
- *Green*—Distressing or mild symptoms, but ambulatory and conversing well. Care required but can be delayed.
- *White*—Ambulatory without symptoms, any minor injuries are amenable to self-care.

Because no deaths occurred, no victims were coded *Black*.

■ Physical Examination

Triage has been completed for an estimated 75% of those waiting for care at Hospital 1. Physical findings observed in each patient category are as follows:

- *Red*—45 patients, and all are unconscious; 11 are having multiple convulsions; 43 are having large- and small-muscle fasciculations. Breathing is labored, and rhonchi are present throughout the lung fields in all 45 victims; respiratory paralysis appears to be imminent in 28 cyanotic patients. CPR is being performed on one patient by an anesthesiologist who was called in for assistance. In the other victims, HRs are less than 40 bpm. Profuse diaphoresis is present, and bowel sounds are hyperactive; vomitus and fecal staining are present on the clothing of some of the victims. Miosis is present in approximately half of the patients.
- *Yellow*—36 patients; these victims have a decreased level of consciousness and severe muscle weakness but respond somewhat to stimuli. All are unable to communicate except for brief responses and sometimes not at all. Facial fasciculations are present in six, but none have experienced a witnessed convulsion. Wheezing is heard on auscultation, and patients complain of shortness of breath. None appear cyanotic. HRs are not less than 40 bpm, but it has been too chaotic to record individual rates consistently. Vomiting, hyperactive bowel sounds, and fecal incontinence are common. Moderate diaphoresis is noted. Miosis is present in 10 patients; communication difficulties make it impossible to assess if visual changes are present.
- *Green*—86 patients; victims are ambulating and conversing. Wheezing and rhonchi are absent and only four complain of chest tightness. Nausea is present in all, but no one has had more than one or two episodes of vomiting. Ten victims have miosis and are complaining of blurry vision. Tearing, runny noses, and mild-moderate diaphoresis are noted. Vital signs were not obtained at this time because nurses are overwhelmed.
- *White*—75 patients; victims are ambulating and conversing, although many are visibly distraught. Fifty-two patients are asymptomatic but are extremely concerned and demand to receive an antidote because they are sure they are going to die. Twenty-five victims complain of nausea, headache, and dizziness. Diaphoresis, tearing, and runny noses are absent. No vomiting or fecal incontinence has occurred in this group.

■ Next Steps

The clinical pharmacist at Hospital 1 contacted the poison center to report patient numbers and the signs and symptoms being observed. The poison center relates that victims from all four hospitals are showing a similar toxidrome pattern. The poison center has been in communication with the on-scene incident commander to review additional information from the concert venue. The category of chemical threat agent most likely involved and antidote and treatment recommendations are reviewed with the clinical pharmacist, who then reports this information to the lead physician. The poison center faxes information to the hospital ED and pharmacy to ensure that the antidote and dosing information are readily available.

The lead physician prioritized the Red group for entry into the ED for immediate care. He assigned the Yellow group to be managed in a medical tent sent up near the ED entrance, approximately 50 yards away from the triage area. The Green group was assigned to be managed as healthcare professionals become free. Those in the White group are moved to a location 200 yards from the triage area with a portable curtain erected to put them out of the line of sight of the other victims. The lead physician called for the behavioral health disaster response team to provide supportive mental health services to the White group. A clinical pharmacist will be there to answer questions about the incident. A nurse will be with the White group to observe for the onset of any new symptoms.

The ED clinical pharmacist contacted the clinical pharmacist in charge of the pharmacy's disaster plan to report the number of victims requiring antidotal and supportive therapies. The initial supply of pharmaceuticals is transported to the ED. Another cart of pharmaceuticals is on its way to the area serving the Yellow group. The pharmaceutical cart for the Green group will be ready in the next 5 minutes. Disaster plan of Hospital 1 has been activated and will be used to obtain additional antidotes, supportive therapies, and supplies. The ED clinical pharmacist and the clinical pharmacist in the pharmacy department will communicate with each other to coordinate antidote needs and availability.

■ Laboratory Findings

Immediate resuscitative measures on the 45 victims are taking precedence at this time. A team of phlebotomists has been called to the ED to begin drawing blood samples. Hand-printed labels are used to mark the vials to save time. Physicians use clinical judgment to monitor patient status.

■ Radiology Findings

Diffuse pulmonary edema is observed on plain film chest X-rays obtained on the victim who was receiving CPR and has now been intubated.

QUESTIONS

Collect Information

1. What subjective and objective information about the event indicates exposure to a chemical agent?

Assess the Information

2.a. Which category of chemical threat agent is most likely to be involved? Describe how you made this decision.

2.b. To initiate antidotal therapies, is it important to know which specific chemical agent in this chemical agent category is involved? Why or why not?

Develop a Care Plan

3.a. What are the goals of pharmacotherapy for each group (Red, Yellow, Green, and White)?

3.b. How would your goals change if there were 5 victims instead of 300 victims presenting to your hospital with an exposure to a chemical threat agent?

3.c. What nondrug measures are required and available to manage these patients?

3.d. What feasible pharmacotherapeutic alternatives are available for treating these patients?

3.e. Provide adult and pediatric doses by route for each chemical threat agent antidote required in this case scenario.

3.f. If a patient's condition worsens and seizure activity occurs, what class of medications should be used for this chemical-induced seizure?

3.g. Which clinical and/or laboratory findings determine whether or not an individual will require the antidote(s)?

3.h. Suppose there are 100 patients in your hospital's ED meeting the criteria for the antidote(s), and you only have enough antidote(s) to treat 25 patients. How do you decide who receives the antidote?

Implement the Care Plan

4.a. What information would you share with the patients about immediate adverse effects of each of the antidotes?

4.b. Describe how care should be coordinated with other healthcare providers.

Follow-Up: Monitor and Evaluate

5.a. Outline a monitoring plan to assess whether the pharmacotherapy treatment for these patients is successful.

5.b. Develop a plan for follow-up that includes appropriate timeframes to assess progress toward achievement of the goals of therapy.

5.c. How long might it take for patients to recover from the ocular effects of the chemical exposure? Incorporate this information into your educational efforts.

■ CLINICAL COURSE

At Hospital 1, 21 patients die from the exposure and 24 remain in critical condition. Critically ill patients are transferred to the ICUs, and half of the telemetry floor beds have been temporarily converted into additional ICU beds.

■ FOLLOW-UP QUESTION

1. What is the initial and ongoing source of antidotes for use after a chemical terrorist event at hospital pharmacies in the United States?

■ SELF-STUDY ASSIGNMENTS

1. Research information on the Strategic National Stockpile Program and the CHEMPACK program. Evaluate the difference in response times and focus for both programs.

2. Research information on your county and state threat preparedness plan. Review the expectations of healthcare professionals according to the plans. Identify gaps in the plan that you may be able to assist in correcting by working with your local health department or state threat preparedness planning agency.

CLINICAL PEARL

Most chemical agents that could be used for a terrorist attack would likely be exploded or released as a gas or vapor in order to increase the extent of the exposure and allow for rapid systemic entry into victims. A general rule of thumb for chemical exposures is that the higher the concentration (or total dose), the faster the onset of symptoms; the lower the concentration (or total dose), the slower the onset of symptoms.

REFERENCES

1. Henretig FM, Kirk MA, McKay Jr CA. Hazardous chemical emergencies and poisonings. N Engl J Med. 2019;380:1638–1655.

2. Agency for Toxic Substances and Disease Registry; Medical Management Guidelines for Nerve Agents: Tabus (GA); Sarin (GB); Soman (GD); and VX [Internet]. Chamblee, GA November 4, 2021.

3. Leikin JB, Thomas RG, Walter FG, Klein R, Meislin HW. A review of nerve agent exposure for the critical care physician. Crit Care Med. 2002;30:2346–2354.

4. Broderick JE, Kaplan-Liss E, Bass E. Experimental induction of psychogenic illness in the context of a medical event and media exposure. Am J Disaster Med. 2011;6(3):163–172.

5. Hick LH, Rubinson, L, O'Laughlin DT, Farmer JC. Clinical review: allocating ventilators during large-scale disasters—problems, planning, and process. Crit Care. 2007;11(3):217.

6. Schwartz MD, Sutter ME, Eisnor D, Kirk MA. Contingency medical countermeasures for mass nerve-agent exposure: use of pharmaceutical alternatives to community stockpiled antidotes. Disaster Med Public Health Prep. 2019;13(3):605–612.

7. Atropen Auto-Injector [package insert]. Columbia, MD, Meridian Technologies Inc, November 2005. Available at: *https://www.meridianmeds.com/sites/default/files/atropen_uspi_2005.pdf*. Accessed November 4, 2021.

8. Pralidoxime Chloride Injection Auto-Injector [package insert]. Columbia, MD, Meridian Technologies Inc, October 2003. Available at: *https://www.meridianmeds.com/sites/default/files/pralidoxime_chloride_uspi_2016.pdf*. Accessed November 4, 2021.

9. DuoDote [package insert]. Columbia, MD, Meridian Technologies Inc, April 2010. Available at: *https://www.meridianmeds.com/sites/default/files/atnaa_uspi_2010.pdf*. Accessed November 4, 2021.

10. Diazepam Autoinjector [package insert]. Columbia, MD, Meridian Technologies Inc, July 2005. Available at: *https://www.meridianmeds.com/sites/default/files/pi/Diazepam_PI.pdf*. Accessed November 4, 2021.

12

HYPERTENSION

Lost Shaker of Salt .... Level II

Julia M. Koehler, PharmD, FCCP

Mark Lutz, MPAS, PA-C

LEARNING OBJECTIVES

After completing this case study, the reader should be able to:

- Classify blood pressure according to current hypertension (HTN) guidelines and discuss the correlation between blood pressure (BP) and risk for cardiovascular morbidity and mortality.

- Identify medications that may cause or worsen HTN.

- Discuss complications (eg, target organ damage) that may occur as a result of uncontrolled and/or long-standing HTN.

- Establish goals for the treatment of HTN and choose appropriate lifestyle modifications and antihypertensive regimens based on patient-specific characteristics, comorbid disease states, and current HTN guidelines.

- Provide appropriate patient counseling for antihypertensive drug regimens.

PATIENT PRESENTATION

■ Chief Complaint

"I'm here to see my new doctor for a checkup. I'm just getting over a cold. Overall, I'm feeling fine, except for occasional headaches. I know that my blood pressure runs high. My other doctor prescribed a low-salt diet for me, so I got rid of my salt shaker!"

■ HPI

A 64-year-old black man presents for establishment of care with a new provider and for evaluation and follow-up of his medical problems. He generally has no complaints, except for occasional mild headaches. He states that he is aware that his blood pressure is uncontrolled and has attempted to reduce his salt intake by not adding extra salt to his food.

■ PMH

HTN × 14 years
Type 2 diabetes mellitus (DM) × 16 years
BPH
CKD

■ FH

Father died of acute MI at age 73. Mother died of multiple myeloma at age 69. Father had HTN and dyslipidemia. Mother had HTN and DM.

■ SH

Has never smoked; reports moderate amount of alcohol intake (one to two drinks per day). He watches his intake of carbohydrates and has attempted to reduce his sodium intake. He does not exercise regularly. He works at Wal-Mart and has healthcare insurance through his employer. Lives alone.

■ Meds

Hydrochlorothiazide/triamterene 25 mg/37.5 mg PO Q AM
Insulin glargine 36 units subcutaneously daily
Insulin lispro 12 units subcutaneously TID with meals
Doxazosin 2 mg PO Q HS
Mucinex D® two tablets Q 12 H PRN cough/congestion
Naproxen 220 mg PO Q 8 H PRN HA

■ All

PCN—rash

■ ROS

Patient states that overall he is doing well and recovering from a cold with symptoms of nasal congestion, sore throat, and cough that have nearly resolved. He has noticed no major weight changes over the past few years. He complains of occasional headaches, which are usually relieved by naproxen, and he denies blurred vision and chest pain. He denies shortness of breath, although he admits to being "out of shape." He denies experiencing any hemoptysis or epistaxis; he also denies nausea, vomiting, abdominal pain, cramping, diarrhea, constipation, or blood in stool. He denies urinary frequency but states that he used to have more difficulty urinating until his physician started him on doxazosin a few months ago. He has no history of arthritic symptoms and denies joint or musculoskeletal pain.

■ Physical Examination

Gen

WDWN, black man; moderately overweight; in no acute distress

VS

BP 162/90 mm Hg (sitting; repeat 164/92 mm Hg), HR 76 bpm (regular), RR 16/min, T 37°C; Wt 95 kg, Ht 6′2″

HEENT

TMs clear; mild sinus drainage; AV nicking noted; no hemorrhages, exudates, or papilledema

Neck

Supple without masses or bruits, no thyroid enlargement or lymphadenopathy

Lungs

Lung fields CTA bilaterally. No wheezes or crackles.

Heart

RRR; normal S_1 and S_2. No S_3 or S_4.

Abd

Soft, NTND; no masses, bruits, or organomegaly. Normal BS.

Genit/Rect

Enlarged prostate

Ext

No CCE; no apparent joint swelling or signs of tophi

Neuro

No gross motor-sensory deficits present. A & O × 3.

■ Labs

Na 138 mEq/L	Ca 9.7 mg/dL	*Fasting lipid panel*
K 4.7 mEq/L	Mg 2.3 mEq/L	Total Chol 161 mg/dL
Cl 99 mEq/L	A1C 6.1%	LDL 79 mg/dL
CO_2 27 mEq/L	Alb 3.4 g/dL	HDL 53 mg/dL
BUN 22 mg/dL	Hgb 13 g/dL	TG 144 mg/dL
SCr 2.2 mg/dL	Hct 40%	
Glucose 110 mg/dL	WBC $9.0 \times 10^3/mm^3$	
	Plts $189 \times 10^3/mm^3$	

■ UA

Yellow, clear, SG 1.007, pH 5.5, (+) protein, (–) glucose, (–) ketones, (–) bilirubin, (–) blood, (–) nitrite, RBC 0/hpf, WBC 1–2/hpf, neg bacteria, one to five epithelial cells.

■ ECG

Abnormal ECG: normal sinus rhythm; left atrial enlargement; left axis deviation; LVH

■ ECHO (6 Months Ago)

Mild LVH, estimated EF 45%

■ Assessment

HTN, uncontrolled
CKD, evidence of proteinuria
Type 2 DM, controlled on current insulin regimen
BPH, symptoms improved on doxazosin

QUESTIONS

Collect Information

1.a. What subjective and objective information indicates the presence of HTN in this patient?

1.b. What evidence of target organ damage or clinical cardiovascular disease (CVD) does this patient have?

1.c. What is this patient's 10-year atherosclerotic cardiovascular disease (ASCVD) risk?

Assess the Information

2.a. How would you classify this patient's HTN, according to current HTN guidelines?

2.b. Create a list of the patient's drug therapy problems and prioritize them. Include assessment of medication appropriateness, effectiveness, safety, and patient adherence.

Develop a Care Plan

3.a. What are the goals of pharmacotherapy for hypertension in this case?

3.b. What nondrug therapies might be useful for this patient's hypertension?

3.c. What feasible pharmacotherapeutic options are available for treating this patient's HTN?

3.d. Create an individualized, patient-centered, team-based care plan to optimize medication therapy for this patient's HTN and other drug therapy problems. Include specific drugs, dosage forms, doses, schedules, and durations of therapy.

Implement the Care Plan

4.a. What information should be provided to the patient to enhance adherence, ensure successful therapy, and minimize adverse effects?

4.b. Describe how care should be coordinated with other healthcare providers.

Follow-Up: Monitor and Evaluate

5. Explain how to monitor and evaluate the care plan for medication appropriateness, effectiveness, safety and patient adherence by using clinical and laboratory data, patient feedback, and other information.

■ SELF-STUDY ASSIGNMENTS

1. Describe the major causes of secondary HTN and the methods by which those could be ruled out in this patient.

2. Outline the changes, if any, that you would make to the pharmacotherapeutic regimen for this patient if he had a history of each of the following comorbidities or characteristics:
   - Severe chronic obstructive lung disease
   - Major depression
   - Ischemic heart disease with a history of MI
   - Cerebrovascular accident
   - Peripheral arterial disease
   - Gout
   - Migraine headache disorder
   - Liver disease
   - Renovascular disease (bilateral or unilateral renal artery stenosis)
   - Heart failure with reduced EF

3. Describe how you would explain to a patient how to use a digital home BP monitor such as the one shown in Fig. 12-1.

CLINICAL PEARL

The majority of hypertensive patients will require two or more BP-lowering medications to achieve recommended BP goals. For patients with resistant hypertension, including those who require

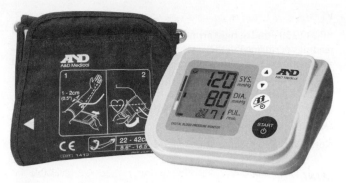

FIGURE 12-1. The LifeSource UA-767 Plus—One-Step Plus Memory digital home blood pressure monitor. (Photo courtesy of A&D Medical, Milpitas, California.)

more than three antihypertensives to achieve a goal blood pressure of <130/80 mm Hg, consideration can be given to either addition or intensification of diuretic therapy, including a possible switch to chlorthalidone or indapamide, or to a loop diuretic for those with poor kidney function or those already receiving treatment with minoxidil.

REFERENCES

1. Welton PK, Carey RM, Aronow WS, et al. 2017 ACC/AHA/AAPA/ABC/ACPM/AGS/APhA/ASH/ASPC/NMA/PCNA guideline for the prevention, detection, evaluation, and management of high blood pressure in adults: a report of the American College of Cardiology/American Heart Association Task Force on Clinical Practice Guidelines. J Am Coll Cardiol. 2018;71:e127–e248. doi: 10.1016/j.jacc.2017.11.006.

2. Salerno SM, Jackson JL, Berbano EP. Effect of oral pseudoephedrine on blood pressure and heart rate: a meta-analysis. Arch Intern Med. 2005;165:1686–1694.

3. American Diabetes Association. Standards of medical care in diabetes—2022. Diabetes Care. 2022;45(1 Suppl):S1–S259.

4. KDIGO clinical practice guideline for the management of blood pressure in chronic kidney disease. Kidney Int Suppl. 2021;99:S1–S87.

5. The SPRINT Research Group. A randomized trial of intensive versus standard blood-pressure control. N Engl J Med. 2015;373:2103–2116. doi: 10.1056/NEJMoa1511939.

6. Neter JE, Stam BE, Kok FJ, et al. Influence of weight reduction on blood pressure: a meta-analysis of randomized controlled trials. Hypertension. 2003;42:878–884.

7. Whelton PK, He J, Cutler JA, et al. Effects of oral potassium on blood pressure. Meta-analysis of randomized controlled clinical trials. JAMA. 1997;277:1624–1632.

8. Flack JM, Sica DA, Bakris GL, et al. Management of high blood pressure in blacks: an update of the International Society on Hypertension in Blacks Consensus Statement. Hypertension. 2010;56:780–800. doi: ahajournals.org/doi/10.1161/HYPERTENSIONAHA.110.152892.

9. Heart Outcomes Prevention Evaluation Study Investigators. Effects of an angiotensin-converting enzyme inhibitor, ramipril, on cardiovascular events in high-risk patients. N Engl J Med. 2000;342:145–153.

10. Heart Outcomes Prevention Evaluation Study Investigators. Effects of ramipril on cardiovascular and microvascular outcomes in people with diabetes mellitus: results of the HOPE study and the MICRO-HOPE substudy. Lancet. 2000;355:253–259.

11. The ALLHAT Officers and Coordinators for the ALLHAT Collaborative Research Group. Major cardiovascular events in hypertensive patients randomized to doxazosin vs chlorthalidone: the Antihypertensive and Lipid-Lowering Treatment to Prevent Heart Attack Trial (ALLHAT). JAMA. 2000;283:1967–1975.

13

HYPERTENSIVE CRISIS

I Don't Really Need Those Pills . . . . Level I

James J. Nawarskas, PharmD, BCPS

LEARNING OBJECTIVES

After completing this case study, the reader should be able to:

- Distinguish a hypertensive urgency from a hypertensive emergency.

- Identify treatment goals for a patient with a hypertensive crisis.

- Develop an appropriate treatment plan for a patient with a hypertensive crisis.

- Describe how a pharmacist can help improve antihypertensive medication adherence and the importance of providing this education.

PATIENT PRESENTATION

■ Chief Complaint

"I'm having trouble breathing, and my chest feels tight."

■ HPI

A 59-year-old woman was admitted to the emergency department with a chief complaint of difficulty breathing and chest tightness. She describes shortness of breath that she thinks started a few weeks ago but wasn't really that noticeable at first. Over the last few weeks, she has noticed her ability to perform daily activities to be more and more limited due to shortness of breath. She is fine when she isn't doing much, but simple activities such as walking her dog or going grocery shopping cause her to become short of breath rather quickly. Consequently, she moves around more slowly now when doing routine activities. She initially attributed this to just being "out of shape" but now is more concerned that it may be something else. The chest tightness started yesterday and was initially very mild, occurring when she would walk her dog outside and resolving readily with rest. However, it has since gotten more troublesome and is limiting her daily activities. While the chest discomfort still improves with rest, it no longer completely resolves. She tried to self-medicate by taking two doses (500 mg each) of acetaminophen last night and another dose this morning, but she says that didn't help. She also states that this discomfort is very different from her gastroesophageal reflux pain. While seated in the emergency department, she describes the chest discomfort as a 2 on a scale of 1–10 (highest). She has a past medical history significant for HTN and gastroesophageal reflux. She had been taking lisinopril and hydrochlorothiazide for several years with good blood pressure control, but about 6 months ago, she stopped taking both medicines because she had to make an urgent trip to visit her daughter out of state and ended up staying with her for a couple of months. Since her daughter lives in a rural area with no pharmacy nearby, she never got the medications refilled when she ran out. After several days, the patient noticed that she felt just fine despite not taking the medicines. Consequently, she never resumed them and has not seen her provider since.

■ PMH

HTN × 9 years
Gastroesophageal reflux × 11 years

■ FH

Both parents had HTN. Father had a heart attack in his early 60s and died in his late 70s of a second heart attack; mother died a few years later from a stroke. Two brothers, 57 and 62 years old, are both alive; the elder has HTN and hypercholesterolemia and underwent CABG surgery 2 years ago; the younger has no chronic diseases. One sister who is 60 years old also has HTN.

■ SH

Married for 36 years with four children (two boys, two girls all older than 25 years with no notable medical problems); she works part-time (2–3 days per week) as a cashier at a large department store. She smoked cigarettes rather heavily when she was younger, but cut back to one to two per day when she was raising her children. As her children got older, she gradually increased her cigarette use and is now smoking about one pack per day and has been doing so for about the past 10 years. She drinks alcohol infrequently (maybe once or twice a month), when she is at a social gathering. She denies ever using recreational drugs. She does not exercise and leads a rather sedentary lifestyle. In terms of diet, for breakfast she typically has a cup of coffee, toast with butter, and two eggs. For lunch, she usually eats a ham or turkey sandwich, although on days she works, she typically does not eat lunch at all and compensates by eating a large breakfast. She does munch on snack cakes and chips on breaks during her work shift, however. For dinner, she likes to eat baked chicken and prepares some canned vegetables as a side dish along with a dinner salad with Italian dressing. She admits to the liberal use of salt during breakfast and dinner. She has a high school education. Her husband is alive and well and works as an accountant. Her household income is average middle class. She has good health insurance through her husband's employer.

■ Meds

Famotidine 20 mg PO once daily in the evening (over-the-counter).

Acetaminophen 500 mg as needed for headaches—she takes maybe two doses a month in addition to the doses mentioned in the HPI.

Lisinopril/hydrochlorothiazide 20/12.5 mg PO once daily—stopped approximately 6 months ago.

■ All

NKDA

■ ROS

The patient complains of breathing trouble as mentioned above; no hearing problems. She complains of chest discomfort as mentioned above but denies palpitations and dizziness. She admits to feeling a lack of energy along with her dyspnea, although she never has been very active. She denies nausea, vomiting, or abdominal pain. She denies any swelling in her extremities or weight gain. She denies mental status changes.

■ Physical Examination

Gen

The patient is a middle-aged Hispanic woman appearing to be in moderate distress.

VS

BP 240/130 mm Hg right arm, 232/128 mm Hg left arm (automated readings performed in the emergency department). A manual measurement repeated in the right arm after several minutes yields a BP of 236/134 mm Hg.

P 74, RR 24, T 36.8°C; Wt 80 kg, Ht 5'5"

Skin

Normal tone and temperature, good turgor

HEENT

PERRLA; EOMI; funduscopic exam revealed arterial tortuosity and A/V nicking, but no papilledema

Neck/Lymph Nodes

No JVD, no bruits, no thyromegaly, or lymphadenopathy

Chest

Wheezing with faint crackles in both lung bases

CV

RRR, no murmurs or rubs appreciated; +S_4 heard at apex

Abd

Soft, NT/ND, no guarding, (+) BS, no abdominal bruits appreciated

MS/Ext

No CCE, pulses 2+ radial; 1+ to 2+ in the rest of her upper and lower extremities

Neuro

A & O × 3

■ Labs

Na 140 mEq/L	Hgb 13.2 g/dL	AST 27 IU/L
K 4.8 mEq/L	Hct 43%	ALT 45 IU/L
Cl 100 mEq/L	WBC 6.6 × 10³/mm³	Cholesterol 186 mg/dL
CO_2 28 mEq/L	Plt 222 × 10³/mm³	HDL 42 mg/dL
BUN 30 mg/dL		Triglycerides 142 mg/dL
SCr 2.3 mg/dL		LDL 116 mg/dL
Glu 112 mg/dL		Troponin-I normal

■ UA

Specific gravity 1.010; pH 5.8; negative for blood or protein; negative for recreational drugs

■ Chest X-Ray

Enlarged heart; cephalization of the pulmonary veins with indistinct vascular margins indicative of pulmonary edema

■ ECG

Normal sinus rhythm; LVH by voltage criteria. There are no ST-segment changes, although there does appear to be some T-wave flattening in the anterior leads. No old ECGs are available for comparison.

■ Chest CT

Negative for aortic dissection

■ Assessment

A 59-year-old woman with a long-standing history of HTN and gastroesophageal reflux presents with an extremely elevated blood pressure and signs and symptoms of target organ damage. She admits to not taking any antihypertensive drug therapy for 6 months, which was initially due to difficulty in getting her medications refilled, and then later due to feeling fine despite not taking the medications.

QUESTIONS

Collect Information

1.a. Is this a hypertensive urgency or an emergency? What subjective and objective information helps distinguish a hypertensive urgency from an emergency in this patient?

1.b. What additional information, if any, is needed to help develop a treatment plan for this patient?

Assess the Information

2.a. Assess the severity of this patient's hypertensive crisis based on the subjective and objective information available.

2.b. Create a list of the patient's drug therapy problems and prioritize them. Include assessment of medication appropriateness, effectiveness, safety, and patient adherence.

Develop a Care Plan

3.a. What are the goals of pharmacotherapy for the hypertensive crisis in this case?

3.b. What nondrug therapies might be useful for this patient's hypertensive crisis?

3.c. What feasible pharmacotherapeutic options are available for treating her hypertensive crisis?

3.d. Create an individualized, patient-centered, team-based care plan to optimize medication therapy for this patient's hypertensive crisis and other drug therapy problems. Include specific drugs, dosage forms, doses, schedules, and durations of therapy.

3.e. How would the treatment goals differ if this patient presented with the same BP but was asymptomatic with normal laboratory findings and no acute changes on ECG or physical examination?

Implement the Care Plan

4.a. What information should be provided to the patient to enhance adherence, ensure successful therapy, and minimize adverse effects?

4.b. Describe how care should be coordinated with other healthcare providers.

Follow-Up: Monitor and Evaluate

5. Explain how to monitor and evaluate the care plan for medication appropriateness, effectiveness, safety and patient adherence by using clinical and laboratory data, patient feedback, and other information.

■ CLINICAL COURSE

Once the blood pressure is lowered to an acceptable level, the inpatient provider consults with you regarding chronic antihypertensive therapy for this patient.

■ FOLLOW-UP QUESTIONS

1. Do you recommend this patient resume her lisinopril/HCTZ as prescribed, or would you recommend alternative drug therapy? Rationalize your answer. If you would recommend alternative drug therapy, which drug(s) would you recommend and why?

2. What nonpharmacologic measures can this patient incorporate as part of an overall treatment plan for her chronic hypertension?

■ SELF-STUDY ASSIGNMENTS

1. You are a pharmacist working in a community pharmacy that has a designated patient care center equipped with a manual blood pressure cuff. Describe your approach in dealing with a patient who reports that the automated blood pressure monitor in the waiting area of the pharmacy provided him or her with extremely high blood pressure measurements.

2. Use an algorithm or flow diagram to illustrate your approach to dealing with a patient who is nonadherent to antihypertensive therapy. After you do so, read the article: Can drugs work in patients who do not take them? The problem of nonadherence in resistant hypertension (Curr Hypertens Rep. 2015;17:69). Then redesign your approach if necessary.

3. Develop an evidence-based treatment algorithm for the use of various oral antihypertensive agents for the treatment of a hypertensive urgency.

CLINICAL PEARL

Rates of medication nonadherence for patients with treatment-resistant hypertension and hypertensive crisis are 50% to 80%, making medication nonadherence the single most important issue for improving blood pressure control and avoiding hypertension-associated morbidity and mortality. Medication adherence assessment therefore needs to be a routine part of every ambulatory care encounter for a patient with hypertension.

REFERENCES

1. Whelton PK, Carey RM, Aronow WS, et al. 2017 ACC/AHA/AAPA/ABC/ACPM/AGS/APhA/ASH/ASPC/NMA/PCNA guideline for the prevention, detection, evaluation, and management of high blood pressure in adults: a report of the American College of Cardiology/American Heart Association Task Force on Clinical Practice Guidelines. Hypertension. 2018;71:e13–e115.

2. Paini A, Aggiusti C, Bertacchini F, et al. Definitions and epidemiological aspects of hypertensive urgencies and emergencies. High Blood Press Cardiovasc Prev. 2018;25:241–244.

3. van den Born BH, Lip GYH, Brguljan-Hitij J, et al. ESC Council on hypertension position document on the management of hypertensive emergencies. Eur Heart J Cardiovasc Pharmacother. 2019;5:37–46.

4. Ramos AP, Varon J. Current and newer agents for hypertensive emergencies. Curr Hypertens Rep. 2014;16:450.

5. Umemura S, Arima H, Asayama K, et al. The Japanese Society of Hypertension Guidelines for the Management of Hypertension (JSH 2019). Hypertens Res. 2019;42:1235–1481.

6. Park SK, Lee D-Y, Kim WJ, et al. Comparing the clinical efficacy of resting and antihypertensive medication in patients of hypertensive urgency: a randomized, control trial. J Hypertens. 2017;35:1474–1480.

7. Varounis C, Katsi V, Nihoyannopoulos P, Lekakis J, Tousoulis D. Cardiovascular hypertensive crisis: recent evidence and review of the literature. Front Cardiovasc Med. 2017;3:51.

8. Varon J. Treatment of acute severe hypertension: current and newer agents. Drugs. 2008;68:283–297.
9. Muiesan ML, Salvetti M, Amadoro V. An update on hypertensive emergencies and urgencies. J Cardiovasc Med. 2015;16:372–382.
10. Hebert CJ, Vidt DG. Hypertensive crises. Prim Care Office Pract. 2008;35:475–487.

14

DYSLIPIDEMIA

Afraid of Another Attack .... Level II

Joel C. Marrs, PharmD, MPH, FAHA, FASHP, FCCP, FNLA, BCACP, BCCP, BCPS, CLS

LEARNING OBJECTIVES

After completing this case study, the reader should be able to:

- Identify patients who require treatment for dyslipidemia.

- Stratify individual patients for risk of coronary heart disease (CHD) and stroke.

- Determine appropriate LDL and non-HDL goals and thresholds based on individual risk factors.

- Recommend a cholesterol management strategy that includes therapeutic lifestyle changes (TLC), drug therapy, patient education, and monitoring parameters.

PATIENT PRESENTATION

■ Chief Complaint

"I am here to see if I need additional medications."

■ HPI

A 52-year-old man presents to pharmacotherapy for optimization of risk reduction therapy clinic by referral from his primary care provider following an ST-elevation myocardial infarction (STEMI) 6 months ago. He reports good adherence to his medications since having his heart attack.

■ PMH

Obesity (BMI 30.5 kg/m²)
Dyslipidemia × 6 years
HTN × 10 years
Chronic kidney disease (stage 3) × 5 years
CAD, s/p STEMI 6 months ago (drug-eluting stents placed in right circumflex and left anterior descending arteries)
GERD × 5 years

■ FH

Father: age 72 with MIs at age 50 and again at age 60.
Mother: age 70 with no major medical conditions noted.
Patient has one older brother age 55 with HTN and a history of one MI at the age of 48.
He has no children.

■ SH

Patient is married and lives with his wife.
College graduate, works as an accountant.
Admits to drinking one to two beers most days of the week and has never used tobacco.
Exercise regimen has increased since his MI; currently rides the bike at the gym for 30 minutes 2–3 days a week.

■ Meds (per medication fill history)

Carvedilol 25 mg PO BID
Atorvastatin 80 mg PO once daily
Aspirin 81 mg PO once daily
Clopidogrel 75 mg PO once daily
Pantoprazole 40 mg PO once daily
Lisinopril 40 mg PO daily
Chlorthalidone 25 mg PO daily
Acetaminophen 500 mg, one to two tablets PO PRN every 6 hours for pain
Garlic capsules

■ All

No known drug allergies

■ ROS

Patient states that he had a heart attack about 6 months ago and was put on a number of medications after that happened. He saw his PCP last month who said he should be seen in the pharmacotherapy clinic for evaluation of his cardiovascular risk reduction medications. He reports he has been adherent to his medication regimen over the last 6 months. He went to cardiac rehab for the first 3 months after his MI but has just been going to the gym to ride the bike two to three times a week now. He denies unilateral weakness, numbness/tingling, or changes in vision. He denies CP and only has SOB if he really pedals hard on the bike for longer than 15 minutes. He denies changes in bowel or urinary habits. He denies any lower extremity edema.

■ Physical Examination

Gen

Obese man in NAD

VS

BP 136/84, P 64, RR 18, T 38.2°C; Wt 102.3 kg, Ht 6'0"

Skin

Warm and dry to touch, normal turgor, (–) for acanthosis nigricans

HEENT

PERRLA; EOMI; funduscopic exam deferred; TMs intact; oral mucosa clear

Neck/Lymph Nodes

Neck supple, no lymphadenopathy, thyroid smooth and firm without nodules

Chest

CTA bilaterally, no wheezes, crackles, or rhonchi

CV

RRR, no MRG, normal S_1 and S_2; no S_3 or S_4

Abd

(+) BS, no hepatosplenomegaly

Genit/Rect

Deferred

Ext

No pedal edema, pulses 2+ throughout

Neuro

No gross motor-sensory deficits present

■ Labs (Fasting)

Na 140 mEq/L	Ca 8.2 mg/dL	*Fasting lipid profile*
K 4.6 mEq/L	Mg 2.1 mEq/L	TC 190 mg/dL
Cl 103 mEq/L	AST 45 units/L	HDL 40 mg/dL
CO$_2$ 23 mEq/L	ALT 40 units/L	LDL 121 mg/dL
BUN 19 mg/dL	T. bili 0.5 mg/dL	TG 145 mg/dL
SCr 1.6 mg/dL	T. prot 7.1 g/dL	
Glucose 119 mg/dL		
Hgb 12.0 mg/dL		
Hct 36%		

■ Assessment

An obese man presents to pharmacotherapy clinic for follow-up about further optimization of this cardiovascular risk reduction therapy. He had a STEMI 6 months ago and has a significant family history of cardiovascular disease. He has uncontrolled dyslipidemia treated with atorvastatin and uncontrolled HTN treated with carvedilol, lisinopril, and chlorthalidone. He reports no drug allergies and rides the bike at the gym 2–3 days a week. He reports using acetaminophen, but no NSAIDs for occasional aches and pains. Patient is interested in what can be done to lower his risk of another heart attack as his dad has had two and his brother has had one. He consistently drinks one to two beers a day but has no history of tobacco use.

QUESTIONS

Collect Information

1.a. What subjective and objective information indicates the presence of dyslipidemia?

1.b. What additional information is needed to fully assess this patient's dyslipidemia?

Assess the Information

2.a. Assess the severity of dyslipidemia based on the subjective and objective information available.

2.b. Create a list of the patient's drug therapy problems and prioritize them. Include assessment of medication appropriateness, effectiveness, safety, and patient adherence.

2.c. What economic, psychosocial, cultural, racial, and ethnic considerations are applicable to this patient?

Develop a Care Plan

3.a. What are the goals of pharmacotherapy for dyslipidemia in this case?

3.b. What nondrug therapies might be useful for this patient's dyslipidemia?

3.c. What feasible pharmacotherapeutic options are available for treating dyslipidemia?

3.d. Create an individualized, patient-centered, team-based care plan to optimize medication therapy for this patient's dyslipidemia and other drug therapy problems. Include specific drugs, dosage forms, doses, schedules, and durations of therapy.

Implement the Care Plan

4.a. What information should be provided to the patient to enhance adherence, ensure successful therapy, and minimize adverse effects?

4.b. Describe how care should be coordinated with other healthcare providers.

Follow-Up: Monitor and Evaluate

5. Explain how to monitor and evaluate the care plan for medication appropriateness, effectiveness, safety and patient adherence by using clinical and laboratory data, patient feedback, and other information.

■ CLINICAL COURSE: ALTERNATIVE THERAPY

The patient is already taking garlic capsules, but he is not sure about the type or dose. Because you are making changes to his current prescription regimen, you need to investigate the advisability of continuing the garlic. Because he is taking a statin drug as indicated, he should not take red yeast rice, a common supplement used for dyslipidemia, because it contains mevacolin K, a lovastatin analog, and would be duplicative therapy. Would fish oil be a possible option for him? See Section 19 in this Casebook for questions about the use of garlic and fish oil for treatment of dyslipidemia.

■ SELF-STUDY ASSIGNMENTS

1. Describe how this patient's other drug/disease interaction issues that are unrelated to dyslipidemia should be managed.

2. What changes, if any, would you make to the pharmacotherapy regimen for this patient if he had presented at the initial visit with each of the following characteristics?

   • Cirrhosis of the liver

   • Stage 5 chronic kidney disease receiving hemodialysis

   • Significant alcohol use

   • Posttransplant

   • Human immunodeficiency virus

CLINICAL PEARL

Icosapent ethyl in a dose of 4 g per day added to statin therapy in patients with established ASCVD has demonstrated reduction in the composite outcome of cardiovascular death, nonfatal myocardial infarction, nonfatal stroke, coronary revascularization, or unstable angina in the REDUCE-IT trial. Addition of icosapent ethyl to statin therapy in patients with moderately elevated triglycerides (135–499 mg/dL) and established ASCVD may be warranted in addition to other lipid-lowering therapy (eg, ezetimibe, PCSK9 inhibitors) for secondary prevention.

REFERENCES

1. Grundy SM, SM, Stone NJ, Bailey AL, et al. 2018 AHA/ACC/AACVPR/ AAPA/ABC/ACPM/ADA/AGS/APhA/ASPC/NLA/PCNA guideline on the management of blood cholesterol: a report of the American College of Cardiology/American Heart Association Task Force on Clinical Practice Guidelines. J Am Coll Cardiol. 2019;73(24):3168–3209.

2. Whelton PK, Carey RM, Aronow WS, et al. 2017 ACC/AHA/AAPA/ ABC/ACPM/AGS/APhA/ASH/ASPC/NMA/PCNA guideline for the prevention, detection, evaluation, and management of high blood pressure in adults. Hypertension. 2018 June;71(6):e13–e115.

3. Eckel RH, Jakicic JM, Ard JD, et al. 2013 AHA/ACC guideline on lifestyle management to reduce cardiovascular risk: a report of the American College of Cardiology American/Heart Association Task Force on Practice Guidelines. Circulation. 2014;129:S76–S99.

4. Jensen MD, Ryan DH, Apovian CM, et al. 2013 ACC/AHA/TOS guideline for the management of overweight and obesity in adults: a report of the American College of Cardiology/American Heart Association Task Force on Practice Guidelines, and The Obesity Society. J Am Coll Cardiol. 2014;63:2985–3023.

5. Cannon CP, Blazing MA, Giugliano RP, et al. Ezetimibe added to statin therapy after acute coronary syndromes. N Engl J Med. 2015;372:2387–2397.

6. Sabatine MS, Giugliano RP, Keech AC, et al. Evolocumab and clinical outcomes in patients with cardiovascular disease. N Engl J Med. 2017;376:1713–1722.

7. Schwartz GG, Steg PG, Szarek M, et al. Alirocumab and cardiovascular outcomes after acute coronary syndrome. N Engl J Med. 2018;379:2097–2107.

8. Bhatt DL, Steg PG, Miller M, et al. Cardiovascular risk reduction with icosapent ethyl for hypertriglyceridemia. N Engl J Med. 2019;380: 11–22.

15

STABLE ISCHEMIC HEART DISEASE

An Uphill Battle . . . . Level III

Regan M. Wade, PharmD, BCPS

David M. Kaylor, PharmD

LEARNING OBJECTIVES

After completing this case study, the reader should be able to:

- Identify modifiable risk factors for ischemic heart disease (IHD) and discuss the potential benefit to be gained by their modification in an individual patient.

- Optimize medical therapy in a patient with persistent angina considering response to current therapy and the presence of comorbidities.

- Assess clinical response to antianginal therapy by identifying relevant monitoring parameters for efficacy and adverse effects.

- Propose appropriate counseling points and follow-up recommendations for both stable and symptomatic patients with angina.

PATIENT PRESENTATION

■ Chief Complaint

"Doc, these drugs just aren't working for my chest pain anymore."

■ HPI

A 72-year-old man with coronary artery disease presents with frequent angina. He is an avid golfer and prefers to walk the course, but this is becoming progressively more difficult for him. He has had two coronary artery bypass operations in the past. A coronary angiogram performed 1 month ago revealed significant disease in the RCA proximal to his graft, but this was considered high risk for angioplasty. His dose of isosorbide mononitrate was increased at that time from 60 to 120 mg once daily. This had no effect on his angina. He is still using about 30 nitroglycerin tablets a week, and these do relieve his chest pain. He reports that most often the chest discomfort comes on with activity, such as walking up slight inclines on the golf course. The discomfort is located in the center of his chest and rated 3–4/10 on average. He reports that the chest discomfort slowly fades as he slows his activity. He also complains of occasional lightheadedness with a pulse around 50 bpm and SBP near 100 mm Hg.

■ PMH

Acute anterior wall MI with CABG surgery in 2009
Posterior lateral MI in 1990 and PTCA to the circumflex at that time
Dyslipidemia
Chronic low back pain
Depression

■ FH

Noncontributory for premature CAD

■ SH

Retired dairy farmer, lives with wife, drinks occasionally, previous smoker—quit in 1998

■ Meds

Carvedilol 6.25 mg PO twice daily
Lisinopril 5 mg PO once daily
Aspirin 325 mg PO once daily
Isosorbide mononitrate, extended-release 120 mg PO once daily
Diltiazem, extended-release 240 mg PO once daily
St. John's wort 300 mg PO three times daily
Celecoxib 200 mg PO once daily
Simvastatin 40 mg PO once daily
Nitroglycerin 0.4 mg SL PRN

■ All

NKDA

■ ROS

No fever, chills, or night sweats. No recent viral illnesses. No shortness of breath; occasional cough with cold weather. No nausea, vomiting, diarrhea, constipation, melena, or hematochezia. No dysuria or hematuria. No myalgias or arthralgias.

Physical Examination

Gen

Pleasant, cooperative man in no acute distress

VS

BP 105/68, P 50, RR 22, T 36.4°C, Ht 5'11", Wt 93 kg, waist circumference 43 in

Skin

Intact, no rashes or ulcers

HEENT

PERRL; EOMI; oropharynx is clear

Neck

Supple, no masses; no JVD, lymphadenopathy, or thyromegaly

Lungs

Bilateral air entry is clear. No wheezes.

CV

RRR, S_1, S_2 normal; no murmurs or gallops; PMI palpated at left fifth ICS, MCL

Abd

Soft, NT/ND; bowel sounds normoactive

Genit/Rect

Heme (–) stool

Ext

No CCE; pulses 2+ throughout

Neuro

A&O × 3, CN II–XII intact; speech is fluent; no motor or sensory deficit; no facial asymmetry; tongue midline.

Labs

Na 137 mEq/L	Hgb 11.8 g/dL	*Fasting lipid profile*
K 4.8 mEq/L	Hct 35.1%	Chol 202 mg/dL
Cl 103 mEq/L	Plt 187 × 10³/mm³	LDL 121 mg/dL
CO_2 21 mEq/L	WBC 7.9 × 10³/mm³	HDL 38 mg/dL
BUN 24 mg/dL	MCV 77 μm³	Trig 215 mg/dL
SCr 1.2 mg/dL	MCHC 29 g/dL	
Glu 98 mg/dL	Trop I 0.02 ng/mL × 2	

ECG

Sinus rhythm, first-degree AVB, 50 bpm, old AWMI, no ST–T wave changes noted, QT 406 milliseconds

Assessment

A 72-year-old man with poorly controlled angina on multiple medications, who is a poor candidate for angioplasty.

QUESTIONS

Collect Information

1.a. What subjective and objective information indicates the presence of chronic angina?

1.b. What additional information is needed to fully assess this patient's chronic angina?

Assess the Information

2.a. Assess the severity of the patient's chronic angina based on the subjective and objective information available.

2.b. Create a list of the patient's drug therapy problems and prioritize them. Include assessment of medication appropriateness, effectiveness, safety, and patient adherence.

Develop a Care Plan

3.a. What are the goals of pharmacotherapy for chronic angina in this case?

3.b. What nondrug therapies might be useful for this patient's chronic angina?

3.c. What feasible pharmacotherapeutic options are available for treating chronic angina?

3.d. Create an individualized, patient-centered, team-based care plan to optimize medication therapy for this patient's chronic angina and other drug therapy problems. Include specific drugs, dosage forms, doses, schedules, and durations of therapy.

Implement the Care Plan

4.a. What information should be provided to the patient to enhance adherence, ensure successful therapy, and minimize adverse effects?

4.b. Describe how care should be coordinated with other healthcare providers.

Follow-Up: Monitor and Evaluate

5. Explain how to monitor and evaluate the care plan for medication appropriateness, effectiveness, safety and patient adherence by using clinical and laboratory data, patient feedback, and other information.

■ CLINICAL COURSE

The patient improved hemodynamically following a switch from diltiazem to amlodipine. However, due to continued frequent episodes of angina, his amlodipine was titrated to 10 mg once daily. He returned to cardiology clinic today, stating that his angina frequency has improved somewhat on the maximum dose of amlodipine but is still bothersome to him. His cardiologist decided to add ranolazine 500 mg twice daily to his regimen in an attempt to further decrease his angina frequency.

■ SELF-STUDY ASSIGNMENTS

1. Summarize the potential role of L-arginine in the treatment of chronic angina.

2. Describe the potential role of allopurinol in the treatment of chronic angina.

CLINICAL PEARL

The 2017 COMPASS trial evaluated rivaroxaban 2.5 mg twice daily with low-dose aspirin in patients with coronary artery disease leading to a new FDA-approved indication for rivaroxaban in reducing the risk of major cardiovascular events. This may impact health care in the United States by potentially increasing the number of patients receiving anticoagulants.

REFERENCES

1. Fihn SD, Gardin JM, Abrams J, et al. 2012 ACCF/AHA/ACP/AATS/PCNA/SCAI/STS guideline for the diagnosis and management of patients with stable ischemic heart disease. J Am Coll Cardiol. 2012;60: e44–e164.

2. Grundy S, Stone N, Bailey A, et al. 2018 AHA/ACC/AACVPR/AAPA/ABC/ACPM/ADA/AGS/APhA/ASPC/NLA/PCNA guideline on the management of blood cholesterol. J Am Coll Cardiol. 2019;73(24): 3168–3209.

3. Smith SC, Benjamin EJ, Bonow RO, et al. AHA/ACCF secondary prevention and risk reduction therapy for patients with coronary and other atherosclerotic vascular disease: 2011 update. J Am Coll Cardiol. 2011;58:2432–2446.

4. Boden WE, Finn AV, Patel D, et al. Nitrates as an integral part of optimal medical therapy and cardiac rehabilitation for stable angina: review of current concepts and therapeutics. Clin Cardiol. 2012;35:263–271.

5. Bangalore S, Steg PG, Deedwania P, et al. β-Blocker use and clinical outcomes in stable outpatients with and without coronary artery disease. JAMA. 2012;308:1340–1349.

6. Antithrombotic Trialists' Collaboration. Collaborative meta-analysis of randomised trials of antiplatelet therapy for prevention of death, myocardial infarction, and stroke in high risk patients. BMJ. 2002;324:71–86.

7. CAPRIE Steering Committee. A randomised, blinded, trial of clopidogrel versus aspirin in patients at risk of ischaemic events (CAPRIE). Lancet. 1996;348:1329–1339.

8. Heart Outcomes Prevention Evaluation Study Investigators. Effects of an angiotensin-converting-enzyme inhibitor, ramipril, on cardiovascular events in high-risk patients. N Engl J Med. 2000;342:145–153.

9. Eikelboom JW, Connolly SJ, Bosch J, et al. Rivaroxaban with or without aspirin in stable cardiovascular disease. N Engl J Med. 2017;377(14):1319–1330.

10. Nidorf SM, Fiolet ATL, Mosterd A, et al. Colchicine in patients with chronic coronary disease. N Engl J Med. 2020;383:1838–1847.

16

ACUTE CORONARY SYNDROME: ST-ELEVATION MYOCARDIAL INFARCTION

I Can't Handle the Pressure . . . . Level III

Kelly C. Rogers, PharmD, BCCP, FCCP, FACC

Robert B. Parker, PharmD, FCCP

LEARNING OBJECTIVES

After completing this case study, the reader should be able to:

• Determine the goals of pharmacotherapy for patients with ST-segment elevation myocardial infarction (STEMI).

• Discuss interventional strategies for patients with STEMI and understand the pharmacotherapeutic agents used with interventions.

• Design a comprehensive medication management plan for the management of STEMI and describe how the selected drug therapy achieves the therapeutic goals.

• Identify appropriate parameters to assess the recommended drug therapy for both efficacy and adverse effects.

• Provide appropriate education to a patient who has suffered STEMI.

PATIENT PRESENTATION

■ Chief Complaint

"This is the worst pain I have ever felt in my life."

■ HPI

A 68-year-old man has been admitted to the ED complaining of chest pressure/pain lasting 20–30 minutes occurring at rest. He describes the pain as substernal, crushing, and pressure-like that radiates to his jaw and is accompanied by nausea and diaphoresis. The pain first started approximately 6 hours ago after he ate breakfast and was unrelieved by antacids or SL NTG × 3. He also states that he has been experiencing intermittent chest pain over the past 3–4 weeks with minimal exertion.

■ PMH

HTN
Type 2 DM
Dyslipidemia
CAD with PCI with a drug-eluting stent (DES) 3 years ago

■ FH

Father died from heart failure at age 75 and mother is alive at age 88 with HTN and type 2 DM.

■ SH

(+) Tobacco × 20 years but quit when he received his DES 3 years ago; drinks beer usually on weekends; denies illicit drug use

■ Meds

Aspirin 81 mg PO daily
Metoprolol tartrate 25 mg PO BID
Atorvastatin 40 mg PO QHS
Metformin 1000 mg PO BID
SL NTG PRN CP

■ All

NKDA

■ ROS

Positive for some baseline CP on exertion for the past 3–4 weeks, now with CP at rest

■ Physical Examination

Gen

WDWN man, A&O × 3, still with ongoing chest pain, somewhat anxious

VS

BP 145/92, P 89, RR 18, T 37.1°C; Wt 95 kg, Ht 5'10"

HEENT

PERRLA, EOMI, fundi benign; TMs intact

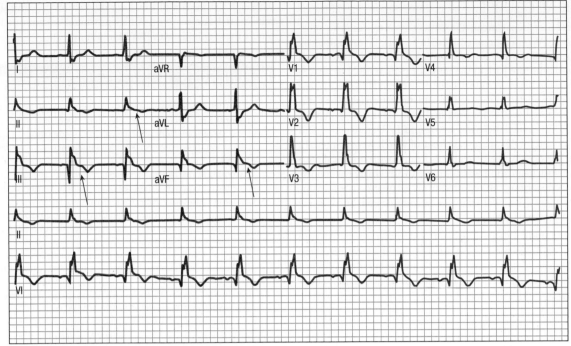

FIGURE 16-1. ECG taken on arrival in the emergency department showing ST-segment elevation (arrows) in leads II, III, and aVF, consistent with acute inferior myocardial infarction. Right bundle branch block is also present in leads V₁–V₃.

Neck

No bruits; mild JVD; no thyromegaly

Lungs

Few dependent inspiratory crackles; bibasilar rales; no wheezes

CV

Normal S_1 and S_2, no MRG

Abd

Soft, nontender; liver span 10–12 cm; no bruits

Genit/Rect

Deferred

MS/Ext

Normal ROM; muscle strength on right 5/5 UE/LE; on left 4/5 UE/LE; pulses 2+; no femoral bruits or peripheral edema

Neuro

CNs II–XII intact; DTRs decreased on left; negative Babinski sign

▇ Labs

Na 134 mEq/L	Ca 9.8 mg/dL	Hgb 14.0 g/dL	*Fasting lipid profile*
K 4.4 mEq/L	Mg 2.0 mg/dL	Hct 44%	T. chol 159 mg/dL
Cl 102 mEq/L	PO_4 2.4 mg/dL	WBC 5.0 × 10³/mm³	Trig 92 mg/dL
CO_2 23 mEq/L	AST 22 units/L	Plt 268 × 10³/mm³	LDL 105 mg/dL
BUN 15 mg/dL	ALT 30 units/L	PT 12.5 s	HDL 36 mg/dL
SCr 1.0 mg/dL	Alk Phos 75 units/L	aPTT 32.4 s	A1C 8.3%
Glu 140 mg/dL	Troponin I 8.6 ng/mL	INR 1.0	NT-pro-BNP 400 pg/mL

▇ ECG

ST-segment elevation of 2–3 mm in leads II, III, and aVF (Fig. 16-1)

▇ Assessment

Acute inferior STEMI

QUESTIONS

Collect Information

1. What subjective and objective findings in this patient are consistent with acute STEMI?

Assess the Information

2.a. What risk factors for the development of coronary artery disease are present in this patient?

2.b. Create a list of this patient's drug therapy problems and prioritize them. Include assessment of medication appropriateness, effectiveness, safety, and patient adherence.

Develop a Care Plan

3.a. What are the goals of pharmacotherapy for STEMI in this case?

3.b. What pharmacotherapeutic options are available for reperfusion in STEMI?

3.c. What nonpharmacologic options are available for reperfusion in STEMI?

3.d. What is the role of anticoagulant therapy during primary PCI, and how should these therapies be monitored?

3.e. What is the role of antiplatelet therapy before, during, and after PCI, and how should these therapies be monitored?

3.f. Create an individualized, patient-centered, team-based care plan to optimize medication therapy for the initial (first 24–48 hours) management of this patient's STEMI. Include specific drugs, dosage forms, doses, schedules, and durations of therapy.

■ CLINICAL COURSE

In the emergency department, the patient received aspirin, morphine, oxygen, IV unfractionated heparin (UFH), IV nitroglycerin, and oral metoprolol. An interventional cardiologist was consulted and discussed with the patient the need for primary PCI to restore blood flow to the heart. Within 1 hour of his arrival to the ED, the patient was transported to the cardiac catheterization lab. The catheterization revealed a 60–70% proximal stenosis in the RCA with thrombus. Additionally, there was a 40% mid-LAD obstruction and 20–30% distal circumflex disease, neither of which were stented. In the catheterization lab, the patient was loaded with oral ticagrelor 180 mg, and anticoagulation was continued with UFH. The following day, the echocardiogram reported an LVEF of 35%. The remainder of the patient's hospital stay was uncomplicated, and he was discharged 4 days post-MI.

3.g. Create an individualized, patient-centered, team-based care plan to optimize medication therapy for the post-discharge management of this patient's CAD and other drug therapy problems. Include specific drugs, dosage forms, doses, schedules, and durations of therapy.

Implement the Care Plan

4.a. What information should be provided to the patient to enhance adherence, ensure successful therapy, and minimize adverse effects?

4.b. Describe how care should be coordinated with other healthcare providers.

Follow-Up: Monitor and Evaluate

5. Explain how to monitor and evaluate the care plan for medication appropriateness, effectiveness, safety and patient adherence by using clinical and laboratory data, patient feedback and other information.

■ SELF-STUDY ASSIGNMENTS

1. It is not uncommon for patients with coronary atherosclerotic disease to have concomitant comorbid conditions such as diabetes mellitus. Review recent clinical trials that demonstrate improvement in cardiovascular outcomes with sodium-glucose cotransporter 2 (SGLT2) inhibitors.

2. A patient comes into your pharmacy with a prescription for clopidogrel 75 mg daily and a bottle of aspirin. He tells you that he received a drug-eluting stent in one of his coronary arteries. He states that he was told to stop taking aspirin 3 months after his stent was placed. He asks you how long he is supposed to take the clopidogrel. Based on recent clinical trials and considering the guideline recommendations on duration of dual-antiplatelet therapy, how should you respond to this patient?

3. In patients with ACS undergoing PCI, current guidelines suggest ticagrelor or prasugrel as reasonable alternatives over clopidogrel for dual antiplatelet therapy in combination with aspirin. Review recent data comparing the efficacy and safety of ticagrelor versus prasugrel in patients with ACS managed with PCI.

CLINICAL PEARL

Opioids such as morphine or fentanyl are frequently administered to patients with ACS undergoing PCI. Numerous small studies show that these agents delay the absorption of clopidogrel, ticagrelor, and prasugrel resulting in decreased inhibition of platelet activity.

Although the impact of this drug interaction on clinical outcomes remains to be determined, clinicians should be cautious about combining these opioids with P2Y12 inhibitors.

REFERENCES

1. O'Gara PT, Kushner FG, Ascheim DD, et al. 2013 ACCF/AHA guideline for the management of ST-elevation myocardial infarction: a report of the American College of Cardiology Foundation/American Heart Association Task Force on Practice Guidelines. Circulation. 2013;127: e362–e425.

2. Lawton JS, Tamis-Holland JE, Bangalore S, et al. 2021 ACC/AHA/SCAI guideline for coronary artery revascularization: a report of the American College of Cardiology/American Heart Association Joint Committee on Clinical Practice Guidelines. J Am Coll Cardiol. 2022;79:e21–e129.

3. Heidenreich PA, Bozkurt B, Aguilar D, et al. 2022 AHA/ACC/HFSA guideline for the management of heart failure: a report of the American College of Cardiology/American Heart Association Joint Committee on Clinical Practice Guidelines. J Am Coll Cardiol. 2022 Mar;24: S0735-1097(21)08395-9.

4. Grundy SM, Stone NJ, Bailey AL, et al. 2018 AHA/ACC/AACVPR/ AAPA/ABC/ACPM/ADA/AGS/APhA/ASPC/NLA/PCNA guideline on the management of blood cholesterol: executive summary: a report of the American College of Cardiology/American Heart Association Task Force on Clinical Practice Guidelines. J Am Coll Cardiol. 2019;73(24): 3168–3209.

5. Lloyd-Jones DM, Morris PB, Ballantyne CM, et al. 2016 ACC expert consensus decision pathway on the role of non-statin therapies for LDL-cholesterol lowering in the management of atherosclerotic cardiovascular disease risk: a report of the American College of Cardiology Task Force on Clinical Expert Consensus Documents. J Am Coll Cardiol. 2016;68:92–125.

6. Whelton PK, Carey RM, Aronow WS, et al. 2017 ACC/AHA/AAPA/ ABC/ACPM/AGS/APhA/ASH/ASPC/NMA/PCNA guideline for the prevention, detection, evaluation, and management of high blood pressure in adults: a report of the American College of Cardiology/American Heart Association Task Force on Clinical Practice Guidelines. J Am Coll Cardiol. 2018;71:e127–248.

7. Das SR, Everett BM, Birtcher KK, et al. 2018 ACC expert consensus decision pathway on novel therapies for cardiovascular risk reduction in patients with type 2 diabetes and atherosclerotic cardiovascular disease: a report of the American College of Cardiology Task Force on Expert Consensus Decision Pathways. J Am Coll Cardiol. 2018;72(24):3200–3223.

17

PERIPHERAL ARTERIAL DISEASE

Tracy J. Costello, PharmD, BCPS

Tracy L. Sprunger, PharmD, BCPS

LEARNING OBJECTIVES

After completing this case study, the reader should be able to:

- Identify risk factors for peripheral arterial disease (PAD).

- Describe the symptoms and diagnosis of PAD.

- Recommend appropriate nonpharmacologic treatment strategies for PAD, including risk factor modification, exercise, and revascularization.
- Design an appropriate pharmacologic treatment plan for a patient with PAD.
- Provide appropriate education to a patient with PAD.

PATIENT PRESENTATION

■ Chief Complaint

"I am having pain in both legs and in my left foot."

■ HPI

A 56-year-old woman with hypertension, diabetes, dyslipidemia, and a history of bilateral leg weakness for the previous year. She reports to her primary care provider today with increased numbness and weakness when she walks. She reports that it is painful to walk even for 4–5 minutes and that her legs are often weak and "give out." She is concerned because she lives alone and is responsible for walking her dog. Her symptoms tend to get better when she is able to rest and prop her feet up.

■ PMH

HTN
Diabetes
Dyslipidemia

■ FH

Mother died of a stroke at the age of 67; father died of pneumonia at the age of 62.

■ SH

Works as a biller in a dentist's office; has one child; lives alone; smokes 1 ppd × 25 years; denies ETOH and illicit drug use; has one dog at home

■ Meds

Aspirin 81 mg PO daily
Atenolol 50 mg PO daily
Empagliflozin 10 mg PO daily
Metformin 1000 mg PO BID
Simvastatin 20 mg PO daily
Hydrochlorothiazide 25 mg PO daily

■ All

NKDA

■ ROS

The patient complains of lower extremity muscle aches and muscle weakness. Denies chest pains, palpitations, syncope, and orthopnea. Denies nausea, vomiting, diarrhea, constipation, change in bowel habits, abdominal pain, or melena. Denies transient paralysis, seizures, syncope, and tremors.

■ Physical Examination

Gen

Woman in NAD. She appears older than her stated age.

VS

BP 149/87, P 73, RR 17, T 98.2°F; Wt 85 kg, Ht 5′4″

Skin

Distal to midshin with shiny-appearing skin, skin atrophy, and lack of hair growth. No evidence of skin breakdown or ulceration.

HEENT

PERRLA; conjunctivae and lids normal; TM intact; normal dentition, no gingival inflammation, no labial lesions; tongue normal, posterior pharynx without erythema or exudate

Neck/Lymph Nodes

Supple, no masses, trachea midline; no carotid bruits; no lymphadenopathy or thyromegaly

Lungs/Thorax

No rales, rhonchi, or wheezes; no intercostal retractions or use of accessory muscles

CV

RRR, S_1, S_2 normal; no murmurs, rubs, or gallops; no thrill or palpable murmurs, no displacement of PMI

Abd

Soft, nontender, no masses, bowel sounds normal; no enlargement or nodularity of liver or spleen

Genit/Rect

Deferred

MS/Ext

Normal gait; no clubbing, cyanosis, petechiae, or nodes; normal ROM and strength, good stability, and no joint enlargement or tenderness; pedal pulses 1+, symmetric

Neuro

CN II–XII grossly intact; DTRs 2+, no pathologic reflexes; sensory and motor levels intact

■ Labs

Na 137 mEq/L	Hgb 12.7 g/dL	WBC 6.3 × 10³/mm³
K 3.9 mEq/L	Hct 34.4%	AST 22 IU/L
Cl 97 mEq/L	Plt 313 × 10³/mm³	ALT 30 IU/L
CO₂ 24 mEq/L	TSH 1.12 mIU/L	
BUN 12 mg/dL	TC 224 mg/dL	
SCr 1.0 mg/dL	TG 220 mg/dL	
Glu 99 mg/dL	LDL 140 mg/dL	
A1C 6.3%	HDL 40 mg/dL	

■ Lower Extremity Arterial Doppler

Ankle–brachial index (ABI)—right: 0.53; left: 0.62

■ Assessment

A 56-year-old woman with a significant smoking history presents with uncontrolled hypertension, dyslipidemia, and new symptoms of intermittent claudication (IC).

QUESTIONS

Collect Information

1.a. What subjective and objective information indicates the presence of peripheral arterial disease?

1.b. What additional information is needed to fully assess this patient's peripheral arterial disease?

Assess the Information

2.a. Assess the severity of peripheral arterial disease based on the subjective and objective information available.

2.b. Create a list of the patient's drug therapy problems and prioritize them. Include assessment of medication appropriateness, effectiveness, safety, and patient adherence.

Develop a Care Plan

3.a. What are the goals of pharmacotherapy for peripheral arterial disease in this case?

3.b. What nondrug therapies might be useful for this patient's peripheral arterial disease?

3.c. What feasible pharmacotherapeutic options are available for treating peripheral arterial disease?

3.d. Create an individualized, patient-centered, team-based care plan to optimize medication therapy for this patient's peripheral arterial disease and other drug therapy problems. Include specific drugs, dosage forms, doses, schedules, and durations of therapy.

3.e. What alternatives would be appropriate if the initial care plan fails or cannot be used?

Implement the Care Plan

4.a. What information should be provided to the patient to enhance adherence, ensure successful therapy, and minimize adverse effects?

4.b. Describe how care should be coordinated with other healthcare providers.

Follow-Up: Monitor and Evaluate

5. Explain how to monitor and evaluate the care plan for medication appropriateness, effectiveness, safety and patient adherence by using clinical and laboratory data, patient feedback and other information.

■ SELF-STUDY ASSIGNMENTS

1. Review the recommendations for dual antiplatelet therapy for the treatment of PAD. Would a patient benefit from combination therapy?

2. Perform a literature search to determine the role of warfarin and direct oral anticoagulant agents for the management of PAD.

CLINICAL PEARL

Although cilostazol has antiplatelet effects, it is currently not recommended for the prevention of atherosclerotic events or the treatment of atherosclerotic disease.

REFERENCES

1. Gerhard-Herman MD, Gornik HL, Barrett C, et al. 2016 ACCF/AHA guideline on the management of patients with lower extremity peripheral artery disease. Circulation. 2017;135:e726–e779.

2. American Diabetes Association. Standards of medical care in diabetes—2022 Diabetes Care. 2022;45(Suppl 1):S1–S264.

3. ACC/AHA/AAPA/ABC/ACPM/AGS/APhA/ASH/ASPC/NMA/PCNA guideline for the prevention, detection, evaluation, and management of high blood pressure in adults: a report of the American College of Cardiology/American Heart Association Task Force on Clinical Practice Guidelines. J Am Coll Cardiol. 2018;71:e127–e248.

4. Grundy SM, Stone NJ, Bailey AL, et al. 2018 AHA/ACC/AACVPR/AAPA/ABC/ACPM/ADA/AGS/APhA/ASPC/NLA/PCNA guideline on the management of blood cholesterol. J Am Coll Cardiol. 2019;73(24):3168–3209.

5. Apovian CM, Aronne LJ, Bessesen DH, et al. Pharmacological management of obesity: an endocrine society clinical practice guideline. J Clin Endocrinol Metab. 2015;100:342–362.

6. Bonaca MP, Scirica BM, Creager MA, et al. Vorapaxar in patients with peripheral artery disease: results from TRA2 P-TIMI 50. Circulation. 2013;127:1522–1529.

7. Eikelboom JW, Connolly SJ, Bosch J, et al; for the COMPASS Investigators. Rivaroxaban with or without aspirin in chronic cardiovascular disease. N Engl J Med. 2017;377(14):1319–1330.

18

HEART FAILURE WITH REDUCED EJECTION FRACTION

Cross My Heart and Hope to Live . . . . Level III

Julia M. Koehler, PharmD, FCCP

Alison M. Walton, PharmD, BCPS

LEARNING OBJECTIVES

After completing this case study, the reader should be able to:

• Recognize the signs and symptoms of heart failure.

• Develop a pharmacotherapeutic plan for treatment of heart failure with reduced ejection fraction (HF*r*EF).

• Outline a monitoring plan for heart failure that includes both clinical and laboratory parameters.

PATIENT PRESENTATION

■ Chief Complaint

"I've been more short of breath lately. I can't *seem* to walk as far as I used to, and either my feet are growing, or my shoes are shrinking!"

HPI

A 68-year-old black woman presents to her primary care provider for evaluation of her shortness of breath and increased swelling in her lower extremities. She reports that her shortness of breath has been gradually increasing over the past 4 days. She has noticed that her shortness of breath is particularly worse when she is lying in bed at night, and she has to prop her head up with three pillows in order to sleep. She also reports exertional dyspnea that is usual for her, but especially worse over the past couple of days.

PMH

Hypertension × 20 years
CHD with history of MI 8 years ago (PCI performed and bare metal stents placed in LAD and RCA)
Heart failure (NYHA FC III)
Type 2 DM × 25 years
CKD (stage 3b)

FH

Father died of lung cancer at age 71; mother died of MI at age 73.

SH

Reports occasional alcohol intake. States she has been trying to follow her low-cholesterol and low-sodium diet. Former smoker (35 pack-year history; quit approximately 10 years ago).

Meds

Valsartan 160 mg PO BID
Furosemide 40 mg PO BID
Carvedilol 3.125 mg PO BID
Pioglitazone 30 mg PO once daily
Dulaglutide 1.5mg subcutaneously once weekly
Spironolactone 25 mg PO once daily
Atorvastatin 40 mg PO once daily
Aspirin 81 mg PO once daily

All

Lisinopril (cough)

ROS

Approximate 7-kg weight gain over the past week. No fever or chills. Denies any recent chest pain, palpitations, or dizziness. Reports worsening shortness of breath with exertion and three-pillow orthopnea. No abdominal pain, nausea, constipation, or change in bowel habits. Denies joint pain or weakness.

Physical Examination

Gen

68-year-old black woman in moderate respiratory distress

VS

BP 134/76 (sitting; repeat 138/78), HR 65, RR 24, T 37°C, O_2 sat 90% RA, Ht 5'5", Wt 79 kg (Wt 1 week ago: 72 kg)

Skin

Diaphoretic; no unusual lesions noted

HEENT

PERRLA; lips mildly cyanotic; dentures

Neck

(+) JVD at 30° (7 cm); no lymphadenopathy or thyromegaly

Lungs/Thorax

Crackles bilaterally, 2/3 of the way up; no expiratory wheezing

Heart

(+) S_3; displaced PMI

Abd

Soft, mildly tender, nondistended; (+) HJR; no masses, mild hepato-splenomegaly; normal BS

Genit/Rect

Guaiac (−), genital examination not performed

MS/Ext

3+ pitting pedal edema bilaterally; radial and pedal pulses are of poor intensity bilaterally

Neuro

A & O × 3, CNs intact; no motor deficits

Labs

Na 131 mEq/L	Hgb 13 g/dL	Mg 1.9 mEq/L	A1C 6.8%
K 4.2 mEq/L	Hct 40%	Ca 9.3 mg/dL	
Cl 99 mEq/L	Plt 192 × 10^3/mm³	Phos 4.3 mg/dL	
CO_2 28 mEq/L	WBC 9.1 × 10^3/mm³	AST 34 IU/L	
BUN 32 mg/dL		ALT 27 IU/L	
SCr 1.7 mg/dL (baseline SCr 1.5 mg/dL)			
eGFR 36 mL/min/1.73 m²			
Glucose 132 mg/dL			
BNP 776 pg/mL (BNP drawn 2 months prior: 474 pg/mL)			

ECG

Q waves in leads II, III, and AVF; hypokinetic inferior wall; evidence of LVH

Chest X-Ray

PA and lateral views (Fig. 18-1) show evidence of congestive failure with cardiomegaly, interstitial edema, and some early alveolar edema. There is a small right pleural effusion. No evidence of infiltrates; evidence of pulmonary edema suggestive of congestive heart failure; enlarged cardiac silhouette.

Echocardiogram

LVH, reduced global left ventricular systolic function, estimated EF 20%; evidence of impaired ventricular relaxation, stage 1 diastolic dysfunction

Assessment

Admit to hospital for acute exacerbation of heart failure

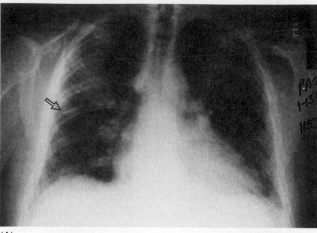

(A)

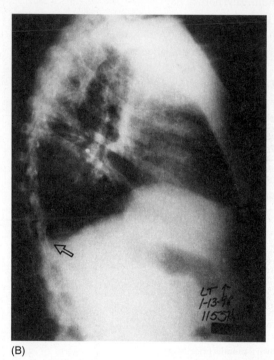

(B)

FIGURE 18-1. *A.* PA CXR demonstrates increased vascular markings representative of interstitial edema, with some early alveolar edema. The *arrow* points out fluid lying in the fissure of the right lung. Note the presence of cardiomegaly. *B.* Lateral view of CXR. *Arrow* points out the presence of pulmonary effusion.

QUESTIONS

Collect Information

1.a. What subjective and objective information indicates the presence of heart failure?

1.b. What additional information is needed to fully assess this patient's heart failure?

Assess the Information

2.a. Assess the type and severity of heart failure based on the subjective and objective information available.

2.b. Create a list of this patient's drug therapy problems and prioritize them. Include assessment of medication appropriateness, effectiveness, safety, and patient adherence.

Develop a Care Plan

3.a. What are the goals of pharmacotherapy for heart failure in this case?

3.b. What nondrug therapies might be useful for this patient's heart failure?

3.c. What feasible pharmacotherapeutic options are available for treating an acute exacerbation of heart failure and for chronic management of heart failure with reduced ejection fraction?

3.d. Create an individualized, patient-centered, team-based care plan to optimize medication therapy for this patient's heart failure and other drug therapy problems. Include specific drugs, dosage forms, doses, schedules, and durations of therapy.

Implement the Care Plan

4.a. What information should be provided to the patient to enhance adherence, ensure successful therapy, and minimize adverse effects?

4.b. Describe how care should be coordinated with other healthcare providers.

Follow-Up: Monitor and Evaluate

5. Explain how to monitor and evaluate the care plan for medication appropriateness, effectiveness, safety and patient adherence by using clinical and laboratory data, patient feedback and other information.

■ SELF-STUDY ASSIGNMENTS

1. Develop a table illustrating the recommended target doses for ACE inhibitors, angiotensin II receptor blockers, an angiotensin receptor-neprilysin inhibitor, and β-blockers in patients with heart failure with reduced EF.

2. Research the topic of diuretic resistance, and be able to describe the phenomenon and methods used to overcome it.

CLINICAL PEARL

The presence of pitting edema is associated with a substantial increase in body weight; it typically takes a weight gain of 10 lb to result in the development of pitting edema.

REFERENCES

1. Heidenreich PA, Bozkurt B, Aguilar D, et al. 2022 AHA/ACC/HFSA guideline for the management of heart failure: a report of the American College of Cardiology/American Heart Association Joint Committee on Clinical Practice Guidelines. J Cardiac Fail. 2022;28:E1–E167. doi: 10.1016/j.cardfail.2022.02.010.

2. McMurray JV, Packer M, Desai AS, et al for the PARADIGM-HF Investigators and Committees. Angiotensin-neprilysin inhibition versus enalapril in heart failure. N Engl J Med. 2014;371:993–1004.

3. Packer M, Anker SD, Butler J, et al for the EMPEROR-Reduced Trial Investigators. Cardiovascular and renal outcomes with empagliflozin in heart failure. N Engl J Med. 2020;383:1413–1424. doi: 10.1056/NEJMoa2022190.

4. McMurray JJV, Solomon SD, Inzucchi SE, et al for the DAPA-HF Trial Committees and Investigators. Dapagliflozin in patients with heart failure and reduced ejection fraction. N Engl J Med. 2019;381:1995–2008. doi: 10.1056/NEJMoa1911303.

5. Taylor AL, Ziesche S, Yancy C, et al for the African-American Heart Failure Trial Investigators. Combination of isosorbide dinitrate and hydralazine in blacks with heart failure. N Engl J Med. 2004;351:2049–2057.

6. Swedberg K, Komajda M, Bohm M, et al. Ivabradine and outcomes in chronic heart failure (SHIFT): a randomised placebo-controlled study. Lancet. 2010;367:875–885.

7. Page RL, O'Bryant CL, Cheng D, et al. Drugs that may cause or exacerbate heart failure: a scientific statement from the American Heart Association. Circulation. 2016;134:e32–e69.

8. American Diabetes Association. Cardiovascular disease and risk management: standards of medical care in diabetes—2022. Diabetes Care. 2022;45(1 Suppl):S144–S174.

19

HEART FAILURE WITH PRESERVED EJECTION FRACTION

A Balancing Act. . . . . Level II

Joel C. Marrs, PharmD, MPH, FAHA, FASHP, FCCP, FNLA, BCACP, BCCP, BCPS, CLS

Sarah L. Anderson, PharmD, FASHP, FCCP, BCACP, BCPS

LEARNING OBJECTIVES

After completing this case study, the reader should be able to:

- Recognize the signs and symptoms of heart failure with preserved ejection fraction (HFpEF).

- Develop a pharmacotherapeutic plan for treatment of HFpEF.

- Outline a monitoring plan for HFpEF that includes both clinical and laboratory parameters.

- Initiate, titrate, and monitor guideline-directed medical therapy (GDMT) in HFpEF when indicated.

PATIENT PRESENTATION

■ Chief Complaint

"Why can't we get my weight stabilized?"

■ HPI

A 67-year-old man who presents to the ED with shortness of breath and bilateral lower extremity edema. He reports his symptoms started approximately 3 weeks ago. He noted that he was gaining about 1–2 lb daily and gained approximately 25 lb of weight over the month prior to admission. He attempted to use his albuterol/ipratropium MDI for relief of his shortness of breath symptoms at home without improvement. As his symptoms of edema and shortness of breath worsened, he called his primary care physician, who increased his furosemide dose over the phone to 80 mg twice daily more than 1 week ago. In the ED, he was noted to be hypoxic with an increased oxygen need from 2 to 4 L by nasal cannula. He was given one dose of IV furosemide 80 mg with minimal improvement in his symptoms and then admitted to the medicine service for further evaluation and management.

■ PMH

CAD (s/p STEMI 10 years ago)
COPD × 5 years
HFpEF × 6 years (last hospitalization 4 months ago)
Dyslipidemia × 15 years
HTN × 25 years
Type 2 DM × 5 years

■ FH

Father is alive at age 88 with type 2 DM; mother is alive at age 87 and has HTN and dyslipidemia; two brothers (age 60 and 64) are alive, and both have type 2 DM and HTN.

■ SH

History of tobacco use (40 pack-year history) but quit 5 years ago. Denies any alcohol or substance abuse. Lives alone.

■ Meds

Albuterol/ipratropium MDI, two puffs inhaled Q 6 H PRN
Aspirin 81 mg PO daily
Clopidogrel 75 mg PO daily
Lisinopril 40 mg PO daily
Carvedilol 12.5 mg PO BID
Furosemide 80 mg PO BID (previously 40 mg PO BID)
Amlodipine 5 mg PO daily
Metformin 1000 mg PO BID
Nitroglycerin 0.4 mg SL q 5 minutes PRN chest pain
Potassium chloride 20 mEq PO daily
Rosuvastatin 20 mg PO daily
Seasonal influenza vaccine (previous year)

■ All

NKDA

■ ROS

Gen

Patient reports a recent 25-lb weight gain over the past month

CV

No complaints of chest pain

Resp

Reports an increase in shortness of breath from baseline over the last month and dyspnea on exertion

GI

No recent changes noted in bowel habits

GU

No complaints

MS

No complaints of MS pain or weakness

Neuro

No complaints

■ Physical Examination

Gen

Patient with 25-lb weight gain over past month with increased shortness of breath

VS

BP 150/82, P 64 (regular), RR 26, T 36.9°C; Wt 102 kg (usual weight 90 kg), Ht 5'10", oxygen saturation of 95% on 4-L nasal cannula

Skin

Chronic venous stasis changes on bilateral lower extremities and 3+ edema to the knees bilaterally

HEENT

PERRLA, EOMI, fundi were not examined. Normocephalic, atraumatic. Nasal cannula in place.

Neck

(+) JVD at 30° (6 cm). No carotid bruit is appreciated. No lymphadenopathy or thyromegaly.

Lungs/Thorax

Respirations are even. Crackles noted in the bilateral lung bases.

Heart

RRR. No murmurs, rubs, or gallops.

Abd

Obese with a nontender, nondistended abdomen; hypoactive bowel sounds

Genit/Rect

Guaiac (–), genital examination not performed

MS/Ext

3+ pitting pedal edema bilaterally; radial and pedal pulses are of poor intensity bilaterally; grip strength even

Neuro

A&O × 3; CNs intact; DTR intact

■ Labs

Na 138 mEq/L	Hgb 15.3 g/dL	Mg 1.7 mEq/L	CK 20 IU/L
K 4.0 mEq/L	Hct 47.2%	Ca 9.1 mg/dL	CK-MB 0.8 IU/L
Cl 103 mEq/L	Plt 298 × 10³/mm³	AST 60 IU/L	PT 12.6 s
CO₂ 26 mEq/L	WBC 6.4 × 10³/mm³	ALT 60 IU/L	INR 1.1
BUN 30 mg/dL	Troponin I 0.5 ng/mL	Alk phos 80 IU/L	TSH 1.12 mIU/L
SCr 1.2 mg/dL		GGT 24 IU/L	A1C 7.5%
Glucose		T. bili 0.2 mg/dL	
108 mg/dL			
BNP 2000 pg/mL			

■ ECG

Sinus rate of 66; QRS 0.08; no ST–T wave changes; low voltage

■ CXR

PA and lateral views show evidence of interstitial edema and some early alveolar edema.

■ Assessment

Decompensated heart failure with pulmonary and lower extremity edema

■ CLINICAL COURSE

The patient was admitted to a telemetry unit. The patient has a known history of HFpEF (EF 52%) per an echocardiogram from 6 months ago. A 2D echocardiogram was obtained today to evaluate the patient's current LV and valvular function. Results revealed evidence of impaired ventricular relaxation and elevated left atrial filling pressures consistent with grade III diastolic dysfunction. EF was estimated at 53%; there was no evidence of mitral stenosis or pericardial disease. A dilated inferior vena cava suggests increased right atrial pressure. Moderate pulmonary HTN is evident.

QUESTIONS

Collect Information

1.a. What subjective and objective information indicates the presence of HFpEF?

1.b. What additional information is needed to fully assess this patient's HFpEF?

Assess the Information

2.a. Assess the severity of HFpEF based on subjective and objective information available.

2.b. Create a list of the patient's drug therapy problems and prioritize them. Include assessment of medication appropriateness, effectiveness, safety, and patient adherence.

2.c. What economic, psychosocial, cultural, racial, and ethnic considerations are applicable to this patient?

Develop a Care Plan

3.a. What are the goals of pharmacotherapy for HFpEF in this case?

3.b. What nondrug therapies might be useful for this patient's HFpEF?

3.c. What feasible pharmacotherapeutic options are available for treating this patient's HFpEF?

3.d. Create an individualized, patient-centered, team-based care plan to optimize medication therapy for this patient's HFpEF and other drug therapy problems. Include specific drugs, dosage forms, doses, schedules, and durations of therapy.

Implement the Care Plan

4.a. What information should be provided to the patient to enhance adherence, ensure successful therapy, and minimize adverse effects?

4.b. Describe how care should be coordinated with other healthcare providers.

Follow-Up: Monitor and Evaluate

5. Explain how to monitor and evaluate the care plan for medication appropriateness, effectiveness, safety and patient adherence by using clinical and laboratory data, patient feedback and other information.

SELF-STUDY ASSIGNMENTS

1. Describe the common causes of HFpEF.

2. Describe how you would evaluate and monitor this patient's quality of life.

3. Evaluate whether evidence exists to support the role of ARNIs in HFpEF.

CLINICAL PEARL

Patients with HF often have co-morbid type 2 DM. In recent years, there has been demonstrated benefit for the role of SGLT2 inhibitors in further reducing risk of CV events in patients with established CVD and type 2 DM. Now evidence also exists regarding the benefit of SGLT2 inhibitors in reducing the risk of CV death and hospitalizations for HF in patients with heart failure with reduced ejection fraction (HFrEF) (dapagliflozin and empagliflozin) and HFpEF (empagliflozin), regardless of whether the patient has diabetes. The 2022 AHA/ACC/HFSA heart failure guideline recommends SGLT2 inhibitors as GDMT in patients with HFrEF and also recommends the use of SGLT2 inhibitors for patients with heart failure with mildly reduced ejection fraction (HFmrEF) and HFpEF.

REFERENCES

1. Tang WH, Francis GS, Morrow DA, et al. National Academy of Clinical Biochemistry Laboratory Medicine Practice Guidelines: clinical utilization of cardiac biomarker testing in heart failure. Circulation. 2007;116:e99–e109.

2. Heidenreich PA, Bozkurt B, Aguilar D, et al. 2022 AHA/ACC/HFSA guideline for the management of heart failure: a report of the American College of Cardiology/American Heart Association Joint Committee on Clinical Practice Guidelines. Circulation. 2022;145(18):e895–e1032. doi: 10.1161/CIR.0000000000001063.

3. Grundy SM, Stone NJ, Bailey AL, et al. 2018 AHA/ACC/AACVPR/AAPA/ABC/ACPM/ADA/AGS/APhA/ASPC/NLA/PCNA guideline on the management of blood cholesterol: a report of the American College of Cardiology/American Heart Association Task Force on Clinical Practice Guidelines. J Am Coll Cardiol. 2019;73(24):e285–e350.

4. Basaraba JE, Barry AR. Pharmacotherapy of heart failure with preserved ejection fraction. Pharmacotherapy. 2015;35:351–360.

5. Hernandez AF, Hammill BG, O'Connor CM, Schulman KA, Curtis LH, Fonarow GC. Clinical effectiveness of beta-blockers in heart failure: findings from the OPTIMIZE-HF (organized program to initiate lifesaving treatment in hospitalized patients with heart failure) registry. J Am Coll Cardiol. 2009;53:184–192.

6. Nichols GA, Reynolds K, Kimes TM, Rosales AG, Chan WW. Comparison of risk of re-hospitalization, all-cause mortality, and medical care resource utilization in patients with heart failure and preserved versus reduced ejection fraction. Am J Cardiol. 2015;116:1088–1092.

7. Pitt B, Pfeffer MA, Assmann SF, et al. Spironolactone for heart failure with preserved ejection fraction. N Engl J Med. 2014;370:1383–1392.

8. Solomon SD, McMurray JJV, Anand IS, et al. Angiotensin–neprilysin inhibition in heart failure with preserved ejection fraction. N Engl J Med. 2019;381:1609–1620.

9. Anker SD, Butler J, Filippatos G, et al. Empagliflozin in heart failure with a preserved ejection fraction. N Engl J Med. 2021;385:1451–1461.

10. Mentz RJ, Wojdyla D, Fiuzat M, et al. Association of beta-blocker use and selectivity with outcomes in patients with heart failure and chronic obstructive pulmonary disease (from OPTIMIZE-HF). Am J Cardiol. 2013;111:582–587.

20

ACUTELY DECOMPENSATED HEART FAILURE

Don't Be Such a Busy Body .... Level II

Kena J. Lanham, PharmD, BCPS, BCGP, BCCP

LEARNING OBJECTIVES

After completing this case study, the reader should be able to:

- Identify the signs and symptoms of acutely decompensated heart failure (ADHF).

- Classify a patient into the appropriate hemodynamic subset based on symptoms and clinical presentation.

- List goals of therapy for treating ADHF.

- Develop a pharmacotherapeutic plan for treating a patient with ADHF in the hemodynamic subset presented.

- Outline a monitoring plan for treating a patient with ADHF in the hospital.

PATIENT PRESENTATION

■ Chief Complaint

"I can no longer lie down flat, because I can't breathe, and I've gained 5 pounds in 3 days."

■ HPI

A 64-year-old woman with a history of ischemic cardiomyopathy with last known EF 25% (ECHO 1.5 years ago) presents to the emergency department with approximately 2–3 days of increasing shortness of breath and reports having gained approximately 5 lb over the past 3 days. The patient also notes increasing leg swelling over the same time period. Over the past week, the patient has noted increasing bloating in her abdomen and has felt slightly nauseated. She states that she had been on torsemide many years ago but for an unknown reason was switched to furosemide.

■ PMH

CAD (status post myocardial infarction × 2 in early 2000s; CABG in 2000, PCI in May 2002)
Dyslipidemia
Mild osteoarthritis

■ FH

Both her mother and father died of MI in their 60s.

■ SH

Patient is a happily married, retired school teacher and is fully functional with ADLs. The patient drinks alcohol occasionally (two to three drinks per week) and has a 30 pack-year history, but quit smoking approximately 12 years ago.

■ Meds

Aspirin 81 mg orally once daily
Carvedilol 12.5 mg orally BID

Fluticasone nasal spray 50 mcg one spray BID
Lasix 80 mg orally BID
Valsartan 80 mg orally twice daily
Meloxicam 15 mg orally daily PRN joint pain
Nitroglycerin 0.4 mg sublingually PRN chest pain
Atorvastatin 40 mg orally QHS

■ All

NKDA

■ ROS

The patient denies any fevers, chills, sweats, or coughs. The patient's diet has not changed recently, is mindful of salt intake, but admits nonadherence to her medication regimen for the past 2 days, stating, "I have been too busy to take my medicine." No significant chest pain or any additional coronary intervention procedures since 2002. All others negative.

■ Physical Examination

Gen

A 64-year-old obese woman in mild respiratory distress

VS

BP 186/92 mm Hg, P 68 bpm, RR 32 on admission (16 currently), oxygen saturation 86–92%; T 97.5°F; Ht 5′3″; Wt 87.4 kg

Skin

Warm and diaphoretic

HEENT

NC/AT with trachea midline

Neck/Lymph Nodes

Neck supple, (+) JVD, no bruits, no thyromegaly

Lungs/Thorax

Crackles in the bases bilaterally

CV

Regular rate and rhythm without any murmurs, gallops, or rubs

Abd

Soft, nondistended, nontender

Genit/Rect

Deferred

MS/Ext

Extremities reveal 2+ pitting edema; all pulses palpable

Neuro

A&O × 3, CNs intact

■ Labs

Na 131 mEq/L	BNP 2867 pg/mL
K 3.7 mEq/L	Troponin 0.03 ng/mL
Cl 101 mEq/L	WBC $8.7 \times 10^3/mm^3$
CO_2 20 mEq/L	Hgb 14.1 g/dL
BUN 24 mg/dL	Hct 42.3%
SCr 1.7 mg/dL	Plt $226 \times 10^3/mm^3$
Glu 96 mg/dL	A1C 6.5%
Ca 9.6 mg/dL	

■ Chest X-Ray

Interstitial infiltrates throughout, tiny pleural effusions bilaterally; mild cardiomegaly; implanted defibrillator leads are at the right atrial appendage and right ventricular apex. No focal pneumonia, pneumothorax, or evidence of frank pulmonary edema.

■ ECG

Sinus rhythm with occasional premature ventricular complexes; no acute ischemia indicated

■ Assessment

Congestive heart failure exacerbation due to medication non-adherence; poorly controlled hypertension. Admit for medical management.

QUESTIONS

Collect Information

1.a. What subjective and objective information indicates the presence of ADHF?

1.b. What additional information is needed to fully assess this patient's ADHF?

Assess the Information

2.a. Assess the severity of ADHF based on the subjective and objective information available.

2.b. Create a list of the patient's drug therapy problems and prioritize them. Include assessment of medication appropriateness, effectiveness, safety, and patient adherence.

Develop a Care Plan

3.a. What are the goals of pharmacotherapy for ADHF in this case?

3.b. What nondrug therapies might be useful for alleviating this patient's symptoms and preventing a recurrence of ADHF?

3.c. What feasible pharmacotherapeutic options are available for treatment of this patient's ADHF?

3.d. Create an individualized, patient-centered, team-based care plan to optimize medication therapy for this patient's heart failure and other drug therapy problems. Include specific drugs, dosage forms, doses, schedules, and durations of therapy.

Implement the Care Plan

4.a. What information should be provided to the patient to enhance adherence, ensure successful therapy, and minimize adverse effects?

4.b. Describe how care should be coordinated with other healthcare providers.

Follow-Up: Monitor and Evaluate

5. Explain how to monitor and evaluate the care plan for medication appropriateness, effectiveness, safety and patient adherence by using clinical and laboratory data, patient feedback and other information.

■ SELF-STUDY ASSIGNMENTS

1. Review the current heart failure treatment guidelines, and create a table highlighting the patient characteristics that necessitate

hospital admission versus those that are conducive to treatment in the outpatient setting.

2. List all Heart Failure National Hospital Inpatient Quality Measures (core measures) that must be fulfilled prior to discharge.

3. Review the available literature on prognostic indicators in heart failure, and create a list of prognostic indicators for readmission or mortality in patients with heart failure.

4. Contrast the pharmacotherapeutic plan developed in this case with that of a pharmacotherapeutic plan for a patient presenting with heart failure with preserved EF.

CLINICAL PEARL

Close follow-up after discharge is crucial as the patient transitions from hospital acute care to outpatient continuing care to ensure adherence to the prescribed medication and dietary regimens. The healthcare provider must be vigilant in securing the continued access of the newer agents shown to improve mortality and morbidity, such as ARNIs and SGLT-2 inhibitors, as they present a challenge with their significantly higher costs compared to the older agents.

REFERENCES

1. Heidenreich PA, Bozkurt B, Aguilar D, et al. 2022 AHA/ACC/HFSA guideline for the management of heart failure: a report of the American College of Cardiology/American Heart Association Joint Committee on Clinical Practice Guidelines. J Am Coll Cardiol. 2022;79(17):e263–e421.
2. Bumetanide Package Insert. Deerfield, IL, Baxter Healthcare, 2009.
3. Furosemide Package Insert. Lake Forest, IL, Hospira Incorporated, 2004.
4. Torsemide Package Insert. Somerset, NJ, Meda Pharmaceuticals, 2009.
5. Felker GM, Lee KL, Bull DA, et al. Diuretic strategies in patients with acute decompensated heart failure. N Engl J Med. 2011;364:797–805.

21

DEEP VEIN THROMBOSIS

Trouble From Deep Within . . . . Level II

Brecon Powell, PharmD

LEARNING OBJECTIVES

After completing this case study, the reader should be able to:

- Define acute deep vein thrombosis (DVT), and discuss its pathophysiology.
- Discuss the clinical presentation of patients with a DVT.
- Develop a pharmacotherapeutic care plan for the management of a patient with a DVT.
- Educate a patient receiving anticoagulation therapy for the treatment of a DVT.

PATIENT PRESENTATION

Chief Complaint

"I'm having pain in my leg."

HPI

A 51-year-old man who presents to his primary care physician because of pain in his right leg. He states that he awoke with the pain 3 days ago and that it has been continuous, although it hurts more when he walks. The pain is located behind his right knee and extends down into his calf. He rates the pain intensity as 3/10 at this time. The patient denies CP and SOB. He denies recent travel, immobility, and leg injury. The patient started atorvastatin 40 mg daily for treatment of dyslipidemia approximately 3 months prior to this visit. He stopped the atorvastatin 3 days ago because he thought it might be causing his leg pain, but the pain has continued.

PMH

Hypertension
Dyslipidemia
Graves disease with thyroid ablation
Gout
Left ankle fracture 9 years ago that required a cast but no surgery
Remote history of depression

PSH

Left herniorrhaphy about 10 years ago. Pilonidal cyst excision in remote past.

FH

Father died at age 81 of liver failure. Mother, one brother, and son all alive and well. No family history of venous thromboembolism or clotting disorders.

SH

Married, one adult child. Drinks one to two alcoholic beverages daily. Smokes ½ pack per day of cigarettes but trying to quit. Denies illicit drug use.

Meds

Allopurinol 300 mg PO once daily
Lisinopril 10 mg PO once daily
Levothyroxine 150 mcg PO once daily
Aspirin 81 mg PO daily
Atorvastatin 20 mg PO once daily (discontinued 3 days ago)

All

NKDA

ROS

Constitutional: No chills, no fatigue.
Eyes: No eye pain or changes in vision.
ENT: No sore throat.
Skin: No pigmentation changes, no nail changes.
Cardiovascular: No CP, palpitations, or syncope.
Respiratory: No cough, SOB, wheezing, or stridor.
GI: No abdominal pain, nausea, diarrhea, or vomiting.
Musculoskeletal: No neck pain, back pain, or injury.
Neurologic: No dizziness, headache, or focal weakness.
Psychiatric/behavioral: Remote history of depression. Not a current problem.

■ Physical Examination

Gen

Somewhat overweight man in NAD. Cooperative, A&O × 3, normal affect.

VS

BP 125/76, P 75 regular, RR 16, T 98.3°F, O$_2$ sat 97%/RA; Wt 220 lb, Ht 6'0"

Skin

Warm, dry, normal color. No rash or induration.

HEENT

Pupils equal and reactive to light. EOM intact. Mucous membranes moist and pink.

Neck

Normal range of motion with no meningeal signs

Lungs/Thorax

Breath sounds normal, no respiratory distress

CV

RRR, no rubs, murmurs, or gallops

Abd

Nontender, no masses, no distension, no peritoneal signs

MS/Ext

Upper extremities: Normal by inspection, no CCE, normal ROM. Lower extremities: Right calf tight, warm to touch, and tender with 1+ pretibial pitting edema. LLE without redness, warmth, and swelling. Lower extremity pulses and sensation are normal bilaterally. Normal ROM.

Neuro

Glasgow coma scale of 15, no focal motor deficits, no focal sensory deficits

■ Labs

Na 140 mEq/L	WBC 5.9 × 10³/μL	AST 16 IU/L
K 3.9 mEq/L	RBC 4.28 × 10⁶/μL	ALT 20 IU/L
Cl 103 mEq/L	Hgb 13.5 g/dL	Alk phos 67 IU/L
CO$_2$ 27 mEq/L	Hct 39.3%	GGT 20 IU/L
BUN 10 mg/dL	Platelets 175 × 10³/μL	Lipid panel (fasting)
SCr 0.84 mg/dL	CK 117 IU/L	TC 180 mg/dL
Glucose 88 mg/dL	INR 1.0	HDL 30 mg/dL
Uric acid 5.0 mg/dL	PT 11.4 seconds	Trig 250 mg/dL
	aPTT 34.8 seconds	LDL 100 mg/dL

Lower extremity venous duplex ultrasonography: Acute DVT of right distal superficial femoral, popliteal, and peroneal veins. No compression or flow in these vessels.

(**Note to reader:** *The "superficial femoral vein" is actually a deep vein, in spite of its name. Use of the name "femoral vein" is preferred because it is less confusing. However, the name "superficial femoral vein" is still encountered, as it is in this patient's venous duplex report.*)

■ Assessment

Acute DVT in right distal femoral, popliteal, and peroneal veins

QUESTIONS

Collect Information

1.a. What subjective and objective information indicates the presence of DVT?

1.b. What additional information is needed to fully assess this patient's DVT?

Assess the Information

2.a. Assess the severity of an acute DVT based on the subjective and objective information available.

2.b. Create a list of the patient's drug therapy problems and prioritize them. Include assessment of medication appropriateness, effectiveness, safety, and patient adherence.

Develop a Care Plan

3.a. What are the goals of pharmacotherapy for DVT in this case?

3.b. What nondrug therapies might be useful for this patient's DVT?

3.c. What feasible pharmacotherapeutic options are available for treating this patient's DVT?

3.d. To keep medication costs low, the clinician and patient agree to start warfarin therapy to manage the patient's DVT. Design a treatment plan for the initial management of this patient's DVT and other drug therapy problems. Include specific dosage forms, doses, schedules, and durations of therapy.

Implement the Care Plan

4.a. What information should be provided for this patient to enhance adherence, ensure successful therapy, and minimize adverse effects?

4.b. Describe how care should be coordinated with other healthcare providers.

Follow-Up: Monitor and Evaluate

5. Explain how to monitor and evaluate the care plan for medication appropriateness, effectiveness, safety and patient adherence by using clinical and laboratory data, patient feedback and other information.

■ CLINICAL COURSE (PART 1)

The patient presents to his PCP 3 days after his first visit. He has been administering his injections and taking warfarin 5 mg daily, as instructed. He continues to experience RLE pain and swelling, but these symptoms are somewhat improved. He denies new CP or SOB. He reports no missed warfarin doses, no changes in his other medications, a diet with consistent vitamin K intake, no change in his alcohol intake, and no acute health problems. He denies bruising and bleeding, other than minor bruising related to his injections. His INR is 1.7.

■ FOLLOW-UP QUESTION

1.a. Identify the patient's anticoagulation therapy-related problem(s), and design treatment and monitoring plans for managing each problem you identify.

■ CLINICAL COURSE (PART 2)

The patient presents to his PCP's office approximately 2 months after his acute DVT episode. He reports that he experienced an

TABLE 21-1	Thrombophilia Test Results	
Test	Result	Reference Interval
Antithrombin III (% activity)	101	85–118
Protein C (% activity)	122	72–220
Protein S (% activity)	111	50–168
Factor V Leiden mutation	Negative	Normal: negative
Prothrombin G-20210-A mutation	Negative	Normal: negative
Anticardiolipin antibodies IgG (GPL units)	5.0	0.0–15.0
Anticardiolipin antibodies IgM (MPL units)	<4.7	0.0–12.5
Thrombin time (s)	15.5	13.0–20.0
DRVVT (s)	63.2	35.0–47.0
DRVVT confirm (s)	36.3	—
DRVVT ratio	1.74	1.10–1.41
StaClot LA	Positive	Normal: negative
Homocysteine, plasma (µmol/L)	10.0	3.7–13.9

episode of very dark brown, "cola"-colored urine 2 days before this visit. He has had no recurrences. The patient denies dysuria, back or groin pain, and blood in his bowel movements. His current dose of warfarin is 2.5 mg on Monday, Wednesday, Friday, and Saturday, and 5 mg on Tuesday, Thursday, and Sunday. Physical examination reveals no CVA tenderness. His INR is 2.3.

■ FOLLOW-UP QUESTION

1.b. Identify the patient's anticoagulation therapy-related problem(s), and design treatment and monitoring plans for managing each problem you identify.

■ CLINICAL COURSE (PART 3)

Three months after his initial presentation, you see the patient in the new anticoagulation clinic at his primary care physician's office. He is currently taking warfarin 2.5 mg on Monday, Wednesday, Friday, and Saturday, and 5 mg on Tuesday, Thursday, and Sunday. His INR is 4.3. The patient's INR 4 weeks ago was 2.3 on the same warfarin dose. The patient has not experienced any symptoms suggesting DVT recurrence or PE occurrence. He states that he has not had any problem with bleeding, has not missed doses or taken extra doses of warfarin in the last month, and has not changed his diet or alcohol intake. His medications have been unchanged, except for a switch from atorvastatin 20 mg daily to rosuvastatin 10 mg daily for the treatment of his dyslipidemia approximately 2–3 weeks ago. You note that the thrombophilia tests given in Table 21-1 were completed prior to the initiation of anticoagulation therapy.

The laboratory summarizes the results in Table 21-1 as consistent with the presence of lupus anticoagulants.

■ FOLLOW-UP QUESTION

1.c. Identify this patient's anticoagulation therapy-related problem(s), and design a treatment and monitoring plan for each problem

that you identify. Be sure to specify the anticipated duration of his anticoagulation therapy.

■ SELF-STUDY ASSIGNMENTS

1. Create a summary of antiphospholipid syndrome, including its definition, clinical presentation, and management.

2. Summarize the existing literature regarding the effects of various statins on response to warfarin. Does warfarin alter the effect of statins?

CLINICAL PEARL

Current guidelines propose long-term anticoagulation (up to 3 months) over anticoagulation for a shorter period of time. Longer treatment courses (eg, 6, 12, or 24 months) or extended therapy (no scheduled stop date) are recommended for patients with a proximal DVT, isolated distal DVT, or PE provoked by surgery/nonsurgical transient risk factors. Extended therapy is recommended in patients with an unprovoked proximal DVT of the leg or PE, or second unprovoked VTE with a low or moderate risk of bleed. Use of anticoagulation should be reassessed annually in all patients who receive extended anticoagulation therapy.

ACKNOWLEDGMENT

This case is based on the patient case written for the 11th edition by Sally A. Arif, PharmD, BCPS-AQ Cardiology and Tran Tran, PharmD, BCPS.

REFERENCES

1. Kearon C, Akl EA, Ornelas J, et al. Antithrombotic therapy for VTE disease: CHEST Guideline and Expert Panel Report. Chest. 2016;149(2):315–352.

2. Robertson L, Kesteven P, McCaslin JE. Oral direct thrombin inhibitors or oral factor Xa inhibitors for the treatment of deep vein thrombosis. Cochrane Database Syst Rev. 2015;6:CD010956.

3. Schulman S, Kearon C, Kakkar AK; for the RE-COVER Study Group. Dabigatran versus warfarin in the treatment of acute venous thromboembolism. N Engl J Med. 2009;361(24):2342–2352.

4. Schulman S, Kakkar AK, Goldhaber SZ; for the RE-COVER II Trial Investigators. Treatment of acute venous thromboembolism with dabigatran or warfarin and pooled analysis. Circulation. 2014;129(7):764–772.

5. Garcia DA, Baglin TP, Weitz JI, Samama MM. Parenteral anticoagulants: Antithrombotic Therapy and Prevention of Thrombosis, 9th ed: American College of Chest Physicians Evidence-Based Clinical Practice Guidelines. Chest. 2012;141(Suppl):e24S–e43S.

6. Van Dongen CJ, MacGillavry MR, Prins MH. Once versus twice daily LMWH for the initial treatment of venous thromboembolism. Cochrane Database Syst Rev. 2005;3:CD003074.

7. Stern A, Abel R, Gibson GL, et al. Atorvastatin does not alter the anticoagulant activity of warfarin. J Clin Pharmacol. 1997;37:1062–1064.

8. Simonson SG, Martin PD, Mitchell PD, et al. Effect of rosuvastatin on warfarin pharmacodynamics and pharmacokinetics. J Clin Pharmacol. 2005;45(8):927–934.

9. Tripodi A, de Groot PG, Pengo V. Antiphospholipid syndrome: laboratory detection, mechanisms of action and treatment. J Intern Med. 2011;270(2):110–122.

22

PULMONARY EMBOLISM

HIT Can Happen .... Level III

Kristen L. Longstreth, PharmD, BCPS

Mary E. Fredrickson, PharmD, BCPS

LEARNING OBJECTIVES

After completing this case study, the reader should be able to:

- Identify the signs, symptoms, and risk factors associated with pulmonary embolism (PE).

- Evaluate a patient for heparin-induced thrombocytopenia (HIT).

- Select an appropriate anticoagulant for the treatment of PE complicated by HIT.

- Monitor anticoagulation therapy for the treatment of PE complicated by HIT.

- Educate a patient on anticoagulation therapy.

PATIENT PRESENTATION

■ Chief Complaint

"I'm having chest pain, and I can't catch my breath."

■ HPI

A 70-year-old woman arrives at the hospital's emergency department by ambulance transfer from her home. The patient is S/P right TKR (postoperative day 10) for severe osteoarthritis. She was discharged from the hospital's orthopedic nursing unit 4 days ago with a prescription for enoxaparin for DVT prophylaxis. The patient was scheduled to receive physical therapy at a local rehabilitation center; however, she canceled therapy due to pain. She has been inactive at home except for completing her activities of daily living with the assistance of her husband. This morning, the patient developed sharp chest pain and shortness of breath while watching television. She denies nausea, vomiting, and diaphoresis. The patient has a nonproductive cough. She is anxious and complains of pain in her right knee and right lower extremity.

■ PMH

HTN × 30 years
Dyslipidemia × 25 years
Chronic stable angina × 2 years (negative regadenoson stress test 2 months ago)
CKD secondary to previously uncontrolled HTN, stage 4 (baseline creatinine 1.8–2.0 mg/dL)
Osteoarthritis
Obesity
S/P TKR right leg (postoperative day 10)

■ FH

Father died at age 74 (lung CA)
Mother died at age 89 (MI)
No siblings

■ SH

The patient is retired. She lives at home with her husband. Prior to surgery, she avoided most physical activity due to severe osteoarthritis. Negative for tobacco abuse. Denies alcohol use.

■ Meds

Home medications

Aspirin 81 mg PO once daily
Metoprolol succinate 100 mg PO daily
Amlodipine 10 mg PO once daily
Hydralazine 50 mg PO TID
Rosuvastatin 20 mg PO once daily
Nitroglycerin 0.4 mg sublingually PRN chest pain
Sevelamer carbonate 1600 mg PO TID with meals
Enoxaparin 30 mg subcutaneously Q 24 hours
Oxycodone sustained release 20 mg PO Q 12 hours
Oxycodone immediate release 5 mg PO Q 6 hours PRN pain
Docusate 100 mg PO QHS
Sennosides 17.2 mg PO QHS

■ All

Lisinopril (angioedema)

■ ROS

Positive for shortness of breath and nonproductive cough. Positive for sharp chest pain at rest. The pain does not radiate and is not reproducible by touch. No palpitations, diaphoresis, nausea, vomiting, or diarrhea. The patient denies headache, fever, and chills. Pain rated by patient as 9/10 in chest and 7/10 in right knee and lower extremity.

■ Physical Examination

Gen

Moderate respiratory distress

VS

BP 128/68, P 101, RR 21, T 36.9°C; Wt 85 kg, Ht 5′4″, O$_2$ sat 88% on RA

Skin

Warm and dry; no rashes

HEENT

Head: atraumatic; PERRLA; EOMI

Neck/Lymph Nodes

No carotid bruits; no lymphadenopathy; no thyromegaly

Lungs/Thorax

CTA; no wheezing or crackles

Breasts

WNL

CV

Tachycardia with regular rhythm; normal heart sounds; no MRG

Abd

Obese, soft; NT/ND; +BS; no organomegaly

Genit/Rect

WNL

MS/Ext

S/P TKR right leg; right lower extremity ROM limited with slight redness, warmth, and edema; pain in right knee and right lower extremity

Neuro

A&O × 3; no focal deficits noted; cranial nerves intact

■ Labs (Nonfasting)

Na 140 mEq/L	Mg 2.1 mEq/L	T. chol 135 mg/dL	D-dimer 975 ng/mL
K 4.5 mEq/L	Phos 4.4 mg/dL	LDL 67 mg/dL	Cardiac enzymes,
Cl 105 mEq/L	Ca 8.9 mg/dL	HDL 42 mg/dL	time 1245
CO_2 26 mEq/L	Alb 3.5 g/dL	TG 130 mg/dL	CK 67 IU/L
BUN 35 mg/dL	AST 18 IU/L	Hgb 12.1 g/dL	CK-MB 1.1 IU/L
SCr 1.8 mg/dL	ALT 12 IU/L	Hct 36.5%	Troponin I
Glu 106 mg/dL	Alk Phos	Plt 72 × 10^3/mm^3	0.03 ng/mL
A1C 5.5%	57 IU/L	WBC 6 × 10^3/mm^3	

■ ECG

Sinus tachycardia. No T wave or ST changes present.

■ Venous Doppler Ultrasound of Right Lower Extremity

Occlusive DVT from the right popliteal vein to the right common femoral vein

■ Chest X-Ray

No evidence of acute cardiopulmonary disease

■ Assessment

1. Chest pain, SOB—history of chronic stable angina; R/O ACS, R/O PE
2. Right lower extremity DVT
3. Thrombocytopenia—R/O HIT
4. S/P TKR right leg for severe osteoarthritis (postoperative day 10)—not infected, pain not controlled
5. CKD—stage 4, creatinine at patient's baseline
6. HTN—stable on current regimen
7. Dyslipidemia—stable on current regimen

QUESTIONS

Collect Information

1.a. What subjective and objective information is consistent with a diagnosis of PE for this patient?

1.b. What risk factors for PE are present for this patient?

1.c. What additional information is needed to fully assess this patient?

■ CLINICAL COURSE (PART 1)

The patient is admitted to a telemetry nursing unit within the hospital for treatment of the DVT and further workup for chest pain and shortness of breath (Table 22-1). A V/Q scan is ordered. The patient's medical chart from the previous admission is reviewed to obtain a more complete medication and laboratory history (Table 22-2).

TABLE 22-1	Cardiac Enzymes (Second Set; Time: 1905)
CK 45 IU/L	
CK-MB 0.7 IU/L	
Troponin I 0.02 ng/mL	

While completing the admission medication reconciliation, a hospital provider discontinues enoxaparin and restarts the patient's other home medications. The provider also orders the following: consult pharmacist to dose and monitor fondaparinux and warfarin; morphine 2 mg IV Q 6 hours PRN severe pain (pain score of 7–10).

■ V/Q SCAN

Multiple segmental perfusion defects, indicating a ventilation–perfusion mismatch and high probability of PE (Fig. 22-1).

Assess the Information

2.a. Assess the severity of the patient's PE based on the subjective and objective information available.

2.b. Create a list of the patient's drug therapy problems and prioritize them. Include assessment of medication appropriateness, effectiveness, safety, and patient adherence.

2.c. Discuss the process to confirm or rule out a suspected diagnosis of HIT.

■ CLINICAL COURSE (PART 2)

A heparin-induced platelet antibody ELISA is drawn and sent to an outside laboratory. An order is written to avoid all heparin (including heparin catheter flushes). Prior to initiating anticoagulation, a baseline aPTT (32.7 seconds; hospital laboratory's normal range is 25–40 seconds), PT (10.8 seconds), and INR (1.0) are obtained to assist with anticoagulation dosing. The nursing unit notifies the pharmacist of the consultation order to dose and monitor fondaparinux and warfarin.

Develop a Care Plan

3.a. What are the goals of pharmacotherapy for the treatment of PE?

3.b. What additional goals of pharmacotherapy exist for a patient with HIT?

3.c. What pharmacotherapeutic options are available to initiate anticoagulation for the treatment of PE in this patient?

TABLE 22-2	Pertinent Medication and Laboratory History from the Previous Admission		
TKR	Plt 239 × 10^3/mm^3	Hgb 12.2 g/dL	
Postoperative day 1	Plt 233 × 10^3/mm^3	Hgb 11.9 g/dL	Enoxaparin 30 mg subcutaneously Q 24 hours started
Postoperative day 2	Plt 227 × 10^3/mm^3		
Postoperative day 3	Plt 229 × 10^3/mm^3		
Postoperative day 4	Plt 221 × 10^3/mm^3	Hgb 12.0 g/dL	
Postoperative day 5	Plt 234 × 10^3/mm^3		
Postoperative day 6	Plt 141 × 10^3/mm^3	Hgb 12.0 g/dL	Discharged from hospital on enoxaparin 30 mg subcutaneously Q 24 hours

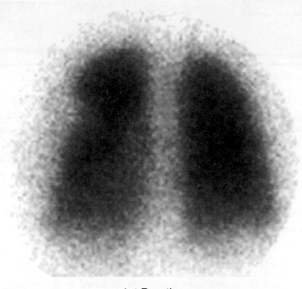

(A)   1st Breath

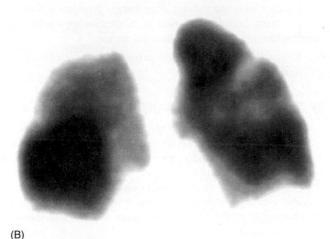

(B)

FIGURE 22-1. Ventilation–perfusion lung scan. (A) Normal ventilation; (B) multiple segmental perfusion defects, indicating a ventilation–perfusion mismatch and high probability of PE. (Reproduced with permission from Rao RK. Pulmonary embolic disease. In: Crawford MH, ed. *Current Diagnosis and Treatment in Cardiology.* 5th ed. New York, NY: McGraw-Hill Education, 2017:389.)

3.d. What non-anticoagulant therapies (pharmacotherapeutic and nondrug) are available for the treatment of PE? Is this patient an appropriate candidate for any of these therapeutic options?

3.e. Create an individualized, patient-centered, team-based care plan to optimize medication therapy for this patient's anticoagulation and other drug therapy problems. For the patient's anticoagulation therapy, the provider prefers to use a parenteral anticoagulant to begin treatment due to higher quality evidence. Select an appropriate parenteral anticoagulant and calculate the initial dose and therapeutic range for this patient.

Implement the Care Plan

4.a. Describe how care should be coordinated with other healthcare providers to transition the patient to warfarin, discontinue parenteral anticoagulation, and determine the appropriate length of warfarin therapy for this patient.

4.b. What information should be provided to the patient to enhance adherence, ensure successful therapy, and minimize adverse effects?

Follow-Up: Monitor and Evaluate

5.a. Explain how to monitor and evaluate this patient's care plan for medication appropriateness, effectiveness, safety and patient adherence by using clinical and laboratory data, patient feedback and other information.

5.b. If a diagnosis of HIT is confirmed, document a plan regarding the future use of heparin and low-molecular-weight heparin therapy in this patient.

■ CLINICAL COURSE (PART 3)

The results of the heparin-induced platelet antibody ELISA were reported as positive with an optical density (OD) of 1.20 (the hospital's laboratory reports OD values greater than 0.40 as positive for heparin-induced antibodies). The patient's INR has been therapeutic for 72 hours on warfarin. The parenteral anticoagulant was discontinued yesterday, and the patient will be discharged home today.

■ SELF-STUDY ASSIGNMENTS

1. Determine the appropriate frequency of platelet count monitoring when therapeutic or prophylactic anticoagulation with unfractionated heparin, low-molecular-weight heparin, or fondaparinux is used in medical or postoperative patients.

2. Investigate the sensitivity and specificity of the various activation and antigen assays available to confirm the diagnosis of HIT.

3. Compare the effects of bivalirudin and argatroban on INR measurement and warfarin monitoring.

4. Describe the role of platelet transfusion in the management of HIT.

CLINICAL PEARL

The optimal duration of anticoagulation in a patient with HIT who does not have evidence of thrombosis (isolated HIT) is unknown. Anticoagulation with a non-heparin anticoagulant should be continued at a minimum until the platelet count has recovered to at least $150 \times 10^3/mm^3$ and stabilized. Some clinicians will also continue anticoagulation for at least 4 weeks to prevent HIT-related thrombosis.

REFERENCES

1. Witt DM, Clark NP, Vazquez SR. Venous thromboembolism. In: DiPiro JT, Yee GC, Posey L, Haines ST, Nolin TD, Ellingrod V, eds. Pharmacotherapy: A Pathophysiologic Approach, 12e. McGraw Hill; 2021. Accessed October 4, 2022. https://accesspharmacy.mhmedical.com/content.aspx?3097&sectionid=268553772

2. Cuker A, Arepally GM, Chong BH, et al. American Society of Hematology 2018 guidelines for management of venous thromboembolism: heparin-induced thrombocytopenia. Blood Adv. 2018;2(22):3360–3392.

3. Stevens SM, Woller SC, Kreuziger LB, et al. Antithrombotic therapy for VTE disease: second update of the CHEST Guideline and Expert Panel Report. CHEST. 2021; doi: 10.1016/j.chest.2021.07.055.

4. Tritschler T, Kraaijpoel N, Le Gal G, Wells PS. Venous thromboembolism: advances in diagnosis and treatment. JAMA. 2018;320(15):1583–1594.

5. Lexicomp Online, Lexi-Drugs Online, Hudson, OH: Wolters Kluwer Clinical Drug Information, Inc.; 2021. Available at: *https://wolterskluwercdi.com/lexicomp-online/*. Accessed November 7, 2021.

6. Salter BS, Weiner MM, Trinh MA, et al. Heparin-induced thrombocytopenia: a comprehensive clinical review. J Am Coll Cardiol. 2016;67:2519–2532.

7. Kang M, Alahmadi M, Sawh S, Kovacs MJ, Lazo-Langner A. Fondaparinux for the treatment of suspected heparin-induced thrombocytopenia: a propensity score-matched study. Blood 2015;125(6):924–929.

8. Crowther, M. Management of heparin-induced thrombocytopenia. In: Leung L, Tirnauer J, eds. *UptoDate*. 2021. Accessed November 2021. Available from *https://www.uptodate.com/contents/management-of-heparin-induced-thrombocytopenia?search=management%20of%20hit&source=search_result&selectedTitle=1~150&usage_type=default&display_rank=1*.

9. Barlow A, Barlow B, Reinaker T, Harris J. Potential role of direct oral anticoagulants in the management of heparin-induced thrombocytopenia. Pharmacotherapy 2019;39(8):837–853.

10. Bristol-Myers S. Coumadin medication guide. Food and Drug Administration; 2017. Available at: *https://www.accessdata.fda.gov/drugsatfda_docs/label/2017/009218s118lbl.pdf#page=30*. Accessed November 14, 2021.

23

CHRONIC ANTICOAGULATION

Crossing the "Bridge" .... Level II

Mikayla L. Spangler, PharmD, BCPS

Beth Bryles Phillips, PharmD, FCCP, FASHP, BCPS, BCACP

LEARNING OBJECTIVES

After completing this case study, the reader should be able to:

- List the goals of anticoagulant therapy for periprocedural management of anticoagulation.

- Appropriately assess a patient's response to chronic warfarin therapy.

- Evaluate thromboembolic risk for patients receiving warfarin therapy and determine the need for bridging therapy.

- Develop a patient-specific pharmacotherapeutic plan for warfarin therapy and periprocedural management of anticoagulation.

- Educate patients appropriately about administration of low-molecular-weight heparins (LMWH) and chronic warfarin therapy.

PATIENT PRESENTATION

Chief Complaint

"I am scheduled to have a colonoscopy, and my physician said to talk to you about what to do with my warfarin."

HPI

A 53-year-old man with a past medical history of severe mitral regurgitation status post (S/P) mitral valve replacement (MVR) 5 years ago presents for follow-up of chronic anticoagulation. He reports that he is scheduled for a colonoscopy with possible polypectomy 2 weeks from today. His physician has been recommending the colonoscopy for routine screening since he turned 50, but he has been reluctant to schedule it. He realized the need for the procedure after a friend was diagnosed with colon cancer. Although no biopsy is planned, his physician explained that he should be off warfarin in case a biopsy is needed. He reports taking one and one-half of a peach-colored warfarin tablet every Tuesday and Saturday, and one whole peach-colored tablet on the other days of the week. He uses a medication box and has not missed any warfarin doses during the last month. He denies any bleeding, excessive bruising, severe headaches, abdominal pain, numbness, tingling, or inability to move one side of his body. His diet with respect to green, leafy vegetables has been consistent. He states that he has been taking ibuprofen 800 mg TID for the last 2.5 weeks for knee pain related to osteoarthritis. He reports drinking one alcoholic beverage, such as beer, Scotch whiskey, or tequila, every night before dinner. He confirms taking all other medications on his medication list and has not started any other new prescription, over-the-counter or alternative therapies.

PMH

Mitral regurgitation S/P MVR with St. Jude's mechanical cardiac valve 5 years ago
Hypertension
Osteoarthritis of the knee
Obesity

FH

Father—colon polyps removed when he was in his 50s but is currently alive and well in his 80s.
Mother—hypertension and is 79 years of age.
Brother—healthy.
He is married and has two children who are alive and well.

SH

(+) ETOH—one serving of alcohol each evening before dinner; (–) smoking

Meds

Amlodipine 10 mg daily
Ibuprofen 200 mg one to two tablets PO TID PRN for osteoarthritis pain
Aspirin 81 mg PO daily
Warfarin 7.5 mg PO Tuesday, Saturday; 5 mg 5 days per week

All

Penicillin—bumps, rash/hives

Physical Examination

VS

BP 116/78, HR 76, RR 14, T 36.5°C; Wt 96.4 kg, Ht 5′9″

Labs

Date	INR	Warfarin dose
Today	2.9	7.5 mg Tuesday, Saturday; 5 mg 5 days per week
1 month ago	2.7	7.5 mg Tuesday, Saturday; 5 mg 5 days per week
2 months ago	3.2	7.5 mg Tuesday, Saturday; 5 mg 5 days per week
3 months ago	2.6	7.5 mg Tuesday, Saturday; 5 mg 5 days per week

Assessment

S/P MVR requiring chronic anticoagulation with target INR 3.0 (range, 2.5–3.5)
Therapeutic INR (target 3.0; range, 2.5–3.5)
Periprocedural management of anticoagulation needed
High-dose ibuprofen use for recent osteoarthritis flare

QUESTIONS

Collect Information

1. What subjective and objective information is relevant for a patient with a mechanical cardiac valve requiring chronic anticoagulation?

Assess the Information

2.a. Provide an assessment of this patient's anticoagulation therapy based on the subjective and objective information available.

2.b. Create a list of the patient's drug therapy problems and prioritize them. Include assessment of medication appropriateness, effectiveness, safety, and patient adherence.

2.c. What economic considerations are applicable to this patient?

Develop a Care Plan

3.a. What are the goals of pharmacotherapy for anticoagulation in this case?

3.b. What are the most important non-pharmacologic considerations for this patient?

3.c. What feasible pharmacotherapeutic options are available for periprocedural management of anticoagulation?

3.d. Create an individualized, patient-centered, team-based care plan for this patient's anticoagulation therapy and other drug therapy problems. Include specific drugs, dosage forms, doses, schedules, and durations of therapy.

3.e. What alternatives would be appropriate if the initial care plan fails or cannot be used?

Implement the Care Plan

4.a. What information should be provided to the patient to enhance adherence, ensure successful therapy, and minimize adverse effects?

4.b. Describe how care should be coordinated with other healthcare providers.

Follow-Up: Monitor and Evaluate

5. Explain how to monitor and evaluate the care plan for medication appropriateness, effectiveness, safety and patient adherence by using clinical and laboratory data, patient feedback and other information.

■ CLINICAL COURSE

On his return to the clinic 1 week after the colonoscopy, he reports that the procedure went well, and he has taken his usual weekly dose of warfarin therapy and continues on bridging therapy. The INR is 2.5, and he is in need of further instructions regarding warfarin and bridging therapy.

■ FOLLOW-UP QUESTION

1. Based on this information, what are your recommendations for warfarin and LMWH therapy?

■ SELF-STUDY ASSIGNMENTS

1. Research the options for bridging in patients with a history of heparin-induced thrombocytopenia, and create a table highlighting the various management options.

2. Research the data on LMWH dosing in morbidly obese patients, and write a one-page paper summarizing how LMWH should be dosed in such patients.

CLINICAL PEARL

Dosing LMWH in obese patients can present challenges due to product availability of dosage strengths. Doses may need to be rounded up or down to the nearest available syringe and the availability of dosage forms may also determine whether enoxaparin may be administered once or twice daily.

REFERENCES

1. Nishimura RA, Otto CM, Bonow RO, et al. 2017 AHA/ACC focused update of the 2014 AHA/ACC guideline for the management of patients with valvular heart disease: a report of the American College of Cardiology/American Heart Association Task Force on Clinical Practice Guidelines. Circulation. 2017;135:e1159–e1195.

2. Whitlock RP, Sun JC, Fremes SE, Rubens FD, Teoh KH. Antithrombotic and thrombolytic therapy for valvular disease: antithrombotic therapy and prevention of thrombosis, 9th ed: American College of Chest Physicians Evidence-Based Clinical Practice Guidelines. Chest. 2012;141:e576S–e600S.

3. Douketis JD, Spyropoulos AC, Spencer FA, et al. Perioperative management of antithrombotic therapy. Chest. 2012;141:e326S–e350S.

4. Spyropoulos AC, Al-Badri A, Sherwood MW, Douketis JD. Periprocedural management of patients receiving a vitamin K antagonist or a direct oral anticoagulant requiring an elective procedure or surgery. J Thromb Haemost. 2016;14:875–885.

5. Vazquez S. Drug-drug interactions in an era of multiple anticoagulants: a focus on clinically relevant drug interactions. Hematology. 2018;132:339–347.

6. Cuker A, Arepally GM, Chong BH, et al. American Society of Hematology 2018 guidelines for management of venous thromboembolism: heparin-induced thrombocytopenia. Blood Adv. 2018;2(22):3360–3392.

7. Baron TH, Kamath PS, McBane RD. Management of antithrombotic therapy in patients undergoing invasive procedures. N Engl J Med. 2013;368:2113–2124.

8. Garcia DA, Baglin TP, Weitz JI, Samama MM. Parenteral anticoagulants. Chest. 2012;141:e24S–e43S.

9. Garwood CL, Gortney JS, Corbett TL. Is there a role for fondaparinux in perioperative bridging? Am J Health Syst Pharm. 2011;68:36–42.

24

STROKE

One Stroke Off Par .... Level II

Erin Berry, PharmD, BCPS

LEARNING OBJECTIVES

After completing this case study, the reader should be able to:

- Identify risk factors for ischemic stroke.

- Discuss the role of thrombolytics in the management of acute ischemic stroke.

- Formulate an appropriate patient-specific drug regimen for the treatment of an acute ischemic stroke.

- Discuss the approach to multi-disease state management for the secondary prevention of ischemic stroke, including the management of hypertension, dyslipidemia, and the use of antiplatelet agents.

- Educate a patient regarding secondary stroke prevention strategies.

PATIENT PRESENTATION

■ Chief Complaint
"My dad is having trouble talking and seems to be losing feeling in his left arm and leg."

■ HPI
A 57-year-old man is brought to the ED by his son at 10 AM after experiencing left arm numbness, slurred speech, and dizziness. The patient's son states that the two of them were enjoying their typical Saturday morning golf outing at the country club when his father dropped his golf club and went down on one knee. They both verify that this was around 9:30 AM, as it was just as they were teeing off on hole 6. After noticing that his father's words were "slow and deliberate," the son immediately called 9-1-1. While in the ED, the patient began to experience left extremity weakness accompanied by a left-sided facial droop.

■ PMH
HTN, diagnosed 10 years ago
Dyslipidemia

■ FH
Both parents alive and relatively healthy. Sister, age 62, also has HTN. Son, age 31, has type 1 DM.

■ SH
Married, lives with wife and two children. Two other children grown and out of the house. Occasional recreational beer or wine consumption. Denies tobacco use.

■ Meds
Simvastatin 10 mg PO daily
Chlorthalidone 25 mg PO daily

■ All
Shellfish (hives)

■ ROS
Mild blurry vision, but no double vision, loss of vision, or oscillopsia

■ Physical Examination
Gen
Slender man lying in bed in no acute distress, responsive with occasionally slurred speech

VS
BP 192/98, P 70, RR 19, T 98.6°F, O_2 sat 97% on RA; Wt 80 kg, Ht 6'0"

Skin
Warm, dry

HEENT
PERRLA, EOMI; no nystagmus, exudates, hemorrhages, or papilledema; mild left-sided facial droop. Normal hearing acuity bilaterally.

Neck
(–) Carotid bruits, (–) lymphadenopathy

Chest
Lungs clear to auscultation bilaterally

CV
RRR, S_1 and S_2 normal, no S_3 or S_4

Abd
Soft, nontender, nondistended, (+) BS

GU
Deferred

MS/Ext
RUE: 5/5; RLE 4/5; LUE: 2/5; LLE: 3/5. No abnormal or involuntary movements. Strong peripheral pulses and brisk capillary refill; no CCE; DTR: 2+ throughout, normal Babinski reflex.

Neuro
Awake, A&O × 3. No aphasia, agnosia, or apraxia. Attention, concentration, and vocabulary are all excellent. No impairment of facial sensation noted with light touch bilaterally. Moderate left facial weakness, as noted by the presence of left-sided facial droop. Mild dysarthria. Shoulder shrug is symmetrical, and tongue is midline on protrusion. Can easily touch chin to chest, and there are no other signs of meningismus.

■ Labs

Na 140 mEq/L	WBC $5.9 \times 10^3/mm^3$	*Fasting lipid profile*
K 4.2 mEq/L	Hgb 16.4 g/dL	Total cholesterol 200 mg/dL
Cl 103 mEq/L	Hct 49.6%	LDL-C 118 mg/dL
CO_2 28 mEq/L	Plt $310 \times 10^3/mm^3$	Triglycerides 160 mg/dL
BUN 10 mg/dL	aPTT 25.3 s	HDL-C 50 mg/dL
SCr 0.6 mg/dL	Trop I 0.01 ng/mL	
Glu 98 mg/dL		

■ Additional Tests
Head CT scan: right-sided middle cerebral artery infarct; no evidence of hemorrhage (Fig. 24-1)
Carotid Dopplers: normal blood flow bilaterally, no appreciable ischemia or stenosis
Angiogram: not performed
Echocardiogram: no evidence of LV thrombus, ejection fraction 55–60%; overall unremarkable
EKG: normal sinus rhythm (Fig. 24-2)

■ Assessment
Acute ischemic stroke secondary to atherosclerosis and ischemic disease in a patient with HTN, dyslipidemia, and no prior history of stroke or transient ischemic attack

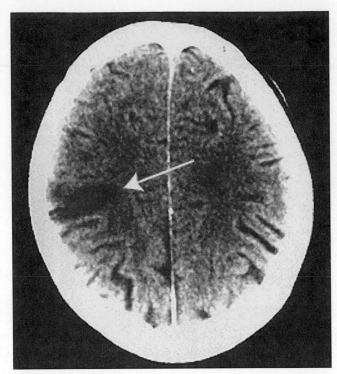

FIGURE 24-1. Head CT scan without contrast negative for hemorrhage and showing right-sided middle cerebral artery infarct.

■ CLINICAL COURSE

It is now 11:00 AM, and you are seeing the patient with the rest of the neurology team.

QUESTIONS

Collect Information

1.a. What subjective and objective information indicates the presence of an acute ischemic stroke?

1.b. What additional information is needed to fully assess this patient's ischemic stroke and to determine a treatment approach?

Assess the Information

2.a. Assess the severity of this patient's stroke, using the National Institute of Health Stroke Severity Scale, based on the subjective and objective information available.

2.b. Create a list of the patient's drug therapy problems and prioritize them. Include assessment of medication appropriateness, effectiveness, safety, and patient adherence.

Develop a Care Plan

3.a. What are the goals of pharmacotherapy for ischemic stroke in this case?

3.b. What nondrug therapies might be useful for this patient's ischemic stroke?

3.c. What feasible pharmacotherapeutic options are available for the treatment of acute ischemic stroke?

3.d. Create an individualized, patient-centered, team-based care plan to optimize medication therapy for this patient's acute stroke and other drug therapy problems. Include specific drugs, dosage forms, doses, schedules, and durations of therapy.

Implement the Care Plan

4.a. What information should be provided to the patient to enhance adherence, ensure successful therapy, and minimize adverse effects?

4.b. Describe how care should be coordinated with other healthcare providers.

Follow-Up: Monitor and Evaluate

5. Explain how to monitor and evaluate the care plan for medication appropriateness, effectiveness, safety and patient adherence by using clinical and laboratory data, patient feedback and other information.

■ SELF-STUDY ASSIGNMENTS

1. Explain which patients are candidates to receive aspirin instead of warfarin or direct oral anticoagulants for the prevention of stroke in the setting of atrial fibrillation.

2. Read the CHANCE trial and explain when, and for how long, treatment with combination of aspirin and clopidogrel is indicated post-stroke or transient ischemic attack.

3. Write a one-page report summarizing the findings of clinical trials utilizing tenecteplase for the treatment of acute ischemic stroke.

CLINICAL PEARL

Initially, elevated blood pressures often decrease, without the use of antihypertensive therapy, within the first few days after an ischemic stroke. When initiating antihypertensive therapy after an acute ischemic stroke, caution should be used to not reduce blood pressure too aggressively unless clinically indicated. This approach to blood pressure management in the acute stroke setting is referred to as "permissive hypertension."

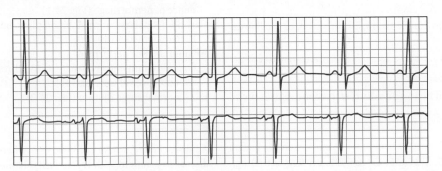

FIGURE 24-2. ECG showing normal sinus rhythm.

ACKNOWLEDGMENT

This case is based on the patient case written for the 11th edition by Alexander J. Ansara, PharmD, BCPS AQ Cardiology.

REFERENCES

1. AHA/ACC/AACVPR/AAPA/ABC/ACPM/ADA/AGS/APhA/ASPC/NLA/PCNA guideline on the management of blood cholesterol: executive summary: a report of the American College of Cardiology/American Heart Association Task Force on Clinical Practice Guidelines. J Am Coll Cardiol. 2019;73(24):3168–3209.
2. Powers WJ, Rabinstein AA, Ackerson T, et al. Guidelines for the early management of patients with acute ischemic stroke: 2019 update to the 2018 guidelines for the early management of acute ischemic stroke: a guideline for healthcare professionals from the American Heart Association/American Stroke Association. Stroke. 2019 Dec;50(12):e344–e418. doi: 10.1161/STR.0000000000000211. Epub 2019 Oct 30. Erratum in: Stroke. 2019 Dec;50(12):e440–e441.
3. Nogueira RG, Jadhav AP, Haussen DC, et al; DAWN Trial Investigators. Thrombectomy 6 to 24 hours after stroke with a mismatch between deficit and infarct. N Eng J Med. 2018;378:11–21.
4. Ricotta JJ, AbuRahma A, Ascher E, et al. Updated society for vascular surgery guidelines for the management of extracranial carotid disease: executive summary. J Vasc Surg. 2011;54:832–836.
5. National Institute of Neurological Disorders and Stroke r-tPA Stroke Study Group. Tissue plasminogen activator for acute ischemic stroke. N Engl J Med. 1995;333:1581–1587.
6. Hacke W, Kaste M, Bluhmki E, et al. Thrombolysis with alteplase 3 to 4.5 hours after acute ischemic stroke. N Eng J Med. 2008;359:1317–1329.
7. Logallo N, Novotny V, Assmus J, et al. Tenecteplase versus alteplase for management of acute ischaemic stroke (NOR-TEST): a phase 3, randomised, open-label, blinded endpoint trial. Lancet Neurol. 2017;16:781–788. doi: 10.1016/S1474-4422(17)30253-3.
8. Chinese Acute Stroke Trial Collaborative Group (CAST). Randomized placebo-controlled trial of early aspirin use in 20,000 patients with acute ischemic stroke. Lancet. 1997;349:1641–1649.
9. International Stroke Trial Collaborative Group (IST). A randomized trial of aspirin, subcutaneous heparin, both, or neither among 19435 patients with acute ischaemic stroke. Lancet. 1997;349:1569–1581.
10. Wang Y, Wang Y, Zhao X, et al; CHANCE Investigators. Clopidogrel with aspirin in acute minor stroke or transient ischemic attack. N Engl J Med. 2013;369:11–19.

25

VENTRICULAR ARRHYTHMIA

Crash in the Heart of the Parking Lot .... Level III

Kwadwo Amankwa, PharmD, BCPS

LEARNING OBJECTIVES

After completing this case study, the reader should be able to:

- Describe risk factors for the development of drug-induced torsades de pointes (TdP).
- Differentiate TdP from other cardiac arrhythmias.
- Select appropriate first-line therapy for acute treatment of TdP.

- Recommend appropriate dosing, common adverse effects, and monitoring parameters for pharmacologic agents used to treat TdP.
- Discuss long-term approaches for the prevention of drug-induced TdP.

PATIENT PRESENTATION

■ Chief Complaint

"I was not feeling well, and I think I passed out."

■ HPI

The patient is a 55-year-old woman who experienced syncope while parking her car in the parking lot of the neighborhood grocery store. There were no injuries from the accident, and she was brought to the ED for evaluation. She reports being in her usual state of relatively good health until she developed a "cold" approximately 4 days before admission. She called her primary care physician complaining of her upper respiratory tract symptoms, and the physician called in a prescription for erythromycin 500 mg QID for 10 days to her pharmacy. She took the first dose on the morning of admission. She started feeling that something was wrong on her way to the grocery store approximately 1 hour after taking the second dose of erythromycin. She reports symptoms of lightheadedness, shortness of breath, as well as palpitations while driving. She passed out while parking, and her car collided with another car with minimal impact, damage, or injury. On medic arrival, she was awake and alert but looked shaken. She was transported to the ED without further events. While being evaluated in the ED, she had another syncopal episode. ACLS protocol was initiated, and a rhythm strip showed TdP.

■ PMH

CAD S/P PCI 3 years prior to present admission
Heart failure (EF 30%)
Dyslipidemia
Paroxysmal atrial fibrillation
GERD

■ SH

She lives with her husband and does not smoke or drink alcohol.

■ Meds

Carvedilol 3.125 mg PO BID
Atorvastatin 80 mg PO at bedtime
Furosemide 40 mg PO BID (recently increased from 40 mg PO once a day due to increased edema)
Warfarin 4 mg PO once daily
Amiodarone 200 mg PO BID
Centrum silver PO once daily
Omeprazole 20 mg PO once daily
Sacubitril/Valsartan 24/26 mg PO BID
Aspirin 81 mg PO once daily
Erythromycin 500 mg PO QID (taken on the day of admission)

■ All

NKDA

■ ROS

The patient has no complaints other than those mentioned in the HPI.

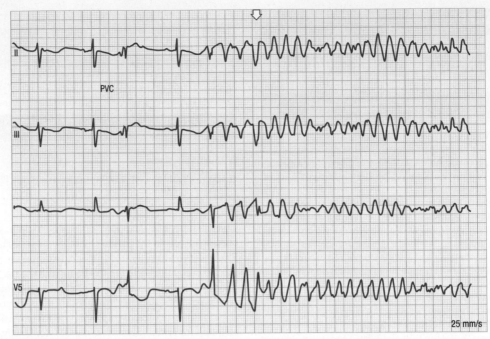

FIGURE 25-1. Electrocardiogram showing torsades de pointes.

■ Physical Examination

Gen

The patient is awake on an ED bed in moderate distress.

VS

BP 104/50, P 98 (200 during syncope), RR 30, T 36.3°C; Ht 5′7″, Wt 90 kg

Skin

Warm and dry; no rashes seen

HEENT

NC/AT. PERRLA. EOMI. Oropharynx is clear.

Neck/Lymph Nodes

Supple; no JVD or bruits; no lymph nodes palpated

Lungs/Thorax

CTA bilaterally

Breasts

Deferred

CV

RRR with no murmurs or gallops

Abd

NTND; no rebound or guarding; (+) bowel sounds

Genit/Rect

Deferred

MS/Ext

Trace edema in the lower extremities; pulses intact

Neuro

A&O × 3

■ Labs

Na 140 mEq/L	Hgb 12.1 g/dL	WBC 12 × 10³/mm³
K 2.8 mEq/L	Hct 35%	
Cl 100 mEq/L	RBC 3.88 × 10⁶/mm³	
CO₂ 29 mEq/L	Plt 200 × 10³/mm³	
BUN 36 mg/dL	MCV 90.5 μm³	
SCr 1.4 mg/dL	MCHC 34.4 g/dL	
Glu 110 mg/dL	INR 2.3	
Mg 1.2 mg/dL		

■ ECG

NSR, QTc 605 milliseconds; rhythm strip from oscilloscope during syncope: TdP (Fig. 25-1)

■ Assessment

A 55-year-old woman S/P syncopal episodes from drug-induced TdP; upper respiratory tract symptoms; drug-induced electrolyte imbalance.

QUESTIONS

Collect Information

1.a. What subjective and objective information indicates the presence of TdP?

1.b. What additional information is needed to fully assess this patient's TdP?

Assess the Information

2.a. What risk factors predisposed this patient to TdP?

2.b. Create a list of the patient's drug therapy problems and prioritize them. Include assessment of medication appropriateness, effectiveness, safety, and patient adherence.

Develop a Care Plan

3.a. What are the short-term goals of pharmacotherapy TdP in this case?

3.b. What nondrug therapies may be useful for this patient's TdP?

3.c. What feasible pharmacotherapeutic options are available for the acute treatment of TdP?

3.d. Create an individualized, patient-centered, team-based care plan to optimize medication therapy for this patient's TdP and other drug therapy problems. Include specific drugs, dosage forms, doses, schedules, and durations of therapy.

Implement the Care Plan

4.a. What information should be provided to the patient to enhance adherence, ensure successful therapy, and prevent recurrence of TdP?

4.b. Describe how care should be coordinated with other healthcare providers.

Follow-Up: Monitor and Evaluate

5. Explain how to monitor and evaluate the care plan for medication appropriateness, effectiveness, safety and patient adherence by using clinical and laboratory data, patient feedback and other information.

■ CLINICAL COURSE

The patient was treated with a magnesium infusion, and she converted to normal sinus rhythm. The erythromycin was stopped. Potassium and magnesium were replaced, and the patient was admitted for further electrophysiology workup.

■ SELF-STUDY ASSIGNMENTS

1. List the most common drug classes associated with TdP.

2. List 10 commonly used medications that have a potential to cause TdP.

CLINICAL PEARL

There is a need for increased pharmacovigilance regarding drug-induced arrhythmias in the outpatient setting because many pharmacologic agents and/or conditions that cause QT prolongation and TdP are present in the outpatient population.

REFERENCES

1. Schwartz PJ, Woosley RL. Predicting the unpredictable. J Am Coll Cardiol. 2016;67:1639–1650.

2. Woosley RL, Heise CW, Gallo T, Tate J, Woosley D, Romero KA. QT drugs list, AZCERT, AZ. Available at: www.CredibleMeds.org. Accessed December 11, 2021.

3. Niedrig D, Maechler S, Hoppe L, et al. Drug safety of macrolide and quinolone antibiotics in a tertiary care hospital: administration of interacting co-medication and QT prolongation. Eur J Clin Pharmacol. 2016;72:859–867.

4. Owens RC, Nolin TD. Antimicrobial-associated QT interval prolongation: pointes of interest. Clin Infect Dis. 2006;43:1603–1611.

5. Tisdale JE. Ventricular arrhythmias. In: Tisdale JE, Miller DA, eds. Drug-Induced Diseases: Prevention, Detection and Management. 3rd ed. Bethesda, MD: American Society of Health-Systems Pharmacists; 2018:523–568.

6. Al-Khatib SM, Stevenson WG, Ackerman MJ, et al. 2017 AHA/ACC/HRS guideline for management of patients with ventricular arrhythmias and the prevention of sudden cardiac death: executive summary. Circulation. 2018:138:e210–e271.

7. Berul CI. Acquired QT syndrome. In: Asirvatham S, Zimetbaum PJ, eds. UpToDate. Available at: http://www.uptodateonline.com. Accessed December 13, 2021.

8. Roden DM. Predicting drug-induced QT prolongation and torsades de pointes. J Physiol. 2016;594:2459–2468.

9. Tilton JJ, Sanoski C, Bauman JL. The arrhythmias. In: DiPiro JT, Yee GC, Posey L, Haines ST, Nolin TD, Ellingrod V, eds. Pharmacotherapy: A Pathophysiologic Approach, 11e. McGraw Hill; 2020. Available at: https://accesspharmacy.mhmedical.com/content.aspx?bookid=2577&sectionid=233592457. Accessed February 14, 2022.

26

ATRIAL FIBRILLATION

Go Easy on My Beating Heart .... Level III

Virginia H. Fleming, PharmD, BCPS

LEARNING OBJECTIVES

After completing this case study, the reader should be able to:

• Describe the cornerstones of atrial fibrillation (AF) treatment.

• Determine therapeutic goals for managing AF in patients with heart failure.

• Recommend an optimal agent for anticoagulation in AF patients with heart failure.

PATIENT PRESENTATION

■ Chief Complaint

"Lately, I feel like my heart has been racing a bit. It really doesn't bother me that much, but I wanted to have it checked out to be sure."

■ HPI

A 64-year-old man with heart failure and a history of persistent AF presents to his primary care physician complaining of palpitations that he first noticed 7 days ago. He reports that he is aware of the palpitations but that he has remained relatively asymptomatic. There has not been a noticeable change in his level of fatigue or exercise capacity during his normal daily activities. The patient was diagnosed with heart failure 6 years ago. For the past few years, his baseline exercise capacity would be described as slight limitation of physical activity with some symptoms during normal daily activities but asymptomatic at rest. He has a history of AF that was cardioverted to NSR, and he has been on amiodarone to maintain NSR for the past 8 months. In the office today, his ECG shows that he is in AF (Fig. 26-1).

■ PMH

Hypertension
Persistent AF (previously in NSR with amiodarone therapy)

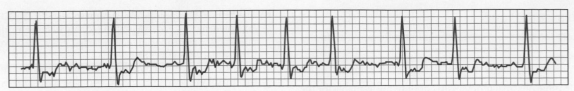

FIGURE 26-1. Rhythm recorded in the patient's physician's office that depicts AF with a ventricular response rate of 110 bpm. AF is characterized by the absence of atrial "p" waves with varying distances between QRS complexes. AF is sometimes referred to as an irregularly irregular rhythm: irregular because it is not NSR; irregular because it produces an irregular ventricular response rate or peripheral pulse.

Heart failure with reduced ejection fraction (LVEF 35%)
Obstructive sleep apnea (AHI 28 events/hr), alleviated with CPAP therapy

■ FH

Both parents are deceased. Father died of an AMI at age 64. Mother died of breast cancer at age 70.

■ SH

Works as an accountant. He is married with two healthy children. He does not smoke but occasionally drinks "a few beers on the weekends."

■ Medications

Carvedilol 6.25 mg PO BID
Digoxin 0.0625 mg PO once daily
Amiodarone 400 mg PO once daily
Furosemide 40 mg PO once daily
KCl 20 mEq PO once daily
Lisinopril 10 mg PO once daily
Warfarin 5 mg PO once daily
Spironolactone 25 mg PO once daily
CPAP therapy (8 cm H_2O) at night

■ Allergies

NKDA

■ ROS

Reports no change in level of fatigue, some exercise intolerance; no headache, lightheadedness, chest pain, angina, or fainting spells; 2+ pitting edema

■ Physical Examination

Gen

Cooperative, well-nourished man in no apparent distress

VS

BP 158/92, P 110 (irregular), RR 20, T 36.3°C, Wt 82.3 kg, Ht 5′11″

Skin

Cool to touch, normal turgor and color

HEENT

PEERLA, EOMI; funduscopic exam reveals mild arteriolar narrowing but no hemorrhages, exudates, or papilledema

Neck

Large and supple, no carotid bruits; no lymphadenopathy or thyromegaly, (−) JVD

Lungs/Thorax

Inspiratory and expiratory rales bilaterally, no rhonchi

CV

Pulse 110 bpm and irregular; normal S_1, S_2, (+) S_3, no S_4

Abd

NT/ND, (+) BS; no organomegaly, (−) HJR

Genit/Rect

Normal male anatomy; stool heme (−)

MS/Ext

Pulses 1+ weak, full ROM, no clubbing or cyanosis; mild edema (2+)

Neuro

A&O × 3; CN II–XII intact; DTR 2+, negative Babinski

■ Labs

Na 140 mEq/L	Hgb 12.0 g/dL	Ca 8.5 mg/dL
K 4.0 mEq/L	Hct 35.8%	Mg 2.1 mEq/L
Cl 105 mEq/L	Plt 212 × 10³/mm³	Dig 0.8 ng/mL
CO_2 24 mEq/L	WBC 9.5 × 10³/mm³	
BUN 22 mg/dL	Polys 65%	
SCr 1.1 mg/dL	Bands 2%	
Glu 109 mg/dL	Lymphs 30%	
INR 2.3	Mono 3%	

■ ECG

Persistent AF, ventricular rate 110 bpm (see Fig. 26-1)

■ Echo

Evidence of systolic dysfunction (LVEF 35%) and moderate left atrial enlargement (5.2 cm). No thrombus seen.

■ Chest X-Ray

Enlarged cardiac silhouette; no evidence of acute pulmonary infection or edema

■ Assessment

Persistent AF, previously in NSR on amiodarone therapy: mildly symptomatic, appropriately anticoagulated with warfarin therapy. Ventricular response rate not controlled.
HF: mildly symptomatic, standard meds not at target doses; candidate for sacubatril/valsartan.
HTN: not controlled; optimize therapy for blood pressure control.
OSA: controlled on CPAP therapy.

QUESTIONS

Collect Information

1.a. What subjective and objective information indicates the presence of persistent atrial fibrillation (AF) with HFrEF?

1.b. What additional information is needed to fully assess this patient's AF?

Assess the Information

2.a. Assess the severity of the patient's AF based on the subjective and objective information available. How would you evaluate the effectiveness of his current medication regimen?

2.b. Create a list of this patient's drug therapy problems and prioritize them. Include assessment of medication appropriateness, effectiveness, safety, and patient adherence.

Develop a Care Plan

3.a. What are the goals for pharmacotherapy for AF in this case?

3.b. What are the goals for pharmacotherapy for this patient's comorbid disease states or conditions?

3.c. What nondrug therapies might be useful for this patient?

3.d. What feasible pharmacotherapeutic options are available for rhythm control in AF? What feasible pharmacotherapeutic options are available for rate control in AF?

3.e. Create an individualized, patient-centered, team-based care plan to optimize medication therapy for this patient's AF and other drug therapy problems. Include specific drugs, dosage forms, doses, schedules, and durations of therapy.

Implement the Care Plan

4.a. What information should be provided to the patient to enhance adherence, ensure successful therapy, and minimize adverse effects?

4.b. Describe how care should be coordinated with other healthcare providers.

Follow-Up: Monitor and Evaluate

5. Explain how to monitor and evaluate the care plan for medication appropriateness, effectiveness, safety and patient adherence by using clinical and laboratory data, patient feedback and other information.

■ ADDITIONAL CASE QUESTIONS

1. How effective is amiodarone therapy in maintaining NSR long-term in patients with AF?

2. What factors may hinder preservation of NSR for this patient?

3. The patient has persistent AF. How is this different than permanent AF?

■ SELF-STUDY ASSIGNMENTS

1. Recommend a management strategy/plan for this patient if he returned in 2 weeks transitioned to rivaroxaban for anticoagulation, with a heart rate of 85 bpm, and no symptoms of tachycardia but with 2+ pitting edema and a 1.2-kg gain in body weight.

2. List the drugs that have been demonstrated to improve mortality in the setting of heart failure and AF.

CLINICAL PEARL

In treating AF with concomitant heart failure with reduced ejection fraction, rate control (aimed at a goal of <80 bpm) plus anticoagulation is a viable treatment option over maintaining NSR with antiarrhythmic therapy. A more lenient rate control goal of <110 bpm is an option for patients with AF whose ejection fraction is preserved.

REFERENCES

1. January CT, Wann LS, Alpert JS, et al. 2014 AHA/ACC/HRS guideline for the management of patients with atrial fibrillation: executive summary. A report of the American College of Cardiology/American Heart Association Task Force on Practice Guidelines and the Heart Rhythm Society. J Am Coll Cardiol. 2014;64(21):2246–2280.

2. January CT, Wann LS, Calkins H, et al. 2019 AHA/ACC/HRS focused update of the 2014 AGA/ACC/HRS guideline for the management of patients with atrial fibrillation: a report of the American College of Cardiology/American Heart Association Task Force on Clinical Practice Guidelines and the Heart Rhythm Society in Collaboration with the Society of Thoracic Surgeons. 2019;140(2); e125–e151.

3. Shelton RJ, Clark AL, Goode K, et al. A randomized, controlled study of rate versus rhythm control in patients with chronic atrial fibrillation and heart failure: (CAFE-II Study). Heart. 2009;95(11):924–930.

4. Roy D, Talajic M, Nattel S, et al. Rhythm control versus rate control for atrial fibrillation and heart failure. N Engl J Med. 2008;358:2667–2677.

5. Heidenreich PA, Bozkurt B, Aguilar D, et al. 2022 AHA/ACC/HFSA guideline for the management of heart failure: a report of the American College of Cardiology/American Heart Association Joint Committee on Clinical Practice Guidelines. J Am Coll Cardiol. 2022;Apr 1:[Epub ahead of print] e1–e159. Available at https://www.jacc.org/doi/pdf/10.1016/j.jacc.2021.12.012. Accessed April 14, 2022.

6. Maddox TM, Januzzi JL, Allen LA, et al. 2021 update to the 2017 ACC expert consensus decision pathway for optimization of heart failure treatment: answers to 10 pivotal issues about heart failure with reduced ejection fraction: a report of the American College of Cardiology Solution Set Oversight Committee. J Am Coll Cardiol. 2021;77(6):772–810.

7. Van Gelder IC, Groenveld HF, Crijns HJ, et al; RACE II Investigators. Lenient versus strict rate control in patients with atrial fibrillation. N Engl J Med. 2010;362(15):1363–1373.

8. Lip GYH, Banerjee A, Boriani G, et al. Antithrombotic therapy for atrial fibrillation. CHEST Guideline and Expert Panel Report. Chest. 2018;154(5):1121–1201.

9. Ruff, CT, Giugliano RP, Braunwald E, et al. Comparison of the efficacy and safety of new oral anticoagulants with warfarin in patients with atrial fibrillation: a meta-analysis of randomized trials. Lancet. 2014;383(9921):955–962.

27

CARDIAC ARREST

Staying Alive .... Level III

Vishal Ooka, PharmD, BCCCP

Sarah Hittle, PharmD, BCCCP

LEARNING OBJECTIVES

After completing this case study, the reader should be able to:

- Discuss possible causes for cardiac arrest.

- Analyze medications used to treat cardiac arrest.

- List the pharmacologic actions of medications used in cardioversion.

- Outline the Advanced Cardiac Life Support (ACLS) guidelines.

- Identify appropriate parameters to monitor a patient who has had circulation restored after cardiac arrest.

PATIENT PRESENTATION

■ Chief Complaint

"I feel like I can't breathe."

■ HPI

A 68-year-old woman presented to the emergency department Monday morning with shortness of breath and weakness. She reported these symptoms began along with a decreased oral intake on Thursday of last week, which ultimately led to her missing her scheduled dialysis session prior to the weekend.

■ PMH

ESRD requiring hemodialysis Monday, Wednesday, and Friday
Endometriosis
HTN
Dyslipidemia
Type 2 DM

■ PSH

Hysterectomy in 1985

■ FH

Mother had HTN and died of an AMI at age 69; no information available for father; one brother is alive with HTN and DM at age 73.

■ SH

Former smoker; quit 8 years ago; previously 1.5 ppd

■ Meds PTA

Atorvastatin 20 mg PO daily
Metoprolol tartrate 50 mg PO twice daily
Sevelamer 800 mg PO TID with meals
Lisinopril 20 mg PO daily
Epoetin alfa 10,000 units subcutaneously three times a week
Insulin glargine 40 units subcutaneously daily
Insulin lispro 5 units subcutaneously with meals

■ All

Sulfa

■ ROS

Difficulty breathing

■ Physical Examination

Gen

68-Year-old woman exhibiting weakness and labored breathing

VS

BP 98/60, P 112, RR 24, O_2 saturation 81% on 4L NC; T 37.9°C; dry Wt 90 kg; Ht 5'4"

Skin

Cold

HEENT

PERRLA; EOMI; no hemorrhages, exudates, or papilledema; oral mucosa clear

Neck/Lymph Nodes

Supple with no JVD or bruits; no lymphadenopathy or thyromegaly

Chest

Mild bibasilar rales with decreased breath sounds

CV

Tachycardic; S_1, S_2 normal; no S_3 or S_4; no murmurs or rubs

Abd

Obese, soft, nontender; (+) BS

Genit/Rect

Stool heme (−)

MS/Ext

3+ pitting edema, age-appropriate strength, and ROM

Neuro

A&O × 3, GCS 15

■ Labs

Na 135 mEq/L	Mg 2 mg/dL	Hgb 8.3 g/dL
K 6.3 mEq/L	Phos 6.5 mg/dL	Hct 28%
Cl 106 mEq/L	Alb 1.8 g/dL	Plt 229 × 103/mm³
CO_2 20 mEq/L		WBC 9.9 × 103/mm³
BUN 55 mg/dL		PMNs 79%
SCr 4.6 mg/dL		Bands 1%
Glu 55 mg/dL		Lymphs 17%
Ca 6.7 mg/dL		Monos 3%

■ ECG

Sinus tachycardia at a rate of 112 bpm

■ Clinical Course

The patient's clinical condition deteriorated shortly after presentation to the ED, at which time she was subsequently intubated for respiratory failure. The patient was noted to have multifocal PVCs with a disorganized rhythm on the monitor and no pulse was detected. A code was called.

■ Assessment

68-Year-old patient with a complex medical history presents to the ED and develops cardiac arrest after missing a hemodialysis session.

QUESTIONS

Collect Information

1. Discuss possible causes for the development of PEA, and identify which potential causes are present in this patient.

Assess the Information

2a. Create a list of this patient's drug therapy problems and prioritize them. Include assessment of medication appropriateness, effectiveness, and safety.

■ CLINICAL COURSE

See Table 27-1 for a record of cardiopulmonary resuscitation (CPR) events and orders.

2.b. Assess the appropriateness of the treatment used to resuscitate this patient (see Table 27-1).

TABLE 27-1	Cardiopulmonary Resuscitation Record of Events and Orders				
Time	**BP**	**Rhythm**	**Pulse**	**Defib. (J)**	**Treatment Given**
0220	56/?	PEA	No pulse Chest compressions	None	Epi 1 mg IVP IO placement Labs ordered: potassium, ABG, lactate
0221	46/?	PEA	No pulse	None	Resume compressions Regular insulin 10 units IVP Sodium bicarbonate 50 mEq IVP Calcium chloride 1 g IVP
0223	73/?	Bradycardia (Fig. 27-1)	Pulse detected HR 50	None	Epi 1 mg IVP D50 1 amp
0225	88/?	VF (Fig. 27-2)	No pulse Chest compressions	360	Vasopressin 40 units IVP
0227	?/133	SVT (Fig. 27-3)	No pulse Chest compressions	360	Chest compressions resumed
0229	160/84	Sinus tach	Pulse detected HR 180	None	

Key: ?, not recorded; ABG, arterial blood gas; BP, blood pressure; Defib., defibrillation; D50, dextrose 50%; Epi, epinephrine; HR, heart rate; IO, intraosseous; IVP, intravenous push; PEA, pulseless electrical activity; Sinus tach, sinus tachycardia; SVT, supraventricular tachycardia; VF, ventricular fibrillation.

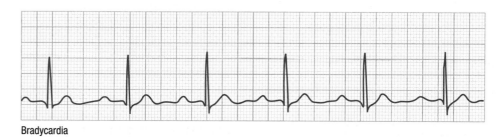

Bradycardia

FIGURE 27-1. Electrocardiogram showing bradycardia. (Reproduced with permission from acls-algorithms.com, Jeffery Media Productions, LLC.)

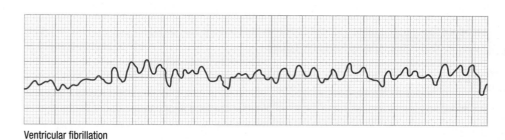

Ventricular fibrillation

FIGURE 27-2. Electrocardiogram showing ventricular fibrillation. (Reproduced with permission from acls-algorithms.com, Jeffery Media Productions, LLC.)

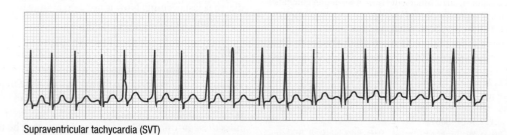

Supraventricular tachycardia (SVT)

FIGURE 27-3. Electrocardiogram showing supraventricular tachycardia. (Reproduced with permission from acls-algorithms.com, Jeffery Media Productions, LLC.)

Develop a Care Plan

3.a. What are the short-term goals of pharmacotherapy for PEA in this case?

3.b. What nonpharmacologic maneuvers should be taken immediately in a patient with PEA?

3.c. What pharmacotherapeutic options are available for the acute treatment of PEA?

3.d. Create an individualized, patient-centered, team-based care plan to optimize medication therapy, maintain the patient's stability, and optimize neurological function following the return of spontaneous circulation (ROSC).

Implement the Care Plan

4. Describe how care should be coordinated with other healthcare professionals.

Follow-Up: Monitor and Evaluate

5. Explain how to monitor and evaluate the care plan for medication appropriateness, effectiveness and safety using the clinical and laboratory data.

■ SELF-STUDY ASSIGNMENTS

1. Search the Internet for commercially available automated external defibrillator (AED) devices. Explain how such a device would be used by a layperson during a cardiac arrest that occurred in the home or workplace.

2. Perform a literature search to determine the odds of surviving a cardiac arrest while hospitalized.

3. List medications that can be administered via the intraosseous route in an emergent situation.

4. Investigate the effects of targeted temperature management following cardiac arrest on patient outcomes.

CLINICAL PEARL

During a cardiac arrest, it is important to identify the underlying cause of the arrest through a rapid assessment of the H's (hypovolemia, hypoxia, hydrogen ion [acidosis], hyper-/hypokalemia, hypothermia, hypoglycemia) and T's (toxins, tamponade, tension pneumothorax, thrombosis).

REFERENCES

1. International Liaison Committee on Resuscitation. Part 3: adult basic and advanced life support. 2020 American Heart Association guidelines for cardiopulmonary resuscitation and emergency cardiovascular care. Circulation. 2020;142(Suppl 2):S366–S468.

2. Link MS, Berkow LC, Kudenchuk PJ, et al. 2015 American Heart Association update for cardiopulmonary resuscitation and emergency cardiovascular care. Circulation. 2015;132(Suppl 2):S444–S464.

3. Vanden Hoek TL, Morrison LJ, Shuster M, et al. Part 12: cardiac arrest in special situations: 2010 American Heart Association guidelines for cardiopulmonary resuscitation and emergency cardiovascular care. Circulation. 2010;122:S829–S861.

4. Neumar RW, Otto CW, Link MS, et al. Part 8: advanced life support: 2010 American Heart Association guidelines for cardiopulmonary resuscitation and emergency cardiovascular care. Circulation. 2010;122:S729–S767.

5. Ong ME, Tiah L, Leong BS, et al. A randomized, double-blind, multicentre trial comparing vasopressin and adrenaline in patients with cardiac arrest presenting to or in the emergency department. Resuscitation. 2012;83:953–960.

6. Gueugniaud PY, David JS, Chanzy E, et al. Vasopressin and epinephrine vs. epinephrine alone in cardiopulmonary resuscitation. N Engl J Med. 2008;359:21–30.

7. Mukoyama T, Kinoshita K, Nagao K, et al. Reduced effectiveness of vasopressin in repeated doses for patients undergoing prolonged cardiopulmonary resuscitation. Resuscitation. 2009;80:755–761.

8. Devlin JW, Skrobik Y, Celine G, et al. Clinical practice guidelines for the management of pain, agitation/sedation, delirium, immobility and sleep disruption in adult patients in the ICU. Crit Care Med. 2018;46:e825–e873.

28

HYPOVOLEMIC SHOCK

A Glass Half Full . . . . Level II

Yvonne C. Huckleberry, PharmD, BCPS, FCCM

Brian J. Kopp, PharmD, BCPS, BCCCP, FCCM

Brian L. Erstad, PharmD, FCCP, MCCM, FASHP

LEARNING OBJECTIVES

After completing this case study, the reader should be able to:

- Develop a plan for implementing fluid or medication therapies for treating a patient in the initial stages of shock.

- Outline the major parameters used to monitor hypovolemic shock and its treatment.

- List the major disadvantages of using only isolated hemodynamic recordings, such as blood pressure measurements, for monitoring the progression of shock.

- Compare and contrast fluids and medications used for treating hypovolemic shock.

PATIENT PRESENTATION

■ Chief Complaint

"I'm beat. I have vomited four times in the last 24 hours and had diarrhea last evening. Now is not a great time to get sick since I'm in college and have finals next week."

■ HPI

Four days prior to admission, a 20-year-old college student had abdominal pain that he attributed to a flare-up in his Crohn disease due to the stress of final examinations. He has an infliximab infusion scheduled for next week; he has them every 8 weeks and does not miss these infusions. However, he admits that he forgets to take his oral medications now that he lives away from his family. When he has Crohn disease pain, he does not feel like eating since this worsens his stomach pain. Furthermore, he has vomiting and diarrhea, which are aggravated by food intake. Per the recommendation of his community pharmacist, the patient purchased a commercially available rehydration solution and attempted to drink the small but frequent volumes recommended by his pharmacist, but he could not keep up with fluid losses. His primary care physician referred him to the local hospital for rehydration and further evaluation.

■ PMH

Crohn disease, diagnosed 4 years ago
Ankylosing spondylitis, diagnosed 3 years ago

■ FH

Noncontributory

■ SH

Does not smoke or use illicit drugs; admits to occasional ETOH use at parties

■ Meds

Infliximab 300 mg by IV infusion over 3 hours every 8 weeks
Azathioprine 100 mg PO daily
Fish oil (unknown strength) one capsule PO BID
Multivitamin one tablet PO daily
Whey shakes for protein supplementation, one shake PO daily

■ All

NKDA

■ ROS

The patient has had a recent increase in weight over the past month (6 kg), although this has decreased by 2 kg in the past few days. Hearing is intact with no vertigo. No dizziness or fainting episodes. No chest pain or dyspnea, but heart has been "racing." Has had one episode of diarrhea and four episodes of vomiting with abdominal pain in the past 24 hours. No musculoskeletal pain or cramping.

■ Physical Examination

Gen

Thin, somewhat anxious man in mild distress

VS

BP 84/58 (baseline 122/78), but possible orthostatic changes not determined, HR 132 (baseline 80), RR 16, T 38.2°C; admission Wt 60 kg, Ht 5′10″

Skin

Pale color (including nail beds) and dry, but not cyanotic; no lesions

HEENT

Normal scalp/skull; conjunctivae pale and dry with clear sclerae; PERRLA, dry oral mucosa; remainder of ophthalmologic exam not performed

Neck/Lymph Nodes

Supple, no lymphadenopathy or thyromegaly

Lungs/Thorax

Clear by palpation and auscultation

CV

RRR; S$_1$ and S$_2$ normal; apical pulse difficult to palpate; no MRG

Abd

Perigastric pain on light palpation, no hepatosplenomegaly or masses; bowel sounds present

Genit/Rect

Normal male genitalia; no hemorrhoids or fistulas noted; stool heme (−)

MS/Ext

No deformities with normal ROM of joints except for hips and knees (somewhat limited ROM); no edema, ulcers, or tenderness

Neuro

Mild muscular atrophy with weak grip strength; CN II–XII intact; 2+ reflexes throughout; Babinski downgoing

■ Labs

Na 149 mEq/L	Hgb 11.9 g/dL	Phos 2.9 mg/dL
K 3.3 mEq/L	Hct 34.3%	AST 35 IU/L
Cl 112 mEq/L	Plt 151 × 10³/mm³	ALT 23 IU/L
CO$_2$ 30 mEq/L	WBC 13 × 10³/mm³	T. bili 1.1 mg/dL
BUN 32 mg/dL	PT 12.1 s	Alk phos 83 IU/L
SCr 1.4 mg/dL[a]	aPTT 33 s	CRP 16 mg/dL
Glu 105 mg/dL	Albumin 3.3 g/dL	ESR 48 mm/hr

[a]Baseline SCr 1.1 mg/dL.

■ Other Test Results

CXR negative. I/O 1200/150 (urinary catheter) for first 6 hours of hospitalization. Results pending for ABG with lactate level, blood and urine cultures, gastroenteric pathogens on stool culture, O & P, and *Clostridium difficile* titer.

■ Assessment

Volume depletion, acute kidney injury, Crohn disease exacerbation, possible acid–base disorder, possible infectious process in setting of immunosuppression, medication nonadherence.

QUESTIONS

Collect Information

1.a. What subjective and objective information indicates the presence of hypovolemic shock and acute kidney injury?

1.b. What additional information is needed to fully assess this patient's hypovolemic shock and acute kidney injury?

Assess the Information

2.a. Assess the severity of hypovolemic shock and acute kidney injury based on the subjective and objective information available.

2.b. Create a list of the patient's drug-related problems and prioritize them. Include assessment of medication appropriateness, effectiveness, safety, and patient adherence.

Develop a Care Plan

3.a. What are the goals of pharmacotherapy for hypovolemic shock and acute kidney injury in this case?

3.b. What nondrug therapies might be useful for this patient?

3.c. What feasible pharmacotherapeutic options are available for treating hypovolemic shock and addressing the associated laboratory alterations?

3.d. Create an individualized, patient-centered, team-based care plan to optimize medication therapy for this patient's hypovolemic shock and other drug therapy problems. Include specific drugs, dosage forms, doses, schedules, and durations of therapy.

Implement the Care Plan

4.a. What information should be provided to the patient to enhance adherence, ensure successful therapy, and minimize adverse effects?

4.b. Describe how care should be coordinated with other healthcare providers.

Follow-Up: Monitor and Evaluate

5. Explain how to monitor and evaluate the care plan for medication appropriateness, effectiveness, safety, and patient adherence by using clinical and laboratory data, patient feedback, and other information.

■ CLINICAL COURSE

No evidence of infection was found. All cultures were negative, and the elevated temperature abated within 12 hours of admission. However, the patient had a complicated clinical course since he received treatment with hypotonic fluids early in his hospital course, which provided inadequate intravascular expansion to correct his hypovolemic shock. After approximately 24 hours, the patient had to be admitted to the ICU for hypotension and acute kidney injury.

■ FOLLOW-UP QUESTION

1. Explain why hypotonic IV fluids such as 5% dextrose are not indicated in a patient with overt hypovolemia, who is going into shock.

■ SELF-STUDY ASSIGNMENTS

1. Search the literature and discuss the results of comparative trials involving crystalloids and colloids for plasma expansion.

2. Write a two-page report that compares the advantages and limitations of each type of fluid for the plasma expansion indication.

CLINICAL PEARL

Isotonic or near-isotonic IV crystalloid solutions are indicated in patients with extracellular fluid depletion, who cannot receive oral rehydration solutions due to the severity of presentation or inability to absorb adequate volumes. Isotonic solutions replenish the extracellular space and have minimal intracellular distribution.

REFERENCES

1. Kidney Disease. Improving Global Outcomes (KDIGO) Acute Kidney Injury Work Group. Clinical Practice Guideline for Acute Injury. Kidney Int Suppl. 2012;2:1–138.

2. Evans L, Rhodes A, Alhazzani W, et al. Surviving sepsis campaign: international guidelines for management of sepsis and septic shock 2021. Intensive Care Med. 2021;47:1181–1247.

3. Krajewski ML, Raghunathan K, Paluszkiewicz SM, et al. Meta-analysis of high- versus low-chloride content in perioperative and critical care fluid resuscitation. Br J Surg. 2015;102:24–36.

4. Semler MW, Self WH, Wanderer JP, et al. Balanced crystalloids versus saline in critically ill adults. N Engl J Med. 2018;378:829–839.

5. Self WH, Semler MW, Wanderer JP, et al. Balanced crystalloids versus saline in noncritically ill adults. N Engl J Med. 2018;378:819–828.

6. Zampieri FG, Machado FR, Biondi RS, et al. Effect of intravenous fluid treatment with a balanced solution vs 0.9% saline solution on mortality in critically ill patients: the BaSICS randomized clinical trial. JAMA. 2021;326:1–12.

7. Finfer S, Micallef S, Hammond N, et al. Balanced multielectrolyte solution versus saline in critically ill adults. N Engl J Med. 2022;386(9):815–826. doi: 10.1056/NEJMoa2114464.

8. Hammond NE, Zampieri FG, Di Tanna GL, et al. Balanced crystalloids versus saline in critically ill adults—a systematic review with meta-analysis. NEJM Evid. 2022;1(2). doi: 10.1056/EVIDoa2100010.

9. Finfer S, Bellomo R, Boyce N, et al; SAFE Study Investigators. A comparison of albumin and saline for fluid resuscitation in the intensive care unit. N Engl J Med. 2004;350:2247–2256.

10. Levitov A, Frankel HL, Blaivas M, et al. Guidelines for the appropriate use of bedside general and cardiac ultrasonography in the evaluation of critically ill patients-part II: cardiac ultrasonography. Crit Care Med. 2016;44:1206–1227.

29

ACUTE ASTHMA

A Little Influenza, a Big Asthma Attack .... Level I

Rebecca S. Pettit, PharmD, MBA, BCPS, BCPPS, FCCP

LEARNING OBJECTIVES

After completing this case study, the reader should be able to:

- Recognize the signs and symptoms of an acute asthma exacerbation.

- Formulate therapeutic endpoints based on the initiation of a pharmacotherapy plan used to treat the acute asthma symptoms.

- Identify appropriate dosage form selection based on the patient's age, ability to take medication, or adherence to technique.

- Determine an appropriate home pharmacotherapy plan, including discharge counseling, as the patient nears discharge from a hospital setting.

PATIENT PRESENTATION

■ Chief Complaint

"My daughter has had a bad fever, and now she is having trouble breathing, and albuterol doesn't help."

■ HPI

An 8-year-old girl presents to the ED with a 2-day history of fevers, malaise, and nonproductive cough. The mother gave acetaminophen and ibuprofen to help control the fever. Mother stated that "a lot of other kids in her class have been sick this fall, too." The patient started having trouble breathing the morning of admission, and the mother gave her albuterol, 2.5 mg via nebulization twice within an hour. She still sounded wheezy to the mother after the albuterol and stated it was "hard to breathe." She was previously well-controlled regarding asthma symptoms. Previous clinic notes reported symptoms during the day only with active play at school or at home and rare nighttime symptoms. She uses PRN albuterol to help with symptoms after playing. Her assessment in the emergency department revealed labored breathing, such that she could only complete four- to five-word sentences. She had subcostal retractions, tracheal tugging with tachypnea at 54 breaths/min. Her other vital signs were a heart rate of 160 bpm, blood pressure of 115/59, temperature of 38.8°C, and a weight of 22.7 kg. The initial oxygen saturation was 88%, and she was started on oxygen at 1 L/min via nasal cannula. Bilateral expiratory and inspiratory wheezes were noted on examination. A chest X-ray revealed a right lower lobe consolidation consistent with pneumonia and possible effusion. After receiving three albuterol/ipratropium nebulizations, her breath sounds and oxygenation did not improve, so she was started on albuterol via continuous nebulization at 10 mg/hr and her oxygen was titrated to 3 L/min. She was also given a dose of 25 mg IV methylprednisolone and a dose of 600 mg IV magnesium sulfate. She was then transferred to the PICU for further treatment and monitoring.

■ PMH

Asthma; last hospitalization 4 years ago, and has had two courses of oral corticosteroids in the past year. Before this exacerbation mother reports she used her albuterol 3–4 times per week due to daytime symptoms and wakes up coughing about 2 nights per week.

■ FH

Asthma on father's side of the family

■ SH

Lives with mother, father, and two siblings, both of whom have asthma. There are two cats and a dog in the home. Father is a smoker but states that he tries to smoke outside and not around the kids. She is in the second grade and is very active on the playground.

■ Meds

Albuterol 2.5 mg nebulized Q 4–6 H PRN wheezing
Fluticasone propionate 44 mcg MDI one puff BID
Acetaminophen 160 mg/5 mL—10 mL PO Q 4 H PRN fever
Ibuprofen 100 mg/5 mL—10 mL PO Q 6 H PRN fever

■ All

NKA

■ ROS

(+) Fever, cough, increased work of breathing

■ Physical Examination

Gen

Alert and oriented but in mild distress with difficulty breathing

VS

BP 125/69, P 120, T 37.9°C, RR 40, O$_2$ sat 94% on 3 L/min nasal cannula

Skin

No rashes, no bruises

HEENT

NC/AT, PERRLA

Neck/LN

Soft, supple, no cervical lymphadenopathy

Chest

Wheezes throughout all lung fields, still with subcostal retractions

CV

RRR, no m/r/g

Abd

Soft, NT/ND

Ext

No clubbing or cyanosis

Neuro

A&O, no focal deficits

■ Labs

Na 141 mEq/L	WBC $34.2 \times 10^3/mm^3$
K 3.1 mEq/L	Neut 91%
Cl 104 mEq/L	Lymph 5%
CO_2 29 mEq/L	Mono 4%
BUN 16 mg/dL	RBC $5.07 \times 10^6/mm^3$
SCr 0.52 mg/dL	Hgb 13 g/dL
Glu 154 mg/dL	Hct 41%
	Plt $310 \times 10^3/mm^3$

Respiratory viral panel nasal swab: positive for influenza A

■ Chest X-Ray

RLL consolidation

■ Assessment

Asthma exacerbation with viral pneumonia

QUESTIONS

Collect Information

1.a. What subjective and objective information indicates the presence of an asthma exacerbation?

1.b. What additional information is needed to fully assess this patient's asthma exacerbation?

Assess the Information

2.a. Assess the severity of the asthma exacerbation based on the subjective and objective information available.

2.b. Create a list of the patient's drug therapy problems and prioritize them. Include assessment of medication appropriateness, effectiveness, safety, and patient adherence.

Develop a Care Plan

3.a. What are the goals of pharmacotherapy for the asthma exacerbation in this case?

3.b. What nondrug therapies might be useful for this patient's asthma exacerbation?

3.c. What feasible pharmacotherapeutic options are available for treating this patient's asthma exacerbation?

3.d. Create an individualized, patient-centered, team-based care plan to optimize medication therapy for this patient's asthma exacerbation and other drug therapy problems. Include specific drugs, dosage forms, doses, schedules, and durations of therapy.

Implement the Care Plan

4.a. What information should be provided to the patient to enhance adherence, ensure successful therapy, and minimize adverse effects?

4.b. Describe how care should be coordinated with other healthcare providers.

Follow-Up: Monitor and Evaluate

5. Explain how to monitor and evaluate the care plan for medication appropriateness, effectiveness, safety, and patient adherence by using clinical and laboratory data, patient feedback, and other information.

■ CLINICAL COURSE

Within 48 hours of initiation of the treatment plan for management of the acute exacerbation, she was stable enough to transfer to the general pediatric floor. Her vital signs were BP 103/70, P 82, RR 35, T 37.2°C, and O_2 sat 99% on 1 L/min nasal cannula. Mother states that she is able to speak in full sentences now and no longer seems to have trouble breathing.

■ FOLLOW-UP QUESTIONS

1. Should any cough and cold products be used for asthma symptoms? Why or why not?

2. What information should be given to patients/families regarding influenza?

3. What information can be given to families who are concerned about giving their child "steroids" for asthma treatment (either in an acute asthma exacerbation or for controller therapy)?

■ SELF-STUDY ASSIGNMENTS

1. Research the efficacy of systemic corticosteroids for treatment of acute asthma exacerbation when given intravenously versus orally (enterally).

2. Discuss the differences in acute asthma exacerbation symptoms in an adult patient versus a pediatric patient, and describe when you would refer a patient (or family) to the physician or emergency department based on an individualized asthma action plan.

3. Discuss the appropriate use of IV magnesium in an acute asthma exacerbation.

CLINICAL PEARL

Patients of any age can use metered dose inhalers with the use of a proper spacer with or without a mask.

REFERENCES

1. Basnet S, Mander G, Andoh J, et al. Safety, efficacy, and tolerability of early initiation of noninvasive positive pressure ventilation in pediatric patients admitted with status asthmaticus: a pilot study. Pediatr Crit Care Med. 2012;13:393–398.

2. National Asthma Education and Prevention Program Expert Panel report 3: guidelines for the diagnosis and management of asthma. Bethesda, MD, National Institutes of Health, 2007. Available at: *http://www.nhlbi.nih.gov/guidelines/asthma/asthgdln.htm*. Accessed November 10, 2021.

3. 2020 Focused Updates to the Asthma Management Guidelines. Bethesda, MD, National Institutes of Health, 2020. Available at: *https://www.nhlbi.nih.gov/health-topics/all-publications-and-resources/2020-focused-updates-asthma-management-guidelines*. Accessed November 10, 2021.

4. Global Initiative for Asthma (GINA). 2021. Global strategy for asthma management and preventions. Available at: *www.ginasthma.org/*. Accessed November 10, 2021.

5. Andrew T, McGintee E, Mittal MK, et al. High-dose continuous nebulized levalbuterol for pediatric status asthmaticus: a randomized trial. J Pediatr. 2009;155:205–210.

6. Vezina K, Chauhan BF, Ducharme FM. Inhaled anticholinergics and short-acting beta(2)-agonists versus short-acting beta2-agonists alone for children with acute asthma in hospital. Cochrane Database Syst Rev. 2014;7:1–55.

7. Rowe BH, Camargo CA. The role of magnesium sulfate in the acute and chronic management of asthma. Curr Opin Pulm Med. 2008;15:70–76.

8. Kokotajlo S, Degnan L, Meyers R, et al. Use of intravenous magnesium sulfate for the treatment of an acute asthma exacerbation in pediatric patients. J Pediatr Pharmacol Ther. 2014;19(2):91–97.

9. Link HW. Pediatric asthma in a nutshell. Pediatr Rev. 2014;35(7):287–298.

10. Rank MA, Li JT. Clinical pearls for preventing, diagnosing, and treating seasonal and 2009 H1N1 influenza infections in patients with asthma. J Allergy Clin Immunol. 2009;124:1123–1126.

30

CHRONIC ASTHMA

Dust in the Wind .... Level II

Julia M. Koehler, PharmD, FCCP

Meghan M. Bodenberg, PharmD, BCPS

Jennifer R. Guthrie, MPAS, PA-C

LEARNING OBJECTIVES

After completing this case study, the reader should be able to:

- Recognize signs and symptoms of uncontrolled asthma.

- Identify potential causes of uncontrolled asthma, and recommend preventive measures.

- Formulate a patient-specific therapeutic plan (including drugs, route of administration, and appropriate monitoring parameters) for management of a patient with chronic asthma.

- Develop a self-management action plan for improving control of asthma.

PATIENT PRESENTATION

Chief Complaint

"I think the dust is getting to me!"

HPI

A 17-year-old girl presents to her primary care provider for follow-up and evaluation regarding her asthma. During her visit, she reports having had to use her albuterol MDI approximately 3–4 days per week over the past 2 months; however, over the past week, she admits to using albuterol once daily. She reports being awakened by a cough at night once a week during the past month. She states she especially becomes short of breath when she visits her father's custom cabinetry workshop and when she exercises (although she admits that her shortness of breath is not always brought on by exercise and sometimes occurs when she is not actively exercising). In addition to her albuterol MDI, which she uses PRN, and she also has a fluticasone MDI, which she uses "most days of the week." She indicates that her morning peak flows have been running around 300 L/min (personal best = 400 L/min) over the past several weeks.

PMH

Asthma (previously documented as "mild persistent") diagnosed at age 7; no prior history of intubations; hospitalized once in the past year for asthma exacerbation; one visit to the ED in the past 6 months; treated with oral systemic corticosteroids during last hospitalization and at ED visit.

Migraine headache disorder (without aura; diagnosed at age 15); currently taking prophylactic medication; has had only one migraine attack in the last year.

FH

Mother, age 49, nonsmoker with HTN, migraine HA disorder, and asthma; father, age 50, smoker with HTN and type 2 DM; brother, age 21, smoker, healthy; twin sister, age 17, nonsmoker, healthy

SH

No alcohol or tobacco use. Single, not sexually active. Lives at home with parents (father is a cabinet maker), twin sister, and two cats. Brother is currently away at college.

Meds

Flovent HFA 44 mcg, two puffs BID

Proventil HFA two puffs Q 4–6 H PRN shortness of breath, cough, wheezing

Propranolol 80 mg PO BID

Maxalt-MLT 5 mg PO PRN acute migraine

All

PCN (rash)

ROS

Denies fever, chills, headache, eye discharge or redness, rhinorrhea, sneezing, sputum production, chest pain, palpitations, dizziness, or confusion

Physical Examination

Gen

Well-developed, well-nourished white female appearing stated age in NAD

VS

BP 110/68, HR 78, RR 16, T 37°C; Wt 58 kg, Ht 5′5″

HEENT

PERRLA; mild oral thrush present on tongue and buccal mucosa

Neck/Lymph Nodes

Supple; no lymphadenopathy or thyromegaly

Lungs/Thorax

No intercostal retractions or accessory muscle use with respirations; good air movement; mild expiratory wheezes bilaterally

CV

RRR; no MRG

Abd

Soft, NTND; (+) BS

Ext

Normal ROM; peripheral pulses 3+; no CCE

Neuro

A&O × 3. No focal deficits.

■ Labs

Na 136 mEq/L	Hgb 14 g/dL	WBC $6.0 \times 10^3/mm^3$
K 3.6 mEq/L	Hct 42%	PMNs 56%
Cl 99 mEq/L	RBC $5.0 \times 10^6/mm^3$	Bands 1%
CO_2 27 mEq/L	Plts $192 \times 10^3/mm^3$	Eosinophils 3%
BUN 18 mg/dL		Basophils 2%
SCr 0.6 mg/dL		Lymphocytes 33%
Glu 98 mg/dL		Monocytes 5%
Ca 9.3 mg/dL		

■ Assessment

A 17-year-old girl with uncontrolled chronic asthma and mild oral thrush.

QUESTIONS

Collect Information

1.a. What subjective and objective information indicates the presence of uncontrolled chronic asthma?

1.b. What additional information is needed to fully assess this patient's asthma? (Consider factors that may have contributed to this patient's uncontrolled asthma.)

Assess the Information

2.a. Assess this patient's level of asthma control based on the subjective and objective information available.

2.b. Create a list of the patient's drug therapy problems and prioritize them. Include assessment of medication appropriateness, effectiveness, safety, and patient adherence.

Develop a Care Plan

3.a. What are the goals of pharmacotherapy for asthma in this case?

3.b. What nondrug therapies might be useful for this patient's asthma?

3.c. What feasible pharmacotherapeutic options are available for treating this patient's chronic asthma?

3.d. Create an individualized, patient-centered, team-based care plan to optimize medication therapy for this patient's asthma and other drug therapy problems. Include specific drugs, dosage forms, doses, schedules, and durations of therapy.

3.e. What alternatives would be appropriate if the initial care plan fails?

Implement the Care Plan

4.a. What information should be provided to the patient to enhance adherence, ensure successful therapy, and minimize adverse effects?

4.b. Describe how care should be coordinated with other healthcare providers.

Follow-Up: Monitor and Evaluate

5. Explain how to monitor and evaluate the care plan for medication appropriateness, effectiveness, safety, and patient adherence by using clinical and laboratory data, patient feedback, and other information.

■ SELF-STUDY ASSIGNMENTS

1. Review the different types of inhaler devices that could be prescribed for asthma, and prepare a table outlining the steps for correct use of each type of device, as well as device-specific recommendations for priming and cleaning.

2. Review the literature on the impact of chronic inhaled corticosteroid use on the risk for development of osteoporosis, and write a two-page paper summarizing the available published literature on this topic.

CLINICAL PEARL

Patients with asthma who report that taking aspirin makes their asthma symptoms worse may have what is known as aspirin-exacerbated respiratory disease (AERD), or Samter's Triad, which includes the combination of bronchial asthma, nasal polyps, and aspirin intolerance. The leukotriene pathway may play a role in the development of asthma symptoms in such patients, and inhibition of cyclooxygenase by aspirin may shunt the arachidonic acid pathway away from prostaglandin synthesis and toward leukotriene production. Although inhaled corticosteroids are still the preferred anti-inflammatory medications for patients with asthma and known aspirin sensitivity, leukotriene modifiers may also be useful in such patients based on this theoretical mechanism.

REFERENCES

1. Expert Panel Working Group of the National Heart, Lung, and Blood Institute. Focused updates to the asthma management guidelines: a report from the National Asthma Education and Prevention Program Coordinating Committee Expert Panel Working Group. J Allergy Clin Immunol. 2020;146:1217–1270. doi: 10.1016/j.jaci.2020.10.003.

2. Global Initiative for Asthma (GINA). Global strategy for asthma management and prevention. 2021. Available at: *https://ginasthma.org/gina-reports/*. Accessed March 31, 2022.

3. National Asthma Education and Prevention Program. Executive Summary of the NAEPP Expert Panel Report 3: Guidelines for the Diagnosis and Management of Asthma. Bethesda, MD, U.S. Department of Health and Human Services, Public Health Service, National Institutes of Health, National Heart, Lung, and Blood Institute, 2007. Full report. Available at: *https://www.nhlbi.nih.gov/health-topics/guidelines-for-diagnosis-management-of-asthma*. Accessed March 31, 2022.

4. Lemanske RF, Mauger DT, Sorkness CA, et al. Step-up therapy for children with uncontrolled asthma while receiving inhaled corticosteroids. N Engl J Med. 2010;362:975–985.

5. Jorup C, Lythgoe D, Bigaard H. Budesonide/formoterol maintenance and reliever therapy in adolescent patients with asthma. Eur Respir J. 2018;51(1):1701688. doi: 10.1183/13993003.01688-2017.

6. Busse W, Raphael GD, Galant S, et al. Fluticasone Propionate Clinical Research Study Group. Low-dose fluticasone propionate compared with montelukast for first-line treatment of persistent asthma: a randomized clinical trial. J Allergy Clin Immunol. 2001;107:461–468.

7. Busse W, Nelson H, Wolfe J, Kalberg C, Yancey SW, Rickard KA. Comparison of inhaled salmeterol and oral zafirlukast in patients with asthma. J Allergy Clin Immunol. 1999;103:1075–1080.

8. US Food and Drug Administration. FDA requires Boxed Warning about serious mental health side effects for asthma and allergy drug montelukast (Singulair); advises restricting use for allergic rhinitis. FDA Drug Safety Communication, March 4, 2020. Available at: *https://www.fda. gov/drugs/drug-safety-and-availability/fda-requires-boxed-warning-about-serious-mental-health-side-effects-asthma-and-allergy-drug*. Accessed March 31, 2022.

9. Holguin F, Cardet JC, Chung KF, et al. Management of severe asthma: a European Respiratory Society/American Thoracic Society guideline. Eur Respir J. 2020;55:1900588. doi: 10.1183/13993003.0058-2019.

31

CHRONIC OBSTRUCTIVE PULMONARY DISEASE

Treading on Thin Air .... Level II

Sarah L. Anderson, PharmD, FASHP, FCCP, BCACP, BCPS

Joel C. Marrs, PharmD, MPH, FAHA, FASHP, FCCP, FNLA, BCACP, BCCP, BCPS, CLS

LEARNING OBJECTIVES

After completing this case study, the reader should be able to:

- Recognize modifiable risk factors for the development of chronic obstructive pulmonary disease (COPD).

- Interpret spirometry readings and patient-specific factors to evaluate and appropriately classify an individual patient's COPD.

- Identify the importance of nonpharmacologic therapy in patients with COPD.

- Develop an appropriate medication regimen for a patient with COPD based on disease classification.

PATIENT PRESENTATION

Chief Complaint

"My wife says I need to get my lungs checked. Ever since we moved, I'm having a hard time breathing."

HPI

A 59-year-old man who is presenting to a new provider at the family medicine clinic today with complaints of increasing shortness of breath. He points out that he first noticed some difficulty catching his breath at his job 3 years ago. He had been able to carry heavy loads up and down a flight of stairs daily for the past 35 years without any problem. However, his shortness of breath began to make this very difficult. Coincidentally at that time, he accepted a managerial position at his company that significantly reduced his activity level. After taking this position, he no longer noticed any problems, but he admits that he avoids activities that cause him to physically exert himself. He noticed significant shortness of breath again after he moved to Colorado from a lower elevation 2 months ago to be closer to his grandchildren. His shortness of breath is worst when he is outside playing with his grandchildren. He maintained his same managerial position with the move and does not physically exert himself at work. His previous physician had placed him on budesonide/formoterol (Symbicort), two inhalations twice daily 2 years ago. He thinks his physician initiated the medication for the shortness of breath, but he is not entirely sure. He is hoping to get a good medication that will help relieve his shortness of breath because the gardening season is right around the corner, and he enjoys this hobby.

PMH

Coronary artery disease (CAD; MI 7 years ago, resulting in a drug-eluting stent [DES] placement at that time; additional DES placed 2 years ago; normal echocardiogram and stress test 3 months ago)
Chronic bronchitis × 8 years (has had one exacerbation in the past 12 months; received oral antibiotic treatment but was not hospitalized)
Cervical radiculopathy

FH

Father (alive) with COPD (smoked a pipe for 40 years). Mother (alive) with CAD and cerebrovascular disease.

SH

He lives with his wife, who is a nurse. He has a 40 pack-year history of smoking. When he had an MI at age 52, he quit smoking temporarily. At present, he continues to smoke five to six cigarettes per day. He drinks two beers most nights of the workweek and two to three glasses of wine on the weekends.

Meds

Aspirin 81 mg PO once daily
Bupropion SR 150 mg PO twice daily
Clopidogrel 75 mg PO once daily
Budesonide/formoterol 80 mcg/4.5 mcg, two inhalations twice daily
OTC naproxen 220 mg PO every 12 hours PRN neck pain
Rosuvastatin 20 mg PO once daily
Metoprolol succinate 50 mg PO once daily
Seasonal influenza vaccine (previous year)

All

NKDA

ROS

(+) Chronic cough with sputum production; (+) exercise intolerance

Physical Examination

Gen

WDWN man in NAD

VS

BP 110/68, P 60, RR 16, T 37°C; Wt 82 kg, Ht 5'9"; pulse ox 93% on RA

Skin

Warm, dry; no rashes

HEENT

Normocephalic; PERRLA, EOMI; normal sclerae; mucous membranes are moist; TMs intact; oropharynx clear

Neck/Lymph Nodes

Supple without lymphadenopathy

Lungs

Decreased breath sounds; no rales, rhonchi, or crackles

CV

RRR without murmur; normal S_1 and S_2

Abd

Soft, NT/ND; (+) bowel sounds; no organomegaly

Genit/Rect

No back or flank tenderness; normal male genitalia

MS/Ext

No CCE; pulses 2+ throughout

Neuro

A&O × 3; CN II–XII intact; DTRs 2+; normal mood and affect

■ Labs

Na 135 mEq/L	Hgb 13.5 g/dL	AST 40 IU/L	Ca 9.6 mg/L
K 4.2 mEq/L	Hct 41.2%	ALT 19 IU/L	Mg 3.6 mg/L
Cl 108 mEq/L	Plt 195 × 10³/mm³	T. bili 1.1 mg/dL	Phos 2.9 mg/dL
CO₂ 26 mEq/L	WBC 5.4 × 10³/mm³	Alb 3.8 g/dL	
BUN 19 mg/dL			
SCr 1.1 mg/dL			
Glu 89 mg/dL			
NT pro-BNP 0 pg/mL			
Troponin 0 ng/mL			

■ Pulmonary Function Tests (During Clinic Visit Today)

Prebronchodilator FEV_1 = 2.98 L (predicted is 4.02 L)
FVC = 4.5 L
Postbronchodilator FEV_1 = 2.75 L

■ Assessment

This is a normal-appearing 59-year-old man presenting to the clinic with complaints of shortness of breath that is limiting his activity and affecting his quality of life. Given the results of spirometry and patient history, patient has COPD in addition to a history of CAD, daily pain from cervical radiculopathy, and chronic cough. Cardiac pathology as a cause of current symptoms is unlikely, given lack of chest pain and recent normal cardiovascular stress test. The patient states that he is adherent to his current medication regimen.

QUESTIONS

Collect Information

1.a. What subjective and objective information indicates the presence of COPD?

1.b. What additional information is needed to fully assess this patient's COPD?

Assess the Information

2.a. Assess the severity of COPD based on the subjective and objective information available.

2.b. Create a list of the patient's drug therapy problems and prioritize them. Include assessment of medication appropriateness, effectiveness, safety, and patient adherence.

2.c. What economic and psychosocial considerations are applicable to this patient?

Develop a Care Plan

3.a. What are the goals of pharmacotherapy for COPD in this case?

3.b. What nondrug therapies might be useful for this patient's COPD?

3.c. What feasible pharmacotherapeutic options are available for treating COPD?

3.d. Create an individualized, patient-centered, team-based care plan to optimize medication therapy for this patient's COPD and other drug therapy problems. Include specific drugs, dosage forms, doses, schedules, and durations of therapy.

Implement the Care Plan

4.a. What information should be provided to the patient to enhance adherence, ensure successful therapy, and minimize adverse effects?

4.b. Describe how care should be coordinated with other healthcare providers.

Follow-Up: Monitor and Evaluate

5. Explain how to monitor and evaluate the care plan for medication appropriateness, effectiveness, safety, and patient adherence by using clinical and laboratory data, patient feedback, and other information.

■ SELF-STUDY ASSIGNMENTS

1. Describe and compare the expectations for deterioration in pulmonary function in patients with COPD who have quit smoking with those who continue smoking. In particular, emphasis should be placed on expected patterns of change in FEV_1, FVC, and general health over time in years.

2. Research and describe the appropriate use of inhaled corticosteroids for the management of stable COPD. Be able to compare and contrast the benefits and risks of this therapy.

3. Analyze the safety surrounding the use of β-blockers in patients with COPD versus those with asthma.

CLINICAL PEARL

All patients with COPD, regardless of GOLD group, should be prescribed a short-acting rescue bronchodilator for immediate symptom relief. Similarly, all patients in Groups B–D should be prescribed a long-acting bronchodilator. Patients should be educated on proper inhaler technique and the importance of daily use of their long-acting bronchodilator medication.

REFERENCES

1. Global Initiative for Chronic Obstructive Lung Disease (GOLD). Global strategy for the diagnosis, management, and prevention of chronic obstructive pulmonary disease: 2022 report. Available at: *http://www.goldcopd.org*. Accessed February 28, 2022.

2. Nici L, Mammen MJ, Charbek E, Alexander PE, Au DH, Boyd CM, et al. Pharmacologic management of COPD: an official ATS clinical practice guideline. Am J Respir Crit Care Med. 2020;201(9):e56–369.

3. Tang B, Wang J, Luo LL, Li QG, Huang D. Risks of budesonide/formoterol for the treatment of stable COPD: a meta-analysis. Int J Chron Obstruct Pulmon Dis. 2019 Apr 1;14:757–766.

4. Aziz MIA, Tan LE, Wu DBC, et al. Comparative efficacy of inhaled medications (ICS/LABA, LAMA, LAMA/LABA and SAMA) for COPD: a systematic review and network meta-analysis. Int J Chron Obstruct Pulmon Dis. 2018 Oct 9;13:3203–3231.

5. Janson C. Treatment with inhaled corticosteroids in chronic obstructive pulmonary disease. J Thorac Dis. 2020 Apr;12(4):1561–1569.

6. Kew KM, Mavergames C, Walters JA. Long-acting beta2-agonists for chronic obstructive pulmonary disease. Cochrane Database Syst Rev. 2013;10:CD010177.

7. Tashkin DP, Pearle J, Iezzoni D, Varghese ST. Formoterol and tiotropium compared with tiotropium alone for treatment of COPD. COPD. 2009;6:17–25.

8. van Noord JA, Aumann JL, Janssens E, et al. Comparison of tiotropium once daily, formoterol twice daily, and both combined once daily in patients with COPD. Eur Respir J. 2005;26:214–222.

9. Karner C, Cates CJ. Long-acting beta(2)-agonist in addition to tiotropium versus either tiotropium or long-acting beta(2)-agonist alone for chronic obstructive pulmonary disease. Cochrane Database Syst Rev. 2012;4:CD008989.

10. Recommended Immunization Schedule for Adults Aged 19 Years of Older, United States, 2021. Available at: *https://www.cdc.gov/vaccines/schedules/hcp/imz/adult.html*. Accessed February 28, 2022.

32

PULMONARY ARTERY HYPERTENSION

Too Much Pressure .... Level II

Marta A. Miyares, PharmD, BCPS, BCCP, CACP

LEARNING OBJECTIVES

After completing this case study, the reader should be able to:

- Determine risk factors for developing pulmonary artery hypertension (PAH).

- Discuss common signs and symptoms associated with PAH.

- List the pharmacologic agents used to treat PAH.

- List the nonpharmacologic agents used to treat PAH.

- Recommend appropriate pharmacologic and nonpharmacologic education for a patient with PAH.

PATIENT PRESENTATION

■ Chief Complaint

"I felt really dizzy and short of breath, and I suddenly passed out on the bathroom floor."

■ HPI

A 32-year-old woman presents to the ED complaining of episodes of dyspnea and dizziness. While stepping out of the shower this morning, she became very weak and experienced a syncopal episode. She remembers falling to the floor and hitting her head but remembers nothing after that. She was brought to the ED this morning by her sister.

■ PMH

Hypertension × 4 years
Diabetes mellitus × 2 years
Asthma (intermittent)

■ FH

Father died of heart failure at the age of 62. Mother is 57 and was diagnosed with PAH 4 years ago. The patient is single and lives with her sister (her only sibling).

■ SH

Denies tobacco or alcohol use. Admits to heavy cocaine use in her late 20s. Has tried various fad diets (including prescription amphetamines) since she was in college.

■ Meds

Hydrochlorothiazide 12.5 mg PO Q AM
Glyburide 5 mg PO daily with breakfast
Albuterol MDI one to two puffs Q 6 H PRN SOB

■ All

NKDA

■ ROS

Today, the patient says she is comfortable at rest but complains of having experienced increased dyspnea, fatigue, and dizziness with her everyday activities for the past 6 months. She says that these symptoms only mildly limit her physical activity and denies experiencing these symptoms at rest. Over the past 2–3 months, she has developed palpitations and noticeable swelling in her ankles. She denies episodes of syncope before this acute incident. Approximately 9 months ago, she was seen by her family physician for increasing shortness of breath. Her physician believed that her increasing dyspnea was attributed to asthma, so he prescribed an albuterol inhaler for her to use. The patient says that the albuterol inhaler did not improve her shortness of breath.

■ Physical Examination

Gen

Patient is lying in ED bed and appears to be in moderate distress.

VS

BP 128/78, P 120, RR 26, T 37°C; Wt 128 kg, Ht 5′6″, O$_2$ sat 88% on room air

Skin

Cool to touch; no diaphoresis

HEENT

PERRLA; EOMI; dry mucous membranes; TMs intact

Neck/Lymph Nodes

(+) JVD; no lymphadenopathy; no thyromegaly; no bruits

Lungs/Thorax

Clear without wheezes, rhonchi, or rales

Breasts

Deferred

CV

Split S_2, loud P_2, S_3 gallop

Abd

Soft; (+) HJR; liver slightly enlarged; normal bowel sounds; no guarding

Genit/Rect

Deferred

MS/Ext

Full range of motion; 2+ edema to both lower extremities; no clubbing or cyanosis; pulses palpable

Neuro

A&O × 3; normal DTRs bilaterally

■ Labs

Na 138 mEq/L	Hgb 14 g/dL	WBC $8.8 \times 10^3/mm^3$	Mg 2.1 mg/dL
K 3.8 mEq/L	Hct 40%	Neutros 62%	Ca 8.4 mg/dL
Cl 98 mEq/L	RBC $5.1 \times 10^6/mm^3$	Bands 2%	BNP 60 pg/mL
CO_2 28 mEq/L	Plt $311 \times 10^3/mm^3$	Eos 1%	
BUN 12 mg/dL	MCV 84 μm^3	Lymphs 32%	
SCr 0.9 mg/dL	MCHC 34 g/dL	Monos 3%	
Glu 88 mg/dL			

■ ECG

Sinus tachycardia (rate 120 bpm); right-axis deviation; ST-segment depression in right precordial leads; tall P waves in leads 2, 3, and aVF

■ Chest X-Ray

Cardiomegaly; prominent main pulmonary artery; no apparent pulmonary edema

■ Two-Dimensional Echocardiography

Right ventricular and atrial hypertrophy; tricuspid regurgitation; estimated mean pulmonary arterial pressure (mPAP) 55 mm Hg

■ Ventilation/Perfusion Scan

Negative for pulmonary embolism

■ Pulmonary Function Tests

FEV_1 = 1.87 L (61% of predicted)
FVC = 2.10 L (57% of predicted)
FEV_1/FVC = 0.89

■ Assessment

A 32-year-old woman presents with signs/symptoms of PAH (likely familial).

QUESTIONS

Collect Information

1.a. What subjective and objective information indicates the presence of PAH?

1.b. What additional information is needed to fully assess this patient's PAH?

Assess the Information

2.a. Assess the severity of PAH based on the subjective and objective information available.

2.b. Create a list of the patient's drug therapy problems and prioritize them. Include assessment of medication appropriateness, effectiveness, safety, and patient adherence.

Develop a Care Plan

3.a. What are the goals of pharmacotherapy for PAH in this case?

3.b. What nondrug therapies might be useful for this patient's PAH?

3.c. What feasible pharmacotherapeutic options are available for treating PAH?

■ CLINICAL COURSE (PART 1)

After admission into the ED, the patient underwent a right heart catheterization for vasoreactivity testing. The results indicated that after receiving the short-acting vasodilator epoprostenol, the patient did not have significant reductions in mPAP and therefore was deemed a nonresponder. The patient's pulmonologist wants to start the patient on bosentan and asks for your recommendation.

3.d. Create an individualized, patient-centered, team-based care plan to optimize medication therapy for this patient's PAH and other drug therapy problems. Include specific drugs, dosage forms, doses, schedules, and durations of therapy.

■ CLINICAL COURSE (PART 2)

After 3 months of bosentan therapy, the patient's liver function tests (LFTs) are elevated, so the patient's pulmonologist tells the patient to stop the bosentan for 1 month. It has now been 1 month and the patient returns with normal LFTs.

3.e. What alternatives to bosentan would be appropriate to try next?

Implement the Care Plan

4.a. What information should be provided to the patient to enhance adherence, ensure successful therapy, and minimize adverse effects?

4.b. Describe how care should be coordinated with other healthcare providers.

Follow-Up: Monitor and Evaluate

5. Explain how to monitor and evaluate the care plan for medication appropriateness, effectiveness, safety, and patient adherence by using clinical and laboratory data, patient feedback, and other information.

■ SELF-STUDY ASSIGNMENTS

1. Perform a literature search to determine which medications used for the treatment of PAH have been shown to be safe in pregnancy. Identify the risks associated with pregnancy in female patients with PAH.

2. Use primary and tertiary literature to identify the potential visual side effects associated with oral phosphodiesterase inhibitors. Identify the visual side effect that is a medical emergency.

3. Review primary and tertiary literature to compare the advantages and disadvantages of using the vasodilators epoprostenol, treprostinil, and iloprost for PAH.

4. Use two different drug information sources to develop a recommendation for transitioning a patient from intravenous epoprostenol to subcutaneous treprostinil.

CLINICAL PEARL

Calcium channel blockers should only be used in patients with PAH who respond favorably to short-acting vasodilators during right heart catheterization.

REFERENCES

1. McLaughlin VV, Archer SL, Badesch DB, et al. ACCF/AHA 2009 expert consensus document on pulmonary hypertension: a report of the American College of Cardiology Foundation Task Force on Expert Consensus Documents and the American Heart Association developed in collaboration with the American College of Chest Physicians; American Thoracic Society, Inc.; and the Pulmonary Hypertension Association. J Am Coll Cardiol. 2009;53(17):1573–1619.

2. Galiè N, Humbert M, Vachiery JL, et al. 2015 ESC/ERS guidelines for the diagnosis and treatment of pulmonary hypertension: the Joint Task Force for the Diagnosis and Treatment of Pulmonary Hypertension of the European Society of Cardiology (ESC) and the European Respiratory Society (ERS): endorsed by Association for European Paediatric and Congenital Cardiology (AEPC), International Society for Heart and Lung Transplantation (ISHLT). Eur Heart J. 2016 Jan 1;37(1):67–119.

3. Klinger JR, Elliott CG, Levine DJ, et al. Therapy for pulmonary arterial hypertension in adults: update of the CHEST guideline and expert panel report. Chest. 2019 Mar;155(3):565–586.

4. McLaughlin VV, Shah SJ, Souza R, Humbert M. Management of pulmonary arterial hypertension. J Am Coll Cardiol. 2015 May 12;65(18):1976–1997.

5. Običan SG, Cleary KL. Pulmonary arterial hypertension in pregnancy. Semin Perinatol. 2014 Aug;38(5):289–294.

6. Xu QX, Yang YH, Geng J, et al. Clinical study of acute vasoreactivity testing in patients with chronic thromboembolic pulmonary hypertension. Chin Med J. (Engl) 2017 Feb 20;130(4):382–391.

7. Bishop BM, Mauro VF, Khouri SJ. Practical considerations for the pharmacotherapy of pulmonary arterial hypertension. Pharmacotherapy. 2012;32(9):838–855.

8. Montani D, Chaumais MC, Guignabert C, et al. Targeted therapies in pulmonary arterial hypertension. Pharmacol Ther. 2014 Feb;141(2):172–191.

9. Thenappan T, Ormiston ML, Ryan JJ, Archer SL. Pulmonary arterial hypertension: pathogenesis and clinical management. BMJ. 2018 Mar 14;360:j5492.

33

CYSTIC FIBROSIS

Blood, Sweat, Lungs, and Gut . . . . Level III

Kimberly J. Novak, PharmD, BCPS, BCPPS, FPPA

LEARNING OBJECTIVES

After completing this case study, the reader should be able to:

- Identify signs and symptoms of common problems in patients with cystic fibrosis (CF).

- Develop an antimicrobial therapy plan and appropriate monitoring strategy for treatment of an acute pulmonary exacerbation in CF.

- Devise treatment strategies for common complications of CF.

- Provide education on aerosolized medications to patients with CF, including appropriate instructions for dornase alfa and inhaled tobramycin.

PATIENT PRESENTATION

■ Chief Complaint

As reported by patient's father: "My daughter's experiencing shortness of breath, fast breathing, increasing cough and sputum production, and decreased energy, and she has a poor appetite."

■ HPI

The patient is a 7-year-old girl with a lifetime history of CF; she was diagnosed with CF at birth after presenting with meconium ileus. She had been doing well until 4 weeks ago, when she developed cold-like symptoms, with a runny nose, dry cough, sore throat, and subjective fever. She was seen at her local pediatrician's office and prescribed a 5-day course of azithromycin suspension 200 mg/5 mL, 160 mg (10 mg/kg) PO on day 1 and 80 mg (5 mg/kg) PO daily on days 2–5 for possible pneumonia. After completing the antibiotic course, the patient was not feeling any better. Father called the pulmonary clinic regarding her symptoms, and the pulmonologist called in a prescription to a local pharmacy for ciprofloxacin suspension 250 mg/5 mL, 325 mg PO BID (~40 mg/kg per day), and prednisolone syrup 15 mg/5 mL, one teaspoonful PO twice daily. Father was also instructed to perform three chest physiotherapy sessions (vest treatments) per day and increase her hypertonic saline schedule from once per day to twice daily with her vest treatments. The patient now presents to the pulmonary clinic for a follow-up to her outpatient treatment course. She describes worsening shortness of breath and chest pain, lung and sinus congestion, poor appetite, and severe fatigue. Father reports increasing cough productive of very dark green sputum but no fever. The patient has lost 2 lb since her last clinic visit and has missed 7 days of school. Her oxygen saturation is 88% in clinic on room air, and she was immediately placed on 1 L of O_2 by nasal cannula.

■ PMH

CF (Phe508del/G551D)
Significant for seven hospitalizations for acute pulmonary exacerbations of CF and two hospitalizations for distal intestinal obstruction syndrome (DIOS) since her initial NICU stay at birth; last hospitalization was 4 months ago
Sinus surgery × 2, last 1 year ago
Pancreatic insufficiency
Poor nutritional status
Recurrent constipation/DIOS
Pulmonary changes c/w long-standing CF with mild bronchiectasis
Seasonal allergies
Asthma
Broken clavicle previous summer after falling from a tree
ADHD

■ FH

Both parents are alive and generally well (father has hypercholesterolemia). The patient has an older half-brother (age 15) without CF who had a recent bout of gastroenteritis and a younger sister (age 2) with CF who was recently diagnosed with RSV bronchiolitis. Two maternal uncles died at ages 13 and 17 from CF.

■ SH

The patient is in first grade and is enrolled in the gifted program at her school. Family is considering home schooling due to frequent absences in the past school year. Lives with her mother, father, and younger sister approximately 100 miles from the nearest CF center. Her older half-brother visits every other weekend. They have well water and a small mixed-breed family dog; father smokes but only outside of the home. Family is experiencing financial difficulties due to a job layoff and recently lost health insurance. Family identifies non-adherence to some prescribed therapies due to drug cost. Family is in the process of applying for state Medicaid assistance.

■ Meds

Ciprofloxacin suspension 250 mg/5 mL, 325 mg PO BID

Prednisolone syrup 15 mg/5 mL, one teaspoonful PO BID

Aerosolized tobramycin 300 mg BID via nebulizer (every other month, currently "on")

Albuterol 0.083% 3 mL (one vial) BID via nebulizer with vest therapy (currently using TID)

Dornase alfa (Pulmozyme) 2.5 mg via nebulizer once daily with morning vest therapy

Sodium chloride 7% aerosol (Hyper-Sal) 4 mL via nebulizer once daily with evening vest therapy (currently using BID)

Fluticasone propionate (Flovent HFA) 44 mcg, one puff once daily

Budesonide (Rhinocort AQ) one spray each nostril once daily

Saline nasal rinse (neti pot) daily

Loratadine 5 mg PO once daily

Creon 12,000 two caps with meals (1500 units of lipase/kg/meal) and one cap with snacks and supplement shakes (750 units of lipase/kg/snack)

Omeprazole 20 mg PO once daily

Ferrous sulfate 324 mg PO BID

MVW Complete Formulation-D1500 one chewable tablet PO once daily

Children's multivitamin with iron one chewable tablet PO once daily

Polyethylene glycol 17 g PO once daily

Atomoxetine 25 mg PO once daily

Ibuprofen 200 mg PO three to four times daily as needed for chest pain

PediaSure two cans per day

■ All

Codeine (itching), bacitracin cream (rash), strawberries (anaphylaxis)

■ ROS

Patient complains of chest pain when coughing and large amounts of expectorated green sputum. Reduced ability to perform usual daily activities and play because of SOB. No current hemoptysis, constipation, vomiting, or abdominal pain. Reports having three to four loose or partially formed stools each day. Patient usually has a large appetite but has not been able to finish a meal for the past week.

■ Physical Examination

Gen

A shy, thin, cooperative, 7-year-old girl who has shortness of breath with her oxygen cannula removed during the examination

VS

BP 100/65, P 144, RR 45, T 37.8°C; Wt 16 kg, Ht 3′10″; oxygen saturation 95% on 1 L of oxygen; 88% on room air

Skin

Normal tone and color, some eczematous lesions at the elbows

HEENT

EOMI, PERRLA; nares with dried mucus in both nostrils; sinuses tender to palpation; no oral lesions, but secretions noted in the posterior pharynx

Neck/Lymph Nodes

Supple; no lymphadenopathy or thyromegaly

Lungs

Crackles heard bilaterally in the upper lobes greater than in the lower lobes; mild scattered wheezes; chest pain not reproducible with palpation

Breasts

Tanner stage I

CV

Tachycardic, regular rate without murmurs

Abd

Ticklish during examination; (+) bowel sounds; abdomen soft and supple; mild bloating noted, with palpable stool

Genit/Rect

Tanner stage I, deferred internal exam

MS/Ext

Clubbing noted, with no cyanosis; capillary refill <2 seconds

Neuro

Alert and awake though reserved; CNs intact; somewhat uncooperative with the full neurologic examination

■ Labs

Na 149 mEq/L	Hgb 15.4 g/dL	WBC 16.5 × 10³/mm³	AST 30 IU/L
K 4.5 mEq/L	Hct 45.2%	Segs 72%	ALT 20 IU/L
Cl 108 mEq/L	MCV 78 μm³	Bands 10%	LDH 330 IU/L
CO₂ 34 mEq/L	MCH 31.1 pg	Lymphs 10%	GGT 75 IU/L
BUN 18 mg/dL	MCHC 34 g/dL	Monos 2%	T. Prot 7.3 g/dL
SCr 0.45 mg/dL	Ca_i 4.6 mEq/Lᵃ	Eos 6%	Alb 3.1 g/dL
Glu 195 mg/dL	Phos 4.6 mEq/L	Mg 2.1 mg/dL	IgE 85 IU/mL
	ᵃCa_i, ionized calcium.		

■ Virology/Serology Results

Respiratory viral antigen panel: negative
COVID-19 PCR: negative
Influenza A/B PCRs: negative
Bordetella pertussis PCR: negative

■ Sputum Culture Results

Organism A: *Pseudomonas aeruginosa*
　　Sensitive: piperacillin/tazobactam, cefepime, ceftazidime, meropenem, aztreonam, tobramycin, amikacin
　　Intermediate: ciprofloxacin, levofloxacin
　　Resistant: gentamicin

Organism B: *Stenotrophomonas maltophilia*
Sensitive: trimethoprim–sulfamethoxazole, minocycline, moxifloxacin
Resistant: ceftazidime, meropenem, levofloxacin, all aminoglycosides

Organism C: *P. aeruginosa*, mucoid strain
Sensitive: piperacillin/tazobactam, cefepime, ceftazidime, meropenem, aztreonam, tobramycin
Resistant: ciprofloxacin, levofloxacin, gentamicin, amikacin

Organism D: *Staphylococcus aureus*
Sensitive: vancomycin, linezolid, trimethoprim–sulfamethoxazole, minocycline
Resistant: nafcillin, cefazolin, clindamycin, erythromycin

Organism E: *Achromobacter xylosoxidans*
Sensitive: piperacillin/tazobactam, ceftazidime, trimethoprim–sulfamethoxazole, minocycline
Resistant: meropenem, cefepime, ciprofloxacin, all aminoglycosides

■ PFTs

FEV_1 65% of predicted (baseline 90%); FVC 82% of predicted (baseline 95%)

■ Chest X-Ray

Bronchiectatic and interstitial fibrotic changes consistent with CF

■ High-Resolution Chest CT (HRCT)

Interval worsening of bronchiectasis in all lobes; increased mucus plugging in left lower lobe

■ Sinus CT

Panopacification of ethmoid and maxillary sinuses, possible polyp extending into right nasal passage

■ Assessment

A 7-year-old CF patient with failed outpatient management of acute pulmonary exacerbation and sinusitis, also with nutritional failure

QUESTIONS

Collect Information

1.a. What subjective and objective information indicates the presence of an acute pulmonary exacerbation of cystic fibrosis?

1.b. What additional information is needed to fully assess this patient's cystic fibrosis?

Assess the Information

2.a. Assess the severity of this patient's acute pulmonary exacerbation of cystic fibrosis based on the subjective and objective information available.

2.b. Create a list of the patient's drug therapy problems and prioritize them. Include assessment of medication appropriateness, effectiveness, safety, and patient adherence.

2.c. What economic, psychosocial, cultural, racial, and ethical considerations are applicable to this patient?

Develop a Care Plan

3.a. What are the goals of pharmacotherapy for the patient's pulmonary exacerbation in this case?

3.b. What nondrug therapies might be useful for this patient's pulmonary exacerbation?

3.c. What feasible pharmacotherapeutic options are available for treating the patient's cystic fibrosis?

3.d. Create an individualized, patient-centered, team-based care plan to optimize medication therapy for this patient's cystic fibrosis and other drug therapy problems. Include specific drugs, dosage forms, doses, schedules, and durations of therapy.

Implement the Care Plan

4.a. What information should be provided to the patient to enhance adherence, ensure successful therapy, and minimize adverse effects?

4.b. Describe how care should be coordinated with other healthcare providers.

Follow-Up: Monitor and Evaluate

5. Explain how to monitor and evaluate the care plan for medication appropriateness, effectiveness, safety and patient adherence by using clinical and laboratory data, patient feedback, and other information.

■ CLINICAL COURSE

Serum tobramycin concentrations were drawn after the second dose of tobramycin, 160 mg (10 mg/kg/dose) IV Q 24 H. Levels are reported as follows:

- Random level: 7.4 mcg/mL collected 4 hours after the end of the 30-minute infusion
- Random level: 1.4 mcg/mL collected 10 hours after end of the 30-minute infusion
- Based on this new information, evaluate the patient's drug therapy. Calculate the maximum concentration at end of infusion (Cmax), true trough, AUC, elimination rate, half-life, volume of distribution, and clearance (standardized for body surface area [BSA]) of her tobramycin therapy. If necessary, suggest modifications. Assume that the previous doses were administered on time.

■ SELF-STUDY ASSIGNMENTS

1. Investigate aztreonam lysine for inhalation (Cayston) and the unique drug delivery device required for administration (Altera Nebulizer System). How are these products prescribed and dispensed to patients?

2. Analyze the role of azithromycin in the chronic medical management of CF. What is/are the proposed mechanism(s) of action of azithromycin in CF management?

3. Review the recommendations for use of fluoroquinolones in children. What data support these recommendations?

4. Investigate CFTR potentiators and modulators used in chronic CF management: ivacaftor (Kalydeco), lumacaftor–ivacaftor (Orkambi), tezacaftor–ivacaftor (Symdeko), and elexacaftor–tezacaftor–ivacaftor (Trikafta). What clinical outcomes are observed with each of these therapies? What other research is being conducted in the new drug class of CFTR potentiators and modulators?

CLINICAL PEARL

Chronic gastric acid suppression (proton pump inhibitor or histamine-2 receptor antagonist) is often used in CF patients to improve efficacy of pancreatic enzyme replacement therapy regardless of the presence of gastroesophageal reflux symptoms. Due to defective bicarbonate transport in the small intestine and subnormal pH, enteric coating may not dissolve consistently in CF patients. Suppression of gastric acid can subsequently raise small intestine pH through mixing of gastrointestinal fluids.

REFERENCES*

1. Moran A, Pillay K, Becker D, et al. ISPAD clinical practice consensus guidelines 2018: management of cystic fibrosis-related diabetes in children and adolescents. Pediatr Diabetes. 2018 Oct;19(Suppl 27):64–74.

2. Altman K, McDonald CM, Michel SH, Maguiness K. Nutrition in cystic fibrosis: from the past to the present and into the future. Pediatr Pulmonol. 2019 Nov;54(Suppl 3):S56–S73.

3. Mogayzel PJ, Naureckas ET, Robinson KA, et al. Cystic fibrosis pulmonary guidelines. Chronic medications for maintenance of lung health. Am J Respir Crit Care Med. 2013;187(7):680–689.

4. Elborn JS. Cystic fibrosis. Lancet. 2016;388(10059):2519–2531.

5. Chmiel JF, Aksamit TR, Chotirmall SH, et al. Antibiotic management of lung infections in cystic fibrosis. I. The microbiome, methicillin-resistant *Staphylococcus aureus*, gram-negative bacteria, and multiple infections. Ann Am Thorac Soc. 2014;11(7):1120–1129.

6. Patel K, Goldman JL. Safety concerns surrounding quinolone use in children. J Clin Pharmacol. 2016;56(9):1060–1075.

7. Zobell JT, Young DC, Waters CD, et al. Optimization of anti-pseudomonal antibiotics for cystic fibrosis pulmonary exacerbations: VI. Executive summary. Pediatr Pulmonol. 2013;48(6):525–537.

8. Epps QJ, Epps KL, Young DC, Zobell JT. State of the art in cystic fibrosis pharmacology–optimization of antimicrobials in the treatment of cystic fibrosis pulmonary exacerbations: I. Anti-methicillin-resistant *Staphylococcus aureus* (MRSA) antibiotics. Pediatr Pulmonol. 2020 Jan;55(1):33–57.

9. Paranjape SM, Mogayzel PJ, Jr. Cystic fibrosis in the era of precision medicine. Paediatr Respir Rev. 2018;25:64–72.

*Additional cystic fibrosis guidelines and clinical information can be found at www.cff.org.

34

GASTROESOPHAGEAL REFLUX DISEASE

A Burning Question .... Level II

Brian A. Hemstreet, PharmD, FCCP, BCPS

LEARNING OBJECTIVES

After completing this case study, the reader should be able to:

- Describe the clinical presentation of gastroesophageal reflux disease (GERD), including typical, atypical, and alarm symptoms.

- Discuss appropriate diagnostic approaches for GERD, including when patients should be referred for further diagnostic evaluation.

- Recommend appropriate nonpharmacologic and pharmacologic measures for treating GERD.

- Develop a treatment plan for a patient with GERD, including both nonpharmacologic and pharmacologic measures and monitoring for efficacy and toxicity of selected drug regimens.

- Outline a patient education plan for proper use of drug therapy for GERD.

PATIENT PRESENTATION

■ Chief Complaint

"I'm having a lot of heartburn. These pills I have been using have helped a little but it's still keeping me up at night."

■ HPI

A 71-year-old woman presents to the GI clinic with complaints of heartburn four to five times a week over the past 5 months. She also reports some regurgitation after meals that is often accompanied by an acidic taste in her mouth. She states that her symptoms are worse at night, particularly when she goes to bed. She finds that her heartburn worsens, and she coughs a lot at night, which keeps her awake. She has had difficulty sleeping and feels fatigued during the day. She reports no difficulty swallowing food or liquids. She has tried OTC Prevacid 24HR as needed for the past 3 weeks. This has reduced the frequency of her symptoms to 3–4 days per week, but they are still bothering her.

■ PMH

Type 2 DM × 5 years
HTN × 10 years

■ FH

Father died of pneumonia at age 75; mother died of gastric cancer at age 68.

■ SH

Patient is married with three children. She is a retired school bus driver. She drinks one to two glasses of wine 4–5 days per week. She does not use tobacco. She has commercial prescription drug insurance.

■ Meds

Amlodipine 5 mg PO once daily
Hydrochlorothiazide 25 mg PO once daily
Metformin 500 mg PO twice daily
Atorvastatin 20 mg PO daily
Aspirin 81 mg PO daily

■ All

Peanuts (hives)

■ ROS

Reports being tired all the time, (–) SOB or hoarseness; (+) cough at night, (+) frequent episodes of heartburn, sometimes after meals, but is worse at night; (–) N/V; (–) BRBPR or dark/tarry stools; (–) dysuria, nocturia, or frequency

■ Physical Examination

Gen

Well-developed woman in NAD

VS

BP 148/85, P 90, RR 17, T 36°C; Wt 220 lb (100 kg), Ht 5'7" (170 cm)

Skin

No lesions or rashes

HEENT

PERRLA; EOMI; moist mucous membranes; intact dentition; oropharynx clear

Neck/Lymph Nodes

Trachea midline; (–) thyromegaly; (–) lymphadenopathy; (–) JVD

Lungs/Thorax

CTA bilaterally

CV

Tachycardia with irregularly irregular rhythm; no MRG

Abd

Obese; NT/ND; (+) BS; (–) HSM

Genit/Rect

Gyn exam deferred; heme (–) brown stool

MS/Ext

No CVA tenderness

Neuro

A&O × 3, CN II–XII intact, 5/5 upper- and lower-extremity strength bilaterally

■ Labs

Na 138 mEq/L	Hgb 13 g/dL	WBC 8.7 × 10³/mm³	AST 21 IU/L
K 3.8 mEq/L	Hct 39%	Neutros 60%	ALT 24 IU/L
Cl 108 mEq/L	RBC 4.6 × 10⁶/mm³	Bands 1%	Alk Phos 55 IU/L
CO₂ 21 mEq/L	Plt 400 × 10³/mm³	Eos 2%	*Fasting lipid panel*
BUN 18 mg/dL		Lymphs 32%	TC 230 mg/dL
SCr 1.1 mg/dL		Monos 5%	LDL 130 mg/dL
Fasting Glu		A1C 9.0%	TG 170 mg/dL
220 mg/dL			HDL 42 mg/dL
Ca 8.9 mg/dL			
Phos			
4.1 mg/dL			

■ EGD

Grade B esophagitis; normal gastric and duodenal mucosa. Biopsy results of esophagus and stomach are negative for atypical cells and *Helicobacter pylori*.

■ Assessment

A 71-year-old woman presenting with uncontrolled GERD symptoms despite self-treatment with intermittent OTC PPI therapy. EGD reveals erosive esophagitis.

QUESTIONS

Collect Information

1.a. What subjective and objective information indicates the presence of GERD in this patient?

1.b. What additional information is needed to fully assess this patient's GERD?

Assess the Information

2.a. Assess the severity of GERD based on the subjective and objective information available. Are the symptoms typical or atypical in nature? Are any alarm symptoms or features present?

2.b. Create a list of this patient's drug therapy problems and prioritize them. Include assessment of medication appropriateness, effectiveness, safety, and patient adherence.

2.c. What patient or lifestyle factors could be contributing to the development of GERD symptoms in this patient?

2.d. What are other potential complications of long-standing untreated GERD?

Develop a Care Plan

3.a. What are the goals of pharmacotherapy for GERD in this case?

3.b. What lifestyle modifications or nondrug therapies might be useful for this patient's GERD?

3.c. What feasible pharmacotherapeutic alternatives are available to treat this patient's GERD?

3.d. Create an individualized, patient-centered, team-based care plan to optimize medication therapy for this patient's GERD and other drug therapy problems. Include specific drugs, dosage forms, doses, schedules, and durations of therapy.

Implement the Care Plan

4.a. What information should be provided to the patient to enhance adherence, ensure successful therapy, and minimize adverse effects?

4.b. Describe how care should be coordinated with other healthcare providers.

Follow-Up: Monitor and Evaluate

5. Explain how to monitor and evaluate the care plan for medication appropriateness, effectiveness, safety, and patient adherence by using clinical and laboratory data, patient feedback, and other information.

■ CLINICAL COURSE

Four weeks later, the patient returns to the clinic for follow-up. Her symptoms have greatly improved, but she is considering stopping therapy because she heard that "all sorts of bad side effects" can happen to her. She saw on television that she could get osteoporosis and that she should be taking calcium. Someone told her that she may also develop some "nasty infections." She does not think it is worth staying on the medication. She also states that she sometimes has brief episodes of heartburn after meals and wishes to know if she should take more of her medication to manage these symptoms.

■ FOLLOW-UP QUESTIONS

1. Should the patient be placed on calcium and vitamin D supplementation because of her acid-suppressive therapy?

2. How would you address her concerns regarding the potential for developing infections due to acid-suppressive therapy?

3. What recommendations could you give her regarding management of the breakthrough symptoms after meals?

■ SELF-STUDY ASSIGNMENTS

1. *H. pylori* is a common cause of peptic ulcer disease and is often tested for in patients presenting with upper GI complaints. Perform a literature search on the relationship between GERD symptoms and *H. pylori*. What conclusions can you draw from the results of these articles? Should *H. pylori* be tested for and treated in patients with GERD?

2. Clinical practice involves providing care to diverse patient populations. Identify and review tertiary drug references and Internet websites that provide educational materials about GERD or its treatment in languages other than English.

CLINICAL PEARL

PPIs may cause false-negative results in patients undergoing urease-based *H. pylori* testing, such as with the urea breath test or rapid urease test, or stool antigen tests. Ideally, these drugs should be discontinued 2 weeks before performing these diagnostic tests.

REFERENCES

1. Katz PO, Dunbar KB, Schnoll-Sussman FH, Greer KB, Yadlapati R, Spechler SJ. ACG clinical guideline for the diagnosis and management of gastroesophageal reflux disease. Am J Gastroenterol. 2022;117:27–56.

2. Richter JE, Rubenstein JH. Presentation and epidemiology of gastroesophageal reflux disease. Gastroenterology. 2018;154:267–276.

3. Vaezi MF, Pandolfino JE, Vela MF, et al. White paper AGA: optimal strategies to define and diagnose gastroesophageal reflux disease. Gastroenterology. 2017;15:1162–1172.

4. Pandit S, Boktor M, Alexander JS, et al. Gastroesophageal reflux disease: a clinical overview for primary care physicians. Pathophysiology. 2018;25(1):1–11.

5. Nadaleto BF, Herbella FAM, Patti MG. Gastroesophageal reflux disease in the obese: pathophysiology and treatment. Surgery. 2016;159:475–486.

6. Shaheen NJ, Falk GW, Iyer PG, et al. ACG clinical guideline: diagnosis and management of Barrett's esophagus. Am J Gastroenterol. 2016;111:30–50.

7. Sandhu DS, Fass R. Current trends in the management of gastroesophageal reflux disease. Gut Liv. 2018;12:7–16.

8. Gyawali CP, Fass R. Management of gastroesophageal reflux disease. Gastroenterology. 2018;154:302–318.

9. Savarino E, Zentilin P, Marabotto E, et al. A review of pharmacotherapy for treating gastroesophageal reflux disease (GERD). Expert Opin Pharmacother. 2017;18:1333–1343.

10. Gyawali CP. Proton pump inhibitors in gastroesophageal reflux disease: friend or foe. Curr Gastroenterol Rep. 2017;(19)46. doi: 10.1007/s11894-017-0586-5.

35

PEPTIC ULCER DISEASE

Feel the Burn .... Level II

Cynthia Moreau, PharmD, BCACP

LEARNING OBJECTIVES

After completing this case study, the reader should be able to:

- List the options for the evaluation and treatment of a patient with symptoms suggestive of peptic ulcer disease (PUD).
- Identify the desired therapeutic outcomes for patients with PUD.
- Identify the factors that guide selection of a *Helicobacter pylori* eradication regimen and improve adherence with the regimen.
- Compare the efficacy of *H. pylori* treatment regimens
- Create a treatment and monitoring plan for a patient diagnosed with PUD, given patient-specific information.

PATIENT PRESENTATION

■ Chief Complaint

"My stomach has been hurting really badly for the past month or so. It seems to get worse at night."

■ HPI

A 67-year-old woman presents to her primary care physician with complaints of episodic epigastric pain for the past 6 weeks. Her pain is nonradiating. It is sometimes worse with meals, but sometimes eating helps improve the pain. She has been experiencing occasional nausea, bloating, and heartburn. She denies any change in color or frequency of bowel movements. She does not have a history of PUD or GI bleeding. She mentions that she has been having frequent headaches for the past month and has been taking naproxen sodium one to two times daily.

■ PMH

CAD with drug-eluting stent placement × 3 months
Hyperlipidemia × 10 years
Hypertension × 20 years
Postmenopausal; LMP ~13 years ago

■ FH

Her mother died at the age of 75 from lymphoma. Her father is alive and has a history of glaucoma, prostate cancer, and AMI at age 70.

■ SH

She is married and has raised three children; she is not employed outside the home. She has never smoked and drinks one to two glasses of wine most days of the week. She drinks caffeine (coffee) daily.

■ Meds

Clopidogrel 75 mg PO daily
Lisinopril 5 mg PO daily
Metoprolol tartrate 25 mg PO twice daily
Aspirin 325 mg PO daily
Atorvastatin 80 mg PO daily
MVI tablet PO daily
Tums 500 mg PO PRN stomach pain
Naproxen sodium 220 mg PO PRN headache (one to two times daily for the past month)

■ All

Penicillin (hives)

■ ROS

Unremarkable except for complaints noted above

■ Physical Examination

Gen

Slightly overweight woman in moderate distress

VS

BP 110/72 left arm (seated), P 99, RR 16 reg, T 37.2°C; Wt 149.6 lb (68 kg), Ht 5'3" (160 cm)

Skin

Warm and dry

HEENT

Normocephalic; PERRLA; EOMI

Chest

CTA

CV

RRR; S$_1$ and S$_2$ normal; no MRG

Abd

Soft; mild epigastric tenderness; (+) BS; no splenomegaly or masses; liver size normal

Genit/Rect

FOBT negative

Ext

Normal ROM; no cyanosis, clubbing, or edema

Neuro

CN II–XII intact; A&O × 3

■ Labs

Na 142 mEq/L	Hgb 12.5g/dL	Ca 9.5 mg/dL
K 4.7 mEq/L	Hct 36%	Mg 2.2 mEq/L
Cl 98 mEq/L	Plt 320 × 10³/mm³	Phos 3.8 mg/dL
CO$_2$ 30 mEq/L	WBC 7.6 × 10³/mm³	Albumin 5.0 g/dL
BUN 8 mg/dL	MCV 82 μm³	TSH 2.4 μU/mL
SCr 0.7 mg/dL	Retic 0.9%	TC 142 mg/dL
FBG 92 mg/dL	Fe 78 mcg/dL	LDL 64 mg/dL
		HDL 53 mg/dL
		TG 127 mg/dL

■ EGD

The patient's PCP referred her for a nonemergent EGD, which revealed a 5.5 mm superficial ulcer in the superior duodenum. The ulcer base was clear and without evidence of active bleeding (Fig. 35-1). In addition, inflammation of the duodenum was detected and biopsied. Biopsy indicated the presence of inflammation and abundant *H. pylori*–like organisms.

■ Assessment

PUD with duodenal ulcer and positive for infection with *H. pylori*.

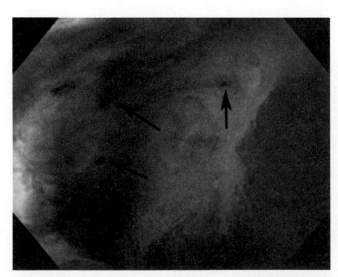

FIGURE 35-1. Endoscopy depicting duodenal ulcer with flat pigmented spots as noted by arrows. Reprinted with permission from Jameson JL, Fauci AS, Kasper DL, et al, eds. *Harrison's Principles of Internal Medicine*. 20th ed. New York, NY: McGraw-Hill Education, 2018.)

QUESTIONS

Collect Information

1.a. What subjective and objective information indicates the presence of PUD?

1.b. What additional information is needed to fully assess this patient's PUD?

Assess the Information

2.a. Assess the severity of PUD based on the subjective and objective information available.

2.b. Create a list of the patient's drug therapy problems and prioritize them. Include assessment of medication appropriateness, effectiveness, safety, and patient adherence.

Develop a Care Plan

3.a. What are the goals of pharmacotherapy for PUD in this case?

3.b. What nondrug recommendations might be useful for this patient's PUD?

3.c. What feasible pharmacotherapeutic options are available for treating this patient's PUD?

3.d. Create an individualized, patient-centered, team-based care plan to optimize medication therapy for this patient's PUD and other drug therapy problems. Include specific drugs, doses, dosage forms, schedules, and durations of therapy.

3.e. What alternatives would be appropriate if the initial care plan fails or cannot be used?

Implement the Care Plan

4.a. What information should be provided to the patient to enhance adherence, ensure successful therapy, and minimize adverse effects?

4.b. Describe how care should be coordinated with other healthcare providers.

Follow-Up: Monitor and Evaluate

5. Explain how to monitor and evaluate the care plan for medication appropriateness, effectiveness, safety, and patient adherence by using clinical and laboratory data, patient feedback, and other information.

■ SELF-STUDY ASSIGNMENTS

1. Describe the advantages and limitations of both endoscopic and nonendoscopic diagnostic tests to detect *H. pylori*.

2. After performing a literature search on *H. pylori* eradication therapy, compare the efficacy of three- and four-drug regimens.

3. Based on the literature search on *H. pylori* eradication therapy, determine whether therapy should be continued for 7–14 days or provided in a sequential order.

CLINICAL PEARL

Rapid urease breath tests for diagnosis of *H. pylori* should not be used for patients who have received bismuth-containing medications, proton pump inhibitors, or antimicrobials within the previous 4 weeks due to the increased risk of a false-negative result.

ACKNOWLEDGMENT

This case is based on the patient case written for the 11th edition by Ashley H. Meredith, PharmD, FCCP, BCACP, BCPS, CDE.

REFERENCES

1. Ierardi E, Losurdo G, La Fortezza RF, Principi M, Barone M, Di Leo A. Optimizing proton pump inhibitors in *Helicobacter pylori* treatment: Old and new tricks to improve effectiveness. World J Gastroenterol. 2019;25(34):5097–5104.

2. Chey WD, Leontiadis GI, Howden CW, Moss SF. Treatment of *Helicobacter pylori* infection. Am J Gastroenterol. 2017;112:212–238.

3. Kenngott S, Olze R, Kollmer M, et al. Clopidogrel and proton pump inhibitor (PPI) interaction: separate intake and a non-omeprazole PPI the solution? Eur J Med Res. 2010;15:220–224.

4. Bouziana SD, Tziomalos K. Clinical relevance of clopidogrel-proton pump inhibitors interaction. World J Gastrointest Pharmacol Ther. 2015;6:17–21.

5. Frelinger AL, Lee RD, Mulford DJ, et al. A randomized, 2-period, crossover design study to assess the effects of dexlansoprazole, lansoprazole, esomeprazole and omeprazole on the steady-state pharmacokinetics and pharmacodynamics of clopidogrel in healthy volunteers. J Am Coll Cardiol. 2012;59:1304–1311.

6. Bhatt DL, Cryer BL, Contant CF, et al. Clopidogrel with or without omeprazole in coronary artery disease. N Engl J Med. 2010;363:1909–1917.

7. Drepper MD, Spahr L, Frossard JL. Clopidogrel and proton pump inhibitors—where do we stand in 2012? World J Gastroenterol. 2012;18:2161–2171.

8. Abraham NS, Hlatky MA, Antman EM, et al. ACCF/ACG/AHA 2010 expert consensus document on the concomitant use of proton pump inhibitors and thienopyridines: a focused update of the ACCF/ACG/AHA 2008 expert consensus document on reducing the gastrointestinal risks of antiplatelet therapy and NSAID use. Circulation. 2010;122:2619–2633.

36

NSAID-INDUCED ULCER DISEASE

To Protect and Serve . . . . Level II

Haley N. Johnson, PharmD, BCPS

Carmen B. Smith, PharmD, BCPS

LEARNING OBJECTIVES

After completing this case study, the reader should be able to:

- Determine whether patients with diabetes who have risk factors for NSAID-induced ulcer disease should remain on aspirin and at what dose.

- Identify the hallmark signs and symptoms of NSAID-induced PUD.

- Recommend appropriate therapy for the treatment of NSAID-induced PUD while considering *Helicobacter pylori* infection and its appropriate diagnosis and follow-up.

- Recommend alternative therapies besides traditional NSAIDs for treatment of pain and inflammation in patients with PUD.

- Educate patients effectively on treatment options for NSAID-induced PUD.

PATIENT PRESENTATION

■ Chief Complaint

"I have had stomach pain, nausea, and bloating in the last 2 weeks."

■ HPI

A 72-year-old woman presents to the emergency department for epigastric pain, early satiety, and nausea for 2 weeks. She normally takes OTC Pepcid for her symptoms, which she states is usually sufficient; however, this time the symptoms persisted. When asked about any recent medication changes, she reports naproxen use the past 2 weeks for osteoarthritis pain.

■ PMH

GERD
OA primarily in right wrist/hand and knees
HTN
Type 2 DM
S/P appendectomy after appendicitis 30 years ago

■ FH

Father died of MI at age 65; mother died of cervical CA in her eighties

■ SH

Retired school teacher; smoked one pack per day for 25 years, quit 9 years ago; admits to drinking alcohol

■ Meds

ASA 325 mg PO once daily
Lisinopril 20 mg PO once daily
Amlodipine 10 mg PO once daily
Metformin 1000 mg PO twice daily
Rosuvastatin 20 mg PO once daily
OTC naproxen 220 mg, one to two tablets PO one to four times daily PRN for OA pain
OTC famotidine 10 mg, one to two tablets twice daily for heartburn

■ All

Codeine (rash); penicillin (rash/hives)

■ ROS

Denies headache or chest pain. Occasional SOB. Positive heartburn. No weakness, polyphagia, polydipsia, or polyuria. Gait slow but steady. Complains of some chronic pain in left knee, which she has been told is from OA.

■ Physical Examination

Gen

The patient is a pleasant woman in mild distress.

VS

BP 126/70, P 86, RR 16, T 36.8°C; Wt 138 lb (62.7 kg), Ht 5′3″ (160 cm)

HEENT

PERRLA; funduscopic exam without hemorrhages, exudates, or papilledema; mild cataracts bilaterally

Neck/Lymph Nodes

Supple; no JVD or thyromegaly; no carotid bruits

Lungs

CTA

CV

RRR, normal S_1, S_2

Abd

Normal BS, moderate epigastric pain on palpation

Genit/Rect

Fecal occult blood test negative

MS/Ext

No skin breakdown or ulcers; mild weakness of RUE; mild deformity of right first finger at MCP joint and swelling of DIP joints on first and second fingers

Neuro

A&O × 3; CN II–XII intact; negative Babinski. Normal sensation in hands bilaterally, decreased pain and vibratory sensation in right foot, normal in left.

■ **Labs**

Na 138 mEq/L	Hgb 8.2 g/dL	*Fasting lipid profile*
K 4.0 mEq/L	Hct 24%	T. Chol 148 mg/dL
Cl 108 mEq/L	Plt 269 × 10³/mm³	LDL-C 70 mg/dL
CO_2 22 mEq/L	WBC 6.0 × 10³/mm³	HDL-C 50 mg/dL
BUN 18 mEq/L	Retic 1.8%	TG 142 mg/dL
SCr 0.9 mg/dL	A1C 6.7%	
Glu 105 mg/dL	TSH 3.06 μIU/mL	

■ **H. pylori Testing**

Rapid urease test of gastric biopsy and serology positive

■ **EGD**

Two small gastric ulcers approximately 6 mm in diameter, both ulcers with clean bases and no active bleeding

■ **Assessment**

The 72-year-old woman presents with peptic ulcer disease secondary to NSAID use and *H. pylori* infection

QUESTIONS

Collect Information

1.a. What subjective and objective information indicates the presence of PUD in this patient?

1.b. What additional information is needed to fully assess this patient's PUD?

Assess the Information

2.a. Assess the severity of PUD based on the subjective and objective information available.

2.b. Create a list of the patient's drug therapy problems and prioritize them. Include assessment of medication appropriateness, effectiveness, safety, and patient adherence.

Develop a Care Plan

3.a. What are the goals of pharmacotherapy for PUD in this case?

3.b. What nondrug therapies might be useful for this patient's PUD?

3.c. What feasible pharmacotherapeutic options are available for treating PUD?

3.d. Create an individualized, patient-centered, team-based care plan to optimize medication therapy for this patient's PUD and other drug therapy problems. Include specific drugs, dosage forms, doses, schedules, and durations of therapy.

3.e. What alternatives would be appropriate if the initial care plan fails or cannot be used?

Implement the Care Plan

4.a. What information should be provided to the patient to enhance adherence, ensure successful therapy, and minimize adverse effects?

4.b. Describe how care should be coordinated with other healthcare providers.

Follow-Up: Monitor and Evaluate

5. Explain how to monitor and evaluate the care plan for medication appropriateness, effectiveness, safety, and patient adherence by using clinical and laboratory data, patient feedback, and other information.

■ **ADDITIONAL CASE QUESTION**

1. Besides the standard PPI or H2RA treatment options, what other pharmacotherapeutic options are available for preventing recurrent PUD in this patient?

■ **SELF-STUDY ASSIGNMENTS**

1. Perform a literature search and assess current information on the efficacy of various agents for secondary prevention of NSAID-induced ulcers. Review expert opinion on the data specific to prevention of aspirin-induced PUD.

2. Review the ASPREE and ASCEND trials examining the cardiac benefits and bleeding risk of low-dose aspirin for primary prevention in elderly and persons with diabetes, respectively.

CLINICAL PEARL

Long-term PPI use has been associated with malabsorption problems (vitamin B_{12} deficiency, reduced pH-dependent calcium absorption leading to osteoporosis), electrolyte abnormalities (hypomagnesemia), and increased infection risk (*Clostridioides difficile* infection, pneumonia).

ACKNOWLEDGMENT

This case is based on the patient case co-written for the 11th edition by Jay L. Martello, PharmD, BCPS.

REFERENCES

1. Chey WD, Leontiadis GI, Howden CW, Moss SF. ACG clinical guideline: treatment of *Helicobacter pylori* infection. Am J Gastroenterol. 2017;112:212–238.

2. Kolasinski SL, Neogi T, Hochberg MC, et al. 2019 American College of Rheumatology/Arthritis Foundation guidelines for the management of osteoarthritis of the hand, hip, and knee. Arthritis Rheumatol. 2020;72(2):220–233.

3. Lanza FL, Chan FKL, Quigley EMM. Guidelines for prevention of NSAID-related ulcer complications. Am J Gastroenterol. 2009;104:728–738.

4. Katz PO, Gerson LB, Vela MF. Guidelines for the diagnosis and management of gastroesophageal reflux disease. Am J Gastroenterol. 2013;108:308–328.

5. Albert MA, Buroker AB, Goldberger ZD, et al. 2019 ACC/AHA guideline on the primary prevention of cardiovascular disease: a report of the American College of Cardiology/American Heart Association Task Force on Clinical Practice Guidelines. Circulation. 2019;140:e596–e646.

37

STRESS ULCER PROPHYLAXIS

A Bloody Good Time............................Level I

Jay L. Martello, PharmD, BCPS

Lena M. Maynor, PharmD, BCPS

LEARNING OBJECTIVES

After completing this case study, the reader should be able to:

- Identify risk factors associated with stress ulcer formation and determine which critically ill patients should receive pharmacologic prophylaxis.

- Recommend appropriate pharmacologic alternatives, including agent, route of administration, and dose for the prevention of stress-induced ulcers.

- Identify and implement monitoring parameters for the recommended stress ulcer prophylaxis regimens.

- Discuss the pharmacologic approaches to the management of stress ulcer–induced bleeding.

PATIENT PRESENTATION

■ Chief Complaint

"My throat is sore."

■ HPI

The patient is a 26-year-old female currently admitted to the surgical intensive care unit (ICU) with traumatic injuries following a motor vehicle accident (MVA) 7 days ago. When EMS arrived in the field, the patient was unresponsive with labored breathing and was intubated prior to transfer to the hospital. On the day of admission, the patient underwent surgical repair of her rib fractures and hemopneumothorax with chest tube placement. The patient was mechanically ventilated until yesterday morning, and the chest tube was removed by interventional radiology earlier this morning. The patient began a clear liquid diet this morning. The patient will be transferred to a step-down unit later today.

■ PMH (Provided by Patient's Mother)

IBS-C × 10 years

S/P cholecystectomy 5 years ago

■ FH

Both mother and father are still alive and in "good health."

■ SH

Patient is a graduate student at a local university. She does not smoke or use illicit drugs. Her mother reports occasional alcohol use.

■ Meds

Lubiprostone 24 mcg PO Q 12 H

Enoxaparin 30 mg Subcut Q 12 H

Pantoprazole 40 mg IV Q 24 H

Acetaminophen 650 mg PO Q 4 H PRN Mild Pain (1–3)

Oxycodone 5 mg PO Q 4 H PRN Moderate Pain (4–6)

Oxycodone 10 mg PO Q 4 H PRN Severe Pain (7–10)

■ All

No known drug allergies

■ ROS

Patient is hoarse from the extubation with a sore throat. Endorses no issues otherwise.

■ Physical Examination

Gen

Young woman; no obvious bleeding on exam

VS

BP 96/64, P 106, RR 24, T 37.3°C; Wt 112 lb (51 kg), Ht 5'11" (180 cm)

Skin

Warm, dry; small, healing lacerations across forehead and chest; ecchymoses present on both legs and arms

HEENT

No blood visible in the nose or ears; no obvious damage to the ears, eyes, or nose

Neck/Lymph Nodes

Supple, no palpable areas of deformity or masses

Lungs

Patient is clear to auscultation, no use of accessory muscles

CV

S_1, S_2 normal; sinus tachycardia with no S_3, S_4

Abd

Firm; decreased bowel sounds

Genit/Rect

No obvious damage to the genital area; otherwise deferred

MS/Ext

(–) CCE, pulses intact

Neuro

Cranial nerves intact; strength 4/5; reflexes normal

■ Labs (Upon ED Presentation)

Na 135 mEq/L	Hgb 10.5 g/dL	PO_4 3.0 mg/dL
K 3.2 mEq/L	Hct 29.2%	Ca 10.2 mg/dL
Cl 101 mEq/L	WBC $8.0 \times 10^3/mm^3$	AST 29 IU/L
CO_2 22 mEq/L	Plt $112 \times 10^3/mm^3$	ALT 22 IU/L
BUN 40 mg/dL		Alk phos 66 IU/L
SCr 1.0 mg/dL		T. bili 0.4 mg/dL
Glu 91 mg/dL		Alb 3.8 g/dL
		INR 1.1

■ ABG

pH 7.43, $PaCO_2$ 48 mm Hg, PaO_2 74 mm Hg, HCO_3^- 23 mEq/L, pulse ox 92%

■ Focused Assessment with Sonography in Trauma (FAST) Exam

No evidence of fluid in the perihepatic, hepatorenal, perisplenic, pericardial, or pelvic spaces

■ CT Abdomen/Pelvis with IV Contrast

There is no evidence for bowel obstruction. The common bile duct does not appear to be dilated. No free fluid present in the abdominal cavity.

■ CT Head with IV Contrast

No midline shift. No evidence for intracranial hemorrhage.

■ Urinalysis

Yellow color, specific gravity 1.026, pH 4.6, ketones negative, protein negative, nitrite negative, bilirubin negative, glucose negative, bacteria 0, WBC 0, RBC 3+, hCG negative

■ Fecal Occult Blood

Negative

■ Assessment

This is a 26-year-old presenting with rib fractures secondary to an MVA s/p operative repair. The patient has improved and is currently appropriate for transfer to the step-down unit.

QUESTIONS

Collect Information

1.a. What subjective and objective information indicates the need for stress ulcer prophylaxis?

1.b. What additional information is needed to fully assess this patient's need for stress ulcer prophylaxis?

Assess the Information

2.a. Assess the patient's risk for a stress ulcer based on the subjective and objective information available.

2.b. Create a list of the patient's drug therapy problems and prioritize them. Include assessment of medication appropriateness, effectiveness, safety, and patient adherence.

Develop a Care Plan

3.a. What are the goals of pharmacotherapy in stress ulcer prophylaxis?

3.b. What nondrug therapies might be useful for this patient?

3.c. What feasible pharmacotherapeutic alternatives are available for stress ulcer prophylaxis?

3.d. Create an individualized, patient-centered, team-based care plan to optimize medication therapy for this patient's stress ulcer prophylaxis and other drug-related problems. Include specific drugs, dosage forms, doses, schedules, and durations of therapy.

Implement the Care Plan

4.a. What information should be provided to the patient to enhance adherence, ensure successful therapy, and minimize adverse effects?

4.b. Describe how care should be coordinated with other healthcare providers.

Follow-Up: Monitor and Evaluate

5. Explain how to monitor and evaluate the care plan for medication appropriateness, effectiveness, safety, and patient adherence by using clinical and laboratory data, patient feedback, and other information.

■ SELF-STUDY ASSIGNMENTS

1. Identify commercially available GI protective products that may be administered via nasogastric or orogastric tube.

2. Identify potential drug interactions and adverse effects with antacids, sucralfate, H_2-receptor antagonists, and proton pump inhibitors.

CLINICAL PEARL

When performing medication reconciliation, always be on the lookout for ulcer prophylaxis agents on the patient's profile. They are often relics from a previous problem that has resolved and are no longer indicated. Patients on ulcer prophylaxis agents without an indication incur increased healthcare costs and are at increased risk for drug interactions and adverse effects, including a greater risk of pneumonia, *Clostridium difficile* infection, hypomagnesemia, and hypocalcemia.

REFERENCES

1. Ye Z, Reintam Blaser A, Lytvyn L, et al. Gastrointestinal bleeding prophylaxis for critically ill patients: a clinical practice guideline BMJ. 2020;368:l6722.
2. Wang Y, Ge L, Ye Z, et al. Efficacy and safety of gastrointestinal bleeding prophylaxis in critically ill patients: an updated systematic review and network meta-analysis of randomized trials. Intensive Care Med. 2020;46:1987–2000.

3. Toews I, George AT, Peter JV, et al. Interventions for preventing upper gastrointestinal bleeding in people admitted to intensive care units. Cochrane Database Syst Rev. 2018;6(6).

4. Huang, HB., Jiang, W., Wang, CY. et al. Stress ulcer prophylaxis in intensive care unit patients receiving enteral nutrition: a systematic review and meta-analysis. Crit Care Med. 2018;22:20.

5. Young PJ, Bagshaw SM, Forbes AB, et al. Effect of stress ulcer prophylaxis with proton pump inhibitors vs histamine-2 receptor blockers on in-hospital mortality among ICU patients receiving invasive mechanical ventilation: The PEPTIC Randomized Clinical Trial. JAMA. 2020;323(7):616–626.

38

CROHN DISEASE

An Inflammatory Situation..................... Level II

Brian A. Hemstreet, PharmD, FCCP, BCPS

LEARNING OBJECTIVES

After completing this case study, the reader should be able to:

- Describe the typical clinical presentation of active Crohn disease (CD), including signs, symptoms, and disease distribution and severity.

- Identify exacerbating factors and potential complications of CD.

- Recommend appropriate pharmacologic treatment for active CD.

- Review major toxicities of drugs commonly used for managing CD.

- Educate a patient on the proper use of medications used to treat CD.

PATIENT PRESENTATION

Chief Complaint

"I'm having occasional diarrhea, sometimes with blood. I also sometimes have a mild, crampy pain in my abdomen. I feel run down lately and have lost a few pounds."

HPI

A 32-year-old man who presents to the clinic with a 3-month history of intermittent episodes of diarrhea. He states that he has been having one to two loose bowel movements a day over this time. This is different from his typical bowel pattern. Over the past 4 weeks, he has also noticed blood in some of his stools. The episodes of diarrhea are frequently accompanied by brief periods of mild, crampy abdominal pain. These symptoms have caused significant problems with his job, as he is a sales representative for a pharmaceutical company and spends a lot of time driving to appointments. He reports a 5-lb unintentional weight loss over this period that he attributes to "not having a great appetite and not wanting to make his abdominal pain worse." He has tried OTC naproxen for the abdominal pain and Pepto-Bismol for the diarrhea, both of which have provided

little relief. He does not recall any exposure to sick contacts. He reports no recent international travel. His PCP referred him to a gastroenterologist.

PMH

Sinusitis (last treated with antibiotics 8 months ago)
Seasonal allergic rhinitis
ACL repair of the right knee 2 years ago due to a skiing accident

FH

Father with DM, mother with HTN. Older sister with CD.

SH

Single. Works as a sales representative for a pharmaceutical company. Occasional alcohol use on the weekends. Smokes 0.5 ppd × 10 years.

Meds

Loratadine 10 mg PO once daily as needed
Naproxen sodium 220 mg PO Q 8–12 H as needed for pain

All

Hydrocodone (GI upset)
Sulfa drugs (severe rash)

ROS

No sick contacts. Heartburn one to two times a week and rhinorrhea one to two times a week in the summer. No cough, SOB, HA, or mental status changes. No knee or joint pain. No jaundice or rashes. No mouth sores.

Physical Examination

Gen

Well-developed man in no apparent distress

VS

Sitting: BP 139/89, P 82; standing: BP 136/70, P 85; RR 17, T 37.9°C; Wt 215 lb (97.7 kg), Ht 5'9" (175 cm)

Skin

No lesions or rashes

HEENT

PERRLA, EOMI, pale conjunctivae, moist mucous membranes, intact dentition, oropharynx clear

Neck/Lymph Nodes

Trachea midline, (−) thyromegaly, (−) lymphadenopathy, (−) JVD

Lungs/Thorax

CTA bilaterally

CV

Regular rate and rhythm, no MRG

Abd

Nontender, nondistended, no rebound or guarding; (+) BS, (−) HSM

Genit/Rect

Prostate size WNL, (–) tenderness, heme (+) stool, no evidence of hemorrhoids

MS/Ext

No CVA tenderness

Neuro

A&O × 3, CN II–XII intact, 5/5 upper and lower extremity strength bilaterally

■ Labs

Na 139 mEq/L	Hgb 12 g/dL	AST 25 IU/L
K 3.0 mEq/L	Hct 37%	ALT 28 IU/L
Cl 100 mEq/L	RBC 2.86 × 10^6/mm^3	Alk phos 50 IU/L
CO$_2$ 26 mEq/L	Plt 400 × 10^3/mm^3	Total bili 1.2 mg/dL
BUN 15 mg/dL	MCV 80 μm^3	Direct bili 0.6 mg/dL
SCr 1.1 mg/dL	WBC 12.7 × 10^3/mm^3	Albumin 4.1 g/L
Glu 104 mg/dL	Neutros 67%	CRP 20 mg/dL
Ca 8.7 mg/dL	Bands 1%	Lipase 15 units/L
Phos 3.9 mg/dL	Eos 2%	ESR 105 mm/hr
	Lymphs 26%	Stool O & P (–)
	Monos 4%	Stool C. diff toxin (–)

■ Radiology

An abdominal X-ray reveals no evidence of obstruction, dilation, or free air.

■ Other

Colonoscopy: reveals a patchy "cobblestone" pattern of inflammation in the terminal ileum. The inflammatory process extends below the intestinal mucosa, and there is evidence of mucosal friability and recent bleeding. A biopsy of the intestinal mucosa reveals leukocyte infiltration and submucosal granulomas consistent with active CD.

■ Assessment

A 32-year-old man presenting with new-onset active CD involving the terminal ileum requiring treatment

QUESTIONS

Collect Information

1.a. What subjective and objective information indicates the presence of CD in this patient?

1.b. What additional information is needed to assess whether this patient has any extraintestinal manifestations of CD?

Assess the Information

2.a. Assess the severity and risk for disease progression and complications of CD in this patient based on the subjective and objective information available.

2.b. Create a list of the patient's drug therapy problems and prioritize them. Include assessment of medication appropriateness, effectiveness, safety, and adherence.

2.c. What factors could lead to the development or exacerbation of CD in this patient?

Develop a Care Plan

3.a. What are the goals of pharmacotherapy for CD in this case?

3.b. What nondrug therapies might be useful for this patient's CD?

3.c. What feasible pharmacotherapeutic alternatives are available for treating this patient's CD symptoms?

3.d. Create an individualized, patient-centered, team-based care plan to optimize medication therapy for this patient's CD and other drug therapy problems. Include specific drugs, dosage forms, doses, schedules, and durations of therapy.

Implement the Care Plan

4.a. What information should be provided to the patient to enhance adherence, ensure successful therapy, and minimize adverse effects?

4.b. Describe how care should be coordinated with other healthcare providers.

Follow-Up: Monitor and Evaluate

5. Explain how to monitor and evaluate the care plan for medication appropriateness, effectiveness, safety, and patient adherence by using clinical and laboratory data, patient feedback, and other information.

■ CLINICAL COURSE

It is now 7 months after the patient's initial presentation. The patient achieved remission after 3 months of initial treatment, after which therapy was discontinued. He has had only a few intermittent episodes of diarrhea and abdominal pain over the last 4 months. However, over the past week, he has had an increase in the frequency of bowel movements to three to four times per day with intermittent blood. He has developed significant abdominal pain, malaise, fever, and dehydration requiring hospitalization. He is admitted to the general medicine floor of the hospital with a recurrence of active moderate to severe CD.

■ FOLLOW-UP QUESTIONS

1. Given this new information, how would you modify the patient's drug therapy?

2. What baseline testing would be required if infliximab, adalimumab, certolizumab, or vedolizumab were to be used in this patient?

■ SELF-STUDY ASSIGNMENTS

1. Search for websites containing information about local support groups in your area to which you may refer patients with CD for help and support.

2. Construct a table outlining the major differences between CD and ulcerative colitis.

3. Review the FDA recommendations for use of the major drug classes for treatment of both active CD and maintenance of remission during pregnancy.

CLINICAL PEARL

Hospitalized patients with active CD are at high risk for venous thromboembolism due to the inflammatory nature of the disease and should be placed on prophylactic therapy for deep vein thrombosis.

REFERENCES

1. Lichtenstein GR, Loftus EV, Isaacs KL, et al. American College of Gastroenterology Clinical Guideline: management of Crohn's disease in adults. Am J Gastroenterol. 2018;113:481–517.

2. American Gastroenterological Association Institute Guidelines for the Identification, Assessment and Initial Medical Treatment in Crohn's Disease Clinical Decision Support Tool. Available at: *https://s3.amazonaws.com/agaassets/pdf/guidelines/IBDCarePathway.pdf*. Accessed November 23, 2021.

3. Gajendran M, Loganathan P, Catinella AP, Hashash JG. A comprehensive review and update on Crohn's disease. Dis Mon. 2018;64(2):20–57.

4. Torres J, Mehandru J, Colombel JF, Peyrin-Biroulet L. Crohn's disease. Lancet. 2017;389:1741–1755.

5. Rogler G, Singh A, Kavanaugh A, Rubin DT. Extraintestinal manifestations of inflammatory bowel disease: Current concepts, treatment, and implications for disease management. Gastroenterology. 2021;161(4):1118–1132. doi:10.1053/j.gastro.2021.07.042.

6. Moja L, Danese S, Fiorino C, et al. Systematic review with network meta-analysis: comparative efficacy and safety of budesonide and mesalazine (mesalamine) for Crohn's disease. Aliment Pharmacol Ther. 2015;41:1055–1065.

7. Coward S, Kuenzig, ME, Hazlewood G, et al. Comparative effectiveness of mesalamine, sulfasalazine, corticosteroids, and budesonide for the induction of remission in Crohn's disease: a Bayesian Network meta-analysis. Inflamm Bowel Dis. 2017;23:461–472.

8. Dorrington AM, Selinger CP, Parkes GC, et al. The historical role and contemporary use of corticosteroids in inflammatory bowel disease. J Crohns Colitis. 2020;14:13161329. doi: 10.1093/ecco-jcc/jjaa053.

9. Baumgart DC, Le Berre C. Newer biologic and small-molecule therapies for inflammatory bowel disease. N Engl J Med. 2021 Sep 30; 385(14):1302–1315. doi: 10.1056/NEJMra1907607.

39

ULCERATIVE COLITIS

Seriously? Four Times a Day? . . . . Level I

Nancy S. Yunker, PharmD, FCCP, BCPS

Alisa K. Escano, PharmD, BCPS

LEARNING OBJECTIVES

After completing this case study, the reader should be able to:

- Identify the common signs and symptoms of ulcerative colitis (UC).

- Evaluate treatment options for an acute episode of UC and recommend a specific treatment plan that includes the medication, dosing regimen, potential side effects, and monitoring parameters.

- Develop a pharmacotherapeutic plan for a patient with UC whose disease is in remission.

- Discuss recent advances in the pharmacotherapy of UC.

PATIENT PRESENTATION

■ Chief Complaint

"I need to see someone. I have ulcerative colitis and I'm having more and more pain and diarrhea. I can't get in to see my gastroenterologist for at least 3 weeks so I came here."

■ HPI

A 32-year-old woman with a history of UC presents to an urgent care center with the chief complaint of a 1.5-week history of abdominal pain associated with cramping, bloody diarrhea, and mucus that she states is typical of her UC flares. She states that she has been having about four bloody bowel movements a day for most of the time, but today she was dizzy when she stood up; she did not have any dizziness while sitting or lying down. She has not traveled outside the country, been hospitalized, or received antibiotics recently. She was diagnosed with UC approximately 3 years ago and has had approximately one exacerbation a year that her gastroenterologist has treated with Pentasa capsules four times a day during each exacerbation. Each time her symptoms have resolved with 4–6 weeks of therapy. She has refused maintenance therapy because she does not want to take a medication four times a day; it is not conducive to her work and social life, and she has refused rectal medications for the same reason. Her last exacerbation was approximately 10 months ago.

■ PMH

UC, diagnosed 3 years ago
Type 1 DM

■ FH

Mother has a history of CAD and lung CA; father has a history of UC, S/P colectomy 18 years ago

■ SH

Works as an office manager; lives with her fiancée; no children; denies tobacco use; drinks one to two glasses of wine every few weeks; acknowledges past marijuana use but states none in the past 10 years

■ Meds

Insulin aspart via insulin pump; settings per endocrinology
Vaccination history is unavailable

■ All

Sulfamethoxazole/trimethoprim (rash)

■ ROS

Negative for chest pain, SOB, dysuria, fever, chills, N/V, myalgias, arthralgias, polyuria, or recent allergic reaction. Positive for mild abdominal soreness, cramping, and intermittent bloody diarrhea with occasional urgency.

■ Physical Examination

Gen

A&O, pleasant, WDWN 32-year-old woman in NAD

VS

At 8 AM:

BP (lying down) 100/58 mm Hg, P 60 bpm

BP (standing) 80/40 mm Hg, P 75 bpm
RR 18/min, T 37.0°C
Wt 145 lb (66 kg), usual weight 150 lb (68 kg); Ht 5′7″ (170 cm); BMI 23.5 kg/m²

Skin

No lesions; warm, adequate turgor

HEENT

PERRLA; EOMI; mucous membranes without lesions or exudates; TMs intact

Lungs

CTA, no rales or rhonchi

CV

RRR, normal S_1 and S_2; no S_3, S_4

Abd

Normal active BS, soft, nondistended; tender to deep palpation but no palpable mass; no liver or spleen enlargement; no rebound tenderness or guarding

Rect

Somewhat tender; heme (+) stool

MS/Ext

No CCE; pulses 2+; normal ROM; strength 5/5 bilaterally

Neuro

A&O × 3; CN II–XII intact; DTRs 2+

Labs

At 10:00 AM:

Na 137 mEq/L	Hgb 13 g/dL	WBC 5.5 × 10³/mm³	AST 22 IU/L
K 3.9 mEq/L	Hct 38%	PMNs 52%	ALT 20 IU/L
Cl 105 mEq/L	Plt 242 × 10³/mm³	Bands 5%	Alk phos 36 IU/L
CO_2 27 mEq/L	MCV 85.3 μm³	Lymphs 36%	T. bili 0.5 mg/dL
BUN 26 mg/dL	MCH 29.1 pg	Basos 1%	PT 12.0 s
SCr 1.0 mg/dL	MCHC 34.1 g/dL	Monos 6%	INR 1.0
Glu 113 mg/dL			Ca 8.9 mg/dL
			Mg 1.9 mEq/L
			PO_4 4.2 mg/dL
			Alb 3.9 g/dL
			A1C 6.2%

Fecal calprotectin: 160 mcg/g

Urinalysis

Color yellow; transparency clear; negative for protein, leukocyte esterase, nitrite, blood, ketones, RBCs, WBCs, and bilirubin; pH 7.0; specific gravity 1.019

Assessment

Lower GI bleeding with a history of UC in a patient who has declined maintenance therapy in the past

D/C with instructions to return if symptoms worsen or contact PCP

QUESTIONS

Collect Information

1.a. What subjective and objective information indicates the presence of active ulcerative colitis?

1.b. What additional information is needed to fully assess the patient's ulcerative colitis?

Assess the Information

2.a. Assess the severity of the ulcerative colitis based on the subjective and objective information available.

2.b. Create a list of the patient's drug therapy problems and prioritize them. Include assessment of medication appropriateness, effectiveness, safety, and patient adherence.

Develop a Care Plan

3.a. What are the goals of pharmacotherapy for ulcerative colitis in this case?

3.b. What nondrug therapies might be useful for this patient's active ulcerative colitis?

3.c. What feasible pharmacotherapeutic alternatives are available for treating ulcerative colitis?

3.d. Create an individualized, patient-centered, team-based care plan to optimize medication therapy for ulcerative colitis and other drug therapy problems. Include specific drugs, dosage forms, doses, schedules, and durations of therapy.

3.e. What alternatives would be appropriate if the initial care plan fails or cannot be used?

Implement the Care Plan

4.a. What information should be provided to the patient to enhance adherence, ensure successful therapy, and minimize adverse effects?

4.b. Describe how care should be coordinated with other healthcare providers.

Follow-Up: Monitor and Evaluate

5. Explain how to monitor and evaluate the care plan for medication appropriateness, effectiveness, safety, and patient adherence by using clinical and laboratory data, patient feedback, and other information.

CLINICAL COURSE

The patient presents to her gastroenterologist for follow-up 1 month after her initial presentation to the urgent care center. She states that her bowel movements are "completely normal," and she no longer has pain. She states that the symptoms started to resolve about 2 weeks after she started treatment. She has had no further complaints of weakness or dizziness. The repeat Hgb today is 12.9 g/dL.

FOLLOW-UP QUESTIONS

1. Considering this new information, what therapeutic intervention(s) and patient education should be provided at this time?
2. What other healthcare maintenance issues should now be addressed in this patient with ulcerative colitis?

CHAPTER 40

SELF-STUDY ASSIGNMENTS

1. Review the literature comparing mesalamine, olsalazine, balsalazide, and sulfasalazine preparations regarding efficacy, adverse effects, and cost; include all currently available mesalamine dosage forms.

2. Perform a literature search to determine what new therapies are being evaluated for UC, including biologics, biosimilars, and small molecules.

3. Review the literature supporting use of cyclosporine, tacrolimus, anti–TNF-α agents in patients with severe, extensive disease poorly responsive to initial corticosteroid treatment.

4. Conduct a literature search to determine how pharmacogenomics is affecting therapy of UC patients.

CLINICAL PEARL

Use of ustekinumab depends on many factors such as insurance reimbursement, cost, and patient preference but based on the limited follow-up data, it appears to have a good safety profile in patients with moderate to severe UC. It may be the preferred agent in biologically naïve, frail patients who are at higher risk for adverse effects from other biologics such as the anti-TNF-α agents and in patients with certain other concomitant diseases such as psoriatic arthritis as it is also labeled for this indication.

REFERENCES

1. Rubin DT, Ananthakrishnan AN, Siegel CA, Sauer BG, Long MD. ACG clinical guideline: ulcerative colitis in adults. Am J Gastroenterol. 2019;114:384–413.

2. Feuerstein JD, Moss AC, Farraye FA. Ulcerative colitis. Mayo Clin Proc. 2019;94:1357–1373.

3. Ko CW, Singh S, Feuerstein JD, Falck-Ytter C, Falck-Ytter Y, Cross RK on behalf of the American Gastroenterological Association Institute Clinical Guidelines Committee. AGA clinical practice guidelines on the management of mild-to-moderate ulcerative colitis. Gastroenterology. 2019;156:748–764.

4. Feuerstein JD, Isaacs KL, Schneider Y, Siddique SM, Falck-Ytter Y, Singh S on behalf of the AGA Institute Clinical Guidelines Committee. AGA clinical practice guidelines on the management of moderate to severe ulcerative colitis. Gastroenterology. 2020;158:1450–1461.

5. Bischoff SC, Escher J, Hebuterne X, et al. ESPEN practical guideline: clinical nutrition in inflammatory bowel disease. Clin Nutr. 2020;39:632–653.

6. Raine T, Bonovas S, Burisch J, et al on behalf of European Crohn's and Colitis Organization (ECCO). ECCO guidelines on therapeutics in ulcerative colitis: medical management. J Crohns Colitis. 2022;16:2–17.

7. Ye B, van Langenberg DR. Mesalazine preparations for the treatment of ulcerative colitis: are all created equal? World J Gastrointest Pharmacol Ther. 2015;6:137–144.

8. Biancone L, Ardizzone S, Armuzzi A, et al. Ustekinumab for treating ulcerative colitis: an expert opinion. Expert Opin Biol Ther. 2020;20:1321–1329.

9. Al-Bawardy B, Shivashankar R, Proctor DD. Novel and emerging therapies for inflammatory bowel disease. Front Pharmacol. 2021;12:651415.

10. Macaluso FS, Liguori G, Galli M. Vaccinations in patients with inflammatory bowel disease. Dig Liver Dis. 2021;53:1539–1545.

40

NAUSEA AND VOMITING

In for a Tune-Up .... Level II

Sasha Haarberg, PharmD, BCOP

LEARNING OBJECTIVES

After completing this case study, the reader should be able to:

- Develop a prophylactic antiemetic regimen based on the anticancer agents' emetic risk that optimizes the management of nausea and vomiting.

- Design an appropriate treatment regimen for anticipatory and breakthrough nausea and vomiting.

- Design a monitoring plan to assess the effectiveness of an antiemetic regimen.

- Discuss with patients and caregivers the reason for antiemetics, their appropriate use, and the management of side effects.

- Recommend appropriate alternative antiemetic strategies based on patient-specific conditions, such as previous response to chemotherapy and side effects.

PATIENT PRESENTATION

■ Chief Complaint

"I have throat cancer and it hurts to swallow."

■ HPI

A 57-year-old man presented to his primary care provider with complaints of pain in the back of his throat and difficulty swallowing. He has had a 14-lb weight loss over the previous 2 months because it has been difficult to eat. Upon physical exam, a mass is felt in his neck. His primary care provider orders a biopsy, and the histopathology reveals squamous cell carcinoma. A PET-CT scan reveals a 3-cm mass in the oropharynx with disease found in multiple cervical lymph nodes. A diagnosis of advanced-stage oropharyngeal cancer is made with the plan to begin systemic chemotherapy and radiation in the outpatient setting.

■ PMH

BPH
Cancer of the oropharynx (p16 negative)
GERD

■ FH

Father died at age 82 of heart and renal failure; mother died at age 68 with emphysema, obesity, MI, hypertension; two sisters, one with diabetes; three adult children, alive and healthy

■ SH

Single and works as a salesman at a car dealership. He has smoked 1–1.5 packs of cigarettes a day starting at the age of 14. He recently stopped smoking because his employer instated a campus-wide no smoking policy. He routinely consumes alcohol, averaging eight to ten alcoholic drinks per week.

■ Meds

Tamsulosin 0.4 mg PO daily
Esomeprazole 40 mg PO daily
Oxycodone ER 10 mg PO Q 12 H
Oxycodone 5 mg PO Q 3 H PRN

■ All

NKDA

■ ROS

Complaints include difficulty swallowing, pain in throat, and weight loss over the past 2 months.

■ Physical Examination

Gen

This is a pleasant man who appears to be in acute distress due to throat pain.

VS

BP 160/82, P 91, RR 20, T 36.6°C; Wt 149.6 lb (68 kg), Ht 6'0″ (183 cm)

Skin

Warm and dry to touch

HEENT

No discharge noted in the external ear canals. Mouth is pink and dry. An abnormal mass is present in the oropharynx.

Neck/Lymph Nodes

Enlarged cervical lymph nodes that are tender to the touch. No JVD or thyromegaly noted.

Lungs/Thorax

Good air movement. No wheezes or rhonchi noted. No spinal abnormalities appreciated.

CV

RRR. No rubs, murmurs, or gallops

Abd

Positive bowel sounds, no hepatosplenomegaly

Genit/Rect

Deferred

MS/Ext

Normal range of motion and equal strength in upper and lower extremities. Positive for 2+ pitting edema in the feet and ankles.

Neuro

Patient A&O × 4. Cranial nerves intact. Gait was not assessed. Patient is very anxious about his diagnosis and treatment.

■ Labs

Na 141 mEq/L	Hgb 12.4 g/dL	T. bili 0.8 mg/dL
K 4.3 mEq/L	Hct 36.3%	Albumin 2.4 g/dL
Cl 106 mEq/L	Plt 148 × 10³/mm³	AST 18 IU/L
CO$_2$ 21 mEq/L	WBC 18.4 × 10³/mm³	ALT 12 IU/L
BUN 21 mg/dL	Neutros 72%	Alk phos 65 IU/L
SCr 0.7 mg/dL	Bands 8%	GGT 40 IU/L
Glu 97 mg/dL	Lymphs 11%	
Mg 1.6 mg/dL	Monos 4%	
	Eos 1%	
	Basos 1%	
	Promyelo 1%	
	Meta 2%	

■ Assessment

The patient has advanced oropharyngeal cancer and is not a candidate for surgical intervention. He would like to proceed with concurrent chemotherapy and radiation, which is planned at the outpatient cancer clinic. He continues to have pain and is anxious about his diagnosis and the chemotherapy he is about to receive. The selected regimen is high-dose cisplatin with concurrent external beam radiation. Orders include:

Palonosetron 0.25 mg IV 30 minutes prior to cisplatin
Dexamethasone 12 mg IV 30 minutes prior to cisplatin
Fosaprepitant 150 mg IV 30 minutes prior to cisplatin on day 1, and then aprepitant 80 mg PO daily on days 2 and 3
Normal saline 1,000 mL with magnesium sulfate 2 g and potassium chloride 20 mEq as pre- and post-cisplatin hydration
Cisplatin 100 mg/m² IV once every 3 weeks administered for 3 cycles
Radiation therapy 2 Gy/day for a total of 70 Gy over 7 weeks
Ondansetron 4 mg PO Q 8 H PRN nausea and vomiting

QUESTIONS

Collect Information

1.a. What subjective and objective information may influence this patient's risk for chemotherapy-induced nausea and vomiting?

1.b. What additional information is needed to fully assess this patient's risk of nausea and vomiting?

Assess the Information

2.a. Assess the emetic risk of this patient's treatment regimen.

2.b. Create a list of this patient's drug therapy problems and prioritize them. Include assessment of medication appropriateness, effectiveness, safety, and patient adherence.

Develop a Care Plan

3.a. What are the goals of pharmacotherapy for nausea and vomiting in this case?

3.b. What nondrug therapies may be useful to prevent this patient's nausea and vomiting?

3.c. What feasible pharmacotherapeutic alternatives are available for the prophylaxis of acute and delayed nausea and vomiting and for the treatment of breakthrough nausea and vomiting?

3.d. Create an individualized, patient-centered, team-based care plan to optimize medication therapy for this patient. Include specific drugs, dosage forms, schedules, and durations of therapy.

Implement the Care Plan

4.a. What information should be provided to the patient to enhance adherence, ensure successful therapy, and minimize adverse effects?

4.b. Describe how care should be coordinated with other healthcare providers.

Follow-Up: Monitor and Evaluate

5. Explain how to monitor and evaluate the care plan for medication appropriateness, effectiveness, safety, and patient adherence by using clinical and laboratory data, patient feedback, and other information.

■ CLINICAL COURSE (PART 1)

You review antiemetics prior to administering the high-dose cisplatin, and the oncologist makes changes based on your recommendations. Following chemotherapy administration, the patient does well for the first 24 hours, but around hour 30, he develops nausea and vomiting. He follows the instructions provided and takes the ondansetron he has at home. He calls the provider's office on day 3 for advice, as he is still experiencing vomiting despite taking the antiemetics. The provider asks about hydration status and learns he has had limited fluid intake over the past 3 days and cannot recall the last time he urinated. He is tired but assumes this is due to the cisplatin therapy.

■ FOLLOW-UP QUESTION

1. What pharmacologic alternatives may be helpful for treatment of breakthrough nausea and vomiting in this patient?

■ CLINICAL COURSE (PART 2)

Five days later, the patient's nausea and vomiting have resolved. He continues to receive concurrent radiation and will return to the clinic to receive cycle 2 of cisplatin.

■ FOLLOW-UP QUESTIONS (CONTINUED)

2. What changes can be made to prevent delayed nausea and vomiting for subsequent chemotherapy cycles?

3. Design a plan to prevent anticipatory nausea and vomiting in this patient for subsequent chemotherapy cycles.

■ CLINICAL COURSE: ALTERNATIVE THERAPY

While discussing his antiemetic regimen, he says, "I remember that my sister used to take ginger to prevent sea sickness when she went on a cruise, and my cousin used ginger when he was having chemotherapy a few years ago. Would that be good for me to try?" See Section 19 in this Casebook for questions about the use of ginger for treatment of nausea and vomiting.

■ SELF-STUDY ASSIGNMENTS

1. Compare the indications, doses, and costs of the 5-HT$_3$ antagonists: dolasetron, ondansetron, granisetron, palonosetron, and the combination product netupitant/palonosetron.

2. Compare the indications, doses, cost, of the NK-1 antagonists: aprepitant, fosaprepitant, rolapitant, or netupitant. Discern the advantages and limitations of each drug.

3. Review the antiemetic regimens that incorporate olanzapine for the prevention of nausea and vomiting.

4. Review various guidelines for antiemetic options for the treatment of refractory nausea and vomiting.

CLINICAL PEARL

For highly emetic chemotherapy regimens, either three or four-drug regimens are widely accepted standard regimens in cancer centers. If dosed appropriately, all 5-HT$_3$ and NK$_1$ receptor antagonists are considered to have equal efficacy. Thus, antiemetic therapy decisions should be based on patient-specific factors, including cost or patient's insurance coverage.

ACKNOWLEDGMENT

This case is based on the patient case written for the 11th edition by Kelly K. Nystrom, PharmD, BCOP and Amy M. Pick, PharmD, BCOP.

REFERENCES

1. Ettinger DS, Berger MJ, Aston J, et al. NCCN Clinical Practice Guidelines in Oncology (NCCN Guidelines') Guideline Antiemesis 1.2021. © 2018 National Comprehensive Cancer Network, Inc. Available at: www.NCCN.org. Accessed November 1, 2021.

2. Navari RM. Managing nausea and vomiting in patients with cancer: what works. Oncology. 2018;32:121–125, 131, 136.

3. Hesketh PJ, Kris MG, Basch E, et al. Antiemetics: ASCO guideline update. J Clin Oncol. 2020;38(24):2782–2797.

4. Jordan K, Jahn F, Aapro M. Recent developments in the prevention of chemotherapy-induced nausea and vomiting (CINV): a comprehensive review. Ann Oncol. 2015;26:1081–1090.

5. Herrstedt J, Roila F, Warr D, et al. Updated MASCC/ESMO consensus recommendations: prevention of nausea and vomiting following high emetic risk chemotherapy. Support Care Cancer. 2017;25:277–288.

6. Roila F, Warr D, Hesketh PJ, et al. 2016 updated MASCC/ESMO consensus recommendations: prevention of nausea and vomiting following moderately emetogenic chemotherapy. Support Care Cancer. 2017;25:289–294.

7. Italian Group for Antiemetic Research. Randomized, double-blind, dose-finding study of dexamethasone in preventing acute emesis induced by anthracyclines, carboplatin, or cyclophosphamide: J Clin Oncol. 2004;22:725–729.

41

DIARRHEA

Diner's Diarrhea . . . . Level I

Marie A. Abate, BS, PharmD

Charles D. Ponte, BS, PharmD, BC-ADM, BCPS, CDCES, CPE, FADCES, FAPhA, FASHP, FCCP, FNAP

LEARNING OBJECTIVES

After completing this case study, the reader should be able to:

- Identify the most likely causes of acute diarrhea.

- Establish primary goals for the treatment of acute diarrhea based on signs, symptoms, and patient history.

- Recommend appropriate nonpharmacologic therapy for patients experiencing acute diarrhea.
- Explain the place of drug therapy in the treatment of acute diarrhea and recommend appropriate products.

PATIENT PRESENTATION

■ Chief Complaint

"I've had very watery bowel movements for a couple of days, along with vomiting. I haven't been able keep anything down and I feel awful."

■ HPI

A 25-year-old woman comes to the Family Medicine Clinic with a complaint of nausea, vomiting, and diarrhea. She had been well until 1.5 days ago, when she began to experience severe nausea that occurred about 6 hours after eating dinner out at a large chain buffet restaurant. She had granola and yogurt for breakfast and a chicken pesto and avocado sandwich for lunch the day her symptoms began. Her boyfriend ate an assortment of seafood and beef dishes while she had salads, chicken stir-fry, and shrimp. He has had no symptoms.

She had eaten several plates of food for dinner along with iced tea. She had a few sips of her boyfriend's soda but did not have any milk or other dairy products. She woke up from sleep with severe nausea and took two tablespoonfuls of Maalox Plus at that time. The nausea persisted, and she began to vomit "several times" with some relief. As the night progressed, she still felt "queasy" and took two Prilosec OTC tablets to settle her stomach. She began to feel dizzy, achy, and warm, and her temperature at the time was 100°F. These complaints continued to persist, and she vomited a few more times. She has not tolerated any solid foods, but she has been able to keep down small amounts of fluid. Since yesterday, she has had four to six liquid stools along with abdominal cramps. She has not noticed any blood or mucus in the bowel movements. Her boyfriend brought her to the clinic because she was becoming weak and lightheaded when she tried to stand up. She denies antibiotic use, laxative use, or excessive caffeine intake. She usually drinks bottled water and has not been traveling outside the country. She often experiences stress-related constipation and occasionally (once every 2 months) has some loose stools alternating with constipation accompanied with abdominal discomfort. A bowel movement usually relieves any associated abdominal pain. She states that this episode is different.

■ PMH

IBS × 2 years
Migraine headaches × 10 years
GERD × 5 years
Depression × 3 years
UTI—6 months ago (treated successfully with ciprofloxacin × 10 days)

■ FH

Noncontributory

■ SH

No current tobacco use; uses marijuana occasionally; drinks wine or a mixed drink socially, usually not more than one glass per week; has about two cups of caffeinated coffee daily. She works as an administrative associate for a local bank. Single, sexually active (one partner, monogamous relationship).

■ Meds

Valproic acid 500 mg PO BID × 6 years
Triphasil oral contraceptive 1 PO at bedtime × 3 years (last taken the evening after the dinner out)
Omeprazole 20–40 mg PO daily as needed
One A Day Women's Formula Multivitamin 1 PO daily
Metamucil one tablespoonful daily
St John's wort two 900 mg tablets daily

■ All

Penicillin → itching, rash on legs, 10 years ago; dust → nasal congestion, watery eyes

■ ROS

Dizzy on standing but no complaints of vertigo; denies headache, sore throat, ear pain, or nasal discharge. Denies coughing or congestion. Frequent bouts of nausea. Frequent loose stools associated with significant cramping. Decreased urination; no dysuria or frequency. Complains of generalized lassitude, mild aching; feels like her heart is skipping beats.

■ PE

Gen

Female, appears ill, in moderate distress

VS

BP 125/82, P 80 (supine), BP 90/60, P 90 (standing), RR 16, T 38°C; Wt 165 lb (75 kg), Ht 5′4″ (162.5 cm)

Skin

Slightly warm to touch, fair skin turgor (mild tenting noted)

HEENT

Dry mucous membranes, non-erythematous TMs, PERRLA, fundi benign, slight erythema in throat

Neck/Lymph Nodes

Without masses, lymphadenopathy, or thyromegaly

Chest

Clear to A&P

CV

RRR without MRG

Abd

Diffuse tenderness, no guarding or rebound, without organomegaly, nondistended, hyperactive bowel sounds

Genit/Rect

Heme (−) stool in the rectal vault; no gross blood

MS/Ext

Normal muscle strength, no CCE

Neuro

A&O × 3; CN II–XII intact; normal reflexes, normal sensory and motor function

■ Labs

Na 135 mEq/L	Hgb 12.0 g/dL	AST 35 IU/L
K 3.2 mEq/L	Hct 35%	ALT 30 IU/L
Cl 97 mEq/L	Plt $350 \times 10^3/mm^3$	T. bili 1.5 mg/dL
CO_2 25 mEq/L	WBC $12.0 \times 10^3/mm^3$	
BUN 25 mg/dL	PMNs 62%	
SCr 1.2 mg/dL	Lymphs 36%	
Glu 90 mg/dL	Monos 2%	

Serum pregnancy test—negative
Stool sample obtained for ova and parasites

■ UA

Clear, dark amber; SG 1.030; pH 6.0; protein (–); glucose (–); acetone (–), bilirubin (–), blood (–); microscopic: 0–2 WBC/hpf, 0–2 RBC/hpf, several hyaline casts

■ Assessment

Probable acute gastroenteritis; R/O other causes
Depression
Migraine headaches
GERD
Irritable bowel syndrome

■ Plan

Admit to observation unit for acute therapy

QUESTIONS

Collect Information

1.a. What subjective and objective information indicates the presence of diarrhea?

1.b. What additional information is needed to fully assess this patient's diarrhea?

Assess the Information

2.a. Assess the severity of the diarrhea based on the subjective and objective information available.

2.b. Create a list of the patient's drug therapy problems and prioritize them. Include assessment of medication appropriateness, effectiveness, safety, and patient adherence.

2.c. What are other possible causes of this patient's diarrhea?

Develop a Care Plan

3.a. What are the goals of pharmacotherapy for diarrhea in this case?

3.b. What nondrug therapies might be useful for this patient's diarrhea?

3.c. What feasible pharmacotherapeutic alternatives are available for treating diarrhea?

3.d. Create an individualized, patient-centered, team-based care plan to optimize medication therapy for the diarrhea and other drug therapy problems. Include specific drugs, dosage forms, doses, schedules, and durations of therapy.

Implement the Care Plan

4.a. What information should be provided to the patient to enhance adherence, ensure successful therapy, and minimize adverse effects?

4.b. Describe how care should be coordinated with other healthcare providers.

Follow-Up: Monitor and Evaluate

5. Explain how to monitor and evaluate the care plan for medication appropriateness, effectiveness, safety, and patient adherence by using clinical and laboratory data, patient feedback, and other information.

■ CLINICAL COURSE

The treatment and monitoring plan you recommended was initiated on admission. The patient's diarrhea slowed by the evening of day 1. The patient had no further episodes of diarrhea or vomiting after midnight. On the morning of day 2, her orthostasis had resolved, her temperature was normal, the IV fluids were stopped, and she received clear liquids by mouth for breakfast and lunch. The patient was discharged during the late afternoon.

■ FOLLOW-UP QUESTIONS

1. How should this patient's contraception be managed after she is rehydrated and returns home?

2. Does the patient need any changes in her prophylactic migraine headache therapy?

3. How should her IBS be managed?

■ SELF-STUDY ASSIGNMENTS

1. Identify the infectious causes of diarrhea. Design an effective pharmacotherapy treatment regimen for each cause.

2. Provide recommendations for the prevention and treatment of traveler's diarrhea.

3. Describe whether antidiarrheal drug products can be safely recommended for use in very young children (<3 years old) or in patients with bloody diarrhea and, if so, the specific products that could be used.

4. Describe when oral rehydration products should be used and recommend a specific product and dosage for young or older patients who present with mild to moderate diarrhea and minimal dehydration.

5. Investigate the relationship between the development of IBS and bacterial gastroenteritis.

CLINICAL PEARL

Broad-spectrum antibiotics (especially clindamycin and the fluoroquinolones) are a common cause of *Clostridioides difficile* colitis. Diarrhea is a common sign of the disease and may begin 3 days after initiating an antibiotic or up to 3 months after a course of antibiotics (the Rule of 3's).

REFERENCES

1. Riddle MS, DuPont HL, Connor BA. ACG clinical guideline: diagnosis, treatment, and prevention of acute diarrheal infections in adults. Am J Gastroenterol. 2016;111:602–622.

2. Acree M, Davis AM. Acute diarrheal infections in adults. JAMA. 2017;318:957–958.

3. DuPont HL. Acute infectious diarrhea in immunocompetent adults. N Engl J Med. 2014;370:1532–1540.

4. Barr W, Smith A. Acute diarrhea. Am Fam Physician 2014;89:180–189.

5. Pulling M, Surawicz CM. Loperamide use for acute infectious diarrhea in children: safe and sound? Gastroenterology. 2008;134:1260–1262.

6. Hanauer SB, DuPont HL, Cooper KM, Laudadio C. Randomized, double-blind, placebo-controlled clinical trial of loperamide plus simethicone versus loperamide alone and simethicone alone in the treatment of acute diarrhea with gas-related abdominal discomfort. Curr Med Res Opin. 2007;23:1033–1043.

7. Sarowska J, Choroszy-Król I, Regulska-Ilow B, Frej-Mądrzak M, Jama-Kmiecik A. The therapeutic effect of probiotic bacteria on gastrointestinal diseases. Adv Clin Exp Med. 2013;22:759–766.

8. Goodman C, Keating G, Georgousopoulou E, Hespe C, Levett K. Probiotics for the prevention of antibiotic-associated diarrhoea: a systematic review and meta-analysis. BMJ Open. 2021;11(8):e043054.

9. Collinson S, Deans A, Padua-Zamora A, et al. Probiotics for treating acute infectious diarrhoea. Cochrane Database Syst Rev. 2020 Dec 8; 12(12):CD003048.

10. Ford AC, Sperber AD, Corsetti M, Camilleri M. Irritable bowel syndrome. Lancet. 2020;396:1675–1688.

42

CONSTIPATION

All Bound Up . . . . Level I

Michelle Fravel, PharmD, BCPS

Beth Bryles Phillips, PharmD, FASHP, FCCP, BCPS, BCACP

LEARNING OBJECTIVES

After completing this case study, the reader should be able to:

- Identify medications that can exacerbate constipation.

- Describe the advantages and disadvantages of each class of laxatives and discuss the appropriate use of each class.

- Recommend an appropriate plan for the treatment of constipation, including lifestyle modifications and drug therapy.

- Educate patients regarding laxative therapy.

PATIENT PRESENTATION

■ Chief Complaint

"I feel just awful ever since starting these pain pills—I think I'd rather be in pain!"

■ HPI

A 64-year-old woman presents to the emergency treatment center complaining of increasing abdominal cramping and nausea for several days and now vomiting for the past several hours. She reports starting Percocet therapy 2 weeks ago for postprocedural pain in association with right TKA. Her last bowel movement was 6 days ago. She began "not feeling well" 4 days ago, with bloating, decreased appetite, decreased thirst, and fatigue. She reports that yesterday, when her cramping was at its worst, she even used a couple of doses of Metamucil, but it did not help. She says she was almost to the point where she thought about trying some powerful laxatives, but she has heard about the addiction they can cause and the last thing she wants is to be addicted to a laxative. She has also tried to just quit taking the pain meds altogether, but she only makes it about

halfway through the morning before the pain becomes unbearable. She reports that she has cut back on the pain pills and is only taking one pill four times a day now, compared two pills four times a day one week ago. On a scale of 1–10, she rates her pain at a 5 today. She does say the pain is improving every day. Her plan is to take one less pain pill every 3 days so that she can successfully taper the meds in about 2 weeks. She reports no fever, CP, or SOB. She states that she typically has daily bowel movements, with no straining, and spends less than 10 minutes, with little effort, having a bowel movement. Her last colonoscopy, performed 2 years ago, was unremarkable.

■ PMH

Hypothyroidism
Type 2 diabetes mellitus
Hypertension
Dyslipidemia
Osteoarthritis status post right TKA 2 weeks ago

■ FH

Her mother is in her 80s and is healthy. Her father died in his 60s from heart disease. She has three brothers and three sisters; one brother has type 2 diabetes. She has two sons who are healthy.

■ SH

She is married and works as a social worker. She quit smoking more than 20 years ago. She does not drink alcohol and does not use illicit drugs.

■ Meds

Levothyroxine 50 mcg PO daily
Lisinopril 20 mg daily
Metformin 1000 mg PO twice daily
Multivitamin/mineral one tablet PO daily
Oxycodone/acetaminophen 5 mg/325 mg one to two tablets Q 4–6 H PRN
Atorvastatin 10 mg PO at bedtime
Verapamil SR 360 mg daily

■ All

NKDA

■ ROS

(+) For constipation, lower abdominal fullness, N/V, right knee pain, (−) for SOB, CP, or fever/chills

■ Physical Examination

Gen

Pleasant woman in distress because of abdominal discomfort; is visibly uncomfortable and holding her stomach during the visit; appears tired

VS

BP 122/60, P 57, RR 16, T 36.2°C; Wt 247 lb (112.4 kg), Ht 5'5" (165 cm); waist circumference 37 in (94 cm); pain rated 5 on scale of 1–10

Skin

Normal skin turgor and color

HEENT

PERRLA and EOM full without nystagmus; no scleral icterus; oral mucosa moist; no ulcerations noted

Neck/Lymph Nodes

Supple, no lymphadenopathy or JVD; no thyromegaly or bruits

CV

Regular, S_1 and S_2 without murmur

Lungs

Normal breath sounds; no crackles or wheezes

Abd

Soft, obese, tender; decreased bowel sounds; stool palpable on left side

Rectal

Stool present in rectal vault; no masses felt; tone fair; push strength fair; nontender

MS/Ext

S/P right TKA; surgical wound healing appropriately; no redness, swelling, exudation; range of motion within normal limits

Neuro

A&O × 3; CNs II–XII symmetric and intact; DTRs 2+

■ Labs

Na 138 mEq/L	Glu 133 mg/dL (fasting)	RBC 6.05 × 10⁶/mm³
K 4.3 mEq/L	A1C 6.4%	Hgb 15.5 g/dL
Cl 101 mEq/L	Ca 9.3 mg/dL	Hct 48%
CO_2 30 mEq/L	TSH 2.70 mIU/mL	MCV 79 μm³
BUN 14 mg/dL	Cholesterol 165 mg/dl	MCH 26 pg
SCr 0.8 mg/dL	LDL 72 mg/dl	MCHC 33%
ACR 327 mg/g	HDL 51 mg/dl	RDW 15.4%
	TG 212 mg/dl	

■ Radiology

X-ray: A plain X-ray of the abdomen showed gas-dilated loops in the colon.

Abdominal CT: scan demonstrated a large amount of stool in the colon and rectal vault.

■ Assessment

Constipation with fecal impaction; secondary symptoms of abdominal discomfort, nausea, and vomiting; etiology likely drug-induced. Disimpaction was successfully performed with no complications. A follow-up PEG-based bowel preparation was successful in clearing bowel and relieving the patient's abdominal pain.

QUESTIONS

Collect Information

1.a. What subjective and objective information indicates the presence of constipation?

1.b. What additional information is needed to fully assess this patient's constipation?

Assess the Information

2.a. Assess the severity of constipation based on the subjective and objective information available.

2.b. Create a list of the patient's drug therapy problems and prioritize them. Include assessment of medication appropriateness, effectiveness, safety, and patient adherence.

2.c. What economic, psychosocial, cultural, racial, and ethical considerations are applicable to this patient?

Develop a Care Plan

3.a. What are the goals of pharmacotherapy for constipation in this case?

3.b. What nondrug therapies might be useful for this patient's constipation?

3.c. What are the pharmacologic options for the treatment of constipation?

3.d. Create an individualized, patient-centered, team-based care plan to optimize medication therapy for this patient's constipation and other drug therapy problems. Include specific drugs, dosage forms, doses, schedules, and durations of therapy.

Implement the Care Plan

4.a. What information should be provided to the patient to enhance adherence, ensure successful therapy, and minimize adverse effects?

4.b. Describe how care should be coordinated with other healthcare providers.

Follow-Up: Monitor and Evaluate

5. Explain how to monitor and evaluate the care plan for medication appropriateness, effectiveness, safety, and patient adherence by using clinical and laboratory data, patient feedback, and other information.

■ CLINICAL COURSE

The recommendations you made were implemented, and the patient returns to your clinic 1 month later. She reports that the drug therapy you recommended resulted in regular bowel function throughout the last 2 weeks of her opioid therapy but expresses she is concerned she'll be "hooked on the laxatives." She does report, however, that her orthopedic physicians have now recommended TKA on the opposite knee. She says that after the last episode with constipation, she just does not think she wants to go through with it.

■ FOLLOW-UP QUESTIONS

1. What regimen would you recommend for preventing opioid-induced constipation in this patient if she chooses to go through with the second TKA procedure?

2. What education would you provide to this patient who has concerns about recurrence of drug-induced constipation?

3. What education would you provide to this patient regarding her concerns about laxative addiction?

■ SELF-STUDY ASSIGNMENTS

1. Suggest pharmacotherapeutic options for the treatment of opioid-induced constipation in a pediatric patient. How does this approach compare with that used in treatment of adults?

2. Perform a literature search to find medications under investigation for the treatment of constipation. What different types of constipation will these new entities be used to treat? What place in therapy will these medications have?

CLINICAL PEARL

Management of medication-related constipation may include discontinuation of the offending agent with initiation of an appropriate alternative or initiation of a medication designed to address medication-related constipation. Failure to recognize medications as contributors to constipation may lead to inappropriate treatment and inadequate relief of constipation symptoms.

REFERENCES

1. Crockett SD, Greer KB, Heidelbaugh JJ, Falck-Ytter Y, Hanson BJ, Sultan S. American Gastroenterological Association Institute guidelines on the medical management of opioid-induced constipation. Gastroenterology. 2019;156:218–226.
2. Paranjpe M, Chin A, Paranjpe I, et al. Self-reported health without clinically measurable benefits among adult users of multivitamin and multimineral supplements: a cross-sectional study. BMJ Open. 2020;10:e039119. doi: 10.1136/bmjopen-2020-039119.
3. Shah BJ, Rughwani N, Rose S. Constipation. Ann Intern Med. 2015;162:ITC1. doi:10.7326/AITC201504070.
4. Freedman MD, Schwartz HJ, Roby R, et al. Tolerance and efficacy of polyethylene glycol 3350/electrolyte solution versus lactulose in relieving opiate induced constipation: a double-blinded placebo-controlled trial. J Clin Pharmacol. 1997;37:904–907.
5. Twycross RG, McNamara P, Schuijt C, et al. Sodium picosulfate in opioid-induced constipation: results of an open-label, prospective, dose-ranging study. Palliat Med. 2006;20:419–423.
6. Wirz S, Nadstawek J, Elsen C, et al. Laxative management in ambulatory cancer patients on opioid therapy: a prospective, open-label investigation of polyethylene glycol, sodium picosulphate and lactulose. Eur J Cancer Care. (Engl) 2012;21:131–140.
7. Mozaffari S, Nikfar S, Abdollahi M. Methylnaltrexone bromide for the treatment of opioid-induced constipation. Expert Opin Pharmacother. 2018;19:1127–1135.
8. Baker D. Formulary drug review: Naldemedine. Hosp Pharm. 2017;52:464–468.
9. Whelton PK, Carey RM, Aronow WS, et al. 2017 ACC/AHA/AAPA/ABC/ACPM/AGS/APhA/ASH/ASPC/NMA/PCNA guideline for the prevention, detection, evaluation, and management of high blood pressure in adults. Hypertension. 2017. doi: 10.1161/HYP.0000000000000065.

43

IRRITABLE BOWEL SYNDROME

Life in the Slow Lane.......................... Level II

Alisa K. Escano, PharmD, BCPS

Nancy S. Yunker, PharmD, FCCP, BCPS

LEARNING OBJECTIVES

After completing this case study, the reader should be able to:

- Determine the signs and symptoms of irritable bowel syndrome (IBS) associated with constipation (IBS-C) and diarrhea (IBS-D).

- Devise patient management strategies for patients with IBS, including pharmacologic and nonpharmacologic options.

- Recommend parameters for monitoring the safety and efficacy of therapy used in patients with IBS.

- Discuss treatment options for IBS-C and IBS-D.

- Evaluate the efficacy of treatment options for patients with IBS.

PATIENT PRESENTATION

■ Chief Complaint

"My IBS is acting up again. I feel all bloated and I really have to strain to have a bowel movement. I have been really uncomfortable for the past 2 months. I added Metamucil capsules to the docusate I was already taking because someone in the past told me that I would probably be able to tolerate the capsules better than Metamucil powder. I haven't seen much improvement in the 8 weeks that I have been using them, plus it is hard to remember to take them three times a day. I have tried to live with this but I really think I need to try something else. Is there anything you can give me?"

■ HPI

A 28-year-old woman presents to her PCP with an 8-month history of hard pellet-like stools and difficulty passing stools. She was diagnosed with IBS when she was 18 years old, her freshman year in college. She has been able to tolerate the minimal symptoms until about 8 months ago when she noticed bloating and a decrease in the number of bowel movements per week. She attributes the worsening symptoms to the stress associated with graduate school and working two jobs. She works as a teaching assistant and as a sales associate in a department store. She states the symptoms worsened since she went back to school, especially during exams. Other than stress, she cannot think of anything else that has changed. She does not remember having any gastroenteritis symptoms in the last year, and she dislikes eating yogurt.

Prior to 8 months ago, she states that she averaged about six stools a week. She estimates that she has had one or two bowel movements a week for the past 8 weeks. She complains of straining to pass her stools and states that she is getting up 60 minutes early in the morning to allow for an attempt to pass a stool and uses the additional time exercising in order to "stimulate her bowels." She also tried eating more bran products but felt like that made the pain and bloating worse, so she stopped. She complains of abdominal pain and bloating almost continuously throughout the day for the past 2 months, although her symptoms are somewhat alleviated by passing a "good stool." She resumed taking docusate 8 months ago. She briefly took senna in addition to the docusate but found that she sometimes had to go to the bathroom at inopportune times and felt that it caused additional cramping. She tried psyllium powder several years ago but hated the taste. She thought about MiraLAX, but her mother took that prior to a GI procedure and said that it caused diarrhea, so the patient is hesitant to try it with all her responsibilities.

■ PMH

Seasonal allergies
Headaches
Anxiety

■ PSH

None

■ FH

Lives alone. Her mother is alive with HTN and her father is alive with hypercholesterolemia. No siblings.

■ SH

No alcohol use or smoking. No travel outside the United States.

■ Meds

Diphenhydramine 25 mg orally Q 6 H for allergy symptoms
Ibuprofen 200 mg, two tablets orally Q 4–6 H PRN headaches, menstrual cramps
Metamucil 0.52 g, four capsules orally three times a day
Docusate 100 mg orally twice daily

■ All

NKDA

■ ROS

Occasional headaches, usually associated with stress or allergy symptoms; occasional nausea, no vomiting; (−) blood in the stool or tarry stools; (+) flatulence and bloating. States that the abdominal symptoms may improve at night before bedtime especially if she uses a heating pad; she is not awakened at night with abdominal pain.

■ Physical Examination

Gen

A&O, WDWN woman appearing slightly anxious

VS

BP 116/78, P 68, RR 18, T 37.0°C; Wt 134 lb (61 kg), Ht 5′6″ (168 cm)

Skin

Dry skin on lower extremities, no rashes noted

HEENT

PERRLA, EOMI, moist mucus membranes, TMs intact

Neck/Lymph Nodes

No thyromegaly, lymphadenopathy, or JVD

Lungs

CTA; no rales or rhonchi

Breasts

Symmetric; no lumps or masses detected; nipples without discharge

CV

RRR, normal S_1 and S_2; no S_3 or S_4

Abd

(+) BS, slightly tender in LLQ, no HSM

Genit/Rect

Vulva normal; no palpable rectal masses; brown stool with no occult blood; no hemorrhoids

MS/Ext

No CCE, pulses 2+, normal ROM, normal strength bilaterally

■ Labs

Na 142 mEq/L	WBC $5.2 \times 10^3/mm^3$
K 4.0 mEq/L	Hgb 14.1 g/dL
Cl 106 mEq/L	Hct 42.4%
CO_2 27 mEq/L	Platelets $210 \times 10^3/\mu L$
BUN 9 mg/dL	
SCr 0.8 mg/dL	
Glu 88 mg/dL	

Serum pregnancy test: negative

■ Assessment

IBS associated with abdominal discomfort, bloating, and constipation

QUESTIONS

Collect Information

1.a. What subjective and objective information indicates the presence of irritable bowel syndrome (IBS) or other problems associated with IBS?

1.b. What additional information is needed to fully assess this patient's IBS?

Assess the Information

2.a. Classify this patient's IBS based on the subjective and objective information available.

2.b. Create a list of the patient's drug therapy problems and prioritize them. Include assessment of medication appropriateness, effectiveness, safety, and patient adherence.

Develop a Care Plan

3.a. What are the goals of pharmacotherapy for IBS in this case?

3.b. What nondrug therapies might be useful for this patient's IBS?

3.c. What feasible pharmacotherapeutic alternatives are available for treating IBS?

3.d. Create an individualized, patient-centered, team-based care plan to optimize medication therapy for the IBS and other drug-related problems. Include specific drugs, dosage forms, doses, schedules, and durations of therapy.

3.e. What alternatives would be appropriate if the initial care plan fails or cannot be used?

Implement the Care Plan

4.a. What information should be provided to the patient to enhance adherence, ensure successful therapy, and minimize adverse effects?

4.b. Describe how care should be coordinated with other healthcare providers.

Follow-Up: Monitor and Evaluate

5. Explain how to monitor and evaluate the care plan for medication appropriateness, effectiveness, safety, and patient adherence by using clinical and laboratory data, patient feedback, and other information.

■ CLINICAL COURSE

The patient returns to the physician 8 weeks later and reports that her symptoms are much improved and that the abdominal pain has resolved. She is happy with her medication regimen, but her friends have suggested that herbal medications may be just as effective. She would like more information about the use of these products for IBS. She also mentions that a friend was recently diagnosed with IBS-D and she wants to know if her friend's treatment will be similar.

■ FOLLOW-UP QUESTIONS

1. What information would you provide regarding the addition or substitution of alternative medications (eg, herbal medications) to this patient's regimen?

2. What therapeutic alternatives are available for the treatment of IBS-D?

■ SELF-STUDY ASSIGNMENTS

1. Conduct a literature search to determine what types of alternative therapies, including probiotics, have been evaluated in IBS. Include a discussion of the scientific rigor of these studies.

2. Conduct an informal survey among friends, family members, coworkers, and fellow students about the incidence of IBS and what therapeutic options they would recommend to a person suffering from IBS.

3. Conduct a search of IBS drug treatment studies on www .clinicaltrials.gov and conduct a literature search to identify new and emerging therapies for IBS. Determine the commercial availability of these agents or potential research trial referral centers.

4. Discuss the hypothesized pathogenesis of IBS including the disorder of the brain–gut axis, disturbed motility, impaired gut barrier function, visceral hypersensitivity, immunologic and infectious causation, genetic factors, psychosocial factors, and dietary alterations.

CLINICAL PEARL

There are many medications that may cause constipation and negatively impact a patient with IBS-C including aluminum-containing antacids, iron, opioids, antihistamines with anticholinergic properties (eg, diphenhydramine and chlorpheniramine), anticholinergics (eg, benztropine), TCAs (eg, amitriptyline), anticonvulsants (eg, carbamazepine), antidiarrheals, antihypertensive agents (eg, clonidine and thiazide diuretics), calcium channel blockers (eg, verapamil), anti-Parkinson agents, psychotherapeutic agents, and vinca alkaloids (eg, vincristine).

REFERENCES

1. Ford AC, Moayyedi P, Chey WD, et al; ACG Task Force on Management of Irritable Bowel Syndrome. American College of Gastroenterology Monograph on the Management of Irritable Bowel Syndrome. Am J Gastroenterol. 2018;113:1–18.

2. Sultan S, Malhotra A. Irritable bowel syndrome. Ann Intern Med. 2017;166:ITC81–ITC96. doi: 10.7326/AITC201706060.

3. Lacy BE, Pimentel M, Brenner DM, et al. ACG clinical guideline: management of irritable bowel syndrome. Am J Gastroenterol. 2021;116:17–44.

4. National Institute for Health and Care Excellence (2008, updated 2017) irritable bowel syndrome in adults: diagnosis and management. (NICE Guideline CG61) Available at: *https://www.nice.org.uk/guidance/cg61*. Accessed November 14, 2021.

5. Chang L, Sultan S, Lembo A, et al. American Gastroenterological Association Institute clinical practice guideline on the pharmacological management of irritable bowel syndrome with constipation. Gastroenterology. 2022;163:118–136.

6. Chey WD, Lembo AJ, Yang Y, Rosenbaum DP. Efficacy of tenapanor in treating patients with irritable bowel syndrome with constipation: A 12-Week, Placebo-Controlled Phase 3 Trial (T3MPO-1). Am J Gastroenterol. 2020;115:281–293

7. Chey WD, Lembo AJ, Yang Y, Rosenbaum DP. Efficacy of tenapanor in treating patients with irritable bowel syndrome with constipation: A 26-Week, Placebo-Controlled Phase 3 Trial (T3MPO-2). Am J Gastroenterol. 2021;116:1294–1303.

8. Kulak-Bejda A, Bejda G, Waszkiewicz N. Antidepressants for irritable bowel syndrome: a systematic review. Pharmacol Rep. 2017;69:1366–1379.

9. Siah KTH, Wong RKM, Ho KY. Melatonin for the treatment of irritable bowel syndrome. World J Gastroenterol. 2014 14;20(10):2492–2498.

10. Lembo A, Sultan S, Chang L, et al. American Gastroenterological Association Institute clinical practice guideline on the pharmacological management of irritable bowel syndrome with diarrhea. Gastroenterology. 2022;163:137–151.

44

PEDIATRIC GASTROENTERITIS

One Thing You Should Try at Home . . . . Level II

Carol Vetterly, Pharm D, BCPPS

Laura M. Panko, MD, FAAP

William McGhee, Pharm D

LEARNING OBJECTIVES

After completing this case study, the reader should be able to:

- Recognize the signs and symptoms of acute viral gastroenteritis with dehydration and accurately assess the severity of the problem.

- Describe the available rotavirus vaccines in the United States, contrast their dosing regimens and product availability, compare their safety and efficacy with the previously available RotaShield® vaccine, and explain their worldwide impact on rotavirus-induced diarrhea.

- Recommend appropriate oral rehydration therapy (ORT) products and treatment regimens for varying degrees of dehydration severity and assess the effectiveness of ORT using clinical parameters.

- Outline education for parents about the limited usefulness of all antidiarrheal products and the role of ondansetron and probiotics in the treatment of acute diarrhea in children.

- Identify the signs and symptoms of severe dehydration that require referral to an ED for immediate IV volume replacement.

PATIENT PRESENTATION

■ Chief Complaint

A 9-month-old girl presents to the Emergency Department (ED) with a 3-day history of fever, vomiting, and diarrhea. Her mother states, "I am worried that she is dehydrated."

HPI

The patient is an otherwise healthy child, last evaluated by her primary care provider at a scheduled well-child appointment 2 weeks prior to her current presentation. No concerns were identified during the appointment. Three days prior to her current ED visit, she developed a tactile fever, confirmed at 100.4°F (38.0°C) rectally, and seemed more tired than usual. Two days before presentation, she awoke from sleep due to an episode of nonbloody, nonbilious emesis. Throughout that day, she had five more episodes of vomiting after attempts at oral intake. She continued to have fatigue and low-grade fevers.

One day prior to presentation to the ED, she had only two episodes of emesis but developed diarrhea. The stools were initially described as slightly formed, but as the day progressed, the stools became watery and voluminous. Her mother estimates that she had five to eight episodes of diarrhea. Her appetite continued to be poor, with refusal of solid foods. On her primary care provider's recommendation, her parents offered her liquids including infant formula and a commercial oral electrolyte solution (ORS) which she refused to drink, instead preferring to drink sips of water and apple juice.

On the morning of presentation to the ED, the patient had another large, watery stool and was more fussy than usual. Her diaper was dry, with no urine output since the night prior to presentation. The family could not accurately assess the number of wet diapers she had in the last 24 hours due to her stooling frequency and consistency. Today, they also noted that her lips appeared dry, and she was not producing tears when crying.

On further history, no sick contacts at home were noted until the day the patient presented to the ED, when her mother developed abdominal discomfort and loose stools. In addition, multiple infants at the daycare the patient attends are experiencing similar symptoms. Her diet normally consists of 24–32 oz of cow's milk-based infant formula per day and a wide variety of solid foods. There has been no exposure to undercooked chicken, beef, or fish. The patient has not had any antibiotic exposure in the past few months.

PMH

The patient was born at 38 weeks via spontaneous vaginal delivery without complications. Her birth weight was 7 lb 10 oz. She required 1 day of phototherapy for hyperbilirubinemia. She was discharged from the newborn nursery on day three of life. She has had monthly viral upper respiratory tract infections and two episodes of otitis media since starting daycare at 3 months of age.

She has no prior hospitalizations or ED visits for illness. Immunizations are up-to-date through her 6 month vaccinations. Development is normal. She is cruising on furniture, speaks three words, and can drink from a training cup.

FH

The patient's mother has a history of mild intermittent asthma. Her father is healthy. She has two older siblings (6 years and 3 years of age), who have no chronic medical conditions.

SH

The patient lives with her parents and two siblings. There are two pet fish in the home but no reptiles or other animal exposures. The patient attends daycare 3 days per week. The family uses city water and has not traveled out of state recently.

Meds

Multivitamin. No prescriptions or over-the-counter medications.

All

NKDA, no food allergies

ROS

Negative for cough, congestion, drooling, noisy breathing, constipation, blood in the stool, abdominal pain, easy bruising, or bleeding. Positive for rash in diaper area and as otherwise noted in the HPI.

Physical Examination

Gen

Patient is ill but nontoxic appearing sitting in her mother's arms quietly. She is very fussy during the examination though could be consoled by her mother.

VS

BP 92/50, P 145, RR 32, T 38.4°C (R), Wt. 18 lb (8.2 kg; 50–75%), Ht 27 in (68 cm, 25%ile), OFC 17 in (43 cm; 50%ile). Wt. at recent well-child check 20 lb (9 kg).

Skin

Pink, no tenting noted, capillary refill 2–3 seconds

HEENT

Anterior fontanelle sunken, eyes moderately sunken, scant tears, nose with clear rhinorrhea, lips and tongue dry, TMs gray and translucent

Neck/Lymph Nodes

Supple, no lymphadenopathy

Lungs/Thorax

Clear, equal breath sounds bilaterally, no increased work of breathing, no wheezes, rales, rhonchi, retractions, or grunting

CV

Tachycardia, 1/6 flow murmur heard in the mid-left sternal border, 2+ radial and femoral pulses bilaterally

Abd

Mildly distended, hyperactive bowel sounds, soft, nontender, no masses or hepatosplenomegaly

Genit/Rect

Normal female genitalia, mild perianal erythema

MS/Ext

Normal muscle bulk, full range of motion of extremities, no peripheral edema

Neuro

Sleepy but arousable, fussy when awake, cranial nerves grossly intact bilaterally, normal strength and tone for age, no focal deficits

Labs

Na 137 mEq/L	Hgb 12.8 g/dL	WBC $14.0 \times 10^3/mm^3$
K 4.4 mEq/L	Hct 41%	Polys 52%
Cl 113 mEq/L	Plt $300 \times 10^3/mm^3$	Bands 5%
CO_2 14 mEq/L		Eos 0%
BUN 23 mg/dL		Basos 3%
SCr 0.4 mg/dL		Lymphs 24%
Glu 80 mg/dL		Monos 16%

Urinalysis: Specific gravity 1.029, 2+ ketones, 1 WBC, 0 RBC, negative for protein

■ Assessment

1. Acute viral gastroenteritis
2. Dehydration with non-gap metabolic acidosis

QUESTIONS

Collect Information

1.a. What subjective and objective information indicates the presence of gastroenteritis and dehydration?

1.b. What additional information is needed to fully assess the patient's gastroenteritis and dehydration?

Assess the Information

2.a. Assess the severity of dehydration based on the subjective and objective information available.

2.b. Create a list of the patient's drug therapy problem(s) and prioritize them. Include assessment of medication appropriateness, effectiveness, safety, and patient adherence.

2.c. What economic, psychosocial, cultural, racial, and ethical considerations are applicable to this case?

Develop a Care Plan

3.a. What are the goals of pharmacotherapy for gastroenteritis and dehydration in this case?

3.b. What nondrug therapies might be useful for this patient's gastroenteritis and dehydration?

3.c. What feasible pharmacotherapeutic alternatives are available for treating this patient's gastroenteritis and dehydration?

3.d. Create an individualized, patient-centered, team-based care plan to optimize medication therapy for this patient's gastroenteritis and dehydration and other drug therapy problems. Include specific drugs, dosage forms, doses, schedules, and durations of therapy.

3.e. What alternatives would be appropriate if the initial care plan fails or cannot be used?

Implement the Care Plan

4.a. What information should be provided to the patient to enhance adherence, ensure successful therapy, and minimize adverse effects?

4.b. Describe how care should be coordinated with other healthcare providers.

Follow-Up: Monitor and Evaluate

5. Explain how to monitor and evaluate the care plan for medication appropriateness, effectiveness, safety, and patient adherence by using clinical and laboratory data, patient feedback, and other information.

■ CLINICAL COURSE

A few months later, the patient returns to her pediatrician for a 1-year well-child visit. Her mother inquires about vaccines to possibly prevent the illness that required the emergency department visit. She asks why the rotavirus vaccine did not prevent her child's diarrheal illness.

■ FOLLOW-UP QUESTIONS

1. Describe the vaccine products available in the United States, including safety and efficacy against rotavirus and the potential for resistance.

2. What information should be provided to the patient's caregiver to explain why the patient experienced acute gastroenteritis despite being fully vaccinated with rotavirus vaccine?

■ SELF-STUDY ASSIGNMENTS

1. Explain the limitations of using probiotics for treating pediatric gastroenteritis, including lack of FDA oversight, purity and standardization of products, lack of recognized treatment regimens, and safety concerns. Write a brief educational document explaining to parents when the use of probiotics should be considered in acute viral gastroenteritis.

2. What role does zinc supplementation have in the treatment of diarrhea in developing countries? Describe the rationale for its use and the most efficient way to administer it.

3. What barriers exist to the widespread implementation of ORT by parents and medical providers? How can these barriers be overcome? (*Hint:* Explore the advantages of ORT vs IV rehydration therapy, including ease of care at home vs hospitalization, insurance issues, and physician reluctance.)

4. Describe the role of the community-based practitioner in the care of patients with pediatric gastroenteritis and dehydration. How would you monitor patient safety and outcome and what you would tell the parents to optimize treatment at home?

CLINICAL PEARL

ORT is the standard of care in the treatment of children with gastroenteritis with mild to moderate dehydration and usually is successful when administered at home. Liquids, including water as well as full-strength juice and soda, are inadequate oral rehydration solutions (ORSs) and have the potential to contribute to diarrhea and the development of electrolyte disturbances. Children with mild symptoms and minimal dehydration may have less treatment failures when diluted apple juice followed by their preferred fluid is used as an alternative to oral electrolytes solution.

REFERENCES

1. Goldman R, Freidman J, Parkin P. Validation of the clinical dehydration scale for children with acute gastroenteritis. Pediatrics. 2008;122:545–549.

2. Freedman S, Willan A, Boutis K, et al. Effect of dilute apple juice and preferred fluids vs electrolyte maintenance solutions on treatment failure among children with mild gastroenteritis. A randomized clinical trial. JAMA. 2016. 315 918: 1966–1974.

3. Florez ID, Nino-Serma LF, Beltran-Arroyave CP. Acute Infectious Diarrhea and Gastroenteritis in Children. Current Infectious Disease Report. 2020; 22 (4). doi: 10.1007/s11908-020-0713-6.

4. Allen SJ, Martinez EG, Gregorio GV, et al. Probiotics for treating acute infectious diarrhoea. Cochrane Database Syst Rev. 2010 Nov 10; 2010(11).

5. Guarino A, Ashkenazi S, Gendrel D, Lo Vecchio A, Shamir R, Szajewska H. European Society for Pediatric Gastroenterology, Hepatology, and Nutrition/European Society for Pediatric Infectious Diseases evidence-based guidelines for the management of acute gastroenteritis in children in Europe: Update. 2014. J Pediatr Gastroenterol Nutr. 2014;59:132–152.

6. Schnadower D, Tarr P, Casper T, Gorelick M, Dean J, O'Connell K, et al. *Lactobacillus rhamnosus* GG versus placebo for acute gastroenteritis in children. N Engl J Med. 2018;379:2015–2016.

7. Freedman S, Hall M, Shah S, et al. Impact of increasing ondansetron use on clinical outcomes in children with gastroenteritis. JAMA Pediatr. 2014;168:321–329.

8. Nunez J, Liu D, Nager A. Dehydration treatment practices among pediatrics-trained and non-pediatrics trained emergency physicians. Pediatric Emergency Care. 2012;28:322–328.

9. Troeger C, Khalil I, Rao P, et al. Rotavirus vaccination and the global burden of rotavirus diarrhea among children younger than 5 years. JAMA Pediatr. 2018;172:958–965. doi: 10.1001/jamapediatrics.2018.1960.

10. American Academy of Pediatrics. Rotavirus infections. In: Kimberlin DW, Brady MT, Jackson MA, Long SS, eds. Red Book: 2018 Report of the Committee on Infectious Diseases. 31st ed. Itasca, IL: American Academy of Pediatrics; 2018:700–704.

45

ASCITES MANAGEMENT IN PORTAL HYPERTENSION AND CIRRHOSIS

Back to Drinking . . . . Level II

Laurel A. Sampognaro, PharmD

Jeffery D. Evans, PharmD

LEARNING OBJECTIVES

After completing this case study, the reader should be able to:

- Identify signs and symptoms of cirrhosis and associated complications.

- Provide pharmacotherapeutic and lifestyle recommendations for managing ascites due to portal hypertension and cirrhosis.

- Develop a patient-specific regimen and monitoring parameters to meet the needs of a patient with ascites, esophageal varices, and hepatic encephalopathy.

- Interpret laboratory values associated with ascites.

- Provide appropriate patient education for the recommended pharmacologic and nonpharmacologic therapy to control complications of cirrhosis, as well as to prevent further complications.

PATIENT PRESENTATION

■ Chief Complaint

"I look like I'm pregnant and it's getting worse."

■ HPI

A 38-year-old man with a history of alcoholic cirrhosis is admitted to the hospital due to an unexplained 8-kg weight gain over the past 6 days, abdominal swelling and pain, shortness of breath, and mild confusion.

■ PMH

Alcoholic cirrhosis diagnosed 2 years ago, Child–Pugh grade A on diagnosis.
Alcohol Use Disorder × 15 years.
EGD performed at time of cirrhosis diagnosis showed no esophageal varices.
Hypertension.

■ FH

Father is alive and well at the age of 70 without significant disease. Mother died at age 47 due to complications of type 1 DM.

■ SH

Recently separated from wife of 10 years and lives alone. Works as a plumber. History of alcohol use disorder but had quit drinking on cirrhosis diagnosis. Admits to heavy alcohol use over the past 2 months since separating from his wife and went on a drinking binge about 1 week ago.

■ Meds

Lisinopril 10 mg once daily

■ All

NKDA

■ ROS

Abdominal discomfort described as occurring throughout the abdomen, shortness of breath, and mild confusion. Patient denies chills or fevers.

■ Physical Examination

Gen

Pleasant, chronically ill man appearing to be in mild distress and fatigued

VS

BP 118/76, P 78, RR 27, T 37.2°C; Wt 94.2 kg, Ht 6′2″

Skin

(+) Palmar erythema, (+) spider angiomata, otherwise normal color

HEENT

PERRL, EOMI, clear sclerae, TMs normal, mucous membranes moist

Neck/Lymph Nodes

Supple, no thyroid nodules

Lung/Thorax

Mild bilateral crackles, decreased breath sounds in right lower lobe likely due to enlarged liver and ascites

Breasts

Nontender without masses

CV

RRR, S_1 and S_2 are normal, no MRG

Abd

Bulging, tender abdomen; hepatomegaly; (+) fluid wave; bowel sounds normal

Genit/Rect

Guaiac negative

MS/Ext

1+ pitting edema in both LE, palmar erythema; no clubbing or cyanosis

Neuro

Mildly confused, forgetful, A&O × 2 (oriented to person and time but does not know at which hospital he is)

■ Labs

Na 135 mEq/L	Hgb 16 g/dL	AST 88 IU/L	Ca 8.5 mg/dL
K 4.1 mEq/L	Hct 47%	ALT 116 IU/L	Mg 1.9 mEq/L
Cl 98 mEq/L	Plt 81 × 10³/mm³	LDH 167 IU/L	Phos 3.5 mg/dL
CO₂ 30 mEq/L	WBC 6.2 × 10³/mm³	T. bili 2.2 mg/dL	TSH 3.6 mIU/L
BUN 19 mg/dL	PT 14.3 seconds	D. bili 0.7 mg/dL	NH₃ 94 mcg/dL
SCr 0.7 mg/dL	PTT 47 seconds	T. prot 7.3 g/dL	HIV (−)
Glu 97 mg/dL	INR 1.33	Alb 2.8 g/dL	

■ Paracentesis

Five liters of fluid removed by paracentesis with an analysis of the fluid performed. The analysis reported a protein level of 1.4 g/dL, PMN 140 cells/mm³, and SAAG 1.4 g/dL. Fluid was sent for culture.

■ EGD

Once stabilized, an EGD was performed, which showed small esophageal varices.

■ Assessment

Worsening cirrhosis; now presenting with ascites and acute encephalopathy

R/O spontaneous bacterial peritonitis (SBP)

QUESTIONS

Collect Information

1.a. What subjective and objective information indicates the presence of ascites and cirrhosis?

1.b. What additional information is needed to fully assess this patient's ascites and cirrhosis?

Assess the Information

2.a. Assess the severity of the ascites and cirrhosis based on the subjective and objective information available.

2.b. Create a list of the patient's drug therapy problems and prioritize them. Include assessment of medication appropriateness, effectiveness, safety, and patient adherence.

Develop a Care Plan

3.a. What are the goals of pharmacotherapy for ascites, portal hypertension, and cirrhosis in this case?

3.b. What nondrug therapies might be useful for this patient's ascites, portal hypertension, and cirrhosis?

3.c. What feasible pharmacotherapeutic alternatives are available for treating the ascites, portal hypertension, and cirrhosis?

3.d. Create an individualized, patient-centered, team-based care plan to optimize medication therapy for this patient's liver disease and other drug therapy problems. Include specific drugs, dosage forms, doses, schedules, and durations of therapy.

3.e. What alternatives would be appropriate if the initial care plan fails or cannot be used?

Implement the Care Plan

4.a. What information should be provided to the patient to enhance adherence, ensure successful therapy, and minimize adverse effects?

4.b. Describe how care should be coordinated with other healthcare providers.

Follow-Up: Monitor and Evaluate

5. Explain how to monitor and evaluate the care plan for medication appropriateness, effectiveness, safety, and patient adherence by using clinical and laboratory data, patient feedback, and other information.

■ CLINICAL COURSE

The culture results for the paracentesis fluid were negative after 3 days.

The patient's mental status began to improve after paracentesis and the administration of lactulose.

■ ADDITIONAL CASE QUESTION

1. What vaccinations should he receive on discharge if he has not had any vaccinations for over 20 years?

■ SELF-STUDY ASSIGNMENTS

1. Identify which pain medications may be used safely in patients with cirrhosis and ascites.

2. Based on this patient's history, what 1-, 2-, and 5-year survival rates would be expected if the patient does not receive a liver transplant?

CLINICAL PEARL

Lactulose is considered by many and mentioned in the guidelines as a first-line agent in the prevention of recurrent hepatic encephalopathy secondary to cirrhosis. However, there is a limited amount of data justifying its use in these patients.

REFERENCES

1. Biggins S, Angeli P, Garcia-Tsao G, et al. Diagnosis, evaluation, and management of ascites, spontaneous bacterial peritonitis and hepatorenal syndrome: 2021 practice guidance by the American Association for the Study of Liver Diseases. Hepatology. 2021;74:1014–1048.

2. Jafri S, Gordon S. Care of the cirrhotic patient. Infect Dis Clin N Am. 2012;26:979–994.

3. Vilstrup H, Amodio P, Bajaj J, et al. Hepatic encephalopathy in chronic liver disease: 2014 practice guideline by the American Association for the Study of Liver Diseases and the European Association for the Study of the Liver. Hepatology. 2014;60:715–735.

4. Garcia-Tsao G, Abraldes J, Berzigotti A, Bosch J. Portal hypertensive bleeding in cirrhosis: risk stratification, diagnosis, and management: 2016 practice guidance by the American Association for the Study of Liver Diseases. Hepatology. 2017;65:310–335.

5. Boregowda U, Umapathy C, Halim N, et al. Update on the management of gastrointestinal varices. World J Gastrointest Endosc. 2019;10(1):1–21.

6. Crabb D, Im G, Szabo G, Mellinger J, Lucey M. Diagnosis and treatment of alcohol-associated liver diseases: 2019 practice guidance from the American Association for the Study of Liver Diseases. Hepatology. 2020;71:306–333.

7. Pedersen J, Bendtsen F, Moller, S. Management of cirrhotic ascites. Ther Adv Chronic Dis. 2015;6(3):124–137.

8. Bernardi M, Maggioli C, Zaccherini G. Human albumin in the management of complications of liver cirrhosis. Crit Care 2012;16(2):211–217.

9. Ge P, Runyon B. The changing role of beta-blocker therapy in patients with cirrhosis. J Hepatol. 2014;60:643–653.

46

ESOPHAGEAL VARICES

Banding the Bleeding. . . . . Level II

Vanessa T. Kline, PharmD, BCPS

Jonathan M. Kline, PharmD, BCPS, CDE

LEARNING OBJECTIVES

After completing this case study, the reader should be able to:

- List nonpharmacologic options for managing patients with bleeding esophageal varices.

- Recommend appropriate pharmacologic therapy for controlling bleeding esophageal varices and adjunctive therapy in the setting of acute variceal bleeding.

- Provide appropriate education for patients receiving therapy for portal hypertension.

PATIENT PRESENTATION

■ Chief Complaint

"I've been throwing up blood, enough to fill my bathroom sink!"

■ HPI

A 55-year-old woman presents to the ED complaining of vomiting blood and bright red blood per rectum. They were in their usual state of health, until shortly after taking a dose of lactulose when they began to feel sick and subsequently vomited a large amount of blood into the bathroom sink. They also report a 2-day history of BRBPR.

■ PMH

Cirrhosis secondary to alcohol use disorder
History of hepatic encephalopathy
Ascites with history of paracentesis
Peptic ulcer disease
Hypertension

■ FH

Father with CAD and CABG; no other history known

■ SH

The patient lives alone and has been able to function independently. Quit drinking 5 years ago. Previously drank 6 beers per weekday and 750 mL of liquor on weekends. Quit smoking 3 years ago (35 pack-year history).

■ Meds

Sucralfate 1 g PO BID
Omeprazole 20 mg PO BID
Bumetanide 1 mg PO BID
Spironolactone 50 mg PO once daily
Propranolol 40 mg PO BID (reports taking sporadically)
Lactulose 20 g PO Q6H (takes only when the patient feels it is needed)
Acetaminophen 650 mg Q6H PRN pain

■ All

NKDA

■ ROS

Negative except for complaints noted in HPI

■ Physical Examination

Gen

Appears older than stated age, lethargic

VS

BP 108/60, P 120, RR 14, T 37.8°C

Skin

Some spider angiomas on abdomen, thick skin, chronic venous stasis changes with lichenification

HEENT

PERRLA; icteric sclerae

Neck/Lymph Nodes

Neck supple; no masses

Lungs/Thorax

Clear to auscultation bilaterally

Breasts

No lumps or masses

CV

Tachycardia, RRR, no M/R/G

Abd

Obese, mildly distended, distant bowel sounds present, difficult to assess for hepatosplenomegaly; dull percussion noted

Rect

Frank blood

Ext

Bilateral 1+ pedal edema

Neuro

Sleepy, moves head occasionally; is arousable and oriented × 3; no asterixis

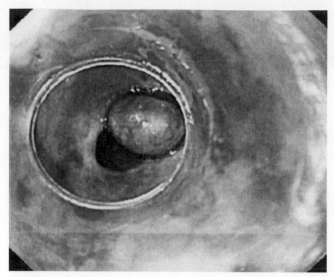

FIGURE 46-1. Endoscopic band ligation of esophageal varices. (Reprinted with permission from Jameson JL, Fauci AS, Kasper DL Hauser SL, Longo DL, Loscalzo J, eds. *Harrison's Principles of Internal Medicine.* 20th ed. New York, NY: McGraw-Hill Education, 2018.)

■ Labs (on Admission)

Na 127 mEq/L	Hgb 7.8 g/dL	AST 104 IU/L
K 4.3 mEq/L	Hct 24.4%	ALT 49 IU/L
Cl 101 mEq/L	WBC 9.2×10^3/mm³	Alk phos 114 IU/L
CO_2 22 mEq/L	Neutrophils 65%	T. bili 4.3 mg/dL
BUN 57 mg/dL	Bands 1%	D. bili 3.3 mg/dL
SCr 1.9 mg/dL	Lymphs 33%	Protein 5.5 g/dL
Glu 155 mg/dL	Monos 1%	Alb 2.5 g/dL
	Plt 68×10^3/mm³	Ca 8.4 mg/dL
	aPTT 42.1 seconds	Phos 4.4 mg/dL
	PT 16.5 seconds	Ammonia 117 mcg/dL
	INR 1.8	

■ EGD

There are several noted varices. One with a red wale sign indicative of recent hemorrhage and one actively bleeding. Two bands were applied. (Fig. 46-1).

■ Assessment

This is a 55-year-old woman with a history of alcoholic cirrhosis who presents with hematemesis secondary to bleeding esophageal varices. Labs show severe anemia, hyponatremia, renal dysfunction, hepatic encephalopathy, hypoalbuminemia, increased serum aminotransferases, and coagulopathy. The patient presents with Child–Pugh class C severity of disease. Will admit to an intensive care unit for further management.

QUESTIONS

Collect Information

1.a. What subjective and objective information indicates the presence of acute cirrhosis complications including bleeding esophageal varices?

1.b. What additional information is needed to fully assess the patient's acute cirrhosis complications including bleeding esophageal varices?

Assess the Information

2.a. Assess the severity of esophageal variceal bleeding based on the subjective and objective information available.

2.b. Create a list of the patient's drug therapy problems and prioritize them. Include assessment of medication appropriateness, effectiveness, safety, and patient adherence.

Develop a Care Plan

3.a. What are the goals of pharmacotherapy for esophageal varices and other complications of cirrhosis in this case?

3.b. What nondrug therapies might be useful for this patient's esophageal varices and other complications of cirrhosis?

3.c. What feasible pharmacotherapeutic alternatives are available for treating the esophageal varices and other complications of cirrhosis?

3.d. Create an individualized, patient-centered, team-based care plan to optimize medication therapy for this patient's esophageal varices and other drug therapy problems. Include specific drugs, dosage forms, doses, schedules, and durations of therapy.

3.e. What alternatives would be appropriate if the initial care plan fails or cannot be used?

Implement the Care Plan

4.a. What information should be provided to the patient to enhance adherence, ensure successful therapy, and minimize adverse effects?

4.b. Describe how care should be coordinated with other healthcare providers.

Follow-Up: Monitor and Evaluate

5. Explain how to monitor and evaluate the care plan for medication appropriateness, effectiveness, safety, and patient adherence by using clinical and laboratory data, patient feedback, and other information.

■ SELF-STUDY ASSIGNMENTS

1. Examine the relative effectiveness of nonpharmacologic therapies versus available pharmacologic treatments for the acute management of variceal bleeding.

2. Describe the effect of fluoroquinolone resistance on use of antibiotics in patients presenting with variceal hemorrhage.

3. Describe the dose-related side effects in patients receiving combination of β-blocker and isosorbide mononitrate therapy.

CLINICAL PEARL

While medication dosing and adjustments in hepatic disease are usually based on the Child–Pugh score, mortality prediction and assessment for hepatic transplantation are done using the Model of End-Stage Liver Disease (MELD) scoring system.

REFERENCES

1. United States Department of Health and Human Services. MELD Calculator—OPTN. Available at: *https://optn.transplant.hrsa.gov/resources/allocation-calculators/meld-calculator/*. Accessed November 7, 2021.

2. Garcia-Tsao G, Abraldes JG, Berzigotti A, Bosch J. Portal hypertensive bleeding in cirrhosis: risk stratification, diagnosis, and management: 2016 practice guidance by the American Association for the Study of Liver Diseases. Hepatology. 2017;65:310–335.

3. Seo YS, Park SY, Kim MY, et al. Lack of difference among terlipressin, somatostatin, and octreotide in the control of acute gastroesophageal variceal hemorrhage. Hepatology. 2014;60:954–963.

4. Satapathy SK, Sanyal AJ. Nonendoscopic management strategies for acute esophagogastric variceal bleeding. Gastroenterol Clin N Am. 2014;43:819–833.

5. Marti-Carvajal AJ, Karakitsiou DE, Salanti G. Human recombinant activated factor VII for upper gastrointestinal bleeding in patients with liver diseases. Cochrane Database Syst Rev. 2012;3:CD004887.

6. Lo GH, Perng DS, Chang CY, Tai CM, Wang HM, Lin HC. A controlled trial of ligation plus vasoconstrictor versus proton pump inhibitor in the control of acute esophageal variceal bleeding. J Gastroenterol Hepatol. 2013;28:684–689.

7. Lo EAG, Wilby KJ, Ensom MHH. Use of proton pump inhibitors in the management of gastroesophageal varices: a systematic review. Ann Pharmacother. 2015;49(2):207–219.

8. Albillos A, Tejedor M. Secondary prophylaxis for esophageal variceal bleeding. Clin Liver Dis. 2014;18(2):359–370.

47

HEPATIC ENCEPHALOPATHY

State of Confusion..............................Level I

Jeffrey T. Wieczorkiewicz, PharmD, BCPS

Carrie A. Sincak, PharmD, BCPS, FASHP

LEARNING OBJECTIVES

After completing this case study, the reader should be able to:

- Identify and correct the precipitating factors associated with the development of hepatic encephalopathy (HE) in a cirrhotic patient.

- Recommend appropriate nonpharmacologic and pharmacologic intervention for a cirrhotic patient who develops HE.

- Design a plan for monitoring the efficacy and adverse effects of recommended treatments for HE.

- Provide patient education for those receiving treatment for HE.

PATIENT PRESENTATION

■ Chief Complaint (from Son)

"My mother says she is dizzy and has felt a little off over the last couple of days."

■ HPI

A 65-year-old woman was brought to the ED by her son because of dizziness and confusion. The patient became increasingly confused over the past 2 days and on admission was alert to person only. The son states she is normally able to converse without difficulty but does require some assistance with ambulation. Over the past 2 days, she has had increasing difficulty with answering questions in conversations. He mentioned that his mother had forgotten to refill her prescription for lactulose when she ran out 1 week ago. His mother

had a scheduled endoscopy 2 days ago and did not take any of her medications the day prior to and the day of the test. She had also told her family that she had "retained a lot of water" and was feeling bad.

■ PMH

ESLD secondary to NASH cirrhosis diagnosed 5 years ago; complicated by ascites

Grade 2 esophageal varices

Hypothyroidism

Colon cancer s/p resection (15 years ago)

■ FH

Not obtainable at this time

■ SH

Retired; lives with her husband; they have one son and two daughters

No history of alcohol use

■ Meds

Folic acid 1 mg PO daily

Furosemide 40 mg PO daily

Lactulose 10 g/15 mL, one tablespoonful PO TID

Levothyroxine 100 mcg PO daily

Multivitamin one tablet PO daily

Pantoprazole 40 mg PO daily

Rifaximin 550 mg PO BID

Thiamine 100 mg PO daily

■ All

No known allergies

■ ROS

Confusion with no loss of consciousness reported. Abdominal pain reported. No change in bowel habits, dysphagia, or odynophagia. Weight gain noted per son.

■ Physical Examination

Gen

Elderly woman in NAD who is disoriented to time and place

VS

BP 134/55, P 82, RR 20, T 36.7°C; Wt 174.7 lb (79.4 kg), Ht 5'0" (152.4 cm)

Skin

Normal skin turgor

HEENT

PERRLA; dry mucous membranes; TMs intact; EOMI; fundi benign; anicteric sclerae; no sinus tenderness

Neck/Lymph Nodes

No masses, thyromegaly or lymphadenopathy

Lungs

Chest symmetric; lungs CTA bilaterally; no wheezes or crackles

CV

S_1 and S_2 normal; RRR with no murmurs

Abd

Nontender; distended abdomen; no splenomegaly; liver edge not identifiable below the costal margin; hypoactive bowel sounds

Rect

Heme (−) stool; no masses

Ext

(+) LE edema; no clubbing or cyanosis

Neuro

Confused; oriented only to person; CNs II–XII intact; DTRs 2+; (+) asterixis

■ Labs

Na 138 mEq/L	Hgb 9.1 g/dL	WBC 6.4 ×	AST 68 IU/L
K 3.3 mEq/L	Hct 29%	$10^3/mm^3$	ALT 25 IU/L
Cl 102 mEq/L	MCV 95 μm³	PMNs 67%	Alk phos 127 IU/L
CO_2 24 mEq/L	MCHC 34 g/dL	Bands 3%	T. bili 1.1 mg/dL
BUN 14 mg/dL	Retic 1.1%	Eos 3%	D. bili 0.3 mg/dL
SCr 1.4 mg/dL	Plt 122 × 10³/mm³	Lymphs 25%	Alb 3.2 g/dL
Glu 118 mg/dL		Monos 2%	NH_3 84 mcg/dL
			Ca 9.1 mg/dL
			Mg 2.7 mg/dL
			Phos 3.3 mg/dL
			PT 14.8 seconds
			aPTT 39.2 seconds
			INR 1.4
			TSH 0.42 μIU/mL

■ Assessment

HE, type C, grade III, episodic, precipitated (by brief noncompliance with maintenance lactulose and rifaximin therapy)

QUESTIONS

Collect Information

1.a. What subjective and objective information indicates the presence of HE in this patient?

1.b. What additional information is needed to fully assess this patient's HE? (See Fig. 47-1.)

Assess the Information

2.a. Assess the severity of HE based on the subjective and objective information available and classify this patient's HE.

2.b. Create a list of the patient's drug therapy problems and prioritize them. Include assessment of medication appropriateness, effectiveness, safety, and patient adherence.

2.c. What precipitating factors could have potentially caused this patient's episode of HE?

Develop a Care Plan

3.a. What are the goals of pharmacotherapy for HE in this case?

3.b. Which nondrug therapies might be useful for this patient's HE?

3.c. What feasible pharmacotherapeutic alternatives are available for treating HE?

3.d. Create an individualized, patient-centered, team-based care plan to optimize medication therapy for HE and other drug therapy problems. Include specific drugs, dosage forms, doses, schedules, and durations of therapy.

Glasgow coma scale		
Eye opening	Spontaneous	4
	To verbal command	3
	To pain	2
	None	1
Verbal responsiveness	Oriented	5
	Confused	4
	Inappropriate words	3
	Incomprehensible sounds	2
	None	1
Motor response	Obeys	6
	Localizes	5
	Withdraws (pain)	4
	Flexion (pain)	3
	Extension (pain)	2
	None	1
	Total: _____	

FIGURE 47-1. Glasgow coma scale (GSC) is a clinical evaluation tool measuring the neurological severity of hepatic encephalopathy. The scale includes an assessment of three separate areas of response: eyes, verbal, and motor. The scores of the individual sections are then added together to reveal the overall severity score. The lowest score (3) indicates the highest level of severity, and the highest score (15) indicates the lowest level of severity. (Reproduced with permission from C.K.Stone, R L. Humphries, *Current Diagnosis & Treatment: Emergency Medicine*, 8th ed. McGraw-Hill Companies Inc, 2018.)

Implement the Care Plan

4.a. What information should be provided to the patient to enhance adherence, ensure successful therapy, and minimize adverse effects?

4.b. Describe how care should be coordinated with other healthcare providers.

Follow-Up: Monitor and Evaluate

5. Explain how to monitor and evaluate the care plan for medication appropriateness, effectiveness, safety, and patient adherence by using clinical and laboratory data, patient feedback, and other information.

■ CLINICAL COURSE

Two days after beginning treatment with the regimen you recommended, the patient is responding positively, and the dose has been titrated appropriately. The dizziness and confusion have subsided, and she is now oriented to time, place, and person with no asterixis detected. The plan is to discharge the patient home tomorrow.

■ SELF-STUDY ASSIGNMENTS

1. Perform a literature search to assess the efficacy and role of rifaximin in the treatment of HE.

2. List the potential advantages and disadvantages of using antibiotics for the treatment of HE.

3. Perform a literature search to determine if protein restriction is appropriate in patients with liver disease, particularly patients with cirrhosis.

CLINICAL PEARL

Medication noncompliance, sedative–hypnotics, other CNS depressants, and narcotics may precipitate HE. A careful medication history is important in patients presenting with the disorder to identify and eliminate reversible causes.

REFERENCES

1. Suraweera D, Sundaram V, Saab S. Evaluation and management of hepatic encephalopathy: current status and future directions. Gut Liver. 2016;10(4):509–519.

2. Weissenborn K. Hepatic encephalopathy: definition, clinical grading and diagnostic principles. Drugs. 2019;79(Suppl 1):S5–S9.

3. Vilstrup H, Amodio P, Bajaj J, et al. Hepatic encephalopathy in chronic liver disease: 2014 practice guideline by American Association for the study of liver diseases and the European Association for the study of the liver. Hepatology. 2014;60:715–735.

4. Kornerup L, Gluud LL, Vilstrup H, et al. Update on the therapeutic management of hepatic encephalopathy. Curr Gastroenterol Rep. 2018;20(5):21.

5. Sharma BC, Sharma P, Lunia MK, Srivastava S, Goyal R, Sarin SK. A randomized, double-blind, controlled trial comparing rifaximin plus lactulose with lactulose alone in treatment of overt hepatic encephalopathy. Am J Gastroenterol. 2013;108(9):1458–1463.

6. Kimer N, Krag A, Moller S, et al. Systematic review with meta-analysis: the effects of rifaximin in hepatic encephalopathy. Aliment Pharmacol Ther. 2014;40:123–132.

7. Mullen KD, Sanyal AJ, Bass NM. Rifaximin is safe and well tolerated for long-term maintenance of remission from overt hepatic encephalopathy. Clin Gastroenterol Hepatol. 2014;12(8):1390–1397.

8. Eltawil KM, Laryea M, Peltekian K, Molinari M. Rifaximin vs conventional oral therapy for hepatic encephalopathy: a meta-analysis. World J Gastroenterol. 2012;18:767–777.

9. Runyon B. Management of adult patients with ascites due to cirrhosis: update 2012. American Association for the study of liver diseases. Available at: https://www.aasld.org/sites/default/files/guideline_documents/adultascitesenhanced.pdf. Accessed November 30, 2021.

48

ACUTE PANCREATITIS

A Sod Story . . . . Level III

Paul M. Reynolds, PharmD, BCCCP

Sterling C. Torian, PharmD

Scott W. Mueller, PharmD, FCCM, FCCP, BCCCP

Robert MacLaren, BSc (Pharm), PharmD, MPH, FCCM, FCCP

LEARNING OBJECTIVES

After completing this case study, the reader should be able to:

- Determine the subjective and objective information (include medical history, signs, symptoms, and laboratory values) commonly associated with acute pancreatitis.

- Evaluate precipitating factors associated with acute pancreatitis.

- Describe the potential etiologies and systemic complications associated with acute pancreatitis.

- Recommend appropriate pharmacologic, nonpharmacologic therapies, and supportive care therapies for patients with acute pancreatitis.

- Given a patient with acute pancreatitis, determine therapeutic goals and a therapeutic plan with appropriate monitoring parameters to assist the healthcare team in realizing desired therapeutic outcomes in a patient with acute pancreatitis.

PATIENT PRESENTATION

■ Chief Complaint

"I've got a really bad pain in my stomach."

■ HPI

A 42-year-old man presents to the ED shortly after midnight because of intense midepigastric pain radiating to his back. He states that the pain started shortly after dinner the night before but has progressively worsened. The pain is unrelated to physical activity, and he began vomiting around midnight tonight.

■ PMH

Alcohol withdrawal seizures 5 months ago, which have not recurred. Hypertension, which is medically controlled.

■ FH

Father died at the age of 56 from an MVA; mother is 72 years old and has type 2 DM and "cholesterol issues," for which she is taking a "statin." One sister, also with "cholesterol issues," taking an unknown medication. The sister also has a remote history of pancreatitis.

■ SH

Divorced with three children. Employed as a groundskeeper at a golf course. Quit smoking 2 weeks ago, endorses a 40 pack-year history of smoking. He states that he used to consume 6–10 beers per day until 5 months ago when he had a withdrawal seizure. He now drinks only on weekends for a total of about 6 beers; he reports sharing a couple of pitchers with 2 friends last night with dinner. Drinks at least 2 cups of coffee each morning.

■ Meds

Hydrochlorothiazide 25 mg once daily for blood pressure
Doxycycline 100 mg twice daily for 10 days for "cellulitis" (day 7 of 7)
Ibuprofen 200 mg OTC several doses per day PRN sore back muscles

■ All

Amoxicillin/clavulanate makes his stomach upset

■ ROS

The patient states that he has been feeling well until last night. Back soreness from unloading pallets of heavy sod 1 week ago has resolved with occasional ibuprofen use. He just finished a course of antibiotics this morning for mild cellulitis that was limited to a 1- × 2-in area of the left lower tibia. He has vomited approximately 6 times since midnight. He has no complaints of diarrhea or blood in the stool or vomitus or knowledge of any prior history of uncontrolled blood sugars or cholesterol.

■ Physical Examination

Gen

The patient is restless and in moderate distress but otherwise is a well-appearing, well-nourished male who looks his stated age.

VS

BP 99/56, P 124, RR 30, T 38.9°C; Wt 89 kg, Ht 5′10″

Skin

Dry with poor skin turgor; location of previous cellulitis appears healed; nontender, (–) erythema, swelling, or warmth

HEENT

PERRLA; EOMI; oropharynx pink and clear; oral mucosa dry

Neck/Lymph Nodes

Supple; no bruits, lymphadenopathy, or thyromegaly

Lungs/Thorax

No external evidence of back injury; (–) spinal/CVA tenderness; normal range of motion; no abnormal breath sounds on auscultation

CV

Sinus tachycardia; no MRG

Abd

Moderately distended with active but diminished bowel sounds; (+) guarding; pain is elicited on light palpation of left upper and midepigastric region. No rebound tenderness, masses, or hepatosplenomegaly.

Rect

Normal sphincter tone; no BRBPR or masses; prostate normal size

MS/Ext

Extremities are warm and well perfused. Good pulses present in all extremities. No clubbing, palmar erythema, or spider angiomata. Cellulitis is no longer evident on lower extremity.

Neuro

A&O × 3; neuro exam benign; CN II–XII intact; strength is equal bilaterally in all extremities. Normal tone and reflexes. No asterixis.

■ Labs

Na 128 mEq/L	Hgb 17 g/dL	AST 342 IU/L	Ca 7.2 mg/dL
K 3.4 mEq/L	Hct 50%	ALT 166 IU/L	Mg 1.7 mEq/L
Cl 105 mEq/L	WBC 15.2 ×	Alk phos 285 IU/L	Phos 2.2 mg/dL
CO_2 18 mEq/L	$10^3/mm^3$	LDH 255 IU/L	Trig 782 mg/dL
BUN 35 mg/dL	Neutros 72%	T. bili 0.6 mg/dL	Repeat trig 1010 mg/dL
SCr 1.5 mg/dL	Bands 4%	Alb 3.2 g/dL	PT 12.8 seconds
Glu 375 mg/dL	Eos 1%	Prealb 25 mg/dL	INR 1.1
	Basos 1%	Amylase 1555 IU/L	aPTT 19.3 seconds
	Lymphs 20%	Lipase 2220 IU/L	
	Monos 2%		BAC 4 mg/dL

■ Other Tests

Negative for presence of serum ketones. Negative for presence of hemoglobin in stool. ASA, acetaminophen, toxic alcohols are negative on serum toxicology screen. Negative viral hepatitis titers and negative for HIV.

■ Arterial Blood Gases

pH 7.31, $PaCO_2$ 38 mm Hg, PaO_2 88 mm Hg, HCO_3^- 17 mEq/L, O_2 sat 98% in room air

■ UA

Color yellow; turbidity clear; SG 1.010; pH 7.2; glucose >1000 mg/dL; bilirubin (–); ketones (–); Hgb (–); protein (–); nitrite (–); crystals (–); casts (–); mucous (–); bacteria (–); urobilinogen: 0.25 EU/dL; WBC 0–5/hpf; RBC 0/hpf; epithelial cells: 0–10/hpf

■ Chest X-Ray

AP view of chest shows the heart to be normal in size. The lungs are clear without any infiltrates, masses, effusions, or atelectasis. No notable abnormalities.

■ Ultrasound

Abdominal: Nonspecific gas pattern; no dilated bowel. Questionable opacity/abnormality of common bile duct. Cannot rule out gallstone/obstruction.

Lower extremity: No signs of deep venous thrombosis.

■ ECG

Sinus tachycardia; rate 140 bpm. No changes from his last ECG (5 months ago), no evidence of myocardial ischemia.

■ Assessment

Acute pancreatitis precipitating hyperglycemia, hypocalcemia, and nonanion gap metabolic acidosis

R/O choledocholithiasis

QUESTIONS

Collect Information

1.a. What subjective and objective information indicates the presence of acute pancreatitis?

1.b. What additional information is needed to fully assess this patient's pancreatitis?

Assess the Information

2.a. Assess the severity of acute pancreatitis based on the subjective and objective information available. Utilize a pancreatitis severity scoring system to complete this assessment.

2.b. Create a list of the patient's drug therapy problems and prioritize them. Include assessment of medication appropriateness, effectiveness, safety, and patient adherence.

2.c. What other etiologies of acute pancreatitis should be considered in this patient?

Develop a Care Plan

3.a. What are the goals of pharmacotherapy for acute pancreatitis in this case?

3.b. What nondrug therapies might be useful for this patient's acute pancreatitis?

3.c. What feasible pharmacotherapeutic alternatives are available for treating acute pancreatitis and associated problems?

3.d. Create an individualized, patient-centered, team-based care plan to optimize medication therapy for this patient's acute pancreatitis and other drug therapy problems. Include specific drugs, dosage forms, doses, schedules, and durations of therapy.

3.e. What alternatives would be appropriate if the initial care plan fails or cannot be used?

Implement the Care Plan

4.a. What information should be provided to the patient to enhance adherence, ensure successful therapy, and minimize adverse effects?

4.b. Describe how care should be coordinated with other healthcare providers.

Follow-Up: Monitor and Evaluate

5. Explain how to monitor and evaluate the care plan for medication appropriateness, effectiveness, safety, and patient adherence by using clinical and laboratory data, patient feedback, and other information.

■ CLINICAL COURSE

A pain control plan is implemented. Partial parenteral nutrition (without lipids) is considered but ultimately withheld as plans are made to initiate enteral nutrition during the daytime (ie, in about 12 hours). After several days of improvement in the hospital, the patient develops a WBC count of $23.4 \times 10^3/mm^3$ with neutrophils 77%, bands 15%, eosinophils 1%, basophils 0%, lymphocytes 3%, and monocytes 4%. He has a temperature of 39.8°C and is noted to be orthostatic (BP 128/76 sitting, 98/60 standing) with a glucose of 480 mg/dL. He has also experienced several episodes of diarrhea and steatorrhea.

Because of these setbacks in the patient's progress, a contrast-enhanced CT scan is obtained. The results demonstrate peripancreatic and retroperitoneal edema. The pancreas itself appears relatively normal except for small nonenhancing areas around the neck of the pancreas, which are suggestive of necrosis.

■ FOLLOW-UP QUESTIONS

1. What potential etiologies might explain this patient's fever and relapsing acute pancreatitis?

2. What are the new treatment goals for this patient?

3. Given this new information, what therapeutic interventions should be considered for this patient?

4. How should these new therapies be monitored for efficacy and adverse effects?

5. When this patient is stable, what information should be provided to him to reduce the likelihood of recurrent pancreatitis?

■ SELF-STUDY ASSIGNMENTS

1. Describe the pathophysiology of autodigestion during acute pancreatitis.

2. Describe the controversies of early enteral nutrition, probiotics, prophylactic antibiotics, and octreotide for management of acute pancreatitis.

3. Summarize published information regarding opioid effects on the sphincter of Oddi.

4. Compose a list of drugs believed to aggravate or cause pancreatitis and assess the level of association for each agent.

CLINICAL PEARL

Empiric antimicrobial therapy is not recommended in patients presenting with acute pancreatitis as studies do not demonstrate beneficial outcomes, including survival or reduced subsequent infection. Unless the patient appears septic or is demonstrating other signs of active infection, antimicrobials should be withheld with the anticipation that symptoms will diminish as the acute pancreatitis resolves.

REFERENCES

1. Leppäniemi A, Tolonen M, Tarasconi A, et al. 2019 WSES guidelines for the management of severe acute pancreatitis. World J Emerg Surg. 2019;14:27.

2. Mederos MA, Reber HA, Girgis MD. Acute pancreatitis. JAMA. 2021;325:382–390.

3. Sinonquel P, Laleman W, Wilmer A. Advances in acute pancreatitis. Curr Opin Crit Care. 2021;27:193–200.

4. Boxhoorn L, Voermans RP, Bouwense SA, et al. Acute pancreatitis. Lancet. 2020;396:726–734.

5. Vege SS, DiMagno MJ, Forsmark CE, Martel M, Barkun AN. Initial medical treatment of acute pancreatitis: American Gastroenterological Association Institute technical review. Gastroenterology. 2018;154:1103–1139.

6. Crockett SD, Wani S, Gardner TB, et al. American Gastroenterological Association Institute guideline on initial management of acute pancreatitis. Gastroenterology. 2018;154:1096–1101.

7. Baron TH, DiMaio CJ, Wany AY, Morgan KA. American Gastroenterology Association clinical practice update: management of pancreatic necrosis. Gastroenterology. 2020;158:67–75.

8. Hines OJ, Pandol SJ. Management of severe acute pancreatitis. BMJ. 2019;367:16227.

9. Kanthasamy KA, Akshintala VS, Singh VK. Nutritional management of acute pancreatitis. Gastroenterol Clin N Am. 2021;50:141–150.

10. Arvanitakis M, Ockenga J, Bezmarevic M, et al. ESPEN guideline on clinical nutrition in acute and chronic pancreatitis. Clin Nutr. 2020;39:612–631.

49

CHRONIC PANCREATITIS

Like a Shot to the Gut . . . . Level II

Jaime L. Gray, PharmD, BCCCP, FCCM

Heather M. Teufel, PharmD, BCCCP

LEARNING OBJECTIVES

After completing this case study, the reader should be able to:

- Identify subjective and objective findings consistent with chronic pancreatitis and acute exacerbations of chronic pancreatitis.

- Evaluate patient-specific data and develop a problem list for patients with acute exacerbations of chronic pancreatitis.

- Discuss therapeutic alternatives and outline a patient-specific plan for pain management during an acute exacerbation of chronic pancreatitis.

- Recommend appropriate pancreatic enzyme replacement therapy for management of steatorrhea in a patient with chronic pancreatitis.

- Determine initial therapy for management of hypertriglyceridemia in a patient with chronic pancreatitis.

PATIENT PRESENTATION

■ Chief Complaint

"I have had pain in my stomach for years, but now I just can't take it anymore. It feels like a shot to the gut."

■ HPI

A 38-year-old woman presents to the ED complaining of stabbing pain in her abdomen with radiation to her back. She has also noticed an increase in loose, foul-smelling stools with an oil-like consistency. The patient has experienced intermittent pain in her abdomen for several years; and has also experienced chronic diarrhea with increased frequency in the 2 weeks. However, her symptoms have worsened following her birthday celebration this past weekend. Concurrent with the pain are nausea and vomiting, which have increased in intensity and frequency in the past week causing decreased oral intake. Patient reports recent unintentional weight loss of 5–10 lbs over the last couple of months. She presents to the ED today as she now has access to health insurance. She did not seek medical attention previously due to the financial implications of being uninsured.

■ PMH

There is no formal past medical history because the patient has not sought medical care since college due to being uninsured. Patient reports being told to watch her cholesterol in high school and recalls receiving the "usual" childhood vaccinations and medical care, but she has not seen a provider in over 10 years.

■ FH

Parents are alive and healthy. She is an only child.

■ SH

Daily alcohol use (reports drinking a couple glasses of wine nightly, with a recent report of heavy drinking last weekend at her birthday celebration).
(+) tobacco use (12 pack years; currently 0.5 pack/day).
Reports occasional marijuana use, but no other illicit drug use.
She is single and not sexually active.
She just started a new job in information technology and has completed a college-level education.

■ Meds

Multivitamin one tablet by mouth daily, has been taking for several years.
Acetaminophen 500–1000 mg by mouth Q 6 H PRN for abdominal pain; frequent daily use.
Loperamide two tablets initially, and then one tablet by mouth PRN diarrhea; she usually takes two to four tablets per day.
Calcium Carbonate 750 mg tablets, 1–2 tablets by mouth PRN nausea and indigestion.
No prescription medications.

■ All

Amoxicillin → rash when she received it as a child for an ear infection, no use since

■ ROS

Decreased oral intake due to nausea and vomiting. No current complaints of indigestion or bloating but does report intermittent feelings of a burning sensation in her throat. Significant abdominal pain and diarrhea as described above. No constipation or fecal incontinence; normal flatus. No blood in the stool. No hemorrhoids. Urine is of normal color, volume, and odor.

■ Physical Examination

Gen

Thin, ill-appearing female, appearing anxious

VS

BP 97/62, P 104, RR 18, T 37.8°C; Wt 115 lb (52 kg), Ht 5′5″ (165 cm), current pain 8 out of 10 on the numerical rating scale

Skin

Normal skin turgor

HEENT

PERRLA, EOMI, oropharynx clear, mucous membranes dry

Neck/Lymph Nodes

Supple; (−) JVD, thyromegaly, lymphadenopathy, or bruits

Lung/Thorax

Audible breath sounds in all lung fields; trachea at midline; normal rate, rhythm, and effort of breathing; (−) vertebral tenderness or deformity

CV

Regular rate and rhythm without gallops or murmur

Abd

Sparse bowel sounds, (+) rebound and guarding

Genit/Rect

No masses, guaiac (−), normal urine output

MS/Ext

Pulses intact bilaterally; good capillary refill; no cyanosis, clubbing, or edema

Neuro

A&O × 3, CN II–XII intact

■ Labs (non-fasting)

Na 140 mEq/L	Hgb 12 g/dL	WBC 8.2 ×	T. bili 1.5 mg/dL
K 4.2 mEq/L	Hct 37%	10³/mm³	Alk phos 140 IU/L
Cl 95 mEq/L	RBC 4.0 × 10⁶/mm³	Neutros 65%	Alb 4.4 g/dL
CO₂ 24 mEq/L	Plt 243 × 10³/mm³	Bands 5%	Prealb 20 mg/dL
BUN 16 mg/dL	MCV 98.2 μm³	Eos 0%	Lipase 203 IU/L
SCr 0.6 mg/dL	MCHC 35 g/dL	Lymphs 28%	Amylase 21 IU/L
Glu 145 mg/dL	LDL 124 mg/dL	Monos 2%	
EtOH level		HDL 27 mg/dL	TC 223 mg/dL
<10 mg/dL		TG 360 mg/dL	

■ CT Abdomen with IV Contrast

Changes consistent with chronic pancreatitis: inflammation of the common bile duct with calcifications seen within the pancreas. No evidence of necrosis or fluid collections (Fig. 49-1).

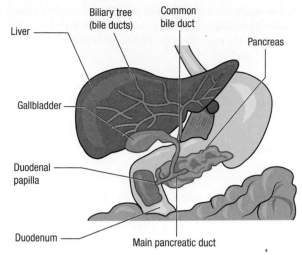

FIGURE 49-1. Anatomic structures depicting joining of common bile duct and the main pancreatic duct before emptying contents into the duodenum. (Source: National Institute of Diabetes and Digestive and Kidney Diseases. Available at: http://www.niddk.nih.gov/health-information/health-topics/diagnostic-tests/ercp/Pages/diagnostic-test.aspx.)

■ Assessment

1. Chronic pancreatitis, toxic metabolic etiology—with acute exacerbation.
2. Elevated triglycerides with other cholesterol numbers out of goal range.
3. Alcohol and smoking cessation education is needed.
4. Routine medical care needed.

QUESTIONS

Collect Information

1.a. What subjective and objective information indicates the presence of chronic pancreatitis?
1.b. What additional information is needed to fully assess this patient's chronic pancreatitis?

Assess the Information

2.a. Assess the severity of chronic pancreatitis based on the subjective and objective information available.
2.b. Create a list of the patient's drug therapy problems and prioritize them. Include assessment of medication appropriateness, effectiveness, safety, and patient adherence.

Develop a Care Plan

3.a. What are the goals of pharmacotherapy for chronic pancreatitis in this case?
3.b. What nondrug therapies might be useful for this patient's chronic pancreatitis?
3.c. What feasible pharmacotherapeutic alternatives are available for treating chronic pancreatitis?
3.d. Create an individualized, patient-centered, team-based care plan to optimize medication therapy for the chronic pancreatitis and other drug therapy problems. Include specific drugs, dosage forms, doses, schedules, and durations of therapy.

3.e. What alternatives would be appropriate if the initial care plan fails or cannot be used?

Implement a Care Plan

4.a. What information should be provided to the patient to enhance adherence, ensure successful therapy, and minimize adverse effects?
4.b. Describe how care should be coordinated with other healthcare providers.

Follow-Up: Monitor and Evaluate

5. Explain how to monitor and evaluate the care plan for medication appropriateness, effectiveness, safety, and patient adherence by using clinical and laboratory data, patient feedback, and other information.

■ ADDITIONAL CASE QUESTION

1. Describe how this patient should be screened for future complications of chronic pancreatitis.

■ SELF-STUDY ASSIGNMENTS

1. What other extrapancreatic diseases are associated with chronic pancreatitis?
2. What psychological factors will impact this patient's adherence to medical therapy or her willingness to seek further treatment given the patient's lack of medical care up to this point? How would this impact your ability to provide care for this patient?

CLINICAL PEARL

Patients with acute complications of chronic pancreatitis that have triglyceride levels >1000 mg/dL require prompt therapy to lower triglyceride levels to prevent necrotizing pancreatitis or other organ failure. Maintaining triglyceride levels within normal range (<150 mg/dL) by use of oral cholesterol medications such as fibrates, statins, or omega-3 fatty acids will help decrease risk of pancreatitis recurrence.

REFERENCES

1. Gardner TB, Adler DG, Forsmark CE, et al. ACG clinical guidelines: chronic pancreatitis. Am J Gastroenterol. 2020;115:322–339.
2. Lohr JM, Dominguez-Munoz E, Rosendahl J, et al. United European Gastroenterology evidence-based guidelines for the diagnosis and therapy of chronic pancreatitis (HaPANEU). United European Gastroenterol J. 2017;5:153–199.
3. Duggan S, O'Sullivan M, Feehan S, Ridgway P, Conlon K. Nutrition treatment of deficiency and malnutrition in chronic pancreatitis: a review. Nutr Clin Pract. 2010;24:362–370.
4. Drewes AM, Bouwense SAW, Campbell CM, et al. Guidelines for the understanding and management of pain in chronic pancreatitis. Pancreatology. 2017;17:720–731.
5. Motov S, Yasavolian M, Likourezos A, et al. Comparison of intravenous ketorolac at three single-dose regimens for treating acute pain in the emergency department: a randomized controlled trial. Ann Emerg Med. 2017;70:177–184.
6. Olesen SS, Bouwense SA, Wilder-Smith OH, van Goor H, Drewes AM. Pregabalin reduces pain in patients with chronic pancreatitis in a randomized, controlled trial. Gastroenterology. 2001;141:536–543.
7. Berry AJ. Pancreatic enzyme replacement therapy during pancreatic insufficiency. Nutr Clin Pract. 2014;29:312–321.

8. Singh VK, Drewes AM. Medical management of pain in chronic pancreatitis. Dig Dis Sci. 2017;62:1721–1728.

9. Talukdar R, Lakhtakia S, Reddy DN, et al. Ameliorating effect of antioxidants and pregabalin combination in pain recurrence after ductal clearance in chronic pancreatitis: results of a randomized, double blind, placebo-controlled trial. J Gastroenterol Hepatol. 2016;31:1654–1662.

10. Garg R, Rustagi T. Management of hypertriglyceridemia induced acute pancreatitis. Biomed Res Int. 2018;1–12.

50

VIRAL HEPATITIS A

My Shot . . . . Level I

Juliana Chan, PharmD, FCCP, BCACP

LEARNING OBJECTIVES

After completing this case study, the reader should be able to:

- Determine which patient populations are at greatest risk for contracting hepatitis A.

- Recommend hepatitis A immunization for appropriate individuals based on current guidelines of the Centers for Disease Control and Prevention (CDC).

- Assess the efficacy and adverse effects of hepatitis A vaccines.

- Outline the benefits of hepatitis A vaccination and the possible adverse effects associated with its use.

PATIENT PRESENTATION

■ Chief Complaint

"I was told to come for a free shot from my neighbors."

■ HPI

A 37-year-old man experiencing homelessness for the last 12 months and was referred by his neighbors to go to the clinic for a "free shot."

■ PMH

HTN
Asthma

■ Surgical History

Several surgeries after a motor vehicle accident that required blood transfusions in the early 90s.

■ FH

Mother with no medical complaints. Father is alive with alcoholic liver disease. One younger sister with DM and older brother with HTN.

■ SH

Divorced since he lost his job during the COVID pandemic in 2020; previously worked as a banker for the past decade. He smoked in his early 20s, one ppd then quit at age 26. He does not drink (or ever drank, due to family history of alcoholism). He had a tattoo placed professionally 2 years ago. There is no history of IV drug use, illicit drug use, or abuse of prescription drugs. Sex, unprotected with multiple partners.

■ Meds

Hydrochlorothiazide 25 mg PO once daily

■ All

Sulfa, ciprofloxacin

■ ROS

Denies weight loss/gain, fevers, chills, headaches, shortness of breath, and coughing. No black stools or obvious blood in stools.

■ Physical Examination

Gen

The patient is in no apparent distress.

VS

BP 126/78, P 72, RR 20, T 36.9°C; Wt 268 lb (121.8 kg), Ht 5'9" (175 cm)

Skin

Warm and dry. Spider angiomas are not present.

HEENT

PERRLA, EOMI; fundi normal; TMs clear. Head is normocephalic and atraumatic; sclerae anicteric.

Neck/Lymph Nodes

Supple; no masses or JVD

Chest

Clear without wheezes, rhonchi, or rales

CV

RRR, S_1, S_2 normal

Abd

(+) Bowel sounds, no masses, nontender, nondistended

Genit/Rect

Rectal exam deferred

MS/Ext

Normal range of motion throughout; no CCE

Neuro

A&O × 3; CN II–XII intact; no focal deficits, negative for asterixis

■ Labs (Nonfasting)

Na 144 mEq/L	Hgb 15.6 g/dL	AST 31 IU/L	HBsAg (−)
K 4.5 mEq/L	Hct 45%	ALT 63 IU/L	anti-HBs (−)
Cl 107 mEq/L	WBC 6.9 × 10³/mm³	Alk phos 67 IU/L	anti-HCV (−)
CO₂ 30 mEq/L	Plt 195 × 10³/mm³	T. bili 1 mg/dL	Total anti-
BUN 16 mg/dL	T. chol 199 mg/dL	PT 13.1 seconds	HAV (−)
SCr 1.2 mg/dL	Trig 219 mg/dL	Alb 4.5 g/dL	
Glu 119 mg/dL	LDL 113 mg/dL		
	HDL 42 mg/dL		

Assessment

This is a 37-year-old man experiencing homelessness with a history of HTN presenting for his hepatitis A virus (HAV) vaccination.

QUESTIONS

Collect Information

1.a. What subjective or objective information indicates the patient's hepatitis A status?

1.b. What additional information is needed to determine the patient's risk for liver disease?

Assess the Information

2.a. Assess for the presence or absence of liver disease based on the subjective and objective information available.

2.b. Create a list of the patient's drug therapy problems and prioritize them. Include assessment of medication appropriateness, effectiveness, safety, and patient adherence.

Develop a Care Plan

3.a. What are the goals of pharmacotherapy for prevention of HAV in this case?

3.b. What nondrug therapies might be useful for this patient's HAV?

3.c. What feasible pharmacotherapeutic alternatives are available for preventing hepatitis A infection?

3.d. Create an individualized, patient-centered, team-based care plan to optimize medication therapy for prevention of hepatitis A and this patient's other drug therapy problems. Include specific drugs, dosage forms, doses, schedules, and durations of therapy.

3.e. What alternatives would be appropriate if the initial care plan fails or cannot be used?

Implement the Care Plan

4.a. What information should be provided to the patient to enhance adherence, ensure successful therapy, and minimize adverse effects?

4.b. Describe how care should be coordinated with other healthcare providers.

Follow-Up: Monitor and Evaluate

5. Explain how to monitor and evaluate the care plan for medication appropriateness, effectiveness, safety, and patient adherence by using clinical and laboratory data, patient feedback, and other information.

■ CLINICAL COURSE

The patient returns to the outreach clinic 10 months later after receiving the recommended hepatitis vaccination dose. Patient states he feels well and had no complaints with the first dose of the vaccine.

■ FOLLOW-UP QUESTION

1. Based on the information provided, how should the vaccination series be completed?

■ STUDY ASSIGNMENTS

1. Compare and contrast the mechanism of action, immunogenicity rate, and adverse effects of the two commercially available hepatitis A vaccines.

2. Determine which vaccines can be given simultaneously with the hepatitis A vaccine.

3. Compare the cost of administering the Havrix and Engerix-B vaccines separately versus the combination product Twinrix for adults and in children.

CLINICAL PEARL

The hepatitis A vaccine is highly effective in preventing hepatitis A infections when given immediately prior to departing to endemic areas. According to the CDC, all children in the United States over 1 year of age should receive the hepatitis A vaccine.

REFERENCES

1. Nelson NP, Weng MK, Hofmeister MG, et al. Prevention of hepatitis A virus infection in the United States: Recommendations of the Advisory Committee on Immunization Practices, 2020. MMWR Recomm Rep. 2020 Jul 3;69(5):1–38. doi: 10.15585/mmwr.rr6905a1. PMID: 32614811.

2. Hepatitis B Questions and Answers for Health Professionals. Available at: https://www.cdc.gov/hepatitis/hbv/hbvfaq.htm#vaccFAQ. Accessed October 15, 2021.

3. Centers for Disease Control and Prevention. Viral Hepatitis Surveillance report, 2019. Available at: https://www.cdc.gov/hepatitis/statistics/2019surveillance/HepA.htm. Accessed October 15, 2021.

4. Hepatitis B. Immunization Action Coalition. Available at: https://www.immunize.org/askexperts/experts_hepb.asp. Accessed October 26, 2021.

51

VIRAL HEPATITIS B

It Runs in the Family . . . . Level II

Juliana Chan, PharmD, FCCP, BCACP

LEARNING OBJECTIVES

After completing this case study, the reader should be able to:

• Outline a pharmacologic and nonpharmacologic regimen for patients with chronic hepatitis B.

• Determine clinical and laboratory endpoints for treatment of chronic hepatitis B.

• Assess the efficacy and adverse effects of chronic hepatitis B treatment with pegylated interferon, entecavir, tenofovir disoproxil, and tenofovir alafenamide.

• Recommend hepatitis B immunization for appropriate individuals based on current guidelines of the Centers for Disease Control and Prevention (CDC).

• Provide patient education on pegylated interferon, entecavir, tenofovir disoproxil, and tenofovir alafenamide treatment.

PATIENT PRESENTATION

■ Chief Complaint

"I'm here for follow up on my hepatitis B."

■ HPI

The patient is a 36-year-old woman with chronic hepatitis B (CHB). She is here for her follow up clinic visit since she was diagnosed with HBV 12 weeks ago.

■ PMH

DM, lifestyle controlled
Chronic hepatitis B
Depression—uncontrolled

■ Surgical History

Tonsillectomy: age 10

■ FH

Mother alive, with HCC secondary to HBV. Father healthy. Older sister with osteopenia.

■ SH

Not in a relationship. Used marijuana at age 20 and tried cocaine once at age 21. She drinks alcohol socially with friends on the weekend. She works at home as an administrative assistant.

■ Meds

St John's wort 300mg daily

■ All

None

■ ROS

Denies any symptoms except for a depressed mood "all of the time" for which she has not seen a mental health provider. Her weight is stable with no loss of appetite. No nausea, vomiting, diarrhea, abdominal pain, or constipation. No melena or hematochezia. No changes in urine or stool color and no history of icteric sclerae.

■ Physical Examination

Gen

The patient is not in acute distress.

VS

BP 124/86, P 82, RR 20, T 37.7°C; Wt 148 lb (67.2 kg), Ht 5′1″ (155 cm)

Skin

Warm and dry; no signs of jaundice. Good turgor.

HEENT

Head is normocephalic, atraumatic. Sclerae are anicteric bilaterally. Neck is supple. No masses or palpable lymphadenopathy. PERRLA. Funduscopic exam normal.

Lungs

Clear to P&A

CV

RRR, S_1, S_2 normal; no S_3 or S_4

Abd

Good bowel sounds, soft, nontender; no evidence of ascites; no palpable hepatosplenomegaly

Rect

Guaiac negative

Ext

Normal range of motion throughout; no C/C/E, no gross lesions, ecchymosis, or peripheral edema

Neuro

CN II–XII intact; DTRs 2+ throughout; negative Babinski

■ Labs

Na 138 mEq/L	Hgb 12.4 g/dL	AST 57 IU/L	HBsAg (+)
K 3.8 mEq/L	Hct 37.3%	ALT 59 IU/L	Anti-HBs (−)
Cl 104 mEq/L	Plt 132 × 10³/mm³	Alk phos 82 IU/L	HBeAg (+)
CO_2 25 mEq/L	WBC 7.3 × 10³/mm³	T. bili 1.2 mg/dL	HBV DNA PCR
BUN 17 mg/dL	T. chol 152 mg/dL	T. prot 7.2 g/dL	Quant 6,641,
SCr 1.1 mg/dL	Trig 138 mg/dL	Alb 3.9 g/dL	119 IU/mL
Glu (nonfasting)		PT 10.3 s	Anti-HBc IgM (−)
93 mg/dL			Anti-HBc total (+)
			Anti-HAV, total (+)
			HBV genotype A

■ Other Tests

Ultrasound of the Abdomen

Findings: There is no ascites. The liver is normal in size with slightly coarsened parenchymal echogenicity without focal lesion. Mild splenomegaly, measuring up to 13 cm. The visualized portions of the abdominal aorta and IVC are unremarkable.

Impression: Coarsened liver echotexture suggestive of underlying liver disease. Mild splenomegaly with no ascites.

■ Assessment

The patient is a 36-year-old woman with chronic hepatitis B and a strong family history of liver cancer.

QUESTIONS

Collect Information

1.a. What subjective and objective information indicates the presence of chronic hepatitis B infection or demonstrates a risk factor for infection?

1.b. What additional information is needed to fully assess this patient's liver disease?

Assess the Information

2.a. Assess the severity of the hepatitis B infection based on the subjective and objective information available.

2.b. Create a list of the patient's drug therapy problems and prioritize them. Include assessment of medication appropriateness, effectiveness, safety, and patient adherence.

Develop a Care Plan

3.a. What are the goals of pharmacotherapy for hepatitis B infection in this case?

3.b. What nondrug therapies might be useful for this patient's hepatitis B infection?

3.c. What feasible pharmacotherapeutic alternatives are available for treating hepatitis B infection?

3.d. Create an individualized, patient-centered, team-based care plan to optimize medication therapy for this patient's hepatitis B infection and other drug therapy problems. Include specific drugs, dosage forms, doses, schedules, and durations of therapy.

Implement the Care Plan

4.a. What information should be provided to the patient to enhance adherence, ensure successful therapy, and minimize adverse effects?

4.b. Describe how care should be coordinated with other healthcare providers.

Follow-Up: Monitor and Evaluate

5. Explain how to monitor and evaluate the care plan for medication appropriateness, effectiveness, safety, and patient adherence by using clinical and laboratory data, patient feedback, and other information.

■ CLINICAL COURSE (PART 1)

The patient tolerated the initial therapy very well with minimal adverse effects. After a year of therapy, her serum HBV DNA is detectable. She also states she has been in a relationship and sexually active. Her lab results since starting HBV treatment are as follows:

Test	12 Weeks After Therapy Started	24 Weeks After Therapy Started	52 Weeks After Therapy Started	1 Year, 3 Months After Therapy Started
AST (IU/L)	51	25	21	35
ALT (IU/L)	56	28	18	33
Alk phos (IU/L)	76	80	83	73
T. bili (mg/dL)	1	1.1	1	0.8
PT (s)	11.2	11.2	10.7	10.1
Alb (g/dL)	3.6	3.5	3.6	3.5
HBsAg	(+)	(+)	(+)	(+)
Anti-HBs	(−)	(−)	(−)	(−)
HBeAg	(+)	(+)	Nonreactive	(+)
HBeAb	(−)	(+)	(+)	(−)
HBV DNA (IU/mL)	95,352	5,226	1,162	2,516

*<29 IU/mL indicates undetectable HBV DNA level.

■ FOLLOW-UP QUESTIONS

1. What laboratory parameters may suggest that a change in HBV therapy is warranted?

2. Based on this new information, develop a drug therapy plan for the patient's hepatitis B. Include specific drugs, dosage forms, doses, schedules, and durations of therapy.

3. What information do you need to provide to the patient, her new partner, and her sister?

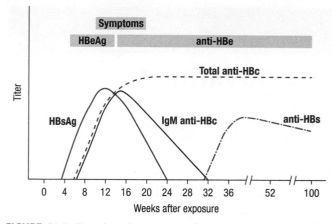

FIGURE 51-1. Typical serologic course of acute hepatitis B virus infection with recovery. *Note:* Serologic markers of infection vary depending on whether the infection is acute or chronic. (Source: Centers for Disease Control and Prevention. Viral Hepatitis Resource Center.)

■ SELF-STUDY ASSIGNMENTS

1. Describe a patient infected with hepatitis B most likely to respond to antiretroviral HBV therapy and how you would monitor for therapeutic efficacy and adverse effects.

2. Compare and contrast the mechanism of action, immunogenicity rate, and adverse effects of the two available hepatitis B vaccines.

3. Determine the cost of the oral antiretroviral HBV agents and pegylated interferon therapy for the treatment of hepatitis B.

4. Review the time course of serologic markers after an acute HBV infection and explain their significance to one of your peers (Fig. 51-1).

CLINICAL PEARL

To eliminate HBV transmission that occurs during infancy and childhood, the Immunization Practices Advisory Committee of the CDC recommends that all newborn infants be vaccinated regardless of the hepatitis B status of the mothers.

REFERENCES

1. Tong MJ, Pan CQ, Han SB, et al. An expert consensus for the management of chronic hepatitis B in Asian Americans. Aliment Pharmacol Ther. 2018;47:1181–1200.

2. Martin P, Nguyen MH, Dieterich DT, et al. Treatment algorithm for managing chronic hepatitis B virus infection in the United States: 2021 update. Clin Gastroenterol Hepatol. 2022;20(8):1766–1775.

3. Terrault NA, Lok ASF, McMahon BJ, et al. Update on prevention, diagnosis, and treatment of chronic hepatitis B: AASLD 2018 hepatitis B guidance. Hepatology. 2018;67:1560–1599.

4. Centers for Disease Control and Prevention. Hepatitis B questions and answers for health professionals. Available at: *https://www.cdc.gov/hepatitis/hbv/hbvfaq.htm#vaccFAQ*. Accessed November 3, 2021.

52

VIRAL HEPATITIS C

The Raging Syndemic .... Level II

Michelle T. Martin, PharmD, FCCP, BCPS, BCACP

LEARNING OBJECTIVES

After completing this case study, the reader should be able to:

- Identify and evaluate the clinical manifestations and laboratory parameters relevant to the assessment and treatment of chronic hepatitis C virus (HCV) infection.

- Design a patient-specific pharmaceutical care plan for a patient with HCV, including drugs, doses, and durations of therapy.

- Develop a plan for monitoring efficacy and adverse effects of the pharmacologic agents used in the management of HCV.

- Identify and evaluate the drug interactions with direct-acting antiviral (DAA) agents used in HCV treatment.

- Provide patient education for patients with chronic HCV regarding their medications, nonpharmacologic interventions/behaviors, and vaccinations.

PATIENT PRESENTATION

■ Chief Complaint

"About 7 months ago, they checked me for HCV when I was in the emergency department (ED). A case worker called me a few days later and said I had HCV and set up a few appointments but I didn't make it to them. I finally went to the appointment last month. I am here today to talk about the test results from last month."

■ HPI

A 25-year-old man who has been linked to the liver clinic after HCV screening in the ED after an admission for an opioid overdose. The ED physician had performed opt-out HCV screening (since the patient had no record of HCV screening in the electronic health record system). The HCV screening was part of the institution's standard practice of screening patients age 18–79 based on American Association for the Study of Liver Diseases (AASLD) recommendations. His HCV antibody test was positive and reflexed to the HCV RNA, which was positive at 1,800,000 international units/mL. A case worker called the patient after his ED visit and linked him to a substance use program, and he was given three appointments with the liver clinic, for which he did not show. The case worker again linked him to care; he then attended the liver clinic appointment 1 month ago, saw the hepatologist, had a FibroScan performed, and labs drawn. He presents today to discuss the results and next steps.

He denies ever having blood transfusion. He reports current use of alcohol and recreational drugs including marijuana and intranasal heroin and cocaine, and he has a history of intravenous heroin use. He had a tattoo placed by a friend at a "tattoo party" while he was in his teens. He denies any jaundice or right upper quadrant pain. He also denies any hepatic encephalopathy or signs or stigmata of chronic liver disease.

■ PMH

Substance use disorder: Began in his late teens.

■ FH

No known family history of liver disease or hepatocellular carcinoma (HCC). Patient is estranged from his parents and has no siblings.

■ SH

The patient earned his high school diploma. He works temporary part-time jobs. He is single and lives with a friend. He uses recreational drugs, including inhaled marijuana one joint three times weekly, alcohol (3–7 drinks 3–5 times weekly), and intranasal heroin and cocaine (1–2 lines daily). He reports that he no longer uses heroin intravenously (last use was 2 years ago).

■ Meds

Omeprazole 20 mg PO daily on occasion × 1 year

■ Allergies and Intolerances

No known drug allergies

■ ROS

He states that his overall health is "fine" despite malnourished appearance. He has fatigue. He does not exercise. The remainder of the review of systems was noncontributory, with no additional pertinent positives or negatives.

■ Physical Examination

Gen

General appearance of an under-nourished man in NAD

VS

BP 128/72, P 88, RR 18, T 37.2°C; Wt 147 lb (66.8 kg), Ht 5'10" (178 cm)

Skin

Intact without xanthomas, hematomas, or ecchymosis. No jaundice or palmar erythema.

HEENT

PERRLA; EOMI; sclerae anicteric; funduscopic exam normal; TM WNL

Neck/Lymph Nodes

Neck supple; no lymphadenopathy or thyromegaly; no carotid bruits

Lungs/Thorax

Clear to auscultation bilaterally. Normal breath sounds.

CV

RRR; S_1, S_2 normal; no S_3 or S_4. No murmurs, rubs, or gallops.

Abd

Soft, NT, ND. Normoactive bowel sounds. No evidence of ascites, no HSM.

MS/Ext

Peripheral pulses 2+ throughout.

Neuro

A&O × 3; CN II–XII intact; DTRs 2+

■ **Labs Obtained in the ED 7 Months Ago**

Anti-HCV (+)

HCV RNA 1,800,000 IU/mL

■ **Labs Obtained at Lab Draw About 1 Month Ago**

Na 141 mEq/L	Hgb 14.1 g/dL	AST 58 IU/L	HBsAg (−)
K 4.2 mEq/L	Hct 39%	ALT 78 IU/L	Anti-HBs (−)
Cl 101 mEq/L	Plt 255 × 10³/mm³	Alk phos 112 IU/L	Anti-HBc (−)
CO₂ 28 mEq/L	WBC 6 × 10³/mm³	T. bili 0.4 mg/dL	Anti-HAV (−)
BUN 15 mg/dL	56% PMNs	Alb 4.1 g/dL	Anti-HCV (+)
SCr 1.1 mg/dL	Bands 1%	GGT 41 IU/L	HCV RNA
Glu 100 mg/dL	Lymphs 36%		1,900,000 IU/mL
	Monos 7%		HCV Genotype 3
	PT 12 seconds		HIV (−)
	INR 1.0		

■ **FibroScan (Performed After Liver Clinic Visit 1 Month Ago)**

2.8 kPa

■ **Assessment/Diagnosis**

Newly diagnosed chronic HCV

QUESTIONS

Collect Information

1.a. What subjective and objective information indicates the presence of HCV?

1.b. What additional information is needed to fully assess this patient's HCV?

Assess the Information

2.a. Assess the severity of HCV based on the subjective and objective information available.

2.b. Create a list of the patient's drug therapy problems and prioritize them. Include assessment of medication appropriateness, effectiveness, safety, and patient adherence.

2.c. What economic, psychosocial, cultural, racial, and ethical considerations are applicable to this patient?

Develop a Care Plan

3.a. What are the goals of pharmacotherapy for HCV in this case?

3.b. What nondrug therapies might be useful for this patient's HCV?

3.c. What feasible pharmacotherapeutic alternatives are available for treating HCV?

3.d. Create an individualized, patient-centered, team-based care plan to optimize medication therapy for this patient's HCV and other drug therapy problems. Include specific drugs, dosage forms, doses, schedules, and durations of therapy.

3.e. What alternatives would be appropriate if the initial care plan fails or cannot be used?

Implement the Care Plan

4.a. What information should be provided to the patient to enhance adherence, ensure successful therapy, and minimize adverse effects?

4.b. Describe how care should be coordinated with other healthcare providers.

Follow-Up: Monitor and Evaluate

5. Explain how to monitor and evaluate the care plan for medication appropriateness, effectiveness, safety, and patient adherence by using clinical and laboratory data, patient feedback, and other information.

■ CLINICAL COURSE (PART 1): WEEK 4 PHONE CALL

The clinician calls the patient to discuss treatment progress. The patient reports feeling more fatigue than at baseline, but he denies other adverse effects. He states that he has missed two doses but has otherwise been adherent to HCV therapy. He is seeing an addiction medicine specialist and is interested in working toward sobriety. He states he might start medication for opioid use disorder (MOUD) and asks about any interactions.

■ FOLLOW-UP QUESTIONS

1. Based on this information, should the therapy continue as planned? Why or why not?

2. Are you concerned about drug interactions with MOUD and his HCV regimen?

3. Outline a plan for vaccinating the patient against other forms of viral hepatitis.

■ CLINICAL COURSE (PART 2): END-OF-TREATMENT PHONE CALL

At the end-of-treatment, the clinician calls the patient and the patient reports feeling "fine." He states he only had slight fatigue in the past few weeks. He states he only missed "a few" doses total during treatment; he has five doses remaining and today was scheduled to be his last dose of therapy.

■ FOLLOW-UP QUESTIONS (CONTINUED)

4. What are the next steps to assess this patient's response to HCV therapy?

5. What other monitoring do you recommend for this patient?

■ SELF-STUDY ASSIGNMENTS

1. Review the AASLD/IDSA simplified guidelines for patients without cirrhosis and the guidelines for treatment-naïve patients with chronic HCV genotype 1 infection and summarize the advantages and disadvantages of the various DAA regimens.

2. Perform a literature search to assess the use of DAAs in patients with ongoing injection drug use or history of substance use.

3. Utilize the University of Liverpool's drug interaction website to assess for the presence and management of additional drug interactions with other DAA options for this patient (e.g., phenobarbital, atorvastatin, oxycodone).

4. Consider limitations of risk-based HCV screening and propose modifications to current practice to identify and diagnose patients with HCV.

CLINICAL PEARL

DAA therapy is associated with potential drug interactions due to some DAAs being substrates, inducers and/or inhibitors of cytochrome P450 (CYP) 3A, P-glycoprotein (P-gp), and organic anion transporting polypeptide (OATP) 1B1 and 2B1. Not all potential drug interactions have been studied and/or listed in the prescribing information. To supplement this information, pharmacokinetic properties of medications can be analyzed for the extent and pathway of metabolism, and drug interaction sources should be assessed. The University of Liverpool's drug interaction website describes many drug interactions with HCV DAAs (*http://www.hep-druginteractions.org*).

REFERENCES

1. Recommendations for testing, managing, and treating hepatitis C. American Association for the Study of Liver Diseases and Infectious Diseases Society of America. Available at: *http://www.hcvguidelines.org/*. Accessed February 15, 2022.

2. Hepatitis C Information for Health Professionals. Division of Viral Hepatitis and National Center for HIV/AIDS, Viral Hepatitis, STD, and TB Prevention. Centers for Disease Control and Prevention Publication. Available at: *http://www.cdc.gov/hepatitis/HCV/index.htm*. Accessed February 15, 2022.

3. Bonder A, Afdhal N. Utilization of FibroScan in clinical practice. Curr Gastroenterol Rep. 2014;16:372.

4. Hep Drug Interactions. University of Liverpool. Available at: *http://www.hep-druginteractions.org*. Accessed February 15, 2022.

5. Deming P, Martin MT, Chan J, et al. Therapeutic advances in HCV genotype 1 infection: insights from the Society of Infectious Diseases Pharmacists. Pharmacotherapy. 2016;36:203–217.

6. Mohammad RA, Bulloch MN, Chan J, et al. Provision of clinical pharmacist services for individuals with chronic hepatitis C viral infection: Joint Opinion of the GI/Liver/Nutrition and Infectious Diseases Practice and Research Networks of the American College of Clinical Pharmacy. Pharmacotherapy. 2014;34:1341–1354.

53

DRUG-INDUCED ACUTE KIDNEY INJURY

Not a Cute Consequence . . . . Level III

Mary K. Stamatakis, PharmD

LEARNING OBJECTIVES

After completing this case study, the reader should be able to:

- Evaluate clinical and laboratory findings in a patient with acute kidney injury (AKI).

- Select pharmacotherapy for treatment of complications associated with AKI.

- Assess appropriateness of aminoglycoside serum concentrations in relation to efficacy and toxicity.

- Develop strategies to prevent drug-induced AKI, including the selection of pharmacologic alternatives that do not adversely affect kidney function.

- Adjust drug dosages based on kidney function to maximize efficacy and minimize adverse events.

PATIENT PRESENTATION

■ Chief Complaint
Not available

■ HPI

A 79-year-old man originally presented to the hospital 1 month ago with symptoms of heart failure that required open heart surgery for mitral valve replacement. He developed mediastinitis and *Serratia* bacteremia (blood cultures × 4 positive for *Serratia marcescens*, sensitive to gentamicin, piperacillin, cefepime, ceftriaxone, and ciprofloxacin; resistance was noted to ampicillin). Therapy was initiated with double coverage including gentamicin and cefepime due to the seriousness of the infection. Today is day 21 of a 6-week course of antibiotic treatment. A gradual increase in his BUN and serum creatinine concentrations from baseline has been noted (Table 53-1), and signs of volume overload are now present.

■ PMH

Acute decompensated heart failure
Mechanical mitral valve replacement surgery 28 days ago
Type 2 DM

Stage 3B CKD
Dyslipidemia
Hypertension
Depression
Osteoarthritis

■ FH
Father had type 2 DM.

■ SH
Denies smoking or alcohol; retired coal miner (11 years ago)

■ Meds

Gentamicin (see Table 53-1 for dosages and serum drug concentrations; gentamicin is currently on hold)
Cefepime 2 g IVPB Q 12 H
Warfarin 5 mg PO once daily
Enalapril 10 mg PO twice daily (currently on hold for the last 4 days)
Metoprolol succinate XL 100 mg PO daily
Furosemide 40 mg PO Q 12 H
Atorvastatin 20 mg PO daily
Escitalopram 10 mg PO daily
Glipizide 10 mg PO daily
Spironolactone 12.5 mg PO daily
Ibuprofen 400 mg PO Q 4–6 H PRN pain (started today for joint pain)

■ All
NKDA

■ ROS

Currently complains of trouble breathing, weakness, general malaise, and pain in right hand. No fever or chills.

■ PE

Gen

Confused-appearing man in mild distress

VS

BP 125/75 mm Hg, P 68 bpm, RR 26, T 37.7°C; current Wt 176 lb (80 kg); admission Wt 165 lb (75 kg), Ht 5'9" (175 cm)

Skin

Surgical incision site healing with no drainage

HEENT

PERRLA, EOMI, poor dentition

Neck/Lymph Nodes

(+) JVD

TABLE 53-1	SCr, BUN, and Serum Gentamicin Concentrations During Hospitalization				
			Gentamicin (mcg/mL)		
Postoperative Day	SCr (mg/dL)	BUN (mg/dL)	Peak[a]	Trough[b]	Gentamicin Dosages
3	1.5	19			140 mg × 1, and then 120 mg Q 12 H
5	1.5	21	6.3	1.1	Continue current regimen
7	1.8	25			
10	2.1	31	6.9	1.8	Continue current regimen
14	2.7	38	8.3	2.5	Decrease to 120 mg Q 24 H
17	3.1	46			
21	3.2	50	9.4	2.7	Gentamicin on hold

BUN, blood urea nitrogen; SCr, serum creatinine.
[a]Serum drug concentrations drawn 30 minutes after a 30-minute infusion.
[b]Serum drug concentrations drawn immediately before a dose.

Chest

Basilar crackles

CV

S_1, S_2 normal, no S_3, irregular rhythm

Abd

Soft, nontender, (+) BS, (−) HSM

Genit/Rect

(−) Masses

MS/Ext

2+ sacral edema; some tenderness and limited motion in right hand

Neuro

A&O to person and place, but not to time

■ Labs (Current)

Na 139 mEq/L	Hgb 9.7 g/dL	Ca 8.6 mg/dL
K 3.7 mEq/L	Hct 29.5%	Mg 2.1 mg/dL
Cl 103 mEq/L	Plt 303 × 10³/mm³	Phos 4.4 mg/dL
CO_2 24 mEq/L	WBC 8.6 × 10³/mm³	INR 2.7
BUN 50 mg/dL	(BUN 19 mg/dL on admission)	
SCr 3.2 mg/dL	(SCr 1.5 mg/dL on admission)	
Glu 119 mg/dL		

■ UA

Color, yellow; character, hazy; glucose (−); ketones (−); SG 1.010; pH 5.0; protein 30 mg/dL; coarse granular casts 5–10/lpf; WBC 0–3/hpf; RBC 0–2/hpf; no bacteria; nitrite (−); osmolality 325 mOsm; urinary sodium 45 mEq/L; creatinine 33 mg/dL, FE_{NA} 3.1%

■ Repeat Blood Cultures Today

Negative

■ Fluid Intake/Output and Daily Weights

Day	I/O	Weight (kg)
3 days ago	3200 mL/900 mL	N/A
2 days ago	2600 mL/1000 mL	76
Yesterday	2800 mL/1300 mL	N/A
Today	N/A	80

■ Assessment

AKI

QUESTIONS

Collect Information

1.a. What subjective and objective information indicates the presence of AKI?

1.b. What additional information is needed to fully assess this patient's AKI?

Assess the Information

2.a. Assess the severity of AKI based on the subjective and objective information available. Assess the stage and category of AKI (prerenal, intrinsic, postrenal), as well as estimation of creatinine clearance.

2.b. Create a list of the patient's drug therapy problems and prioritize them. Include assessment of medication appropriateness, effectiveness, safety, and patient adherence.

Develop a Care Plan

3.a. What are the goals of pharmacotherapy for AKI in this case?

3.b. What nondrug therapies might be useful for this patient's AKI?

3.c. What feasible pharmacotherapeutic alternatives are available for treating AKI?

3.d. Create an individualized, patient-centered, team-based care plan to optimize medication therapy for the AKI and other drug therapy problems. Include specific drugs, dosage forms, doses, schedules, and durations of therapy.

Implement the Care Plan

4.a. What information should be provided to the patient to enhance adherence, ensure successful therapy, and minimize adverse effects?

4.b. Describe how care should be coordinated with other healthcare providers.

Follow-Up: Monitor and Evaluate

5. Explain how to monitor and evaluate the care plan for medication appropriateness, effectiveness, safety, and patient adherence by using clinical and laboratory data, patient feedback, and other information.

■ ADDITIONAL CASE QUESTIONS

1. What risk factors did the patient have for gentamicin-induced AKI?

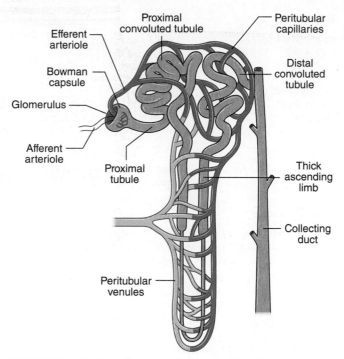

FIGURE 53-1. Nephron. (Reproduced with permission from Jameson JL, Fauci AS, Kasper DL, et al, eds. *Harrison's Principles of Internal Medicine*. 20th ed. New York, NY: McGraw-Hill; 2018.)

2. What therapeutic interventions could have been initiated to decrease the likelihood of developing drug-induced AKI?

■ SELF-STUDY ASSIGNMENTS

1. Create a list of medications that can cause AKI and should be avoided in patients with AKI or in patients at risk for AKI.

2. Using the figure of the nephron (Figure 53-1), indicate where each of the following classes of diuretics exert their effect: carbonic anhydrase inhibitors, loop diuretics, thiazide diuretics, and potassium-sparing diuretics.

CLINICAL PEARL

A "triple whammy" effect on kidney function can be seen what patients are administered the combination of angiotensin-converting enzyme inhibitors/angiotensin receptor antagonists, diuretics, and nonsteroidal anti-inflammatory drugs, especially in the elderly.

REFERENCES

1. Kidney Disease: Improving Global Outcomes (KDIGO) Acute Kidney Injury Work Group. KDIGO clinical practice guideline for acute kidney injury. Kidney Int Suppl. 2012;2:1–138.

2. Frazee EN, Personett HA, Wood-Wentz DM, Herasevich V, Lieske JC, Kashani KB. Overestimation of glomerular filtration rate among critically ill adults with hospital-acquired oliguanuric acute kidney injury. J Pharm Pract. 2016;29:125–131.

3. Lopez-Novoa JM, Quiros Y, Vicente L, Morales AI, Lopez-Hernandez FJ. New insights into the mechanism of aminoglycoside nephrotoxicity: an integrative point of view. Kidney Int. 2011;79:33–45.

4. Wargo KA, Edwards JD. Aminoglycoside-induced nephrotoxicity. J Pharm Pract. 2014;27:573–577.

5. Brater DC. Update in diuretic therapy: clinical pharmacology. Semin Nephrol. 2011;31:483–494.

54

ACUTE KIDNEY INJURY

There's Nothing Cute About It . . . . Level II

Scott Bolesta, PharmD, BCPS, FCCM, FCCP

LEARNING OBJECTIVES

After completing this case study, the reader should be able to:

- Assess a patient with AKI using clinical and laboratory data.

- Classify AKI in a patient.

- Distinguish between AKI resulting from prerenal and that from intrinsic injury.

- Recommend changes to the pharmacotherapeutic regimen of a patient with AKI.

- Justify appropriate therapeutic interventions for a patient with AKI.

PATIENT PRESENTATION

■ Chief Complaint

"I feel really weak."

■ HPI

A 72-year-old man presents to the ED with complaints of severe weakness that started this morning and recent stomach pain for the past week. He was feeling well until he developed stomach pain 1 week ago that worsened with meals. Two days ago, the pain worsened to the point where he avoided eating, and last evening he felt more tired than usual and went to bed early. He had difficulty sleeping due to the pain, and since waking this morning he has been in too much pain and too weak to perform his normal ADLs.

■ PMH

HTN × 30 years
CAD × 20 years
MI × 2 with most recent 2 months ago s/p PCI with drug-eluting stent placement
s/p CABG 20 years ago
HFrEF × 4 years
OA × 5 year

■ FH

Father died of an acute MI at age 52; mother had diabetes mellitus and died of a stroke at the age of 65.

■ SH

Retired and living at home with his wife. Before retirement, the patient was employed as an accountant. No alcohol, no tobacco use.

■ Meds

Aspirin 81 mg PO daily
Amlodipine 10 mg PO once daily

Furosemide 40 mg PO once daily
Metoprolol succinate 50 mg PO once daily
Enalapril 20 mg PO once daily
Prasugrel 10 mg PO daily
Atorvastatin 80 mg PO daily
Naproxen 500 mg PO BID

■ All

NKA

■ ROS

In addition to weakness and stomach pain, the patient complains of feeling cold but denies chills or fever. No changes in vision. Denies SOB, CP, and cough. Complains of feeling lightheaded. Has been having frequent loose black stools over the past 3 days and abdominal pain that has become severe in the past 2 days. Has noted a decrease in the frequency of his urination over the past 24 hours. Denies musculoskeletal pain or cramping.

■ Physical Examination

Gen

Pale man who appears in moderate distress and generally weak and lethargic

VS

BP 89/43 mm Hg (77/32 mm Hg on standing), P 123 bpm, RR 25, T 36.1°C; Wt 171.6 lb (78 kg), Ht 5'9" (175 cm)

Skin

Pale and cool with poor turgor

HEENT

PERRLA; EOMI; fundi normal; conjunctivae pale and dry; TMs intact; tongue and mouth dry

Neck/Lymph Nodes

No JVD or HJR; no lymphadenopathy or thyromegaly

Lungs

No crackles or rhonchi

CV

Tachycardic with regular rhythm; normal S_1, S_2; no S_3; faint S_4; no MRG

Abd

Rigid with guarding, epigastric tenderness, ND; no HSM; hyperactive BS

Genit/Rect

Stool heme (+); slightly enlarged prostate

MS/Ext

Weak pulses; no peripheral edema; mild swelling of MCP joints of both hands

Neuro

A&O × 3; CNs intact; DTRs 2+; Babinski (−)

■ Labs

Na 132 mEq/L	Ca 8.6 mg/dL
K 5.6 mEq/L	Mg 2.1 mg/dL
Cl 97 mEq/L	Phos 4.3 mg/dL
CO_2 22 mEq/L	WBC 8.6×10^3/mm³
BUN 53 mg/dL	Hgb 7.6 g/dL
SCr 1.8 mg/dL	Hct 22.5%
Glu 123 mg/dL	Plt 96×10^3/mm³

■ Assessment

Admit to hospital for evaluation and management of dehydration, evaluation for acute GI bleed, and potential acute kidney injury.

■ Clinical Course

On admission, the patient was resuscitated aggressively with balanced crystalloids given IV and multiple transfusions (4 units of PRBCs). His home medications were held, he was started on a continuous IV pantoprazole infusion of 8 mg/hr, and he underwent an emergent EGD. During endoscopy, a large ulcer in the gastric antrum was found with an exposed spurting artery. Endoscopic therapy was unsuccessful, and the patient was taken to the OR for surgical intervention. He was hypotensive in the OR (BP 70 mm Hg systolic on average) and was started on a norepinephrine infusion to maintain a stable BP. Postoperatively, he remained on mechanical ventilation, and his urine output averaged 35 mL/hr over the first 12 postoperative hours despite continued IV hydration and repeated transfusions in the OR. He also remained on norepinephrine for a continued low BP. On the morning of postoperative day 1, his labs were as follows:

Na 134 mEq/L	Ca 8.2 mg/dL
K 5.4 mEq/L	Mg 2.2 mg/dL
Cl 111 mEq/L	Phos 4.7 mg/dL
CO_2 19 mEq/L	WBC 14.6×10^3/mm³
BUN 49 mg/dL	Hgb 10.3 g/dL
SCr 2.5 mg/dL	Hct 29.8%
Glu 145 mg/dL	Plt 112×10^3/mm³

Urinalysis also showed muddy brown casts, urine sodium of 72 mEq/L, and specific gravity of 1.004. The patient remained on mechanical ventilation and norepinephrine, his urine output had not improved, and his chest radiograph showed diffuse bilateral pulmonary edema with a decrease in O_2 saturation to 86%. An echocardiogram revealed hypokinesis of the anterior portion of the left ventricle and an EF of 25%. The patient was started on dobutamine, and an internal jugular vein catheter was inserted and CVVH-DF was begun.

■ Assessment

A 72-year-old man with an acute UGI bleed, AKI, and volume overload heart failure.

QUESTIONS

Collect Information

1.a. What subjective and objective information indicates the presence of AKI postoperatively?

1.b. What additional information is needed to fully assess this patient's AKI postoperatively?

Assess the Information

2.a. Assess the severity of AKI based on the subjective and objective information available.

2.b. Create a list of the patient's drug therapy problems and prioritize them. Include assessment of medication appropriateness, effectiveness, safety, and patient adherence.

Develop a Care Plan

3.a. What are the goals of pharmacotherapy for AKI in this case?

3.b. What nondrug therapies might be useful for this patient's AKI?

3.c. What feasible pharmacotherapeutic options are available for treating AKI?

3.d. Create an individualized, patient-centered, team-based care plan to optimize medication therapy for the AKI and other drug therapy problems. Include specific drugs, dosage forms, doses, schedules, and durations of therapy.

Implement the Care Plan

4.a. What information should be provided to the patient to enhance adherence, ensure successful therapy, and minimize adverse effects?

4.b. Describe how care should be coordinated with other healthcare providers.

Follow-Up: Monitor and Evaluate

5. Explain how to monitor and evaluate the care plan for medication appropriateness, effectiveness, safety, and patient adherence by using clinical and laboratory data, patient feedback, and other information.

■ CLINICAL COURSE

On postoperative day 5, his pulmonary edema had resolved, he had been weaned off norepinephrine and dobutamine, the dialysis catheter was removed, and he was extubated. His subsequent hospital course was uneventful, and his kidney function gradually improved.

■ SELF-STUDY ASSIGNMENTS

1. Evaluate the evidence regarding the effectiveness of intravenous 0.9% sodium chloride compared to balanced crystalloids (eg, Plasmalyte, Ringer's lactate) in volume resuscitation for outcomes related to kidney function.

2. Write a brief paper that discusses the utilization of intravenous sodium bicarbonate in the setting of AKI in patients who present with shock.

CLINICAL PEARL

Most laboratory markers of kidney function (eg, serum creatinine) in patients with AKI usually lag behind the true change in GFR, often by a day or more. Therefore, adjustment of drug therapy dosing in these patients can be challenging, and often trends in urine output over the previous hours are used to anticipate the need to make dose adjustments.

REFERENCES

1. Kidney Disease: Improving Global Outcomes (KDIGO) Acute Kidney Injury Work Group. KDIGO clinical practice guideline for acute kidney injury. Kidney Inter Suppl. 2012;2:1–138.
2. Semler MW, Self WH, Wanderer JP, et al. Balanced crystalloids versus saline in critically ill adults. N Engl J Med. 2018;378(9):829–839.
3. Prowle JR, Kirwan CJ, Bellomo R. Fluid management for the prevention and attenuation of acute kidney injury. Nat Rev Nephrol. 2014;10:37–47.
4. Palevsky PM. Renal replacement therapy in acute kidney injury. Adv Chronic Kidney Dis. 2013;20:76–84.
5. Ejaz AA, Mohandas R. Are diuretics harmful in the management of acute kidney injury? Curr Opin Nephrol Hypertens. 2014;23:155–160.
6. Kellum JA, Lameire N. Diagnosis, evaluation, and management of acute kidney injury: a KDIGO summary (part 1). Crit Care. 2013;17:204.

55

PROGRESSIVE KIDNEY DISEASE

It Was Only a Matter of Time . . . . Level III

Christie Schumacher, PharmD, BCPS, BCACP, BCCP, BC-ADM, CDCES, FCCP

LEARNING OBJECTIVES

After completing this case study, the reader should be able to:

- Identify risk factors for progression of chronic kidney disease (CKD) in persons with diabetes.

- Design an individualized care plan, including lifestyle modifications and pharmacotherapy, for persons with diabetes and CKD.

- Identify clinical and laboratory parameters used to evaluate progression of CKD and the efficacy and safety of related medication therapy.

- Summarize counseling points for non-pharmacologic and pharmacologic management options for persons with CKD.

PATIENT PRESENTATION

■ Chief Complaint

"I'm here to follow up on the results of my labs."

■ HPI

A 38-year-old woman with type 2 diabetes mellitus (T2DM), hypertension (HTN), and dyslipidemia returns to her primary care physician (PCP) for a follow-up visit. At her routine physical examination 3 months ago, her annual nephropathy screening revealed a urine albumin-to-creatinine ratio (UACR) of 659 mg/g, which was elevated from the previous year's screening that showed a mildly increased UACR of 145 mg/g and an SCr of 1.2 mg/dL. A second spot urine test from 1 week ago showed a persistently elevated UACR of 673 mg/g. She has returned to the office today to review her lab results and presents with no complaints. She brought with her a list of her medications and self-monitoring blood glucose readings.

■ PMH

T2DM × 8 years
HTN × 6 years
Dyslipidemia × 5 years
Seasonal allergies

■ FH

Father had T2DM and cardiovascular disease (CVD) and passed away at age 50 secondary to a myocardial infarction (MI); mother (age 62) has HTN and dyslipidemia; brother (age 31) also has T2DM.

■ SH

The patient is an administrative assistant with prescription drug benefits. She reports occasional alcohol consumption on weekends or when out with friends (one to two alcoholic beverages per month). She smokes one pack per day (ppd); decreased from previously reported two ppd last year. No history of illicit drug use.

■ Meds

Metformin 1000 mg PO twice daily
Semaglutide 0.5 mg subcutaneously every 7 days
Hydrochlorothiazide 25 mg PO daily
Atorvastatin 20 mg PO daily
Mometasone two sprays (100 mcg) in each nostril once daily PRN allergies
Cetirizine 10 mg PO daily PRN allergies
Naproxen 220 mg PO twice daily PRN headaches
Multivitamin PO daily

■ All

NKDA, seasonal allergies to grass and pollen

■ ROS

Occasional headaches, generally associated with menstruation; no c/o polyuria, polydipsia, polyphagia, sensory loss, or visual changes
No chest pain, palpitations, dizziness, edema, fatigue, or SOB

■ Physical Examination

Gen

No acute distress

VS

BP 148/84 mm Hg (R arm), repeat BP 146/82 mm Hg (L arm), HR 82 bpm, RR 18, T 37.5°C; Wt 191 lb (87 kg), Ht 5'6" (168 cm)

Skin

Warm, dry, no rashes

HEENT

PERRLA, EOMI, negative for diabetic retinopathy; no retinal edema or vitreous hemorrhage
TMs intact
Oral mucosa moist with no lesions

Neck/Lymph Nodes

Supple without adenopathy or thyromegaly

Lungs/Thorax

Clear, breath sounds normal

CV

Heart sounds normal, no murmurs, no bruits

Abd

Soft NT/ND

Genit/Rect

Rectal exam deferred; recent Pap smear negative

MS/Ext

No CCE, normal ROM

Neuro

A&O × 3; CNs intact; normal DTRs

■ Labs (1 Week Ago, Fasting)

Na 140 mEq/L	Hgb 12.2 g/dL	Fasting lipid profile
K 3.9 mEq/L	Hct 36.1%	T. chol 212 mg/dL
Cl 107 mEq/L	WBC 9.5 × 10³/mm³	Trig 149 mg/dL
CO₂ 26 mEq/L	Plt 148 × 10³/mm³	LDL 140 mg/dL
BUN 29 mg/dL	Ca 9.4 mg/dL	HDL 42 mg/dL
SCr 1.6 mg/dL	Phos 2.7 mg/dL	Alb 3.4 g/dL
Glu 196 mg/dL	Uric acid 6.2 mg/dL	
A1C 8.2%	eGFR 46.4 mL/min/1.73 m²	

■ UA (1 Week Ago)

pH 5.2, 1+ glucose, (–) ketones, 3+ protein, (–) leukocyte esterase and nitrite; (–) RBC; 3–4 WBC/hpf, UACR 673 mg/g
Urine Hcg: Negative

■ Assessment

A 38-year-old woman with diabetes diagnosed today with CKD and overt macroalbuminuria complicated by inadequately managed co-conditions.

QUESTIONS

Collect Information

1.a. What objective information indicates the presence of CKD in this patient?

1.b. What additional information is needed to fully assess this patient's CKD and other diseases that may contribute to CKD?

Assess the Information

2.a. Assess the severity of CKD based on the subjective and objective information available. Calculate eGFR and CrCl in this patient based on her most recent labs using the CKD-EPI and Cockcroft-Gault equations.

2.b. Create a list of the patient's drug therapy problems and prioritize them. Include assessment of medication appropriateness, efficacy, safety, and patient adherence.

Develop a Care Plan

3.a. What are the goals of pharmacotherapy for CKD in this case?

3.b. What nondrug therapies might be useful for this patient's CKD?

3.c. What feasible pharmacotherapeutic alternatives are available for treating this patient's CKD and other diseases that may contribute to CKD?

3.d. Create an individualized, patient-centered, team-based care plan to optimize medication therapy for this patient's CKD and other drug therapy problems. Include specific drugs, dosage forms, doses, frequency, and durations of therapy.

Implement the Care Plan

4.a. What information should be provided to the patient to enhance adherence, optimize efficacy, and minimize adverse effects?

4.b. Describe how care should be coordinated with other healthcare providers.

Follow-Up: Monitor and Evaluate

5. Explain how to monitor and evaluate the care plan for medication appropriateness, effectiveness, safety, and patient adherence by using clinical and laboratory data, patient feedback, and other information.

■ SELF-STUDY ASSIGNMENTS

1. Discuss the role of diuretic therapy in patients with normal kidney function compared to those with eGFR values <30 mL/min/1.73 m^2.

2. Explain the proposed rationale for the nephroprotective effects of sodium-glucose cotransporter-2 (SGLT2) inhibitors.

3. Describe the role of finerenone, a nonsteroidal mineralocorticoid receptor antagonist, in reducing CKD progression and cardiovascular events in clinical practice.

CLINICAL PEARL

The American Diabetes Association (ADA) recommends that a sodium-glucose cotransporter-2 inhibitor be initiated in patients with T2DM and CKD to reduce chronic kidney disease progression and cardiovascular events.

REFERENCES

1. American Diabetes Association. Standards of medical care in diabetes—2022. Diabetes Care. 2022;45(Suppl 1):S1–S264.
2. Kidney Disease: Improving Global Outcomes (KDIGO) 2020 clinical practice guideline for diabetes management in chronic kidney disease. Kidney Int. 2020;98:S1–S115.
3. Kidney Disease: Improving Global Outcomes (KDIGO) 2012 clinical practice guideline for the evaluation and management of chronic kidney disease. Kidney Int. 2013;3:S1–S150.
4. Kidney Disease: Improving Global Outcomes (KDIGO) 2021 clinical practice guideline for the management of blood pressure in chronic kidney disease. Kidney Int. 2021;99:S1–S87.
5. Whelton PK, Carey RM, Aronow WS, et al. 2017 ACC/AHA/AAPA/ABC/ACPM/AGS/APhA/ASH/ASPC/NMA/PCNA guideline for the prevention, detection, evaluation, and management of high blood pressure in adults: a report of the American College of Cardiology/American Heart Association Task Force on Clinical Practice Guidelines. Hypertension. 2018;71(6):1269–1324.
6. National Kidney Foundation. Frequently asked questions about GFR estimates. Available at: https://www.kidney.org/sites/default/files/docs/12-10-4004_abe_faqs_aboutgfrrev1b_singleb.pdf. Accessed March 11, 2022.
7. Grundy SM, Stone NJ, Bailey AL, et al. 2018 ACC/AHA/AACVPR/AAPA/ABC/ACPM/ADA/AGS/APhA/ASPC/NLA/PCNA guideline on the management of blood cholesterol: a report of the American College of Cardiology Foundation/American Heart Association Task Force on Clinical Practice Guidelines. J Am Coll Cardiol. 2019;73:e285–e350.

56

END-STAGE KIDNEY DISEASE

Urine Trouble . . . . Level II

Katie E. Cardone, PharmD, BCACP, FNKF, FASN, FCCP

LEARNING OBJECTIVES

After completing this case study, the reader should be able to:

• Identify medication-related problems in a patient with end-stage kidney disease (ESKD) maintained on chronic hemodialysis.

• State the desired therapeutic outcomes for ESKD, anemia of chronic kidney disease, and mineral and bone disorder.

• Develop a plan to manage ESKD and associated complications that includes plans for monitoring patient response to changes in therapy.

• Outline a patient education plan to effectively implement medication-related interventions for ESKD.

PATIENT PRESENTATION

■ Chief Complaint

"I'm feeling more tired than usual."

■ HPI

A 50-year-old woman presents to the outpatient dialysis center for her routine HD treatment. Today, the patient is sleeping in her dialysis chair when you arrive at the clinic, which is unusual for her. She is usually awake, reading a magazine, or watching television. She has ESKD secondary to hypertension and has been on HD for 5 years. She has a failed AV fistula and graft and is currently dialyzed via central venous catheter. She has an upcoming appointment with the vascular surgeon to reevaluate her HD access. She also frequently leaves HD 30–60 minutes early against medical advice.

■ PMH

ESKD secondary to HTN
Anuria
HTN
Anemia
Secondary hyperparathyroidism
H/O gestational diabetes 12 years ago
GERD

■ PSH

Cesarean section 12 years ago
Tubal ligation 10 years ago
AV fistula creation 5 years ago (failed)
AV graft creation 3 years ago (failed)

■ FH

Father died of MI at age 60. Mother deceased due to breast cancer. No siblings. Has a 12-year-old son in good health.

■ SH

Married, lives with husband and a 12-year-old son. Occasional social alcohol use. Smokes 1/2 ppd (decreased from one ppd × 10 years). Denies caffeine consumption.

■ Meds

Furosemide 80 mg PO in the morning on non-dialysis days
Metoprolol succinate 50 mg PO QHS
Lisinopril 20 mg PO daily
Calcium acetate 667 mg three caps PO TID with meals
Nephro-Vite PO daily
Omeprazole 20 mg PO daily
Ferrous sulfate 325 mg PO TID
Docusate 100 mg PO daily PRN
Calcium carbonate PO PRN heartburn
Epoetin alfa 10,000 units IV three times weekly with dialysis (dose stable for 3 months)
Iron sucrose 50 mg IV once weekly at dialysis
Calcitriol 0.5 mcg PO three times weekly with dialysis

■ All

NKDA

■ ROS

Complains of feeling tired and weak over the past several weeks. Reports some swelling in feet and lower legs. Also reports constipation, nausea, and heartburn.

■ Physical Examination

Gen

The patient is a WDWN woman in NAD who appears her stated age.

VS

BP 175/88 mm Hg (predialysis); 149/89 mm Hg (postdialysis)
Wt 195 lb (88.6 kg) predialysis; 177 lb (84.0 kg) postdialysis
P 91 bpm, RR 16, T 36.5°C; Ht 5′4″ (163 cm)

Skin

Dry, scaly arms and legs

HEENT

PEERLA, EOMI, TMs intact

Neck/Lymph Nodes

Supple, no adenopathy, no thyromegaly

Lungs/Thorax

Clear, breath sounds normal

CV

RRR, no murmurs, no bruits

Abd

Soft, NT/ND

Genit/Rect

Deferred

Ext

Mild bilateral lower extremity edema

Neuro

CN II–XII intact; A&Ox3

■ Labs

Na 143 mEq/L	Hgb 9.3 g/dL	AST 21 IU/L	Alb 3.0 g/dL
K 4.3 mEq/L	Hct 27.5%	ALT 4 IU/L	Ca 9.7 mg/dL
Cl 95 mEq/L	RBC 2.84 ×	LDH 139 IU/L	Phos 6.7 mg/dL
CO_2 26 mEq/L	$10^6/mm^3$	Alk phos 175 IU/L	iPTH 855 pg/mL
BUN 59 mg/dL	MCV 81.8 m^3	T. bili 0.3 mg/dL	T. sat 12%
SCr 8.9 mg/dL	MCHC 32.4 g/dL		Ferritin
Glu 88 mg/dL	WBC 5.7 × $10^3/mm^3$		99 ng/mL

The nephrologist provided the following dialysis prescription:

Dialyze 3.5 hours per session, three times per week (T, Th, Sat, morning shift)
Estimated dry weight: 83.5 kg
Dialyzer: high-flux polysulfone filter, surface area 1.8 m^2
Blood flow rate: 400 mL/min
Dialysate flow rate: 800 mL/min
Dialysate: bicarbonate
Na 145 mEq/L, K 2.0 mEq/L, Ca 2.5 mEq/L, HCO_3 35 mEq/L
Heparin: 5000 unit IV bolus, and then 1000 units/hr until 1 hour before termination

■ Assessment

A 50-year-old woman with need for management of complications of ESKD.

QUESTIONS

Collect Information

1.a. What subjective and objective information indicates the presence of ESKD and complications of ESKD?

1.b. What additional information is needed to fully assess this patient's ESKD?

Assess the Information

2.a. Assess the severity of ESKD based on the subjective and objective information available.

2.b. Create a list of the patient's drug therapy problems and prioritize them. Include assessment of medication appropriateness, effectiveness, safety, and patient adherence.

Develop a Care Plan

3.a. What are the goals of pharmacotherapy for ESKD and related problems in this case?

3.b. What nondrug therapies might be useful for this patient's ESKD and related problems?

3.c. What feasible pharmacotherapeutic alternatives are available for treating this patient's ESKD-related problems?

3.d. Create an individualized, patient-centered, team-based care plan to optimize medication therapy for this patient's ESKD and other drug-related problems. Include specific drugs, dosage forms, doses, schedules, and durations of therapy.

Implement the Care Plan

4.a. What information should be provided to the patient to enhance adherence, ensure successful therapy, and minimize adverse effects?

4.b. Describe how care should be coordinated with other healthcare providers.

Follow-Up: Monitor and Evaluate

5. Explain how to monitor and evaluate the care plan for medication appropriateness, effectiveness, safety, and patient adherence by using clinical and laboratory data, patient feedback, and other information.

■ SELF-STUDY ASSIGNMENTS

1. The patient develops a sinus infection for which she goes to an urgent care clinic. She is prescribed levofloxacin 500 mg PO daily × 14 days. Evaluate the appropriateness of this prescription for the patient. What changes, if any, would you suggest regarding this prescription?

2. The patient would like a kidney transplant but must first quit smoking to become eligible for transplant. Create a smoking cessation plan for her.

CLINICAL PEARL

ESAs should be used judiciously with the lowest dose possible used due to their association with adverse cardiovascular outcomes in multiple clinical trials. In the face of iron deficiency and low hemoglobin, iron should be replenished before increasing the ESA dose. When ESAs are used in ESKD, hemoglobin concentrations in the normal range for healthy individuals should not be the target. Rather, avoidance of the need for blood transfusions and maintenance of quality of life should be the goal, typically at a lower hemoglobin concentration than the "normal range."

REFERENCES

1. Georgianos PI, Agarwal R. Pharmacotherapy of hypertension in chronic dialysis patients. Clin J Am Soc Nephrol. 2016;11:2062–2075.

2. Kidney Disease: Improving Global Outcomes (KDIGO) Anemia Work Group. KDIGO clinical practice guideline for anemia of chronic kidney disease. Kidney Int Suppl. 2012;2:1–335.

3. Epogen (Epoetin Alfa) [Package Insert]. Thousand Oaks, CA, Amgen Inc., 2018.

4. Kidney Disease: Improving Global Outcomes (KDIGO) CKD-MBD Work Group. KDIGO 2017 clinical practice guideline update for the diagnosis, evaluation, prevention, and treatment of chronic kidney disease-mineral and bone disorder (CKD-MBD). Kidney Int Suppl. 2017;7:1–59.

5. Rottembourg J, Schellekens H. Non biologic complex drug concept: experiences with iron sucrose and low molecular weight heparin. J Blood Lymph. 2014;4:123.

6. Triferic (Ferric Pyrophosphate Citrate) [Package Insert]. Wixom, MI, Rockwell, 2018.

7. Pai AB, Jang SM, Wegrzyn N. Iron-based phosphate binders—a new element in management of hyperphosphatemia. Expert Opin Drug Metab Toxicol. 2016;12:115–127.

57

SYNDROME OF INAPPROPRIATE ANTIDIURETIC HORMONE RELEASE

A Sudden Change of Mind...................... Level I

Kimberly M. Beck, PhD, RPh

Jane M. Gervasio, PharmD, BCNSP, FCCP

LEARNING OBJECTIVES

After completing this case study, the reader should be able to:

- Identify the etiologies of hyponatremia and specifically the syndrome of inappropriate antidiuretic hormone (SIADH) release.

- Assess risk factors for developing hyponatremia and SIADH.

- Evaluate osmotic and fluid status in patients with hyponatremia.

- Recommend and monitor appropriate therapy and alternative treatments for SIADH.

- Discuss treatment options for SIADH, proper administration of selected treatments, and potential side effects.

PATIENT PRESENTATION

■ Chief Complaint

"There's nothing wrong with me, I don't know why she made me come here!"

■ HPI

A 43-year-old man who presents to the ED after several episodes of "weird" behavior, according to his family and friends. He is accompanied by his wife who stated that the patient had been the unrestrained driver in a car accident 3 days earlier. The patient was driving himself home late from work when he swerved off the road and hit a tree. His wife indicates that he hit his head on the steering wheel and lost consciousness for approximately 2 minutes but appeared otherwise unharmed except for a cut on his forehead. The paramedics cleaned and bandaged the patient's lesion and noted that he was combative and disoriented but refused to go to the hospital. The wife states that the patient has not been "acting like himself" since the accident and she had observed him displaying worsening confused and disoriented behavior in the past 24 hours.

■ PMH

Depression for 6 years

■ SH

Lives at home with wife; has two children. Social alcohol use. Denies smoking and use of illicit substances.

■ Meds

Fluoxetine 20 mg by mouth daily for 6 years

All

Penicillin (reaction unknown)

ROS

Difficult to obtain because of decreased mental status. Wife states that he has no medical problems except depression.

Physical Examination

Gen

A&O × 3 but disoriented about recent events. Patient is agitated and confused.

VS

BP 130/84 mm Hg, P 88 bpm, RR 21, T 37°C; Wt 209 lb (95 kg), Ht 5′9″ (175 cm)

Skin

Diaphoretic centrally and very warm; small lesion above left eye

HEENT

NC/AT; EOMI; PERRL; TMs WNL bilaterally

Neck/Lymph Nodes

Supple without lymphadenopathy, masses, goiter, or bruits

Lung/Thorax

Clear to A&P bilaterally

CV

RRR; no MRG

Abd

Soft, NT/ND w/o masses or organomegaly; decreased bowel sounds in all four quadrants

Genit/Rect

Deferred

MS/Ext

Normal ROM; muscle strength 5/5 and equal bilaterally; pulses 2+ throughout; no CCE; capillary refill < 2 seconds

Neuro

CN II–XII intact; DTRs 2/4 and equal bilaterally; sensory intact; (–) Babinski

Labs

Na 112 mEq/L	Ca 9.2 mg/dL	T. chol 167 mg/dL
K 3.9 mEq/L	Phos 2.9 mg/dL	TSH 4.12 μIU/mL
Cl 90 mEq/L	Uric acid 3.2 mg/dL	Serum osmolality 238 mOsm/kg
CO_2 27 mEq/L	AST 87 IU/L	
BUN 16 mg/dL	ALT 59 IU/L	
SCr 0.9 mg/dL	T. bili 0.7 mg/dL	
Glu 115 mg/dL	LDH 256 IU/L	

UA

SG 1.008, pH 6.8, leukocyte esterase (–), nitrite (–), protein (–), ketones (–), urobilinogen nl, bilirubin (–), blood (–), glucose 80 mg/dL, spot urine sodium 125 mEq/L, osmolality 420 mOsm/kg

CT Head

Closed head injury (head trauma)

Assessment

1. Closed head injury
2. SIADH

QUESTIONS

Collect Information

1.a. What subjective and objective information indicates the presence of SIADH?

1.b. What additional information is needed to fully assess this patient's SIADH?

Assess the Information

2.a. Assess the severity of SIADH based on the subjective and objective information available.

2.b. Create a list of the patient's drug therapy problems and prioritize them. Include assessment of medication appropriateness, effectiveness, safety, and patient adherence.

Develop a Care Plan

3.a. What are the goals of pharmacotherapy for SIADH in this case?

3.b. What nondrug therapies might be useful for this patient's SIADH?

3.c. What feasible pharmacotherapeutic alternatives are available for treating SIADH?

3.d. Create an individualized, patient-centered, team-based care plan to optimize medication therapy for this patient's SIADH and other drug therapy problems. Include specific drugs, dosage forms, doses, schedules, and durations of therapy.

Implement the Care Plan

4.a. What information should be provided to the patient to enhance adherence, ensure successful therapy, and minimize adverse effects?

4.b. Describe how care should be coordinated with other healthcare providers.

Follow-Up: Monitor and Evaluate

5. Explain how to monitor and evaluate the care plan for medication appropriateness, effectiveness, safety, and patient adherence by using clinical and laboratory data, patient feedback, and other information.

■ CLINICAL COURSE

After the patient's serum sodium returned to baseline, the team began to discuss his discharge regimen.

FOLLOW-UP QUESTION

1. Identify the appropriate discharge regimen for this patient. Should he continue fluoxetine?

SELF-STUDY ASSIGNMENTS

1. Calculate this patient's serum osmolality and compare this to the measured serum osmolality.

2. What are the risk factors for hyponatremia caused by antidepressants?

3. Perform a literature search to determine which antidepressants are most associated with SIADH. Identify the general progression of antidepressant-induced SIADH.

CLINICAL PEARL

Hyponatremia may result from thiazide and loop diuretic use. Patients present with signs and symptoms of dehydration (poor skin turgor, tachycardia, orthostatic hypotension, oliguria, azotemia, nausea) and potentially low serum potassium and/or magnesium concentrations. Treatment would include normal saline or Lactated Ringer's infusion and discontinuation of offending diuretic.

ACKNOWLEDGMENT

This case is based on the patient case co-written for the 11th edition by Sarah A. Nisly, PharmD, BCPS, FCCP.

REFERENCES

1. Tudor RM, Thompson CJ. Posterior pituitary dysfunction following traumatic brain injury: review. Pituitary. 2019;22:296–304. doi: 10.1007/s11102-018-0917-z.

2. Sterns RH. Treatment of severe hyponatremia. Clin J Am Soc Nephrol. 2018;13:641–649. doi: 10.2215.CJN.10440917.

3. Viramontes TS Truong H, Linnebur SA. Antidepressant-induced hyponatremia in older adults. Consult Pharm. 2016;31:139–150. doi: 10.4140/TCP.n.2016.139.

4. Wilke RA. Potential use of pharmacogenetics to reduce drug-induced syndrome of inappropriate antidiuretic hormone (SIADH). J Pers Med. 2021;11:253. doi: 10.3390/jpm11090853.

5. Mazhar F, Pozzi M, Gentili M, et al. Association of hyponatraemia and antidepressant drugs: a pharmacovigilance-pharmacodynamic assessment through an analysis of the US Food and Drug Administration Adverse Event Reporting System (FAERS) database. CNS Drugs. 2019;33:581–592. doi: 10.1007/s40263-019-00631-5.

6. Hoorn EJ, Zietse R. Diagnosis and treatment of hyponatremia: compilation of the guidelines. J Am Soc Nephrol. 2017;28(5):1340–1349. doi: 10.1681/ASN.2016101139.

7. Der-Nigoghossian C, Lesch C, Berger K. Effectiveness and tolerability of conivaptan and tolvaptan for the treatment of hyponatremia in neurocritically ill patients. Pharmacotherapy. 2017;37:528–534. doi: 10.1002/phar.1926.

8. Morris JH, Bohm NM, Nemecek BD, et al. Rapidity of correction of hyponatremia due to syndrome of inappropriate secretion of antidiuretic hormone following tolvaptan. Am J Kidney Dis. 2018;71:772–782. doi: 10.1053/j.ajkd.2017.12.002.

9. Estilo A, McCormick L, Rahman M. Using tolvaptan to treat hyponatremia: results from a post-authorization pharmacovigilance study. Adv Ther. 2021;38:5721–5736. doi: 10.1007/s12325-021-01947-9.

58

ELECTROLYTE ABNORMALITIES IN CHRONIC KIDNEY DISEASE

Turn Down the 'Lytes . . . . Level II

Lena M. Maynor, PharmD, BCPS

Mary K. Stamatakis, PharmD

LEARNING OBJECTIVES

After completing this case study, the reader should be able to:

• Interpret clinical and biochemical findings in patients with CKD.

• Recommend a patient-specific therapeutic plan for treating electrolyte abnormalities with chronic kidney disease-mineral and bone disorder (CKD-MBD).

• Monitor the effectiveness of the pharmacotherapeutic plan for treating electrolyte abnormalities in CKD.

• Recommend appropriate drug doses in patients undergoing dialysis to minimize the potential for adverse drug events.

PATIENT PRESENTATION

■ Chief Complaint

"I just don't feel like myself."

■ HPI

A 67-year-old man with type 2 DM, HTN, and stage 5 CKD presents to the ED. He receives hemodialysis (HD) three times a week with a high-flux hemodialysis membrane. His wife brought him into the ED this morning after she noticed increased confusion and lethargy, worsening over the past 2–3 days. According to his wife, the patient missed his HD session 2 days ago. She reports no other new symptoms except for increased pain in his feet from his neuropathy for which his PCP increased his gabapentin dose last week.

■ PMH

Type 2 DM × 20 years
HTN × 30 years
Stage 5 CKD; he has been receiving HD for the past 5 years with a high-flux cellulose triacetate membrane; he has no residual renal function
Diabetic neuropathy
Anemia of CKD
Dyslipidemia
CKD-MBD
Uremic pruritus

■ FH

Father with CAD; mother with DM and HTN

■ SH

Retired from a glass factory; on disability; past history of smoking, quit 3 years ago; (–) EtOH for the past 7 years

■ Meds

Gabapentin 300 mg PO BID (increased last week from 300 mg PO at bedtime)
Nephrocaps 1 PO daily
Sodium ferric gluconate 62.5 mg IV once weekly with HD
Metoprolol tartrate 25 mg PO BID
Amlodipine 10 mg PO daily
Lipitor 10 mg PO daily
Glipizide XL 10 mg PO daily
Sitagliptin 25 mg PO daily
Epogen 6000 IU IV three times a week with HD
Calcijex 2 mcg IV three times a week with HD

■ All

NKDA

■ ROS

Increased fatigue and confusion; pain and numbness in lower extremities

■ PE

Gen

Patient somnolent; does not appear to be in distress

VS

BP 168/82 mm Hg, P 82 bpm, RR 14, T 36.8°C; dry body Wt 150 lb (68 kg), Ht 5′11″ (180 cm)

Skin

Normal; intact, warm, and dry

HEENT

NC/AT, PERRLA, EOMI, fundoscopy WNL, oropharyngeal mucosa clear

Neck/Lymph Nodes

Positive JVD; no lymphadenopathy, normal thyroid

Lungs

Crackles in bases bilaterally

CV

Normal S_1 and S_2; no S_3 or S_4

Abd

Soft, NT/ND, no HSM

Genit/Rect

Normal prostate, guaiac-negative stool

MS/Ext

1+ bilateral pedal edema, no clubbing or cyanosis

Neuro

A&O to person only, CN II–XII intact, normal DTRs bilaterally

■ Labs

Na 140 mEq/L	Hgb 11.2 g/dL	Ca 8.4 mg/dL
K 7.1 mEq/L	Hct 34.5%	Mg 2.4 mg/dL
Cl 99 mEq/L	Plt 182 × 10³/mm³	Phos 7.9 mg/dL
CO_2 18 mEq/L	WBC 7.8 × 10³/mm³	AST 12 IU/L
BUN 82 mg/dL		ALT 8 IU/L
SCr 8.2 mg/dL		T. bili 0.9 mg/dL
Glu 118 mg/dL		Alk phos 34 IU/L
		Alb 3.0 g/dL
		Intact PTH 602 pg/mL (last month 595 pg/mL)

■ ABG

pH 7.35, PaO₂ 94, PaCO₂ 38, HCO₃ 20 on room air

■ Chest X-Ray

No infiltrates or effusions

■ ECG

Decreased P waves, widening of the QRS complex, peaked T waves

■ Assessment

A 67-year-old man with type 2 DM, CKD on HD admitted to the hospital with altered mental status and electrolyte abnormalities with plans for emergent hemodialysis.

QUESTIONS

Collect Information

1.a. What subjective and objective information indicates the presence of electrolyte abnormalities?

1.b. What additional information is needed to fully assess this patient's electrolyte abnormalities?

Assess the Information

2.a. Assess the severity of electrolyte abnormalities based on the subjective and objective information available.

2.b. Create a list of the patient's drug therapy problems and prioritize them. Include assessment of medication appropriateness, effectiveness, safety, and patient adherence.

Develop a Care Plan

3.a. What are the goals of pharmacotherapy for the electrolyte abnormalities in this case?

3.b. What nondrug therapies might be useful for this patient's electrolyte abnormalities?

3.c. What feasible pharmacotherapeutic alternatives are available for treating the electrolyte abnormalities?

3.d. Create an individualized, patient-centered, team-based care plan to optimize medication therapy for this patient's electrolyte abnormalities and other drug therapy problems. Include specific drugs, dosage forms, doses, schedules, and durations of therapy.

Implement the Care Plan

4.a. What information should be provided to the patient to enhance adherence, ensure successful therapy, and minimize adverse effects?

4.b. Describe how care should be coordinated with other healthcare providers.

Follow-Up: Monitor and Evaluate

5. Explain how to monitor and evaluate the care plan for medication appropriateness, effectiveness, safety, and patient adherence by using clinical and laboratory data, patient feedback, and other information.

■ SELF-STUDY ASSIGNMENT

1. Determine the need for and timing of screening for complications associated with CKD, such as anemia of CKD and CKD-MBD.
2. Create a list of medications that are associated with hyperkalemia.

CLINICAL PEARL

Erythropoietin can be administered at any time during the dialysis procedure because of its large molecular weight. The molecule is too large to fit through the pores of a dialysis membrane and is therefore not eliminated during the dialysis procedure.

REFERENCES

1. KDIGO 2017 clinical practice guideline update for the diagnosis, evaluation, prevention, and treatment of chronic kidney disease-mineral and bone disorder (CKD-MBD). Kidney Int Suppl. 2017;7:1–59.
2. Alfonzo A, Harrison A, Baines R, et al. Clinical practice guidelines: Treatment of acute hyperkalaemia in adults. Bristol, UK: UK Renal Association; 2020. Available at: *https://ukkidney.org/sites/renal.org/files/RENAL%20ASSOCIATION%20HYPERKALAEMIA%20GUIDELINE%202020.pdf.* Accessed September 17, 2021.
3. Kasai S, Sato K, Murata Y, Kinoshita Y. Randomized crossover study of the efficacy and safety of sevelamer hydrochloride and lanthanum carbonate in Japanese patients undergoing hemodialysis. Ther Apher Dial. 2012;16:341–349.
4. Floege J, Covic AC, Ketteler M, et al. Long-term effects of the iron-based phosphate binder, sucroferric oxyhydroxide, in dialysis patients. Nephrol Dial Transplant. 2015;30:1037–1046.
5. Ganz T, Bino A, Salusky IB. Mechanism of action and clinical attributes of Auryxia® (ferric citrate). Drugs. 2019;79:957–968.

59

HYPERCALCEMIA OF MALIGNANCY

Up, Up, and Away............................ Level II

Laura L. Jung, BS Pharm, PharmD

Lisa M. Holle, BS Pharm, PharmD, BCOP, FHOPA, FISOPP

LEARNING OBJECTIVES

After completing this case study, the reader should be able to:

• Recognize the signs and symptoms of hypercalcemia.
• Evaluate laboratory data and clinical symptoms for assessment and monitoring of hypercalcemia, hypercalcemia treatment, and complications of hypercalcemia.
• Recommend a pharmacotherapeutic plan for the initial treatment of cancer-related hypercalcemia.
• Recognize and develop management strategies for toxicities associated with treatment options for hypercalcemia.

PATIENT PRESENTATION

■ Chief Complaint

"I can't stop throwing up."

■ HPI

A 62-year-old woman presents to her family practitioner today with a 2-day history of nausea and vomiting. She states that her stomach has not felt normal for the past 3–4 days and is painful. Her daughter states that for the past several days, she has complained of constipation, nausea, and extreme thirst, but because she has been vomiting, it has been hard to keep her mother drinking enough liquids. She also reports that her mother stopped taking the sustained-release morphine that was started last week because she thought these were side effects of the morphine. The daughter states that her mom's last bowel movement was 3 days ago despite administration of a stool softener daily. The daughter also reports her mother has gone "downhill" over the past month and spends 80% of her day in bed and the remainder in the recliner.

■ PMH

Stage IV non–small cell lung cancer diagnosed 1.5 years ago. At the time of diagnosis, a CT scan revealed a 3-cm mass in the hilum of the right lung, extensive mediastinal lymphadenopathy, and a moderate right pleural effusion with pleural studding. A transbronchial biopsy identified the mass as adenocarcinoma, epidermal growth factor (EGFR), anaplastic lymphoma kinase (ALK), ROS1, BRAF V600E mutations, negative, and PD-L1 expression positive (30%). Cytology of the pleural effusion also revealed adenocarcinoma. She was treated with the following regimens: (1) pembrolizumab/carboplatin/pemetrexed × 4 cycles; (2) pembrolizumab/pemetrexed maintenance × 6 cycles; (3) docetaxel × 8 cycles; and (4) gemcitabine × 3 cycles. The last CT scan performed yesterday revealed a new tumor 3.5 × 4.2 mm in the left lower lobe and liver metastases.

COPD × 4 years
Dyslipidemia

■ FH

Mother died of NSCLC at age 80 years; father died of MI at 64 years; one sister died of breast cancer at 69 years; one sister and three brothers alive.

■ SH

Tobacco: 2 ppd × 30 years; chronic alcohol use × 30 years EtOH (three to four drinks per day). Worked as an office assistant × 25 years. Lives at home with boyfriend of 16 years; has four grown daughters, ages 47, 44, 39, and 34 years. Had her first child at age 15.

■ Meds

Morphine sulfate sustained-release 30 mg PO Q 12 H (started 1 week ago)
Morphine sulfate oral solution 5 mg PO Q 2 H PRN pain (estimated use two times in the 24 hours before she stopped taking sustained-released)
Docusate sodium 200 mg PO at bedtime PRN
Simvastatin 20 mg PO daily

■ All

Cephalosporins, penicillin

■ ROS

No fever or chills. Daughter has noted that the patient is more tired than usual and is extremely thirsty, which she believes has affected her appetite over the past week. She denies polyuria, chest pain, unusual shortness of breath, dyspnea, or cough. The patient states her pain is 8/10 throughout the day.

■ Physical Examination

Gen

Thin woman in obvious discomfort

VS

BP 95/70 mm Hg, P 105 bpm, RR 16, T 38°C; Wt 110 lb (50 kg), Ht 5'1" (152.5 cm)

Skin

Slightly warm to touch, fair skin turgor (mild tenting noted)

HEENT

PERRLA, EOMI, fundi benign; nonerythematous TMs; oropharynx clear; mucous membranes dry

Neck/Lymph Nodes

Neck supple, slight axillary lymphadenopathy

Lungs

Decreased breath sounds; bilateral wheezes

Breasts

Breasts nontender. No palpable masses or nipple discharge.

CV

RRR, S_1, S_2 normal; ECG shows shortened ST and QT intervals

Abd

Firm, distended, tender; decreased bowel sounds; stool palpable on left side

Genit/Rect

Normal female genitalia; stool heme (–)

MS/Ext

Bilateral lower extremity weakness graded at 4/5; otherwise normal

Neuro

A&O × 3; sensory and motor intact; strength 5/5 upper, 4/5 lower; CN II–XII intact; Babinski (–)

■ Labs

Na 142 mEq/L	AST 63 IU/L	Ca 14.0 mg/dL	WBC 6.8 × 10³/mm³
K 3.5 mEq/L	ALT 35 IU/L	Mg 1.5 mEq/L	Hgb 12.7 g/dL
Cl 109 mEq/L	Alk phos 200 IU/L	Phos 3.5 mEq/L	Hct 40%
CO₂ 22 mEq/L	T. prot 5.1 g/dL	Alb 2.2 g/dL	Plt 174 × 10³/mm³
BUN 40 mg/dL	T. bili 1.6 mg/dL	LDH 160 IU/L	
SCr 1.4 mg/dL	D. bili 0.7 mg/dL		
Glu 100 mg/dL			

■ Chest X-Ray

Osteolytic lesions on the right and left clavicles, masses in right and left lower lobes consistent with NSCLC

■ Assessment

A 62-year-old woman with metastatic NSCLC s/p three different treatment regimens. Poor performance status. Presenting with first episode of possible tumor-induced hypercalcemia with associated complications and uncontrolled pain.

Admit to inpatient oncology service for further management of hypercalcemia, related complications, and pain control.

QUESTIONS

Collect Information

1.a. What subjective and objective information indicates the presence of hypercalcemia of malignancy?

1.b. What additional information is needed to fully assess this patient's hypercalcemia of malignancy?

Assess the Information

2.a. Assess the severity of hypercalcemia of malignancy based on the subjective and objective information available.

2.b. Create a list of the patient's drug therapy problems and prioritize them. Include assessment of medication appropriateness, effectiveness, safety, and patient adherence.

Develop a Care Plan

3.a. What are the goals of pharmacotherapy for hypercalcemia of malignancy in this case?

3.b. What nondrug therapies might be useful for this patient's hypercalcemia of malignancy?

3.c. What feasible pharmacotherapeutic alternatives are available for treating hypercalcemia of malignancy?

3.d. Create an individualized, patient-centered, team-based care plan to optimize medication therapy for this patient's hypercalcemia of malignancy and other drug therapy problems. Include specific drugs, dosage forms, doses, schedules, and durations of therapy.

3.e. What alternatives would be appropriate if the initial care plan fails or cannot be used?

Implement the Care Plan

4.a. What information should be provided to the patient to enhance adherence, ensure successful therapy, and minimize adverse effects?

4.b. Describe how care should be coordinated with other healthcare providers.

Follow-Up: Monitor and Evaluate

5. Explain how to monitor and evaluate the care plan for medication appropriateness, effectiveness, safety, and patient adherence by using clinical and laboratory data, patient feedback, and other information.

■ CLINICAL COURSE

Patient's serum calcium level decreased to 8.8 mg/dL by day 3 with the treatment you recommended. She was discharged from the hospital on day 5 with improvement in her mental status. However, she returned to the hospital on day 10 with a serum calcium level of 15.2 mg/dL. She is very somnolent and lethargic.

CHAPTER 60

■ FOLLOW-UP QUESTIONS

1. What pharmacologic and nonpharmacologic options might be considered at this time and why?

2. How would you monitor the therapy you recommended for efficacy and adverse effects?

■ SELF-STUDY ASSIGNMENTS

1. What nonmalignant disease states can induce hypercalcemia?

2. What treatment(s) can decrease the risk of developing hypercalcemia in patients receiving calcitriol for anticancer therapy?

CLINICAL PEARL

Although denosumab does not need to be dose reduced in renal dysfunction, practitioners should be aware of an increased risk of hypocalcemia, even in HCM patients.

REFERENCES

1. Wagner J, Arora S. Oncologic metabolic emergencies. Hematol Oncol Clin N Am. 2017;31:941–957.

2. Mirrakhimov AE. Hypercalcemia of malignancy: an update on pathogenesis and management. N Am J Med Sci. 2015;7:483–493.

3. Shane E, Berenson JR. Treatment of hypercalcemia. In: Mulder JE, ed. UpToDate. https://www.uptodate.com/contents/treatment-of-hypercalcemia. Accessed October 19, 2021.

4. Goldner W. Cancer-related hypercalcemia. J Oncol Pract. 2016;12:426–432.

5. Bentata Y, El Maghraoui H, Benabdelhak M, et al. Management of hypercalcaemic crisis in adults: current role of renal replacement therapy. Am J Emerg Med. 2018;36:1053–1056.

6. Sternlicht H, Glezerman IG. Hypercalcemia of malignancy and new treatment options. Ther Clin Risk Manag. 2015;11:1779–1788.

7. Zometa [Package Insert]. Novartis Pharmaceuticals Corporation, East Hanover, NJ, 2018.

8. Sensipar [Package Insert]. Amgen Inc, Thousand Oaks, CA. 2019.

9. Non-Small Cell Lung Cancer NCCN Clinical Practice Guidelines in Oncology. V.6.2021. 2021 National Comprehensive Cancer Network, Inc. Available at: NCCN.org. Accessed October 19, 2021.

10. Asonitis N, Kassi E, Kokkinos M, et al. Hypercalcemia of malignancy treated with cinacalcet. Endocrinol Diabetes Metab. 2017;17:pii 17-0118.

60

HYPOKALEMIA AND HYPOMAGNESEMIA

Blinded by the Lytes . . . . Level III

Denise M. Kolanczyk, PharmD, BCPS

LEARNING OBJECTIVES

After completing this case study, the reader should be able to:

• Identify potential causes of electrolyte disorders.

• Select the appropriate route of administration and dose of electrolyte replacement therapy specific for a patient.

• Develop a monitoring plan for efficacy and toxicity in patients receiving electrolyte replacement therapy.

• Outline a patient education plan for a patient receiving electrolyte replacement supplements.

PATIENT PRESENTATION

■ Chief Complaint

"I'm short of breath."

■ HPI

A 45-year-old woman with a history of nonischemic cardiomyopathy presents to the ED with a 3-day history of shortness of breath with mild to moderate exertion. She reports three-pillow orthopnea × 2 days and cough during sleep. Denies chest pain; occasional palpitations. She has some stomach discomfort that she notices after taking her potassium supplement. She reports a 10-lb weight gain in the past week and an increase in her lower extremity edema.

Approximately 1 month ago, she was hospitalized with atypical chest pain and had persistent hypokalemia for which her metolazone 5 mg daily was discontinued. About 2 weeks ago, she visited the ED due to significant fluid retention in her lower extremities. Her potassium was 7.2 mEq/L (hemolyzed sample); it was repeated with a result of 5.5 mEq/L. At that time, her potassium supplement dose was reduced from 80 mEq PO QID to 80 mEq PO BID, and she was instructed to resume metolazone 5 mg PO MWF only.

■ PMH (Per Patient Report and Medical Records)

Nonischemic cardiomyopathy—echo LVEF 25% (11 months ago)
ICD placement 1 month ago
HTN
Asthma
Type 2 DM with peripheral neuropathy
Obesity
Hypothyroidism

■ FH

Both parents are deceased.

■ SH

Lives with husband. No alcohol use. Former smoker—quit 8 years ago. No illicit drugs.

■ Meds

Candesartan 32 mg PO daily
Carvedilol 25 mg PO BID
Spironolactone 25 mg PO daily
Furosemide 80 mg PO BID
Metolazone 5 mg PO MWF
Atorvastatin 20 mg PO daily
Metformin 1000 mg PO BID
Pregabalin 50 mg PO BID
Tiotropium one capsule (18 mcg) inhaled once daily
Fluticasone/salmeterol 500/50 one inhalation BID
Albuterol 90 mcg/actuation 2 inhalations q6 PRN SOB
Magnesium oxide 400 mg PO daily
Potassium chloride 80 mEq PO BID
Levothyroxine 75 mcg PO daily

ALL

NKDA

ROS

Patient reports becoming short of breath for the past 3 days while walking up one flight of stairs or if she walks too quickly on a flat surface. Previously she could walk two flights of stairs before becoming short of breath. She uses three pillows at night to sleep but does not report PND. She reports increased swelling in her lower extremities, abdominal fullness, and early satiety. Additionally, she reports mild nausea when taking her potassium supplement. States that she has not changed her diet but did visit her sister and family 1 week ago and ate foods that are not part of her usual diet (eg, fried chicken, fried vegetables, chips, and dip). Denies ever having an ICD discharge.

Physical Examination

Gen

Appears older than her stated age; obese; mild dyspnea at rest

VS

BP 115/70 mmHg, P 106 bpm, RR 20, T 35.8°C, O_2 sat 88% room air
Wt 192 lb [87.3 kg; baseline weight 184 lb (83.6 kg)], Ht 5′5″ (165 cm)

Skin

Skin warm, dry

HEENT

PERRLA; conjunctivae clear; moist mucous membranes; tongue midline

Neck/Lymph Nodes

Supple; JVP estimated at 14 cm; no carotid bruit; no lymphadenopathy; (+) thyroid nodules

Lungs

Bibasilar rales R > L; occasional wheezes

CV

Tachycardic; normal S_1, S_2; $+S_3$; $-S_4$; 2/6 holosystolic murmur best heard at second left intercostal space

Abd

Obese; good bowel sounds; no bruits; no hepatosplenomegaly, (+) hepatojugular reflux; no evidence of ascites

Genit/Rect

Deferred

Ext

No cyanosis; 3+ pitting edema to knees bilaterally; 2+ pulses bilaterally in upper and lower extremities

Back

No CVA tenderness

Neuro

Alert and oriented × 3; no focal deficits; mild sensory deficit in feet bilaterally; CN II–XII grossly intact

Labs

Na 130 mEq/L	Hgb 10.4 g/dL	Ca 8.3 mg/dL	Alb 3.0 g/dL
K 2.8 mEq/L	Hct 29.3%	Mg 1.3 mEq/L	PT 14 seconds
Cl 93 mEq/L	WBC $4.5 \times 10^3/mm^3$	Phos 3.1 mEq/L	INR 1.2
CO_2 30 mEq/L		AST 100 IU/L	aPTT 21 seconds
BUN 17 mg/dL	Plt $165 \times 10^3/mm^3$	ALT 110 IU/L	CK 30 IU/L
SCr 1.0 mg/dL	BNP 1533 pg/mL	Troponin I	
Glu 143 mg/dL	A1C 7.8%	<0.01 ng/mL	

Chest X-Ray

Bilateral pulmonary edema; moderate R pleural effusion; small L pleural effusion; (+) cardiomegaly

12-Lead ECG

Sinus tachycardia; LBBB; no evidence of acute ischemia

Assessment

A 45-year-old female with a history of nonischemic cardiomyopathy presents with volume overload and electrolyte abnormalities. Admit to inpatient telemetry unit for management.

QUESTIONS

Collect Information

1.a. What subjective and objective information indicates the presence of electrolyte abnormalities?

1.b. What additional information is needed to fully assess this patient's electrolyte abnormalities?

Assess the Information

2.a. Assess the severity of the patient's electrolyte abnormalities based on the subjective and objective information available. Classify this patient's hyponatremia.

2.b. Create a list of the patient's drug therapy problems and prioritize them. Include assessment of medication appropriateness, effectiveness, safety, and patient adherence.

Develop a Care Plan

3.a. What are the goals of pharmacotherapy for the electrolyte abnormalities in this case?

3.b. What nondrug therapies might be useful for this patient's electrolyte abnormalities?

3.c. What feasible pharmacotherapeutic alternatives are available for treating the patient's hypokalemia, hypomagnesemia, and hypervolemic hyponatremia?

3.d. Create an individualized, patient-centered, team-based care plan to optimize medication therapy for this patient's electrolyte abnormalities and other drug-related problems. Include specific drugs, dosage forms, doses, schedules, and durations of therapy.

Implement the Care Plan

4.a. What information should be provided to the patient to enhance adherence, ensure successful therapy, and minimize adverse effects?

4.b. Describe how care should be coordinated with other healthcare providers.

Follow-Up: Monitor and Evaluate

5. Explain how to monitor and evaluate the care plan for medication appropriateness, effectiveness, safety, and patient adherence by using clinical and laboratory data, patient feedback, and other information.

■ CLINICAL COURSE

The medical team implemented the pharmacotherapy plan you recommended. Today is day 4 of hospitalization, and her clinical status is improved. She states she can walk further without becoming short of breath and only needs one pillow to sleep. Additionally, she describes less swelling in her legs. On physical exam, her HR is 73, BP is 108/57 mm Hg, and O_2 saturation is 96% on room air. Her lungs are clear, and she has 1+ edema in her legs. Pertinent laboratory results indicate serum potassium 3.8 mEq/L, SCr 1.2 mg/dL, Mg 1.8 mg/dL, CO_2 26 mEq/L, and Glu 129 mg/dL. Her JVP is 8 cm, and she has no hepatojugular reflex. She is scheduled for discharge today.

■ FOLLOW-UP QUESTION

1. What changes should be made to the patient's medication regimen at hospital discharge to prevent future electrolyte imbalances?

■ SELF-STUDY ASSIGNMENT

1. Describe how a patient's acid–base status can affect serum electrolyte concentrations.

2. Discuss changes to the patient's outpatient management that would optimize outcomes for heart failure and hyperglycemia.

CLINICAL PEARL

Hypokalemia and hypomagnesemia often coexist. In patients refractory to potassium replacement, magnesium concentrations should be evaluated, and any magnesium deficit must be corrected before potassium can be appropriately replaced.

REFERENCES

1. Kraft MD, Btaiche IF, Sacks GS, Kudsk KA. Treatment of electrolyte disorders in adult patients in the intensive care unit. Am J Health-Syst Pharm. 2005;62:1663–1682.

2. Ahmed F, Mohammed A. Magnesium: the forgotten electrolyte—a review on hypomagnesemia. Med Sci. 2019;7:56. doi: 10.3390/medsci7040056.

3. Weir MR, Espaillat R. Clinical perspectives on the rationale for potassium supplementation. Postgrad Med. 2015;127(5):539–548.

4. Cohn JN, Kowey PR, Whelton PK, Prisant M. New guidelines for potassium replacement in clinical practice. A contemporary review by the National Council on Potassium in Clinical Practice. Arch Intern Med. 2000;160:2429–2436.

5. Hollenberg SM, Stevenson LW, Ahmad T, et al. 2019 ACC expert consensus decision pathway on risk assessment, management, and clinical trajectory of patients hospitalized with heart failure: a report of the American College of Cardiology Solution Set Oversight Committee. J Am Coll Cardiol. 2019;74(15):1966–2011.

6. Ferreira JP, Butler J, Rossignol P, et al. Abnormalities of potassium in heart failure. JACC state-of-the-art review. J Am Coll Cardiol. 2020;75(22):2836–2850.

7. American Diabetes Association. Diabetes care in the hospital: Standards of Medical Care in Diabetes—2022. Diabetes Care. 2022;45(Suppl 1):S244–S253.

8. Yancy CW, Januzzi JL Jr, Allen LA, et al. 2017 ACC expert consensus decision pathway for optimization of heart failure treatment: answers to 10 pivotal issues about heart failure with reduced ejection fraction: a report of the American College of Cardiology Task Force on Clinical Expert Consensus Decision Pathways. J Am Coll. 2018;71:201–230.

61

METABOLIC ACIDOSIS

Oh, My Aching Acidosis........................ Level II

Justin M. Schmidt, PharmD, BCPS

LEARNING OBJECTIVES

After completing this case study, the reader should be able to:

• Determine the clinical and laboratory manifestations of metabolic acidosis.

• Differentiate the most probable cause(s) of metabolic acidosis.

• Develop a patient-specific pharmacotherapeutic plan for treating chronic metabolic acidosis.

• Provide medication education for patients with chronic metabolic acidosis.

PATIENT PRESENTATION

■ Chief Complaint

"I just feel so weak all the time."

■ HPI

A 67-year-old woman with progressive CKD due to HTN was referred to the nephrology clinic for management of fatigue. Her fatigue started a couple of years ago but has progressed to the point that it interferes with her gardening and evening walks. She reports occasional muscle cramps (one every 1–2 months) that last a few seconds to minutes and are not associated with exertion. She reports frequent nonadherence to her furosemide when she feels well.

■ PMH

HTN
CKD stage 4
Seasonal allergic rhinitis
Menopause at 53 years old

■ FH

History of CAD in her mother's family (mother had a heart attack at age 60). No known family history of CKD.

■ **SH**

The patient is a retired schoolteacher who lives with her husband of 38 years and has three grown children. She denies alcohol use. There is no history of tobacco habituation or recreational drug use.

■ **Meds**

Amlodipine 5 mg PO daily
Aspirin 81 mg PO daily
Furosemide 40 mg PO daily, taken intermittently for lower extremity edema (reports that she has not taken any for the past few months)
Metoprolol succinate 25 mg PO daily

■ **All**

NKDA

■ **ROS**

Fatigue worsening over the past 2 years. Denies weight changes or changes in appetite. Denies fever/chills. No palpitations, shortness of breath, or chest pain. Denies abdominal pain, nausea/vomiting, and melena. Admits to weakness and reports occasional myalgia but is not experiencing myalgias currently.

■ **PE**

Gen

Pleasant woman in NAD

VS

BP 155/85 mm Hg, P 78 bpm, RR 16, T 37.2°C; Wt 165 lb (75 kg), Ht 5′4″ (162.5 cm)

Skin

Normal color and texture. Intact, warm and dry.

HEENT

No hemorrhages or exudates on funduscopic examination

Neck/Lymph Nodes

JVP 3 cm; carotid pulses 2+ bilaterally; no thyromegaly or lymphadenopathy

Chest

CTA and P

CV

Unable to palpate PMI; regular rate and rhythm; normal S_1 and S_2; no murmurs

Abd

Obese, soft, nontender; normoactive bowel sounds; no organomegaly

MS/Ext

Minimal sternal tenderness

Neuro

No focal cranial nerve deficits; strength 4/5 in all extremities.

■ **Labs**

Na 138 mEq/L	Hgb 12.2 g/dL	AST 13 IU/L
K 4.4 mEq/L	Hct 37 %	ALT 7 IU/L
Cl 112 mEq/L	Plt 225 × 10³/mm³	Alk phos 113 IU/L
CO_2 19 mEq/L	WBC 7.6 × 10³/mm³	GGT 14 IU/L
BUN 37 mg/dL	Ca 8.4 mg/dL	T. bili 0.4 mg/dL
SCr 2.9 mg/dL	Mg 2.2 mg/dL	Alb 3.6 g/dL
Glu 89 mg/dL	Phos 4.3 mg/dL	

eGFR (CKD-EPI) 21 mL/min/1.73 m²

■ **ABG on RA**

pH 7.32; $PaCO_2$ 36 mm Hg; PaO_2 106 mm Hg; bicarbonate 19 mEq/L

■ **Urinalysis macro (dipstick) panel**

Color yellow; appearance clear; SG 1.025; pH 5.2; blood (−); glucose (−); ketones (−); leukocyte esterase (−); nitrite (−); bilirubin (−); urobilinogen 0.5 mg/dL; protein > 300 mg/day

■ **KUB**

No nephrocalcinosis or nephrolithiasis

■ **Assessment**

1. Acidosis
2. CKD
3. Hypertension

QUESTIONS

Collect Information

1.a. What subjective and objective information indicates the presence of metabolic acidosis?

1.b. What additional information is needed to fully assess this patient's metabolic acidosis and related complications?

Assess the Information

2.a. Assess the severity of metabolic acidosis based on the subjective and objective information available.

2.b. Create a list of the patient's drug therapy problems and prioritize them. Include assessment of medication appropriateness, effectiveness, safety, and patient adherence.

2.c. What factors may have contributed to the development of metabolic acidosis?

Develop a Care Plan

3.a. What are the goals of pharmacotherapy for metabolic acidosis in this case?

3.b. What nondrug therapies might be useful for this patient's metabolic acidosis?

3.c. What feasible pharmacotherapeutic alternatives are available for treating metabolic acidosis?

3.d. Create an individualized, patient-centered, team-based care plan to optimize medication therapy for this patient's metabolic acidosis and other drug therapy problems. Include specific drugs, dosage forms, doses, schedules, and durations of therapy.

3.e. What alternatives would be appropriate if the initial care plan fails or cannot be used?

Implement the Care Plan

4.a. What information should be provided to the patient to enhance adherence, ensure successful therapy, and minimize adverse effects?

4.b. Describe how care should be coordinated with other healthcare providers.

Follow-Up: Monitor and Evaluate

5. Explain how to monitor and evaluate the care plan for medication appropriateness, effectiveness, safety, and patient adherence by using clinical and laboratory data, patient feedback, and other information.

■ SELF-STUDY ASSIGNMENTS

1. Differentiate between the bone disease of metabolic acidosis versus that associated with chronic kidney disease and osteoporosis.

2. Discuss the types of metabolic acidoses that may be present in patients with CKD and how they may be differentiated.

CLINICAL PEARL

While the chronic metabolic acidosis associated with CKD is usually not progressive, there is increasing evidence that correction of acidosis is related to decreased progression of CKD. Appropriate oral alkali therapy or dietary intervention may result in improved nutritional status, renal function, and quality of life for patients with CKD.

REFERENCES

1. Ikizler TA, Burrowes JD, Byham-Gray LD, et al. KDOQI clinical practice guideline for nutrition in CKD: 2020 update. Am J Kidney Dis. 2020;76:S1–S107.
2. Kraut JA, Madias NE. Metabolic acidosis of CKD: an update. Am J Kidney Dis. 2016;67:307–317.
3. Kidney Disease: Improving Global Outcomes (KDIGO) CKD Work Group. KDIGO 2012 clinical practice guideline for the evaluation and management of chronic kidney disease. Kidney Int Suppl. 2013;3:1–150.
4. Melamed ML, Raphael KL. Metabolic acidosis in CKD: a review of recent findings. Kidney Med. 2021;3:267–277.
5. Kidney Disease: Improving Global Outcomes (KDIGO) Blood Pressure Work Group. KDIGO 2021 clinical practice guideline for the management of blood pressure in chronic kidney disease. Kidney Int. 2021;99:S1–S87.
6. Goraya N, Simoni J, Jo C, Wesson DE. A comparison of treating metabolic acidosis in CKD stage 4 hypertensive kidney disease with fruits and vegetables or sodium bicarbonate. Clin J Am Soc Nephrol. 2013;8:371–381.
7. Foque D, Pelletier S, Mafra D, Chauveau P. Nutrition and chronic kidney disease. Kidney Int Suppl. 2011;80:348–357.
8. Raphael KL. Approach to the treatment of chronic metabolic acidosis in CKD. Am J Kidney Dis. 2016;67:696–702.
9. McNeil JJ, Wolfe R, Woods RL, et al. Effect of aspirin on cardiovascular events and bleeding in the healthy elderly. N Eng J Med. 2018;379:1509–1518.
10. Kidney Disease: Improving Global Outcomes (KDIGO) CKD–MBD Work Group. KDIGO 2017 clinical practice guideline update for the diagnosis, evaluation, prevention, and treatment of chronic kidney disease–mineral and bone disorder (CKD–MBD). Kidney Int Suppl. 2017;7:1–60.

62

METABOLIC ALKALOSIS

Keep Me in the Loop . . . . Level I

Natalie I. Rine, PharmD, BCPS, BCCCP

LEARNING OBJECTIVES

After completing this case study, the reader should be able to:

- Identify the signs and symptoms of metabolic alkalosis.
- Interpret laboratory findings that are consistent with metabolic alkalosis.
- Describe patient-specific factors that contribute to the development of metabolic disorders.
- Recommend appropriate first-line treatment regimens and alternatives for metabolic alkalosis.
- Formulate a patient-specific pharmacotherapeutic plan for the treatment and monitoring of metabolic alkalosis.

PATIENT PRESENTATION

■ Chief Complaint

"I feel very weak and tired."

■ HPI

A 60-year-old male presents to the ED with complaints of generalized weakness, fatigue, myalgias, and polyuria over the past 2 days. He states that recently he has felt bloated and has been taking extra doses of his "water pill." He also mentioned that he may have eaten something bad because he has thrown up three times since dinner last night.

■ PMH

Hypertension (diagnosed 15 years ago)
HFrEF (diagnosed 3 years ago)
Diabetes, type 2—diet controlled
Dyslipidemia (diagnosed 3 years ago)

■ FH

Mother is alive with a history of HTN and dyslipidemia. Father is alive with HTN. Younger sister is alive with dyslipidemia.

■ SH

Patient reports he does not consume alcohol except a glass of wine "at special occasions." He denies tobacco or illicit drug use. Lives at home with his wife of 35 years and their two dogs.

■ Meds

Lisinopril 20 mg PO once daily
Carvedilol 25 mg PO BID
Furosemide 40 mg PO once daily
Atorvastatin 40 mg PO once daily
Last dose of all medications was this morning 3 hours before arriving at the ED

■ All

Codeine—patient reports "I get short of breath."

■ ROS

Denies unusual weight gain or loss. He denies fever, chills, or night sweats, but reports dizziness that has occurred off and on over the past week in addition to generalized fatigue and weakness. No reported chest pain, palpitations, shortness of breath, or cough. He denies diarrhea, constipation, or change in bowel habits. He reports a recent increase in thirst and urination, but no change in urine color. He reports myalgias and perioral numbness that began recently with the fatigue and weakness.

■ Physical Examination

Gen

The patient is ill-appearing and feels warm to the touch.

VS

BP 93/62 mm Hg, HR 101, RR 20, T 37.9°C; Wt 176 lb (80 kg), Ht 5'7" (170 cm); O_2 sat 96% on RA

Skin

Soft, intact, warm, dry

HEENT

EOMI; PERRLA; no sinus tenderness; dry mucous membranes; no oral lesions; no nasal congestion present

Neck/Lymph Nodes

No JVD or bruits; no lymphadenopathy or thyromegaly

Chest

CTA bilaterally

CV

RRR; normal S_1, S_2; no S_3 or S_4; no murmurs, rubs, gallops

Abd

Soft, NTND; (+) bowel sounds

GU/Rect

WNL

MS/Ext

No CCE; feet are dry and wrinkled

Neuro

A&O × 3. CN II–XII intact.

Labs

Na 132 mEq/L	Hgb 12.4 g/dL	Alb 3.8 g/dL
K 2.9 mEq/L	Hct 36.7%	AST 19 IU/L
Cl 85 mEq/L	Plt 324 × 10³/mm³	ALT 16 IU/L
CO₂ 39 mEq/L	WBC 12.1 × 10³/mm³	Alk phos 62 IU/L
BUN 24 mg/dL	Mg 1.7 mEq/L	T. bili 0.4 mg/dL
SCr 1.1 mg/dL	Phos 3.6 mg/dL	PT 11.3 s
Glu 118 mg/dL	Ca 7.6 mg/dL	INR 0.96
		HgbA1C 5.6%

■ ABG

pH 7.54, $PaCO_2$ 46 mm Hg, PaO_2 86 mm Hg, HCO_3 38.3 mEq/L on RA

■ UA

Urine sodium 18 mEq/L; potassium 33 mEq/L; chloride 9 mEq/L, urine pH 6.1

■ Chest X-Ray

Mild pulmonary congestion, otherwise unremarkable

■ ECG

Sinus tachycardia, rate 101, no acute ST-segment or T-wave changes

■ Assessment

Admit patient for hypotension, flulike symptoms, electrolyte and acid–base abnormalities.

QUESTIONS

Collect Information

1.a. What subjective and objective information indicates the presence of metabolic alkalosis?

1.b. What additional information is needed to fully assess this patient's metabolic alkalosis?

Assess the Information

2.a. Assess the severity of metabolic alkalosis based on the subjective and objective information available.

2.b. Create a list of the patient's drug therapy problems and prioritize them. Include assessment of medication appropriateness, effectiveness, safety, and patient adherence.

2.c. What are possible nondrug-related causes of this patient's metabolic alkalosis?

Develop a Care Plan

3.a. What are the goals of pharmacotherapy for metabolic alkalosis in this case?

3.b. What nondrug therapies might be useful for this patient's metabolic alkalosis?

3.c. What feasible pharmacotherapeutic alternatives are available for treating metabolic alkalosis?

3.d. Create an individualized, patient-centered, team-based care plan to optimize medication therapy for this patient's metabolic alkalosis and other drug-related problems. Include specific drugs, dosage forms, doses, schedules, and durations of therapy.

Implement the Care Plan

4.a. What information should be provided to the patient to enhance adherence, ensure successful therapy, and minimize adverse effects?

4.b. Describe how care should be coordinated with other healthcare providers.

Follow-Up: Monitor and Evaluate

5. Explain how to monitor and evaluate the care plan for medication appropriateness, effectiveness, safety, and patient

adherence by using clinical and laboratory data, patient feedback, and other information.

■ CLINICAL COURSE

The patient was started on IV fluids, and labs were reassessed a few hours later. The patient is observed to have 1+ pitting edema in the lower extremities. Laboratory values are as follows:

Na 140 mEq/L	BUN 14 mg/dL	*ABG*
K 3.8 mEq/L	SCr 0.8 mg/dL	pH 7.46
Cl 103 mEq/L	Mg 2.1 mEq/L	$PaCO_2$ 39 mm Hg
CO_2 30 mEq/L		PaO_2 92 mm Hg
		HCO_3 31 mEq/L

■ FOLLOW-UP QUESTION

1. Based on the new findings, what modifications in therapy are warranted, if any?

■ SELF-STUDY ASSIGNMENTS

1. Prepare a paper on the three phases (initiation, maintenance, and compensation) of the pathogenesis of metabolic alkalosis. Describe the mechanisms behind each phase and the treatments, if appropriate.

2. Describe how assessment of urine electrolytes is useful in the diagnosis and treatment of metabolic alkalosis.

3. Research what medications, dietary supplements, and medical procedures could contribute to metabolic alkalosis.

CLINICAL PEARL

Although most cases of metabolic alkalosis are asymptomatic, the disorder can lead to serious complications from electrolyte abnormalities (eg, tetany, arrhythmias, mental status changes). In addition to assessing arterial blood gas and laboratory tests, it is important to obtain a thorough patient history to identify underlying cause of metabolic alkalosis and treat it appropriately.

REFERENCES

1. Emmett M. Metabolic alkalosis: a brief pathophysiologic review. Clin J Am Soc Nephrol. 2020 Dec 7;15(12):1848–1856.

2. Soifer JT, Kim HT. Approach to metabolic alkalosis. Emerg Med Clin N Am. 2014;32:453–463.

3. Shah N, Shaw C, Forni LG. Metabolic alkalosis in the intensive care unit. Neth J Crit Care. 2008;12(3):113–119.

4. Gennari FJ, Weise WJ. Acid–base disturbances in gastrointestinal disease. Clin J Am Soc Nephrol. 2008;3:1861–1868.

5. Evans L, Rhodes A, Alhazzani W, et al. Surviving sepsis campaign: international guidelines for management of sepsis and septic shock 2021. Crit Care Med. 2021;49:e1063–e1143.

6. Seifter JL. Integration of acid–base and electrolyte disorders. N Engl J Med. 2014;371:1821–1831.

7. Moviat M, Pickkers P, van der Hoeven PHJ, et al. Acetazolamide-mediated decrease in strong ion difference accounts for the correction of metabolic alkalosis in critically ill patients. Crit Care. 2006;10:R14. doi: 10.1186/cc3970.

8. Oh YK. Acid–base disorders in ICU patients. Electrolyte Blood Press. 2010;8:66–71.

63

ALZHEIMER DISEASE

Oh Right! I Keep Forgetting.. . . . . Level II

Amie Taggart Blaszczyk, PharmD, BCPS, BCGP, FASCP

Rebecca J. Mahan, PharmD, BCGP, BCACP, FASCP

LEARNING OBJECTIVES

After completing this case study, the reader should be able to:

- Assess cognitive deficits and noncognitive/behavioral symptoms of Alzheimer disease (AD).

- Evaluate the drug therapy regimens for medications that could interfere with the AD process and future drug therapy recommendations.

- Design a nonpharmacologic plan for a patient with AD based on target symptoms.

- Recommend appropriate pharmacotherapy to manage the cognitive and behavioral symptoms of AD.

- Determine appropriate education and counseling to provide to patients and care partners about AD, the possible benefits and adverse effects of pharmacotherapy for the disorder, and the importance of adherence to therapy.

PATIENT PRESENTATION

■ Chief Complaint

"I'm not sure why we are here. My daughter said I have to move, and I don't want to because there are people stealing from my house and I have to catch them before they take it all. My kids are just worriers."

■ HPI

The patient is a 74-year-old woman who presents to the geriatric care clinic for a routine visit accompanied by her daughter. The patient was diagnosed with AD 3 years ago. Her initial symptoms included forgetting times and dates easily, misplacing and losing items, repeating questions and current events, the inability to answer questions, and increasing difficulty with managing finances. She was initially treated with oral rivastigmine that was eventually discontinued due to intolerable side effects although it worked well to slow her decline. Treatment with donepezil 10 mg at bedtime has been well tolerated for the past 2 years, and she has been

participating more actively in family and social functions. Behavioral problems have been infrequent since diagnosis and have not required treatment. Since her last clinic visit, she began using an over-the-counter medication for sleep.

The patient lives on her own; her daughter and son share the duties of visiting her twice a day. They have been able to maintain a regular routine with their mother's daily activities, nutrition, and financial responsibilities, using lists and notes to help the patient orient herself. Her daughter sets up a medication box weekly for the patient but has recently noticed quite a few pills left in the container at the end of the week. When the daughter asks her mother about them, the patient has thrown the medication bottles at her and tells her "You take them!" The daughter is moving in 1 month to live closer to her own daughter to help with grandchildren and has asked her younger unmarried brother to help take care of their mother. He has agreed to be his mother's caregiver. He lives and works across town and is not sure if he wants to move his mother into his home. There has been discussion about placing the patient in an assisted living or long-term care facility. The patient displays lack of interest, apathy, and tearfulness lately, especially when her children are talking about her care. The daughter asks about her mother's current Alzheimer's medication and her recent increase in agitation and decline in mood. During the appointment, the patient turns to her daughter and asks, "Why are you talking about me?" The daughter reminds her that the appointment is for her Alzheimer's. The patient responds "Oh, right! I keep forgetting."

■ PMH

Osteoarthritis in hands and hip × 6 years
Hypertension × 15 years
AD diagnosed × 3 years

■ FH

Noncontributory, both parents deceased; two children, both of whom live nearby

■ SH

Lives at home; has been widowed for 10 years (husband died of cancer); negative for tobacco use; occasional alcohol use socially, none for ~5 years

■ Meds

Donepezil 10 mg PO at bedtime
Lisinopril 10 mg PO once daily
Protein shakes PRN for weight loss
Acetaminophen 325 mg one to two tablets PO every 6 hours PRN for pain (uses once daily at bedtime)
Diphenhydramine 25 mg at bedtime PRN for sleep (takes nightly for the last month)

■ All

NKDA

■ **ROS**

Endorses trouble getting to sleep and staying asleep in the past secondary to "keeping an eye out for robbers." Weight stable. Displays apathy, tearfulness, and frustration during assessment. Reports occasional knee pain; no c/o heartburn, chest pain, or shortness of breath.

■ **Physical Examination**

Gen

Well-developed woman who appears her stated age

VS

BP 144/82 mm Hg, P 63 bpm, RR 18, T 37°C; Wt 165 lb (74.8 kg), Ht 5'6"

Skin

Intact, normal color, no suspicious moles or spots, normal skin turgor

HEENT

WNL, TMs intact

Neck/Lymph Nodes

Neck supple without thyromegaly or lymphadenopathy

Lungs/Thorax

Clear, normal breath sounds

Breasts

No masses or tenderness

CV

RRR, no murmurs or bruits

Abd

Soft, NT/ND

Genit/Rect

Deferred

MS/Ext

No CCE, Heberden's nodes on both hands, decreased ROM (L) hip

Neuro

Motor, sensory, CNs, cerebellar, and gait normal. MoCA score 16/30, compared to a score of 19/30 last year. Disoriented to season, month, date, and day of week. Appropriate language and visuospatial skills but impaired attention and very poor short-term memory. Unable to remember any of four words after 3 minutes. Able to follow commands.

■ **Labs (Fasting)**

Na 139 mEq/L	Hgb 13.5 g/dL	T. bili 0.9 mg/dL	Vit B$_{12}$ 612 pg/mL
K 3.7 mEq/L	Hct 39.0%	D. bili 0.3 mg/dL	TSH 2.5 mIU/L
Cl 108 mEq/L	AST 25 IU/L	T. prot 7.5 g/dL	Free T$_4$ 0.9 ng/dL
CO$_2$ 25.5 mEq/L	ALT 24 IU/L	Alb 4.5 g/dL	Uric acid 6.8 mg/dL
BUN 16 mg/dL	Alk phos 81 IU/L	Ca 9.7 mg/dL	
SCr 1.4 mg/dL	GGT 22 IU/L	Phos 4.5 mg/dL	
Glu 102 mg/dL	LDH 85 IU/L		

■ **CT Scan (Head, 4 Years Ago)**

Mild to moderate generalized cerebral atrophy

■ **Assessment**

1. Behavioral and psychiatric symptoms of dementia (BPSD), uncontrolled, treated

2. Insomnia/drug–disease interaction, uncontrolled, treated

3. Possible depression, uncontrolled, untreated

4. Progression of AD, controlled, treated

5. Osteoarthritic pain, controlled, treated

QUESTIONS

Collect Information

1.a. What subjective and objective information indicates the presence of the cognitive and noncognitive problems of AD?

1.b. What additional information is needed to fully assess this patient's AD?

Assess the Information

2.a. Assess the severity of AD based on the subjective and objective information available.

2.b. Create and prioritize a list of the patient's drug therapy problems. Include assessment of medication appropriateness, effectiveness, safety, and patient adherence.

2.c. What economic, psychosocial, safety, and ethical considerations are applicable to this patient?

Develop a Care Plan

3.a. What are the goals of pharmacotherapy in this case?

3.b. What nondrug therapies for AD might be useful for this patient?

3.c. What feasible pharmacotherapeutic options are available to treat this patient's AD?

3.d. Create an individualized, patient-centered, team-based care plan to optimize medication therapy for this patient's AD and other drug therapy problems. Include specific drugs, dosage forms, doses, schedules, and durations of therapy.

Implement the Care Plan

4.a. What information should be provided to the patient/care partner to enhance adherence, ensure successful therapy, and minimize adverse effects?

4.b. Describe how care should be coordinated with other healthcare providers.

Follow-Up: Monitor and Evaluate

5. Explain how to monitor and evaluate the care plan for medication appropriateness, effectiveness, safety, and patient adherence by using clinical and laboratory data, patient feedback, and other information. What clinical and laboratory parameters should be used to evaluate the therapy for achievement of the desired therapeutic outcome or to detect or prevent adverse effects?

■ CLINICAL COURSE

The patient's daughter has moved to be closer to her own daughter, and the patient's son accompanies the patient to her next appointment. He mentions his mother's agitation and apathy improved with your recommended drug therapy plan. She remains tearful at times and is now not sleeping well at night. She continues to be fearful of someone coming into her house and insists that some of her things are missing. During the appointment, she gets tearful mentioning "I don't know where my little girl is."

■ FOLLOW-UP QUESTIONS

1. What further evaluation should be done to address the patient's continued tearfulness and sleep problems?

2. Discuss the use of antipsychotic medications for the treatment of BPSD. Include a discussion of the pros and cons of treatment.

3. What is the impact of vitamin B_{12} and thyroid function on the presentation and progression of dementia symptoms?

4. Determine the clinical utility of combination therapy with a cholinesterase inhibitor and memantine. What improvements in clinical condition may be expected? Is the potential benefit worth the risk?

■ SELF-STUDY ASSIGNMENTS

1. Compare and contrast the Global Deterioration Scale and the FAST criteria for determining the staging of AD.

2. Discuss the management of chronic medical conditions and primary prevention strategies in a patient with progressing dementia. What are the pros and cons of treatment relative to the patient's quality of life; cost, side effects, and complexity of the drug regimen; and ethical considerations?

3. Discuss the pros and cons of the approval of aducanumab based on the trial data presented to the FDA. Who are ideal candidates for a trial of this therapy, and what monitoring plan should be put in place to ensure safety and efficacy are being monitored?

4. Investigate the evidence, safety data, and potential issues for valproic acid and the combination product dextromethorphan/quinidine, which are commonly used alternatives to antipsychotics in treating the BPSD.

CLINICAL PEARL

Individuals starting a cholinesterase inhibitor for their dementia should have their pulse monitored closely, as these medications have the potential to decrease heart rate up to 10 bpm. Studies have linked cholinesterase inhibitors to inappropriate pacemaker placement and falls. This is especially important if the patient is on a concomitant medication that can also reduce heart rate (eg, β-blockers).

REFERENCES

1. Krishnan K, Rossetti H, Hynan LS, et al. Changes in Montreal Cognitive Assessment scores over time. Assessment 2017;24(6):772–777.

2. Reus VI, Fochtmann LJ, Eyler AE, et al. The American Psychiatric Association practice guideline on the use of antipsychotics to treat agitation or psychosis in patients with dementia. Am J Psychiatry 2016;173(5):543–546.

3. Cummings JL, Isaacson RS, Schmitt FA, Velting DM. A practical algorithm for managing Alzheimer's disease: what, when, and why? Ann Clin Transl Neurol. 2015;2(3):307–323.

4. Holmes HM, Sachs GA, Shega JW, et al. Integrating palliative medicine into the care of persons with advanced dementia: identifying appropriate medication use. J Am Geriatr Soc. 2008;56:1306–1311.

5. Rabins PV, Rovner BW, Rummans T, et al. Guideline watch (October 2014): practice guideline for the treatment of patients with Alzheimer's disease and other dementias. Focus (Am Psychiatr Publ.) 2017; 15(1):110–128.

6. Campbell N, Boustani M, Limbil T, et al. The cognitive impact of anticholinergics: a clinical review. Clin Interv Aging 2009;4:225–233.

7. Chi S, Yu J-T, Tan M-S, et al. Depression in Alzheimer's disease: epidemiology, mechanisms, and management. J Alz Dis. 2014;42(3):739–755.

8. Ehret MJ, Chamberlin KW. Current practices in the treatment of Alzheimer disease: where is the evidence after the phase III trials? Clin Ther. 2015;37:1604–1616.

9. Sadowsky CH, Galvin JE. Guidelines for the management of cognitive and behavioral problems in dementia. J Am Board Fam Med. 2012;25:350–366.

64

MULTIPLE SCLEROSIS

The One With the Spinal Cord Disease . . . . Level II

Aimee M. Banks, PharmD, BCPS, MSCS

LEARNING OBJECTIVES

After completing this case study, the reader should be able to:

• Recognize the signs, symptoms, and diagnostic criteria of multiple sclerosis (MS).

• Identify the short-term and long-term treatment goals for patients with MS.

• Apply a knowledge of disease-modifying therapies (DMT) for MS to develop an appropriate treatment regimen and care plan.

• Educate patients and healthcare practitioners on the proper storage, administration, adverse effects, and monitoring of disease-modifying therapies for MS.

PATIENT PRESENTATION

■ Chief Complaint

"My legs are numb and weak, and I'm having trouble walking and urinating."

■ HPI

A 26-year-old woman who was in good health until 7 days ago has developed numbness and tingling in her left foot. Over the last 7 days, the numbness extended higher up her leg to her lower abdomen, stopping at the umbilicus, and then going down the right leg. She also developed weakness in both of her legs, is having trouble walking, and is bothered by urinary urgency and incontinence. She presents to the Neurology clinic today, as a referral from her PCP.

PMH

Migraine headaches, since adolescence, which are now well controlled
Depression, now well controlled
Obesity most of her life

FH

African American descent. Both parents are alive and well. She has no siblings and there is no family history of neurologic disease.

SH

Married; employed as an accountant; no children. She has smoked one pack per day for 8 years; use of alcohol is limited to an occasional glass of wine or beer on weekends; no illicit drug use.

Meds

Citalopram 10 mg PO daily for depression
Amitriptyline 50 mg PO QHS for migraine prevention
Acetaminophen, aspirin, and caffeine (Excedrin) two tablets PO PRN headache
Sumatriptan 50 mg PO PRN migraine

All

NKDA

ROS

Unremarkable except that she reports feeling run down and tired most of the day, which she noticed has been ongoing for more than 6 months. No previous history of visual disturbance (eg, pain, blurred, double vision), sensory, motor, bowel, bladder, or gait disturbance.

Physical Examination

Gen

The patient is a Black woman who appears to be slightly anxious but is otherwise in NAD.

VS

BP 120/72 mm Hg, P 88 bpm and regular, RR 20, T 36.6°C; Wt 86.4 kg, Ht 5′2″, BMI 34.7 kg/m^2

Skin

Normal turgor; no obvious lesions, tumors, or moles

HEENT

NC/AT, TMs clear

Neck/Lymph Nodes

Supple, without lymphadenopathy or thyromegaly

CV

RRR; S$_1$, S$_2$ normal; no MRG

Lungs

Clear to A&P

Abd

NTND

Genit/Rect

Deferred

MS/Ext

Normal ROM; pulses 2+ throughout

Neuro

CNs II–XII are intact; no signs of optic neuropathy.

Motor: Tone, bulk, and strength are 5/5 in both arms, with good fine motor movements. In the legs, she has 4/5 strength in an upper motor neuron pattern, with normal tone and bulk.
Sensory: Moderately diminished light touch, pain, and temperature in both legs with a cord level at the umbilicus and decreased vibratory sensation in both great toes. (+) Romberg sign.
Coordination: Finger-to-nose and alternating movements with the hands are normal, as is heel-to-shin bilaterally.
Gait: Mildly unsteady on tandem walking; timed 25-foot walk was 6.2 seconds.
Reflexes: 2/2 in UE, 3/3 in LE; (+) Babinski bilaterally.

The patient is alert, oriented, and cooperative. No Lhermitte's sign is noted.

Labs

Na 140 mEq/L	Alk Phos 63 IU/L	GGT 33 IU/L
K 4.1 mEq/L	AST 22 IU IU/L	ESR 20 mm/hr
Cl 99 mEq/L	ALT 23 IU/L	CRP 1.0 mg/dL
CO$_2$ 23 mEq/L	WBC 5.6	TSH 1.0 µIU/mL
Anion gap 9	RBC 4.8	Vit. B$_{12}$ 510 ng/L21
Glu 109 mg/dL	Hgb 12.8	25(OH) vitamin D 21 ng/mL
BUN 11 mg/dL	Hct 40	Serum ACE 32 mcg/L
SCr 0.85 mg/dL	Plt 265	ANA negative
Ca total 9.4 mg/dL	% Neut 58.7	Lyme serology negative
Protein total 8.1 g/dL	% Lymph 29.2	AQP4 antibody negative
Albumin 4.9 g/dL	% Mono 7.7	MOG antibody negative
Bilirubin 0.7 mg/dL	% Eos 2.2	Anti-JCV antibody negative

Lumbar Puncture

CSF analysis shows opening pressure 140 mm H$_2$O, 10 WBC/µL, 97% lymphocytes; protein 30 mg/dL, glucose 65 mg/dL; IgG index 1.7; 12 oligoclonal bands unique to CSF.

MRI Scan

Thoracic spine MRI with and without injection of contrast material reveals a one-segment long enhancing lesion in the posterior thoracic spine at level T10.
Brain MRI shows multiple areas of T2 and FLAIR hyperintense lesions; four were periventricular, one was in the left cerebellum, two were juxtacortical; and none of the areas enhance after injection of contrast material. A total of 12 T2 and FLAIR lesions were seen in the brain; see Fig. 64-1.

Assessment

A 26-year-old woman with a newly diagnosed relapsing-remitting multiple sclerosis (RRMS), based on clinical presentation plus MRI and CSF results, presenting with the first acute demyelinating event. She has risk factors for a highly active disease course, requiring pharmacotherapy treatment with disease modification, in addition to modifiable risk factors for MS such as vitamin D deficiency, smoking, and obesity.

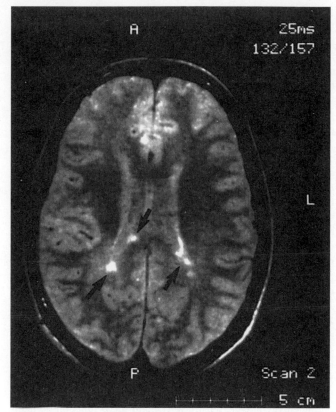

FIGURE 64-1. Brain MRI scan. Arrows highlight typical periventricular white matter lesions seen in multiple sclerosis.

QUESTIONS

Collect Information

1.a. What subjective and objective information indicates the presence of relapsing-remitting multiple sclerosis (RRMS)?

1.b. What additional information is needed to fully assess this patient's RRMS?

Assess the Information

2.a. Assess the severity of this patient's RRMS based on the subjective and objective information available.

2.b. Create a list of the patient's drug therapy problems and prioritize them. Include assessment of medication appropriateness, effectiveness, safety, and patient adherence.

Develop a Care Plan

3.a. What are the goals of pharmacotherapy for RRMS in this case?

3.b. What nondrug therapies for MS might be useful for this patient's RRMS?

3.c. What feasible pharmacotherapeutic options are available for treating RRMS?

3.d. Create an individualized, patient-centered, team-based care plan to optimize medication therapy for this patient's RRMS and other drug therapy problems. Include specific drugs, dosage forms, doses, schedules, and durations of therapy.

3.e. What alternatives would be appropriate if the initial care plan fails or cannot be used?

Implement the Care Plan

4.a. What information should be provided to the patient to enhance adherence, ensure successful therapy, and minimize adverse effects?

4.b. Describe how care should be coordinated with other healthcare providers.

Follow-Up: Monitor and Evaluate

5. Explain how to monitor and evaluate the care plan for medication appropriateness, effectiveness, safety, and patient adherence by using clinical and laboratory data, patient feedback, and other information.

■ SELF-STUDY ASSIGNMENTS

1. Develop appropriate DMT recommendations by applying a knowledge of clinical trial efficacy and safety data in combination with AAN and CMSC practice guidelines.

2. Identify treatment considerations of MS during family planning and pregnancy.

3. Recommend symptomatic treatments for chronic symptoms of MS.

CLINICAL PEARL

Although MS is highly variable in presentation and disease course, several prognostic factors associated with highly active MS can help identify patients who may be at higher risk of unfavorable outcomes. Current guidelines encourage high-efficacy DMTs for patients with highly active MS, those at risk of a poor prognosis, and those with a suboptimal response to other DMTs. DMT selection should be highly individualized and based on patient- and therapy-specific considerations.

ACKNOWLEDGMENT

This case is based on the patient case written for the 11th edition by Sarah N. Fischer, PharmD and Jacquelyn L. Bainbridge, PharmD, FCCP, MSCS.

REFERENCES

1. Thompson AJ, Banwell BL, Barkhof F, et al. Diagnosis of multiple sclerosis: 2017 revisions of the McDonald criteria. Lancet Neurol. 2018;17:162–173.

2. Rush CA, MacLean HJ, Freedman MS. Aggressive multiple sclerosis: proposed definition and treatment algorithm. Nat Rev Neurol. 2015;11:379–389.

3. Ford CC, Morrow SA. CMSC practical guidelines for the selection of disease-modifying therapies in multiple sclerosis: CMSC DMT Guideline Writing Group, 2019. Available at: *https://cmscscholar.org/ blog/2019/03/11/cmsc-practical-guidelines-for-the-selection-of-disease-modifying-therapies-in-ms/*. Accessed January 22, 2022.

4. Le Page E, Veillard D, Laplaud DA, et al. Oral versus intravenous high-dose methylprednisolone for treatment of relapses in patients with multiple sclerosis (COPOUSEP): a randomised, controlled, double-blind, non-inferiority trial. Lancet 2015;386:974–981.

5. Liu S, Liu X, Chen S, Chen S, Xiao Y, Zhuang W. Oral versus intravenous methylprednisolone for the treatment of multiple sclerosis relapses: a meta-analysis of randomized controlled trials. PLoS One 2017;12:e0188644. doi: 10.1371/journal.pone.0188644.

6. Rae-Grant A, Day GS, Marrie RA, et al. Practice guideline recommendations summary: disease-modifying therapies for adults with multiple sclerosis: report of the Guideline Development, Dissemination, and Implementation Subcommittee of the American Academy of Neurology. Neurology 2018;90:777–788.

7. Plavina T, Subramanyam M, Bloomgren G, et al. Anti-JC virus antibody levels in serum or plasma further define risk of natalizumab-associated progressive multifocal leukoencephalopathy. Ann Neurol. 2014;76:802–812.

8. Natalizumab (Tysabri) prescribing information. Cambridge, MA: Biogen Inc., 2021. Available at: https://www.tysabrihcp.com/content/dam/commercial/tysabri/hcp/en_us/pdf/tysabri_prescribing_information.pdf. Accessed January 23, 2022.

65

COMPLEX PARTIAL SEIZURES

An Overdue Visit to a Neurology Clinic . . . . Level II

James W. McAuley, RPh, PhD, FAPhA

LEARNING OBJECTIVES

After completing this case study, the reader should be able to:

- Identify necessary data to collect for patients with complex partial seizures.

- Define potential drug-related problems for antiepileptic drugs.

- List desired therapeutic outcomes for patients with complex partial seizures.

- Based on patient characteristics, choose appropriate pharmacotherapy for treatment of partial seizures, and develop a suitable care plan.

- Identify key issues for a woman of childbearing potential taking antiepileptic drugs.

PATIENT PRESENTATION

■ Chief Complaint

"My family doctor told me I should see a neurologist about my seizures."

■ HPI

PL is a 36-year-old woman referred to the neurology clinic by her PCP for evaluation of her seizures and antiepileptic drug therapy. She is enduring quite a heavy seizure burden. Her last seizure was 10 days ago, which resulted in her falling down her basement stairs. Her seizures started at a very early age, and she said no one has been able to identify why she started having seizures. She remembers having them in grade school and being confused a lot throughout her schooling. She was briefly tried on phenobarbital initially but has been on phenytoin most of her life. She has poor seizure control with no extended seizure-free periods. She has not seen a neurologist for years, if ever. She has not had any neuroimaging studies and provides no previous EEG results.

On speaking with the patient and her husband of 2.5 years, most of her events involve "blackouts" and losing track of time. Occasionally, she has "grand mal" seizures. She is more likely to have a seizure if she gets overly tired or stressed. She has no history of severe head injury with loss of consciousness or other significant risk factors for seizures. She states that at some time in her past, she "felt really bad, almost drunk" on higher doses of phenytoin. She states that she is very adherent, although she has run out of medication more than once. Because she is having seizures, she does not drive and therefore must rely on others for transportation. This lack of independence is a major concern for PL.

Data gathered from reviewing her seizure calendar over the past 2 months (Fig. 65-1) suggest that she is experiencing approximately eight "small" seizures per month (complex partial seizures with no secondary generalization) and one "big" seizure per month (a secondarily generalized tonic–clonic seizure). Her interview details and her overall score on her responses to the QOLIE-31 questions show a significant impact of the seizures on her quality of life. Her scores on the energy/fatigue, seizure worry, and social function domains are especially low in comparison with a cohort of other patients with epilepsy. The score on her NDDI-E was 11, indicating that she had some mood issues, but she was not depressed. On asking if there is anything else the patient would like to discuss, PL and her husband state that they desire to start a family in the near future.

■ PMH

Noncontributory, except as described previously

■ FH

Both parents deceased; one younger brother in good health; no seizure disorder, cancer, or CV disease

■ SH

Married; works in a local restaurant; denies tobacco and alcohol use; finished high school with a "C" average; no children

■ Meds

Phenytoin (Dilantin) 300 mg PO at bedtime

■ All

NKDA

■ ROS

Tired a lot but no problems with balance or double vision

■ Physical Examination

Gen

Pleasant woman showing some anxiety during this initial visit

VS

BP 132/87 mm Hg, P 72 bpm, RR 18, T 36.2°C; Wt 66.8 kg, Ht 5'1"

Patient Instructions: Please record the number and type of seizures you have each day.

S = Small, B = Big, ? = Possible seizure   **Patient: P. Livingston**

March

Sunday	Monday	Tuesday	Wednesday	Thursday	Friday	Saturday
		1	2	3	4	5 S
6	7	8	9	10	11 S	12 S
13	14 S→B	15	16	17	18	19
20	21	22 S, S	23 S	24	25	26
27	28	29	30 S	31		

April

Sunday	Monday	Tuesday	Wednesday	Thursday	Friday	Saturday
					1	2
3	4 S	5	6 S	7 S	8	9
10	11	12	13	14	15 S	16 S, S→B
17	18	19 S	20	21	22	23
24	25 ? S	26	27	28	29 S	30

FIGURE 65-1. Seizure calendar (S = small seizure, B = big seizure, ? = possible seizure).

Skin

Normal color, hydration, and temperature

HEENT

Mild hirsutism; (+) gingival hyperplasia

Neck/Lymph Nodes

(–) JVD; (–) lymphadenopathy

Lungs/Thorax

CTA

Breasts

Deferred

CV

Normal S₁ and S₂, RRR, NSR, normal peripheral pulses

Abd

NT/ND, (+) BS, no HSM

Genit/Rect

Deferred

MS/Ext

Significant burn on palm of right hand. This happened within the last week when she had a seizure while frying eggs on the stovetop. Her husband stated that he witnessed her put hand directly in the frying pan during her seizure.

Neuro

CNs II–XII intact; slight lateral gaze nystagmus noted. Motor: 4/5 muscle strength on left side, 5/5 on right side. DTRs: 2+ RUE, 1+ LUE, 0 RLE, 0 LLE. Sensory: normal light touch and pinprick. Station: normal.

■ Labs

Na 137 mEq/L	Hgb 14.5 g/dL	AST 31 IU/L
K 4.1 mEq/L	Hct 41.7%	ALT 22 IU/L
Cl 100 mEq/L	RBC 4.71 × 10⁶/mm³	Alk phos 187 IU/L
CO₂ 29 mEq/L	MCV 88.6 μm³	GGT 45 IU/L
BUN 9 mg/dL	MCHC 34.7 g/dL	Ca 7.3 mg/dL
SCr 0.6 mg/dL	Plt 212 × 10³/mm³	Alb 3.9 g/dL
Glu 107 mg/dL	WBC 5.4 × 10³/mm³	

■ EEG

Abnormal for bitemporal slowing, which is more significant in the left temporal region, as characterized by polymorphic and epileptiform discharges consistent with a history of seizure disorder

■ Assessment

1. Seizure disorder, uncontrolled with phenytoin
2. Potential adverse drug reactions from phenytoin
3. Woman of childbearing potential without folic acid supplementation
4. Possible osteomalacia secondary to long-term phenytoin therapy

QUESTIONS

Collect Information

1.a. What subjective and objective information indicates the presence of complex partial seizures?

1.b. What additional information is needed to fully assess this patient's complex partial seizures?

Assess the Information

2.a. Assess the severity of complex partial seizures based on the subjective and objective information available.

2.b. Create a list of the patient's drug therapy problems and prioritize them. Include assessment of medication appropriateness, effectiveness, safety, and patient adherence.

2.c. What economic, cultural, racial, ethical, and psychosocial considerations are applicable to this patient?

Develop a Care Plan

3.a. What are the goals of pharmacotherapy in this case?

3.b. What nondrug therapies for complex partial seizures might be useful for this patient?

3.c. What feasible pharmacotherapeutic options are available for treating complex partial seizures?

3.d. Create an individualized, patient-centered, team-based care plan to optimize medication therapy for this patient's complex partial seizures and other drug therapy problems. Include specific drugs, dosage forms, doses, schedules, and durations of therapy.

3.e. What alternatives would be appropriate if the initial care plan fails or cannot be used?

Implement the Care Plan

4.a. What information should be provided to the patient to enhance adherence, ensure successful therapy, and minimize adverse effects?

4.b. Describe how care should be coordinated with other healthcare providers.

Follow-Up: Monitor and Evaluate

5. Explain how to monitor and evaluate the care plan for medication appropriateness, effectiveness, safety, and patient adherence by using clinical and laboratory data, patient feedback, and other information.

■ CLINICAL COURSE

A collective decision was made among the healthcare practitioners, the patient, and her husband to add another antiepileptic drug to her current drug regimen and to see her back in 6 weeks. She was given written and verbal information on this new drug and instructed to call or use the patient portal with any questions, problems, or concerns. She and her husband verbalized an understanding. At her next visit, the patient reported that there had been an initial response to the addition of the new antiepileptic drug (ie, fewer seizures), but she still has some "small" seizures and one "big" seizure per month. There are no recent laboratory data. Her neurologic examination is unchanged. She and her husband would like to further discuss their desire to start a family.

■ FOLLOW-UP QUESTION

1. What is known about long-term effects on cognition and behavior in children exposed to antiepileptic drugs in utero?

■ SELF-STUDY ASSIGNMENTS

1. Outline a plan for assessing this patient's adherence with her medication regimen.

2. What risk factors does this patient have for osteoporosis? What interventions should be made?

3. Would switching this patient from brand Dilantin to generic phenytoin be an appropriate alternative? What are the ramifications of making this change?

4. What role can community pharmacists play in the care of patients with epilepsy?

CLINICAL PEARL

Although epilepsy affects men and women equally, there are many women's health issues, including menstrual cycle influences on seizure activity, drug interactions between contraceptives and antiepileptic drugs, and teratogenicity of antiepileptic drugs.

REFERENCES

1. Taylor RS, Sander JW, Taylor RJ, Baker GA. Predictors of health-related quality of life and costs in adults with epilepsy: a systematic review. Epilepsia 2011;52:2168–2180.
2. Gill SJ, Lukmanji S, Fiest KM, Patten SB, Wiebe S, Jetté N. Depression screening tools in persons with epilepsy: a systematic review of validated tools. Epilepsia 2017;58:695–705.
3. Beghi E. Addressing the burden of epilepsy: many unmet needs. Pharmacol Res. 2016;107:79–84.
4. England MJ, Liverman CT, Schultz AM, Strawbridge LM. Epilepsy across the spectrum: promoting health and understanding. A summary of the Institute of Medicine report. Epilepsy Behav. 2012;25:266–276.
5. Voinescu PE, Pennell PB. Delivery of a personalized treatment approach to women with epilepsy. Semin Neurol. 2017;37:611–623.
6. Meador KJ, Baker GA, Browning N, et al. Fetal antiepileptic drug exposure and cognitive outcomes at age 6 years (NEAD study): a prospective observational study. Lancet Neurol. 2013;12:244–252.
7. Griepp DW, Kim DJ, Ganz M, et al. The effects of antiepileptic drugs on bone health: a systematic review. Epilepsy Res. 2021;173:106619.
8. Mula M, Kanner AM, Schmitz B, Schachter S. Antiepileptic drugs and suicidality: an expert consensus statement from the Task Force on Therapeutic Strategies of the ILAE Commission on Neuropsychobiology. Epilepsia 2013;54:199–203.
9. Long L, Cotterman-Hart S, Shelby J. To reveal or conceal? Adult patient perspectives on SUDEP disclosure. Epilepsy Behav. 2018;86:79–84.
10. Bacci JL, Zaraa S, Stergachis A, Simic G, White HS. Community pharmacists' role in caring for people living with epilepsy: a scoping review. Epilepsy Behav. 2021;117:107850.

66

GENERALIZED TONIC–CLONIC SEIZURES

A Senior Shaken by Seizures .... Level II

Kevin M. Bozymski, PharmD, BCPS, BCPP

LEARNING OBJECTIVES

After completing this case study, the reader should be able to:

- Define epilepsy.
- Differentiate seizure types based on clinical presentation and description.
- Recommend drugs of choice and alternative therapies for different types of seizures.
- Determine appropriate dosing, the most common adverse effects, and monitoring parameters for antiepileptic drugs (AEDs).
- Develop an appropriate pharmacotherapy care plan for a patient with epilepsy.

PATIENT PRESENTATION

■ Chief Complaint

"I had a seizure a few weeks ago and banged up my head."

■ HPI

A 68-year-old man whose seizures are reportedly well-controlled with carbamazepine monotherapy arrives at your clinic. The seizure from 2.5 weeks ago was the patient's first seizure in 20 months. During the seizure, he fell to the floor and sustained a laceration to his occipital region that required staples for closure. The description of his seizures is vague because there have been only six seizures documented since he developed epilepsy 3 years ago. Because the patient lives alone in an assisted living facility, only half of the documented seizures have been witnessed by another individual who could provide a description. Two seizures were witnessed by other residents who described him as "falling to the ground and starting to shake." One seizure occurred in the day room with a facility nurse present documenting that the patient fell to the ground, developed rhythmic extensions to both his legs, became incontinent of urine, and was sleepy and disoriented for 2 hours after the episode.

He has only been treated with carbamazepine. This medication was started by his family practice physician after his second seizure 3 years ago. An EEG was obtained at that time and was unremarkable. Because the seizures are so infrequent, the dose of carbamazepine has never been adjusted.

■ PMH

Tonic–clonic seizures diagnosed 3 years ago
Hypertension
Dyslipidemia
Major depressive disorder (MDD)

■ FH

Mother died at age 74 of "natural causes"; had HTN and MDD for many years. Father died at age 70 of "natural causes"; did not have any known medical illnesses. All his children and grandchildren are alive and well. One son and one daughter have HTN.

■ SH

Retired factory worker; resides in an assisted living facility. He is widowed and has six children and nine grandchildren, whom he sees frequently. He denies past or present tobacco and illicit drug use. He reports a history of regular alcohol use but now only drinks one beer that his grandson brings to him every Saturday evening. He reports adhering to a low-cholesterol diet.

■ Meds

Aspirin 81 mg PO once daily
Atorvastatin 40 mg PO once daily
Carbamazepine XR 200 mg PO twice daily
Lisinopril 20 mg PO once daily
Multivitamin with minerals one tablet PO once daily
Sertraline 100 mg PO once daily

■ All

NKDA
Adverse drug effect history—none

■ Physical Examination

Gen

Exam reveals an elderly man who appears his stated age in NAD.

VS

BP 126/78 mm Hg, HR 72, RR 16, temperature not measured; Ht 5'10", Wt 72.5 kg

HEENT

Normocephalic; scalp: healing 3-cm lesion in the occipital region with corresponding mild tenderness and bruising; PERRL

Neck/LN

No thyromegaly, lymphadenopathy, or carotid bruits

Chest/Lungs

Lungs CTA

CV

RRR, no m/r/g

Abd

Soft, nontender; no HSM; (+) BS

MS/Ext

Normal tone; 5/5 strength in all extremities

Neuro

Awake; A&O × 3; CN II–XII intact, reflexes 2+ and symmetric throughout

■ Labs

Na 127 mEq/L	Hgb 13.5 g/dL	Fasting lipid profile
K 4.7 mEq/L	Hct 41%	T. chol 155 mg/dL
Cl 90 mEq/L	RBC 3.9×10^6/mm³	TG 123 mg/dL
CO_2 25 mEq/L	WBC 5.1×10^3/mm³	HDL-C 39 mg/dL
BUN 10 mg/dL	Diff WNL	LDL-C 91 mg/dL
SCr 0.6 mg/dL	MCV 97 μm³	
Glu 100 mg/dL	Carbamazepine 6 mg/L	

■ EEG at Today's Clinic Appointment

Sleep-deprived EEG unremarkable. Photic stimulation failed to produce any other changes.

■ Patient Health Questionnaire (PHQ-9) at Today's Clinic Appointment

Total score of 3 (2 points for "feeling tired or having little energy," 1 point for "trouble falling or staying asleep, or sleeping too much").

■ Assessment

1. Epilepsy with generalized tonic–clonic (GTC) seizures
2. Hyponatremia
3. Major depressive disorder, controlled
4. Hypertension, controlled
5. Dyslipidemia, controlled

QUESTIONS

Collect Information

1.a. What subjective and objective information indicates the presence of generalized tonic–clonic seizures?

1.b. What additional information is needed to fully assess this patient's generalized tonic–clonic seizures?

Assess the Information

2.a. Assess the severity of the generalized tonic–clonic seizure based on the subjective and objective information available.

2.b. Create a list of the patient's drug therapy problems and prioritize them. Include assessment of medication appropriateness, effectiveness, safety, and patient adherence.

2.c. What economic, psychosocial, cultural, racial, and ethical considerations are applicable to this patient?

Develop a Care Plan

3.a. What are the goals of pharmacotherapy for generalized tonic–clonic seizures in this case?

3.b. What nondrug therapies might be useful for this patient's generalized tonic–clonic seizures?

3.c. What feasible pharmacotherapeutic options are available for treating generalized tonic–clonic seizures?

3.d. Create an individualized, patient-centered, team-based care plan to optimize medication therapy for the generalized tonic–clonic seizures and other drug therapy problems. Include specific drugs, dosage forms, doses, schedules, and durations of therapy.

3.e. What alternatives would be appropriate if the initial care plan fails or cannot be used?

Implement the Care Plan

4.a. What information should be provided to the patient to enhance adherence, ensure successful therapy, and minimize adverse effects?

4.b. Describe how care should be coordinated with other healthcare providers.

Follow-Up: Monitor and Evaluate

5. Explain how to monitor and evaluate the care plan for medication appropriateness, effectiveness, safety, and patient adherence by using clinical and laboratory data, patient feedback, and other information.

■ SELF-STUDY ASSIGNMENTS

1. AEDs may interact with a number of other medications used in the elderly patient population. Considering major medical conditions encountered, research potential interactions with medication classes used to treat those conditions.

2. Perform a literature search to identify articles that have concluded that AEDs can be withdrawn after a certain seizure-free interval.

3. Write a concise paper outlining the current recommendations for assisting a person who is having a seizure.

4. Assume that a patient taking divalproex has poorly controlled seizures and a decision is made to add lamotrigine. Compose a brief pharmacotherapy plan about this AED addition, including any precautions that should be taken.

CLINICAL PEARL

People diagnosed with epilepsy are at greater risk of developing depression and other mood disorders, and AEDs may in turn increase the risk of suicidal ideation or behavior. Clinicians should periodically employ standardized mental health rating scales (such as the PHQ-9) to assess a patient's risk and decrease stigma about discussing mental health concerns.

ACKNOWLEDGMENT

This case is based on the patient case written for the 11th edition by Jennifer A. Donaldson, PharmD, BCPPS.

REFERENCES

1. Leppik IE, Walczak TS, Birnbaum AK. Challenges of epilepsy in elderly people. Lancet 2012;380:1128–1130.
2. Wojewodka G, McKinlay A, Ridsdale L. Best care for older people with epilepsy: a scoping review. Seizure 2021;85:70–89.
3. Bryson AS, Carney PW. Pharmacotherapy for epilepsy in the elderly. J Pharm Pract Res. 2015;45:349–356.
4. Bruun E, Kalviainen R, Keranen T. Outcome of initial antiepileptic drug treatment in elderly patients with newly diagnosed epilepsy. Epilepsy Res. 2016;127:60–65.
5. Beniczky S, Wiebe S, Jeppesen J, et al. Automated seizure detection using wearable devices: a clinical practice guideline of the International League Against Epilepsy and the International Federation of Clinical Neurophysiology. Clin Neurophysiol. 2021;132(5):1173–1184.
6. Glauser T, Ben-Menachem E, Bourgois B, et al. Updated ILAE evidence review of antiepileptic drug efficacy and effectiveness as initial monotherapy for epileptic seizures and syndromes. Epilepsia 2013;54: 551–563.
7. Lattanzi S, Trinka E, Del Giovane C, Nardone R, Silvestrini M, Brigo F. Antiepileptic drug monotherapy for epilepsy in the elderly: a systematic review and network meta-analysis. Epilepsia 2019;60(11): 2245–2254.
8. Berghuis B, van der Palen J, de Haan GJ, et al. Carbamazepine and oxcarbazepine-induced hyponatremia in people with epilepsy. Epilepsia 2017;58(7):1227–1233.

67

STATUS EPILEPTICUS

Tempest in a Tom Collins .... Level II

Kyle A. Weant, PharmD, BCPS, BCCCP, FCCP

LEARNING OBJECTIVES

After completing this case study, the reader should be able to:

- Define status epilepticus and its precipitating causes.

- Identify measures that should be taken in the emergency department for a patient in status epilepticus.

- Recommend appropriate drug treatment for status epilepticus.

- Recommend an optimal care plan for a patient with status epilepticus.

PATIENT PRESENTATION

■ Chief Complaint

As given by a friend of the patient: "I walked back into the room after getting breakfast and he was having a seizure. He kept shaking for a couple of minutes, so I went to get the RA and he said we needed to get him to the ED."

■ HPI

A 20-year-old man brought to the university hospital emergency department (ED) by his college roommate and dormitory resident assistant (RA). The roommate reported that he and the patient went out partying the night before because all the fraternities were throwing rush parties. The roommate left the patient partying at the fraternity house at about 2:00 AM. He heard the patient return to the room at approximately 4:30 AM and he was clearly intoxicated.

■ PMH

Medical records revealed that the patient developed generalized tonic–clonic seizures in childhood. Phenobarbital was initiated and controlled the seizures for many years. Withdrawal of phenobarbital was attempted 10 years ago after several years of being seizure free. The drug was restarted when seizures occurred during the attempted taper. Phenobarbital was replaced, due to sedation and lethargy, with carbamazepine. Phenytoin was added 8 years ago because of frequent and prolonged breakthrough seizures. He has had occasional breakthrough seizures since his admission to the university 2 years ago. Breakthrough seizures are typically associated with his nonadherence with medications or sleep deprivation due to prolonged study sessions. He is routinely followed in the university hospital neurology clinic.

■ FH

Negative for epilepsy; the patient has two siblings, all alive and well. No other information on family history was obtained.

■ SH

Single with no children; no tobacco use; reports drinking up to six beers per week

■ Meds

Carbamazepine 500 mg PO TID
Phenytoin 100 mg PO BID

■ All

NKDA

■ ROS

Unobtainable

■ Physical Examination

Gen

WDWN man who is unarousable, continues to have intermittent jerking of his extremities; clothes are wet from urinary incontinence

VS

BP 150/90 mm Hg, P 150 bpm, RR 25, T 37.5°C; Wt 68.3 kg; Ht 5′7″

Skin

Warm, dry, and pale; nail beds are pale

HEENT

Mucous membranes are dry

Neck/Lymph Nodes

Supple; no thyromegaly or lymphadenopathy

Lungs/Chest

Symmetric, lungs CTA

CV

RRR, no m/r/g

Abd

Soft, no HSM, BS normal in all four quadrants

MS/Ext

Muscle mass normal, full ROM

Neuro

Unarousable; reflexes 3+ bilaterally

■ Labs

Na 136 mEq/L	Hgb 12.8 g/dL	Urine drug screen: pending
K 4.5 mEq/L	Hct 41%	Carbamazepine: pending
Cl 97 mEq/L	Plt 320×10^3/mm³	Phenytoin: pending
CO_2 28 mEq/L	WBC 9.0×10^3/mm³	Ethanol: pending
BUN 16 mg/dL	Diff WNL	
SCr 1.0 mg/dL		
Glu 60 mg/dL		

■ EEG

Baseline from medical record: Diffuse background slowing; no focal changes or epileptiform activity present; photic stimulation failed to produce other changes.

■ Assessment

1. Status epilepticus
2. Generalized tonic–clonic seizures, uncontrolled
3. Medication nonadherence (suspected) with pending drug concentrations
4. Potential alcohol use disorder

QUESTIONS

Collect Information

1.a. What subjective and objective information indicates the presence of status epilepticus?

1.b. What additional information is needed to fully assess this patient's status epilepticus?

Assess the Information

2.a. Assess the severity of the status epilepticus based on the subjective and objective information available.

2.b. Create a list of the patient's drug therapy problems and prioritize them. Include assessment of medication appropriateness, effectiveness, safety, and patient adherence.

Develop a Care Plan

3.a. What are the goals of pharmacotherapy in this case?

3.b. What nondrug therapies for status epilepticus might be useful for this patient?

3.c. What feasible pharmacotherapeutic options are available to treat status epilepticus?

3.d. Create an individualized, patient-centered, team-based care plan to optimize medication therapy for this patient's status epilepticus and other drug therapy problems. Include specific drugs, dosage forms, doses, schedules, and durations of therapy.

3.e. What alternatives would be appropriate if the initial care plan fails or cannot be used?

Implement the Care Plan

4.a. What information should be provided to the patient to enhance adherence, ensure successful therapy, and minimize adverse effects?

4.b. Describe how care should be coordinated with other healthcare providers.

Follow-Up: Monitor and Evaluate

5. Explain how to monitor and evaluate the care plan for medication appropriateness, effectiveness, safety, and patient adherence by using clinical and laboratory data, patient feedback, and other information.

■ SELF-STUDY ASSIGNMENTS

1. There are several drug interactions with phenytoin and carbamazepine. Describe the effects that these drugs have on each other. What, if anything, should be done to compensate for these drug interactions?

2. Antiepileptic medications are available in multiple dosage forms. Prepare a table with what dosage forms may be used via a feeding tube, what dosage forms may help with patient adherence, and what IV to PO, or PO to IV conversions exist for products with an intravenous dosage form.

3. Prepare a two-page paper summarizing the hematologic adverse effects of all the anticonvulsants.

CLINICAL PEARL

Seizures that last longer than 5 minutes are less likely to stop spontaneously and exhibit time-dependent resistance to antiepileptic medications, hence necessitating emergent treatment.

ACKNOWLEDGMENT

This case is based on the patient case written for the 11th edition by Jennifer A. Donaldson, PharmD, BCPPS.

REFERENCES

1. Brophy GM, Bell R, Claassen J, et al. Guidelines for the evaluation and management of status epilepticus. Neurocrit Care 2012;17(1):3–23.

2. Glauser T, Shinnar S, Gloss D, et al. Evidence-based guideline: treatment of convulsive status epilepticus in adults and children: report of the Guideline Committee of the American Epilepsy Society. Epilepsy Curr. 2016;16(1):48–61.

3. Paschal AM, Rush SE, Sadler T. Factors associated with medication adherence in patients with epilepsy and recommendations for improvement. Epilepsy Behav. 2014;31:346–350.

4. Leach JP, Mohanraj R, Borland W. Alcohol and drugs in epilepsy: pathophysiology, presentation, possibilities, and prevention. Epilepsia 2012;53(Suppl 4):48–57.

5. Silbergleit R, Durkalski V, Lowenstein D, et al. Intramuscular versus intravenous therapy for prehospital status epilepticus. N Engl J Med. 2012;366:591–600.

6. Burakgazi E, Bashir S, Doss V, Pellock J. The safety and tolerability of different intravenous administrations of levetiracetam, bolus versus infusion, in intensive care unit patients. Clin EEG Neuro. 2014;45:89–91.

7. McLaughlin K, Carabetta S, Hunt N, et al. Safety of intravenous push lacosamide compared with intravenous piggyback at a tertiary academic medical center. Ann Pharmacother. 2021;55:181–186.

8. Epilepsies: diagnosis and management. National Institute for Health and Care Excellence (NICE), 2021. Available at: https://www-ncbi-nlm-nih-gov.proxy1.library.jhu.edu/books/NBK553536/. Accessed January 12, 2022.

68

ACUTE MANAGEMENT OF THE TRAUMATIC BRAIN INJURY PATIENT

The Agony of Defeat..........................Level III

Denise H. Rhoney, PharmD, FCCP, FCCM, FNCS

Dennis Parker, Jr., PharmD, FCCM

LEARNING OBJECTIVES

After completing this case study, the reader should be able to:

- Discuss the goals of cerebral resuscitation.

- Interpret parameters beneficial in assessing the severity of the brain injury.

- Describe the impact of prior antithrombotic therapy on traumatic brain injury (TBI) and devise an appropriate treatment plan for patients with TBI while on antithrombotic therapy.

- Discuss the therapeutic management of TBI and increased intracranial pressure associated with acute brain injury.

- Recommend appropriate therapy to prevent medical complications after brain injury.

PATIENT PRESENTATION

■ Chief Complaint

Not available—the patient was brought to the ED by EMS as a trauma code 1.5 hours after the accident.

■ HPI

A 28-year-old man who was brought to the ED after suffering a ski accident while on vacation with his wife. His wife reports that he was difficult to arouse at the scene of the accident.

■ PMH (As Per Patient's Wife)

Depression

■ FH

Unknown

■ SH

Unknown

■ ROS

Unobtainable

■ Meds

Sertraline 50 mg PO daily

■ All

NKDA

■ Physical Examination

Skin

Multiple bruises on the face and extremities bilaterally

HEENT

The patient has multiple soft tissue injuries to the face. The left pupil is 4 mm and slowly reactive to direct light, and the right pupil is 2 mm and slowly reactive to light. EOMs are reactive. External inspection of ears and nose reveals no acute abnormalities. There is some dried blood in the mouth. The head has a large open scalp laceration on the forehead with surrounding ecchymoses. Neck is in a cervical collar; therefore, movement was not attempted. There are no gross masses in the neck.

Lungs

Rhonchi and crackles present bilaterally with thick secretions

Heart

Sinus tachycardia with S_1 and S_2 present

Abd

Soft with no masses or tenderness but decreased bowel sounds. There is no gross hepatosplenomegaly.

Ext

No nontraumatic edema is noted.

Neuro

On painful stimuli, opens his eyes spontaneously, no verbal response, and withdraws away from the painful stimuli with a Glasgow Coma Scale score is 9.

VS

BP 87/60 mm Hg, P 126 bpm, RR 30, T 37.9°C; Wt 85 kg, Ht 6′0″

■ Labs

Na 135 mEq/L	Hgb 13.8 g/dL	Ca 8.4 mg/dL	*ABG*
K 3.7 mEq/L	Hct 40.9%	Mg 1.8 mg/dL	pH 7.4
Cl 106 mEq/L	Plt 166 × 10³/mm³	Phos 2.4 mEq/L	HCO_3 22 mEq/L
CO_2 20 mEq/L	WBC 12.0 ×	Alb 4.0 g/dL	$PaCO_2$ 36 mm Hg
BUN 15 mg/dL	10³/mm³		PaO_2 86 mm Hg
SCr 1.1 mg/dL	Diff N/A		O_2 sat 91% on RA
Glu 225 mg/dL			Urine drug
			screen (−)
			Blood alcohol
			<20 mg/dL

■ Portable Chest X-Ray

Right upper lobe atelectasis, no rib fractures

■ Head CT

There is a left parietal open depressed skull fracture. There is an area of hemorrhagic contusion in the left frontal region.

■ Assessment

A 28-year-old man S/P head trauma with skull fracture and hemorrhagic contusion secondary to ski accident with altered mental status. He has mild to moderate respiratory distress and is admitted to the neurointensive care unit for intubation and sedation. He needs therapy to correct his hemodynamic instability and hyperglycemia. Prophylaxis for potential seizure, stress ulcer, and venous thromboembolism may be needed.

QUESTIONS

Collect Information

1.a. What subjective and objective information indicates the presence of a traumatic brain injury?

1.b. What additional information is needed to fully assess this patient's traumatic brain injury?

Assess the Information

2.a. Assess the severity of traumatic brain injury based on the subjective and objective information available.

2.b. Create a list of the patient's drug therapy problems and prioritize them. Include assessment of medication appropriateness, effectiveness, safety, and patient adherence.

Develop a Care Plan

3.a. What are the goals of pharmacotherapy for traumatic brain injury in this case?

3.b. What nondrug therapies for traumatic brain injury might be useful for this patient?

3.c. What feasible pharmacotherapeutic alternatives are available for treating traumatic brain injury?

3.d. Create an individualized, patient-centered, team-based care plan to optimize medication therapy for this patient's traumatic brain injury and other drug therapy. Include specific drugs, dosage forms, doses, schedules, and durations of therapy.

3.e. What alternatives would be appropriate if the initial care plan fails or cannot be used?

Implement the Care Plan

4.a. What information should be provided to the patient to enhance adherence, ensure successful therapy, and minimize adverse effects?

4.b. Describe how care should be coordinated with other healthcare providers.

Follow-Up: Monitor and Evaluate

5. Explain how to monitor and evaluate the care plan for medication appropriateness, effectiveness, safety, and patient adherence by using clinical and laboratory data, patient feedback, and other information.

■ CLINICAL COURSE

While the patient was in the emergency department, it was decided to administer tranexamic acid 1 g infused over 10 minutes followed

Time	Temp (°C)	HR (bpm)	BP (mm Hg)	ICP (mm Hg)	CPP (mm Hg)	BG (mg/dL)	Fluid A (mL)	Fluid B (mL)	Fluid C (mL)	Nutrition	UOP (mL)	Meds given
0600	37.6	85	120/86	18	79	306	80		12	NPO	60	Insulin aspart 8 units
0700		88	128/88	22	77		80		12		105	
0800		89	119/67	15	69		80		12	NPO	100	
0900		85	125/89	16	70		80	100	12		60	Levetiracetam 1000 mg IV
1000	38.2	86	110/65	20	60	288	80		12	NPO	55	Insulin aspart 6 units APAP 325 mg
1100		92	115/79	22	71		80		12		60	Fentanyl 25 mcg × 2
1200		94	129/55	18	62		80		12	NPO	67	
1300		100	100/68	19	60		80		12		100	
1400	38.1	92	113/70	17	67	270	80		12	NPO	55	Insulin aspart 6 units APAP 325 mg
1500		98	130/85	21	79		80		12		70	
1600		89	129/75	18	75		80		12	NPO	60	
1700		94	119/88	20	76		80		12		60	
1800	37.5	85	115/66	22	75	240	80		12	NPO	60	Aspart 2 units
1900		86	124/50	22	53		80		12		80	
2000		83	144/54	16	68		80		12	NPO	60	
2100		89	140/87	24	81		80	100	12		70	Levetiracetam 1000 mg IV
2200	38.6	86	139/84	24	78	220	80		12	NPO	75	Aspart 2 units APAP 325 mg
2300		90	120/86	20	77		80		12		60	
2400		70	132/75	12	82		80		12	NPO	50	
0100		78	140/70	20	73		80		12		110	
0200	37.5	72	135/68	20	70	190	80		12	NPO	120	
0300		79	149/75	19	81		80		12		80	
0400		75	137/68	28	63		80		12	NPO	110	
0500		77	130/68	27	62		80		12		60	

Fluid A = 3% sodium chloride/acetate; Fluid B = levetiracetam IVPB; Fluid C = midazolam infusion (concentration = 1 mg/mL).

HR, heart rate; BP, blood pressure; ICP, intracranial pressure; CPP, cerebral perfusion pressure; BG, blood glucose; UOP, urine output; IVPB, intravenous piggy bag.

FIGURE 68-1. Neurointensive care unit flowsheet. Day 1 (0–24 hours postadmission).

by an intravenous infusion of 1 g over 8 hours. On arrival at the intensive care unit, it was decided to intubate the patient orally using a rapid sequence intubation technique (fentanyl 200 mcg IV followed by lidocaine 100 mg IV, midazolam 2 mg IV, and rocuronium 5 mg IV). The patient was started on 3% sodium/acetate solution at 75 mL/hr and midazolam intravenous infusion at 12 mg/hr. Other medications include levetiracetam 2 g IV load followed by 1 g IV Q 12 H, fentanyl 25 mcg IV Q 1 H PRN, and insulin aspart correction dose protocol as needed hourly. Neurologic examine hourly to monitor for potential elevation in intracranial pressure and need for invasive monitoring.

Over the next 48 hours, pertinent laboratory measurements were normal. See ICU flowsheet for other important parameters for the first 24 hours (Fig. 68-1) and second 24 hours (Fig. 68-2) in the ICU.

■ SELF-STUDY ASSIGNMENTS

1. Discuss a pharmacotherapy plan for a traumatic brain injury patient who presents on antiplatelet therapy prior to admission.

2. Review paroxysmal autonomic instability or "sympathetic storming" and its treatment options and monitoring parameters.

3. Discuss an approach for managing the neurobehavioral sequelae of traumatic brain injury.

4. Describe potential pharmacokinetic alterations that may impact your drug therapy in patients who experience traumatic brain injury.

CLINICAL PEARL

There are only three standards of care for severe brain injury patients: (1) use of corticosteroids is not recommended for improving outcome or reducing ICP; (2) in the absence of increased ICP, chronic prolonged hyperventilation ($PaCO_2 < 25$ mm Hg) should be avoided; and (3) prophylactic use of antiseizure drugs is not recommended for preventing late posttraumatic seizures (>7 days).

Time	Temp (°C)	HR (bpm)	BP (mm Hg)	ICP (mm Hg)	CPP (mm Hg)	BG (mg/dL)	Fluid A (mL)	Fluid B (mL)	Fluid C (mL)	Nutrition	UOP (mL)	Meds given
0600	37.4	85	121/76	19	72	226	80		12	NPO	70	Insulin aspart 4 units IV
0700		78	125/80	20	75		80		12		150	
0800		80	129/66	25	62		80		12	NPO	100	
0900		82	135/87	26	77		80	100	12		200	Levetiracetam 1000 mg IV
1000	38.2	86	120/60	20	60	188	80		12	NPO	350	Insulin aspart 2 units IV APAP 325 mg
1100		95	110/70	28	55		125		12		300	Fentanyl 25 mcg × 2
1200		98	119/65	28	55		125		12	NPO	150	
1300		97	110/78	29	60		125		12		350	
1400	38.3	90	118/77	35	55	286	125		12	NPO	300	Insulin aspart 8 units IV APAP 325 mg
1500		88	135/80	31	67		125		12		500	
1600		89	129/85	28	72		125		12	NPO	350	
1700		77	120/87	20	78		125		12		200	
1800	38.1	80	135/68	23	67	240	125		12	NPO	250	Aspart 2 units IV APAP 325 mg
1900		76	128/60	24	59		125		12		200	
2000		80	141/70	26	68		125		12	NPO	150	
2100		78	140/86	14	90		125	100	12		250	Levetiracetam 1000 mg IV
2200	37.8	80	129/89	24	78	220	125		12	NPO	300	Aspart 4 units IV
2300		80	130/76	18	84		125		12		300	
2400		76	137/70	25	80		125		12	NPO	250	
0100		78	140/80	17	83		125		12		250	
0200	37.9	78	145/78	22	78	190	125		12	NPO	100	Aspart 2 units IV
0300		88	145/70	28	77		125		12		250	
0400		80	127/78	25	76		125		12	NPO	300	
0500		75	138/69	27	75		125		12		250	

Fluid A = 3% sodium chloride/acetate; Fluid B = levetiracetam IVPB; Fluid C = midazolam infusion (concentration = 1 mg/mL).

HR, heart rate; BP, blood pressure; ICP, intracranial pressure; CPP, cerebral perfusion pressure; BG, blood glucose; UOP, urine output; IVPB, intravenous piggy bag.

FIGURE 68-2. Neurointensive care unit flowsheet. Day 2 (24–48 hours postadmission).

REFERENCES

1. Zehtabchi S, Abdel Baki SG, Flaxon L, Nishijima D. Tranexamic acid for traumatic brain injury: a systematic meta-analysis Am J Emerg Med. 2014;32:1503–1509. doi: 10.1016/j.ajem.2014.09.023.

2. CRASH-3 trial collaborators. Effects of tranexamic acid on death, disability, vascular occlusive events and other morbidities in patients with acute traumatic brain injury (CRASH-3): a randomized, placebo-controlled trial. Lancet. 2019;394(10210):1713–1723.

3. Devlin JW, Skrobik Y, Celine G, et al. Clinical practice guidelines for the prevention and management of pain, agitation/sedation, delirium, immobility, and sleep disruption in adult patients in the ICU. Crit Care Med. 2018;46:e825–e873.

4. Carney N, Totten AM, O'Reilly C, et al. Guidelines for the management of severe traumatic brain injury, fourth edition. Neurosurgery. 2017;80:6–15.

5. McClave SA, Martindale RG, Vanek VW, et al. Guidelines for the provision and assessment of nutrition support therapy in the adult critically ill patient: Society of Critical Care Medicine (SCCM) and American Society for Parenteral and Enteral Nutrition (A.S.P.E.N.). J Parenter Enteral Nutr. 2016;40:159–211.

6. Nyquist P, Bautista C, Jichci D, et al. Prophylaxis of venous thrombosis in neurocritical care patients: an evidence-based guideline: a statement for healthcare professionals from the Neurocritical Care Society. Neurocrit Care. 2016; 24:47–60. doi: 10.1007/s12028-015-0221-y.

7. Madden LK, Hill M, May TL, et al. The implementation of targeted temperature management: an evidence-based guideline from the Neurocritical Care Society. Neurocrit Care. 2017;27:468–487.

8. D'Eramo RE, Nadpara PA, Sandler M, et al. Intravenous versus oral acetaminophen use in febrile neurocritical care patients. Ther Hypothermia Temp Manag. 2021. doi.org/10.1089/ther.2021.0019

9. Moheet AM, Livesay SL, Abdelhak T, et al. Standards for neurologic critical care units: a statement for healthcare professionals from the Neurocritical Care Society. Neurocrit Care. 2018;29:145–160. doi.org/10.1007/s12028-018-0601-1

69

PARKINSON DISEASE

Slow and Shaky................................Level III

Mary L. Wagner, PharmD, MS

Jennifer Y. Chen, MD

LEARNING OBJECTIVES

After completing this case study, the reader should be able to:

- Recognize motor and nonmotor symptoms of Parkinson disease (PD).

- Develop an optimal pharmacotherapeutic plan for a patient with PD progressing through different stages of the disease.

- Recommend alternative therapy for a patient experiencing adverse drug effects, drug–drug interactions, and drug–food interactions.

- Educate patients with PD about the disease, pharmacotherapeutic options, and nonpharmacologic treatments.

PATIENT PRESENTATION

■ Chief Complaint

"I'm having problems at work because my tremor makes it difficult to type on the computer, and I am slower with most tasks."

■ HPI

LT is a 63-year-old, right-handed woman who presents to the neurology clinic for tremor. It started in her right thumb 2 years ago but has since progressed to her entire right hand and forearm. It is worse at rest and when she moves, it will initially improve but then come back. She also reports that she is slower overall in most of her tasks and her muscles feel a little stiff. She denies falls or changes to her gait and balance. She also admits to difficulty falling asleep at night, but no difficulty staying asleep. Of note, her partner also reports that she calls out in her sleep and reaches for objects but has not hurt him or herself. Her symptoms have affected her job performance as a graphic designer, resulting in her contemplating early retirement. She also complains of constipation, depressed mood, lack of pleasure in her usual activities, and loss of sense of smell for about 2 years.

■ PMH

Broken left wrist after fall 1 year ago

■ FH

Mother died at age 89 of complications associated with a hip fracture, osteoporosis, and Alzheimer disease (clinical diagnosis without postmortem confirmation); father died from an ischemic stroke at age 58; two daughters are in good health.

■ SH

(–) Alcohol, (–) tobacco, married for 23 years

■ Meds

Calcium carbonate 600 mg PO every morning and night

■ All

None

■ ROS

Smell: Decreased for last 2 years (as above).
Cognition: No changes except occasional word-finding difficulties.
Mood/behavior: Sad with mild apathy and occasional crying spells. No suicidal thoughts, hallucinations, paranoia, anxiety, or vivid dreams.
Speech/swallow: No problems.
Orthostasis: No lightheaded upon standing.
Bladder: Wakes up once per night. No incontinence.
Bowel: Moderate constipation (BM decreased from daily to every other day, uses laxatives about once a month).
Sleep: Insomnia as above; partner reports some dream enactment.
Temperature regulation: No problems, no sweating.
Pain: None.

■ Physical Examination

VS

BP 118/74 mm Hg sitting, 116/70 mm Hg standing, P 70 bpm, RR 13; T 36.8°C; Wt 53 kg, Ht 5′2″

Neuro Exam

Mental status: Patient is awake and alert, speech is fluent and appropriate. MoCA 30/30, PHQ9 10/27 (Score cut-offs of 5-mild, 10-moderate, 15-moderately severe, and 20 represent severe-depression; www.phqscreeners.com).
Cranial nerves: PERRLA, EOMI, face is symmetric but decreased blink rate and facial expression; no dysarthria, but speech with decreased cadence. Tongue is midline, shoulder shrug is 5/5 bilaterally.
Motor:

- Strength: Full strength throughout.

- Tone: Mild rigidity across the right arm, otherwise normal.

- Movements: Mild slowing and hesitations on right fast finger taps (FFTs), hand movements, and rapid alternating movements (RAMs). Toe taps and heel stomps are normal bilaterally.

- Tremor: Mild to moderate rest tremor on the right that re-emerges on posture after 10 seconds. Slight tremor on finger-nose-finger.

- Handwriting sample: Somewhat slow and progressively smaller in size indicating signs of micrographia.

- Other movements: None.

Gait: Rises out of chair easily without pushing off, base is narrow, good stride length, no freezing, normal turns. There is decreased right arm swing with re-emergent tremor. No retropulsion.
Remainder of the neurologic exam normal.
ADLS: She is able to perform all activities without assistance, but she reports problems with typing, dressing, cutting food, and motor coordination (due to decreased hand agility and tremor).
Modified Hoehn-Yahr stage I (unilateral involvement only).

■ Labs

Na 136 mEq/L	Hgb 13.5 g/dL	AST 20 IU/L
K 4.3 mEq/L	Hct 40.5%	ALT 24 IU/L
Cl 101 mEq/L	RBC 4.42 × 10⁶	Alk phos 80 IU/L
CO$_2$ 23 mEq/L	WBC 5.0 × 10³/mm³	GGT 18 IU/L
BUN 12 mg/dL	Plt 395 × 10³/mm³	Ferritin 100 ng/mL
SCr 0.73 mg/dL	Homocysteine 6 μmol/L	TSH 2.0 mIU/L
Glu 83 mg/dL	Vitamin D, 25-hydroxy 18 ng/mL	T$_4$ total 7.5 mcg/dL

■ **Assessment**

1. Parkinson disease, stage 1, newly diagnosed, untreated

2. Depression, untreated and uncontrolled

3. Sleep disturbances, untreated

4. Constipation, untreated and uncontrolled

■ **Clinical Course**

The patient is told that she has PD, and the various treatment options are presented to her. She asks about treatment options that may delay disease progression.

QUESTIONS

Collect Information

1.a. What subjective and objective information indicates the presence of PD?

1.b. What additional information is needed to fully assess this patient's PD?

Assess the Information

2.a. Assess the severity of PD based on the subjective and objective information available.

2.b. Create and prioritize a list of the patient's drug therapy problems. Include assessment of medication appropriateness, effectiveness, safety, and patient adherence.

2.c. What economic, psychosocial, safety, and ethical considerations are applicable to this patient?

Develop a Care Plan

3.a. What are the goals of pharmacotherapy for Parkinson's diseases motor and nonmotor symptoms in this case?

3.b. What nondrug therapies for PD might be useful for this patient?

3.c. What feasible pharmacotherapeutic options are available to treat this patient's PD?

3.d. Create an individualized, patient-centered, team-based care plan to optimize medication therapy for this patient's PD and other drug therapy problems. Include specific drugs, dosage forms, doses, schedules, and durations of therapy.

3.e. What alternatives would be appropriate for this patient's PD symptoms if the initial care plan fails or cannot be used?

Implement the Care Plan

4.a. What information should be provided to the patient/care partner to enhance adherence, ensure successful therapy, and minimize adverse effects?

4.b. Describe how care should be coordinated with other healthcare providers.

Follow-Up: Monitor and Evaluate

5. Explain how to monitor and evaluate the care plan for medication appropriateness, effectiveness, safety, and patient adherence by using clinical and laboratory data, patient feedback, and other information.

■ CLINICAL COURSE—7 YEARS LATER

Her symptoms improved after stating carbidopa-levodopa and she was stable for several years with slight increases in dose. She then started to develop mild wearing off for which rasagiline was added. This initially decreased her off time and she was able to continue working until age 65. In the last 3 years, her motor fluctuations worsened. She takes 1½ tabs of carbidopa-levodopa 25–100 every 4 hours (7:30 AM, 11:30 AM, 3:30 PM, 7:30 PM) but feels the wearing off an hour prior to her next dose and it takes about 30 min to an hour for the medication to work. In addition, she has occasional dose failures and unpredictable off periods. Her off symptoms consist of tremor, slowness, shuffling, and freezing of gait. Sometimes her OFF symptoms are so severe that she cannot move.

Pramipexole was recently added for worsening wearing-off but was discontinued due to compulsive/impulsive behavior. Entacapone was added with only minimal benefit. Of note, she also developed involuntary choreic movements that occur at peak dose. They are embarrassing, but patient prefers these movements than to being off. Amantadine was tried for the movements but caused worsening constipation and a strange pattern on her skin.

She is now 70 years old and no longer working but volunteering a few hours a week at the library and church. Her off symptoms cause difficulty with handling utensils, dressing, turning in bed, and getting out of a chair. Her freezing of gait has also caused occasional falls, which has made her fearful of starting exercise programs.

Her depression symptoms responded to CBT but increased to the point medication was needed. Venlafaxine was used initially used and then switched to mirtazapine for increased appetite and sleep effect. She continues with CBT and mindfulness training. Her sleep, appetite, and mood are adequately controlled. She denies any suicidal thoughts and reports no new problems with mood. However, she has been having occasional illusions, mistaking a tree for a person, or seeing a shadow in the corner of her eye. She retains insight and is redirectable when this occurs and does not find them bothersome. Cognitively, she feels some changes, having more word-finding difficulty and slower at processing but is still independent in her ADLs and instrumental ADLs.

About a month prior to the visit, she purchased coenzyme Q10, kava, and *Mucuna pruriens*/velvet bean (a herbal supplement that contains natural levodopa), thinking they would be a natural way to help her PD.

■ ROS

Cognition: More difficulty with word finding, multitasking, and slow processing but still independent.

Mood/behavior: Depression controlled on mirtazapine.

Speech/swallow: No problems but does not more occasional drooling. Not bothersome.

Orthostasis: Occasional lightheadedness, but no fainting or falls from it.

Bladder: Wakes up once per night. No incontinence.

Bowel: Constipation managed on bowel regimen; has bowel movement every day.

Sleep: Sleeps through night on mirtazapine; occasional calling out.

Vitals: BP 124/74 mm Hg (sitting), 104/70 (standing); and weight 50 kg.

Neuro exam: (she is currently On but starting to wear off)

- Mental status: Patient is awake and alert, speech is fluent and appropriate. MoCA 26/30 (–3 delayed recall but able to get with hints, –1 exact date), PHQ9 5/27.

- Cranial nerves: PERRLA, EOMI, face is symmetric, decreased facial expression in upper and lower face; no dysarthria, but speech slightly soft.

Motor:

- Tone: Mild rigidity across neck and right arm, slight across the left arm. Normal in legs.
- Movements: mild slowing and loss of amplitude on right fast finger taps (FFTs), hand movements, and rapid alternating movements (RAMs). Toe taps with multiple hesitations and moderate loss of amplitude, worse on the right. Heel stomps slightly slow bilaterally.
- Tremor: rare slight rest tremor on the right hand.
- Other movements: mild choreiform dyskinesias of the neck, shoulders, right arm, and right foot.

Gait: She can rise out of chair without use of arms but needs two tries; base is narrow, there is decreased stride length with right leg drag. There is brief freezing on turn. She takes 3 steps back on pull test but does not need to be caught.

Modified Hoehn-Yahr stage 3 (bilateral involvement, mild impairment in balance).

■ MEDS

Calcium carbonate 600 mg PO every morning and night
Carbidopa 25 mg/levodopa 100 mg 1 ½ tabs PO four times daily (7 AM, 12 PM, 5 PM, and 10 PM)
Rasagiline 1 mg PO once daily
Mirtazapine 15 mg PO at bedtime daily
Multivitamin one tablet PO daily
Metamucil one tablespoonful PO twice daily
Polyethylene glycol (PEG) 1 capful daily
Milk of Magnesia 1 tablespoon PRN (she takes about once monthly)
Coenzyme Q10 100 mg PO once daily
Kava 100 mg PO at bedtime
Velvet bean 30 g PO once daily
Calcium 500mg/magnesium 250 mg/vit D 1000 u daily

Previous Medication Tried

Pramipexole—stopped due to increased compulsive behaviors
Entacapone—minimal benefit
Amantadine—worsened constipation

■ LABS

Within normal limits and similar to previous labs: GFR 60 mL/min; ferritin 150 ng/mL

DXA scan (6 years ago) T-score: spine –1.8 and left hip –1.5

■ FOLLOW-UP QUESTIONS

1. List the patient's problems at this visit.
2. List and explain any drugs or foods that could be causing any drug–drug or drug–food interactions.
3. For each of the motor and nonmotor problems identified, what adjustments in drug therapy do you recommend?
4. What information should be provided to the patient to ensure successful therapy, enhance adherence, and minimize adverse effects with medications that have been added since the last visit?

■ SELF-STUDY ASSIGNMENTS[1]

1. Review the pharmacology and efficacy reports of investigational drugs for PD.
2. Investigate the treatment of other nonmotor symptoms of PD such as autonomic dysfunction, dementia, apathy, anxiety, and psychosis and assess which ones can be prodrome symptoms that precede the diagnosis of PD.
3. Investigate the use of deep brain stimulation for the treatment of motor complications in PD.

CLINICAL PEARL

As PD progresses, the timing of medication needs to coincide with symptoms. Evaluate the onset and duration of each dose and make modifications accordingly. Symptoms may worsen when patients are forced to receive medications at predetermined dosing times such as those used in hospitals and nursing homes. Thus, let the patient's symptoms guide the dosing times

ACKNOWLEDGMENT

This case is based on the patient case written for the 11th edition by Mary L. Wagner, PharmD, MS and Yuchen Wang, PharmD.

REFERENCES

1. Bloem BR, Okun MS, Klein C. Parkinson's disease. Lancet. 2021;397 (10291):2284–2303.
2. Bloem BR, Okun MS, Klein C. Parkinson's disease: supplementary appendix. Lancet. 2021;397(10291). Available at: *https://ars-els-cdn-com.proxy1.library.jhu.edu/content/image/1-s2.0-S014067362100218X-mmc2.pdf*. Accessed April 15, 2022.
3. Grimes D, Fitzpatrick M, Gordon J, et al. Canadian guideline for Parkinson disease. CMAJ. 2019;191(36):E989–E1004.
4. de Bie RMA, Clarke CE, Espay AJ, Fox SH, Lang AE. Initiation of pharmacological therapy in Parkinson's disease: when, why, and how. Lancet Neurol. 2020;19(5):452–461.
5. Seppi K, Ray Chaudhuri K, Coelho M, et al; The collaborators of the Parkinson's Disease Update on Non-Motor Symptoms Study Group on behalf of the Movement Disorders Society Evidence-Based Medicine Committee. Update on treatments for nonmotor symptoms of Parkinson's disease-an evidence-based medicine review. Mov Disord. 2019;34(2):180–198. Erratum in: Mov Disord. 2019;34(5):765.
6. Fox SH, Katzenschlager R, Lim SY, et al. International Parkinson and movement disorder society evidence-based medicine review: update on treatment for the motor symptoms of Parkinson's disease. Mov Disord. 2018;33(8):1248–1266.
7. Goetz CG, Poewe W, Rascol O, et al. Movement Disorder Society Task Force report on the Hoehn and Yahr staging scale: status and recommendations. Mov Disord. 2004;19(9):1020–1028.
8. Bega D, Zadik C. Complementary and alternative management of Parkinson's disease: an evidence-based review of Eastern influenced practices. J Mov Disord. 2014;7(2):57–66.
9. Zigmond MJ, Cameron JL, Hoffer BJ, Smeyne RJ. Neurorestoration by physical exercise: moving forward. Parkinsonism Relat Disord. 2012;18(Suppl 1):S147–S150.
10. The Medical Letter, Inc. Drugs for Parkinson's disease. Med Letter Drugs. 2021;63(1618):25–32.

70

CHRONIC PAIN MANAGEMENT

Opioid Medication in Cancer Survivorship ...... Level III

Stephanie Abel, PharmD, BCPS

LEARNING OBJECTIVES

After completing this case study, the reader should be able to:

- Define the goals for pain management in a patient with chronic pain in cancer survivorship.

- Apply the principles and tools discussed when prescribing, assessing, monitoring, and dispensing chronic opioid therapy (COT) in cancer survivorship

- Identify possible presence of risk factors for aberrant behavior surrounding COT in the setting of cancer survivorship.

- Describe strategies to identify and manage aberrant drug-related behavior (ADRB) and risks associated with COT.

- Recommend pharmacotherapy using current guidelines for prescribing COT in patients in cancer survivorship.

PATIENT PRESENTATION

■ Chief Complaint

"I am here to get help with the pain from my cancer. I have been cured for 3 years but am still in so much pain every day. Everything hurts. My pain is 10/10, it is always at a 10/10! I have tried the medications that everyone has prescribed me, but they never seem to work and I'm still in pain and I miss out on so many things. On top of that, we moved here a few months ago because my husband got a good job and the schools are better for our kids, but I don't really know anyone, and it has been so stressful (patient becomes tearful). I am so tired all the time and can't contribute at home or do the things I should be doing."

■ HPI

A 33-year-old woman presents to clinic for chronic pain management from sequelae of her cancer treatment. She has a history of stage 1b2 cervical cancer s/p total abdominal hysterectomy with bilateral salpingo-oophorectomy (TAH-BSO), pelvic radiation, and cisplatin, paclitaxel, and bevacizumab chemotherapy. She has no evidence of disease and has not had active cancer for the past 3 years.

Pain Assessment

Onset/course: since cancer started
Location: bilateral lower extremities, low back, bilateral groin, vagina, rectum
Quality: legs and feet: burning, shooting, stinging; back and bilateral groin: sharp, burning; vagina and rectum: pressure like
Intensity: 10/10
Worse: nothing
Better: higher dose of pain medications
Associated symptoms: numbness and tingling started after chemotherapy

While there are no definitive signs of non-medical use of her opioid medications, she has been calling and asking for early refills of her opioid medications due to overuse since she established care after moving 3 months ago.

■ PMH

History of stage 1b2 cervical cancer (diagnosed 6 years ago, no evidence of disease for past 3 years)
Chronic renal failure with percutaneous nephrostomy tubes (PNT)
Anxiety
Depression

■ FH

Her brother had opioid use disorder and died of an opioid-related overdose 2 years ago.

■ SH

The patient is on disability and lives at home with her husband and two school-aged children. She denies using illicit drugs, alcohol, or tobacco.

■ Meds

Oxycodone IR 30 mg PO Q4H PRN for pain
Morphine ER 160 mg PO Q8H for pain
Gabapentin 800 mg Q8H
Diazepam 5 mg PO TID PRN

■ All

No known drug allergies

■ ROS

Positive for fatigue, depression, pain in lower extremities, groin, low back, vagina, and rectum

■ Physical Examination

Gen

The patient is a 33-year-old woman with negative affect and normal appearance.

VS

BP 120/72 mm Hg, P 76 bpm, RR 15, T 37.5°C; Wt 58 kg, Ht 155 cm

HEENT

PERRLA, EOMI, TMs intact

Neck

Supple, no JVD, no bruits

Resp

CTA and P; no crackles or wheezes

CV

NSR without MRG

Breasts

Negative

Abd

Soft, NT, liver and spleen not palpable, (+) BS, bilateral percutaneous nephrostomy tubes functioning properly without any noted site tenderness or inflammation

Genit/Rect

Positive for bladder incontinence, dyspareunia, pelvic pain, vaginal bleeding, and vaginal discharge

MS/Ext

Tone: normal
Strength: 5/5 in BUE & BLE

Positive for myoclonic jerking in BUE approximately every 60 seconds, pain in lower extremities, groin, low back, vagina, and rectum with hyperalgesia in lower extremities (sensitivity to cold, pressure, touch, vibration) and low back (sensitivity to pressure and vibration)

Neuro

CN II–XII intact, A&O × 3
Normal motor strength in the upper extremities with reflexes 1+ and symmetric and normal sensation extremities, no CCE

■ Labs

Chem 7: SCr 1.4, everything else WNL
LFTs: WNL
CBC: WNL

■ Assessment

1. Cancer-related pain with opioid-induced hyperalgesia
2. Chronic renal failure with PNT and opioid-induced neurotoxicity
3. Possible ADRB
4. Anxiety
5. Depression

QUESTIONS

Collect Information

1.a. What subjective and objective information indicates the presence or severity of chronic cancer-related pain in a cancer survivor?

1.b. What additional information is needed to fully assess this patient's chronic pain?

Assess the Information

2.a. Assess the severity of chronic cancer-related pain based on the subjective and objective information available.

2.b. Create a list of the patient's drug therapy problems and prioritize them. Include assessment of medication appropriateness, effectiveness, safety, and patient adherence.

Develop a Care Plan

3.a. What are the patient's goals of pharmacotherapy in this case?

3.b. What nondrug therapies for chronic cancer-related pain might be useful for this patient?

3.c. What feasible pharmacotherapeutic options are available for treating chronic cancer-related pain in survivorship?

3.d. Create an individualized, patient-centered, team-based care plan to optimize medication therapy for this patient. Include specific drugs, dosage forms, doses, schedules, and durations of therapy.

3.e. What alternatives would be appropriate if the optimal plan fails or cannot be used?

Implement the Care Plan

4.a. What information should be provided to the patient to enhance adherence, ensure successful therapy, and minimize adverse effects?

4.b. Describe how care should be coordinated with other healthcare providers.

Follow-Up: Monitor and Evaluate

5. Explain how to monitor and evaluate the care plan for medication appropriateness, effectiveness, safety, and patient adherence by using clinical and laboratory data, patient feedback, and other information.

■ CLINICAL COURSE

The physician in the clinic decides that the patient is at a very high risk for accidental opioid overdose because of her high total daily opioid dose and concomitant gabapentin and diazepam. The physician also states that her recent urine drug screening (UDS) came back positive for opiates and oxycodone and asks for a consult.

■ FOLLOW-UP QUESTIONS

1. What tools can be employed to monitor for aberrant drug-related behavior?

2. What steps can be taken if the patient begins to exhibit aberrant drug-related behavior, yet has a valid reason to continue opioid medications?

3. Compare and contrast the terms: physical dependence, tolerance, addiction, and withdrawal.

■ SELF-STUDY ASSIGNMENTS

1. Prepare a list of opioids and their corresponding equianalgesic dosing.

2. The use of opioid medication is a controversial topic; often it is driven more by passion than by scientific data. In three to four sentences per viewpoint, discuss this issue from the perspective of (1) a provider and (2) the patient.

CLINICAL PEARL

Opioids are often used in the treatment of cancer-related pain. As cancer survivorship continues to increase, these patients should be evaluated for a decrease in their opioid therapy, addressing any high-risk concomitant medications and managing any long-term adverse effects of opioid therapy.

ACKNOWLEDGMENT

This case is based on the patient case written for the 11th edition by Ernest J. Dole, PharmD, PhC, FASHP, BCPS.

REFERENCES

1. Glare P, Aubrey K, Gulati A, Lee YC, Moryl N, Overton S. Pharmacologic management of persistent pain in cancer survivors. Drugs. 2022;82(3):275–291. doi: 10.1007/s40265-022-01675-6.

2. Cheatle MD, Compton PA, Dhingra L, et al. Development of the revised opioid risk tool to predict opioid use disorder in patients with chronic nonmalignant pain. J Pain. 2019;20(7):842–851. doi: 10.1016/j.jpain.2019.01.011MEDD.

3. Tesarz J, Leisner S, Gerhardt A, et al. Effects of eye movement desensitization and reprocessing (EMDR) treatment in chronic pain patients: a systematic review. Pain Med. 2014;15:247–263.

4. Bhaskar A. Interventional pain management in patients with cancer-related pain. Postgrad Med. 2020;132(Supl 3):13–16. doi: 10.1080/00325481.2020.1807796.

5. Dowell D, Ragan KR, Jones CM, Baldwin GT, Chou R. CDC Clinical Practice Guideline for Prescribing Opioids for Pain — United States, 2022. MMWR Recomm Rep. 2022;71(No. RR-3):1–95. doi: 10.15585/mmwr.rr7103a1.

6. National Comprehensive Cancer Network. National Comprehensive Cancer Network Clinical Practice Guidelines in Oncology. Survivorship. Version 3, 2021. Available at: https://www.nccn.org/login?ReturnURL=https://www.nccn.org/professionals/physician_gls/pdf/survivorship.pdf. Accessed April 15, 2022.

7. Paice JA, Portenoy R, Lacchetti C, et al. Management of chronic pain in survivors of adult cancers: American Society of Clinical Oncology Clinical Practice Guideline. J Clin Oncol. 2016;34(27):3325–3345. doi: 10.1200/JCO.2016.68.5206.

8. Webster LW, Fine PG. Review and critique of opioid rotation practices and associated risks of toxicity. Pain Med. 2012;1:1–9.

9. Argoff CE, Alford DP, Fudin J, et al. Rational urine drug monitoring in patients receiving opioids for chronic pain: Consensus recommendations. Pain Med. 2018;19(1):97–117. doi: 10.1093/pm/pnx285.

10. Jannetto PJ, Langman LJ. Using clinical laboratory tests to monitor drug therapy in pain management patients. J Appl Lab Med. 2018;2(4):471–472. doi: 10.1373/jalm.2017.025304.

71

ACUTE PAIN MANAGEMENT

No Pain, Much Gain............................Level I

Charles D. Ponte, BSc, PharmD, BC-ADM, BCPS, CDCES, CPE, FADCES, FAPhA, FASHP, FCCP, FNAP

LEARNING OBJECTIVES

After completing this case study, the reader should be able to:

- Differentiate acute pain from chronic pain.

- Describe the typical clinical findings associated with acute pain.

- Describe the subjective and objective assessment of pain.

- Identify appropriate nonopioid and opioid analgesics for selected patients with acute pain.

- Choose suitable drug and nondrug therapy for the management of common opioid analgesic side effects.

- Develop an appropriate therapeutic plan (including monitoring parameters) for a patient with acute pain.

PATIENT PRESENTATION

■ Chief Complaint

"My belly hurts, and I can't stand the sight of food."

■ HPI

A 68-year-old man presents to the emergency department with a 2-day history of nausea, vomiting, and epigastric and RUQ abdominal pain. The patient states that the pain began several hours after eating a large platter of extra hot chicken wings with cheese fries and gravy at a local restaurant. The pain intensified and was associated with escalating nausea followed by several episodes of vomiting. The vomiting finally ceased, but the abdominal pain has persisted and is worse after meals. The pain is now dull, constant, and "bores" to his back. Lying up in bed or sitting in a chair seems to relieve some of the pain. Since the initial episode, his appetite has decreased, and he has been avoiding fried or fatty foods. He denies any change in stool color or consistency.

■ PMH

HTN × 20 years; poorly controlled
Dyslipidemia × 23 years
Alcoholic fatty liver disease without cirrhosis × 10 years

■ FH

Father deceased (esophageal varices), age 76; mother deceased (MI), age 83; brother alive and well, age 65; sister with breast cancer and gallbladder disease, age 58

■ SH

He is a retired bar owner and lives with his wife (married for 35 years) on a 10-acre farm a few miles from town. He has two dogs and a cat. He has a 50 pack-year history of smoking and a history of chronic alcohol abuse.

■ ROS

As per HPI; otherwise negative

■ Meds

Atorvastatin 20 mg PO once daily
Hydrochlorothiazide 25 mg PO once daily
Losartan 100 mg PO once daily
Aspirin 81 mg PO once daily
Famotidine 20 mg PO PRN heartburn
MVI one tablet PO once daily

■ All

Doxycycline—abdominal pain
Morphine—hives, mild wheezing, and throat "tightness"

■ Physical Examination

Gen

A pleasant, elderly man in mild to moderate acute distress; appears his stated age

VS

BP 160/95 mm Hg (sitting), P 84 bpm, RR 20, T 37.8°C; pain 6/10; Wt 90 kg, Ht 5′10″

HEENT

PERRLA, fundi with mild AV nicking; TMs intact; mucous membranes moist

Chest

Clear to A&P

Heart

Normal S_1 and S_2; without murmur, rub, or gallop

Abd

Normal bowel sounds, without organomegaly, moderate diffuse epigastric pain with deep palpation with mild guarding

Genit/Rect

Slightly enlarged prostate; guaiac (–) stool

Ext

Good strength throughout, reflexes intact, mild decreased pinprick sensation to both lower extremities; no CCE

■ Labs

Na 138 mEq/L	Hgb 12.6 g/dL	AST 98 U/L
K 3.6 mEq/L	Hct 36%	ALT 77 U/L
Cl 97 mEq/L	Platelets 340 × 10³/mm³	Alk phos 200 U/L
CO₂ 23 mEq/L	WBC 14.0 × 10³/mm³	T. bili 3.4 mg/dL
BUN 15 mg/dL	Neutros 76%	D. bili 2.6 mg/dL
SCr 1.3 mg/dL	Bands 4%	Amylase 435 U/L
Glu 110 mg/dL	Eos 2%	Lipase 367 U/L
	Lymphs 18%	Lipids
		T. chol 210 mg/dL
		HDL 30 mg/dL
		LDL 120 mg/dL
		TG 300 mg/dL

■ Assessment

A 68-year-old man admitted to the emergency department with acute pain due to presumed acute cholecystitis/acute pancreatitis from biliary obstruction or alcohol abuse.

QUESTIONS

Collect Information

1.a. What subjective and objective information indicates the presence of acute pain?

1.b. What additional information is needed to fully assess this patient's acute pain?

Assess the Information

2.a. Assess the severity of acute pain based on the subjective and objective information available.

2.b. Create a list of the patient's drug therapy problems and prioritize them. Include assessment of medication appropriateness, effectiveness, safety, and patient adherence.

2.c. What economic, psychosocial, cultural, racial, and ethical considerations are applicable to this patient?

Develop a Care Plan

3.a. What are the goals of pharmacotherapy in this case?

3.b. What nondrug therapies for acute pain management might be useful for this patient?

3.c. What feasible pharmacotherapeutic options are available to treat this patient's acute pain?

3.d. Create an individualized, patient-centered, team-based care plan to optimize medication therapy for this patient's acute pain and other drug therapy problems. Include specific drugs, dosage forms, doses, schedules, and durations of therapy.

3.e. What alternatives would be appropriate if the initial care plan fails or cannot be used?

Implement the Care Plan

4.a. What information should be provided to the patient to enhance adherence, ensure successful therapy, and minimize adverse effects?

4.b. Describe how care should be coordinated with other healthcare providers.

Follow-Up: Monitor and Evaluate

5. Explain how to monitor and evaluate the care plan for medication appropriateness, effectiveness, safety, and patient adherence by using clinical and laboratory data, patient feedback, and other information.

■ CLINICAL COURSE

The patient was admitted to the hospital for presumed cholecystitis/acute pancreatitis/hepatitis and pain control. An abdominal ultrasound and abdominal CT were ordered. Blood cultures were obtained. Gastroenterology and general surgery services were consulted. The patient was made NPO except for his home medications. A sliding-scale insulin regimen was also ordered.

The drug therapy regimen that a pharmacist recommended for the patient was initiated. At the end of the first hospital day, the patient states that the medication "eases the pain some," but the pain is inadequately controlled. The pain is rated as an 8/10 using a single-dimensional visual analog pain scale. The patient also complains of some nausea and urinary hesitancy.

■ FOLLOW-UP QUESTIONS

1. What is the most likely cause of this patient's inadequate pain control?

2. What are the revised management goals for this patient?

■ SELF-STUDY ASSIGNMENTS

1. Describe the role of NMDA antagonists in the management of pain.

2. Describe the pathophysiology and management of opioid-induced respiratory depression.

3. What types of pain do not typically respond to opioid analgesics?

4. Explain the pathophysiology behind the development of opioid tolerance.

5. Explain the concepts of equianalgesic doses and relative analgesic potency.

6. Explain the WHO analgesic ladder and list representative analgesic classes (or individual agents) associated with each step of the ladder.

7. Describe the advantages and disadvantages of single- and multi-dimensional pain assessment instruments.

CLINICAL PEARL

Analgesic tolerance can be overcome by switching from one opioid to another. Because cross-tolerance is not complete among opioids, use only 50–75% of the equianalgesic dose of an opioid when changing from one drug to another and titrate accordingly.

REFERENCES

1. Caparrotta TM, Antoine DJ, Dear JW. Are some people at increased risk of paracetamol-induced liver injury? A critical review of the literature. Eur J Clin Pharmacol. 2018;74:147–160.

2. Bello AE, Holt RJ. Cardiovascular risk with non-steroidal anti-inflammatory drugs: clinical implications. Drug Saf. 2014;37:897–902.

3. Friedman A, Nabong L. Opioids: pharmacology, pathophysiology, and clinical implications in pain medicine. Phys Med Rehabil Clin N Am. 2020;31:289–303.

4. Swegle JM, Logemann C. Management of common opioid-induced adverse effects. Am Fam Physician 2006;74:1347–1354.

5. Martyn JAJ, Mao J, Bittner EA. Opioid tolerance in critical illness. N Engl J Med. 2019 Jan 24;380(4):365–378.

6. Pastino A, Lakra A. Patient controlled analgesia. In: StatPearls [Internet]. StatPearls Publishing. Available at: *https://www.ncbi.nlm.nih.gov/books/NBK551610/*. Accessed January 2, 2022.

7. Whelton PK, Carey RM, Aronow WS, et al. 2017 ACC/AHA/AAPA/ABC/ACPM/AGS/APhA/ASH/ASPC/NMA/PCNA guideline for the prevention, detection, evaluation, and management of high blood pressure in adults: a report of the American College of Cardiology/American Heart Association Task Force on clinical practice guidelines. J Am Coll Cardiol. 2018;71:e127–e248.

8. Azoulay L, Filion KB, Platt RW, et al. Association between incretin-based drugs and the risk of acute pancreatitis. JAMA Intern Med. 2016;176(10):1464–1473.

9. Pizzimenti V, Giandalia A, Cucinotta D, et al. Incretin-based therapy and acute cholecystitis: a review of case reports and EudraVigilance spontaneous adverse drug reaction reporting database. J Clin Pharm Ther. 2016;41:116–118.

72

PAIN, AGITATION, AND DELIRIUM IN CRITICAL CARE

Dazed and Confused .... Level III

Mojdeh S. Heavner, PharmD, BCPS, BCCCP, FCCM

Jason J. Heavner, MD, FCCP

LEARNING OBJECTIVES

After completing this case study, the reader should be able to:

- Assess pain, agitation, and delirium in the intensive care unit.

- Discuss goals of therapy in the management of pain, agitation, and delirium in the intensive care unit (ICU).

- Design an evidence-based pharmacotherapeutic regimen for managing pain, agitation, and delirium in the ICU.

- Identify patient- and agent-related factors that may affect how the patient is managed for pain, agitation, and delirium in the ICU.

PATIENT PRESENTATION

▪ Chief Complaint

"Trouble breathing" per family

▪ HPI

A 72-year-old woman with a history of dyslipidemia and mild cognitive impairment was brought to the emergency department (ED) because she was acting strange and appeared to have trouble breathing. The day prior, the patient had a cough, shortness of breath, and reported a subjective fever. Today, her family found the patient lying on the floor with labored breathing; she was sleepy and not talking.

Upon arrival to the ED, she was obtunded and required emergent intubation for airway protection. Post-intubation chest radiograph revealed a right lobe consolidation as well as a right-sided moderate pneumothorax. A chest tube was inserted, followed by a swoosh of air. Post-intubation, the patient had progressive hypotension requiring treatment with norepinephrine infusion, vasopressin, and hydrocortisone. She was admitted to the intensive care unit for further management.

▪ PMH

Mild cognitive impairment
Dyslipidemia

▪ FH

Her father had a history of alcohol dependence and died from complications of cirrhosis. The patient's mother had a history of Alzheimer dementia and died from complications of pneumonia. Her two children are healthy.

▪ SH

Married; retired lawyer; never smoker; per family report, she occasionally drinks one glass of wine.

▪ Home Meds

Rosuvastatin 10mg PO nightly
Calcium + vitamin D3 600 mg/20 mcg daily

▪ Current Meds

Piperacillin/tazobactam 3.375 g IV Q 8 H
Norepinephrine 0.1 mcg/kg/min IV infusion
Vasopressin 0.03 units/min
Hydrocortisone 50 mg IV Q 6 H
Midazolam 5 mg/hr IV infusion

▪ All

NKDA

▪ ROS

Unobtainable secondary to patient's critical condition

◼ Physical Examination

Gen

Well developed, intubated, restless

VS

BP 99/58 mm Hg (MAP 72 mm Hg), P 90 bpm, RR 22, T 37.6°C; SpO$_2$ 97% on AC/VC 22 bpm/350 mL/5 cm H$_2$O/50%; Wt 64.4 kg, Ht 5′5″, BMI 23.6 kg/m^2

Skin

Normal turgor; mottling over knees and lower extremities

HEENT

NC/AT; sclera anicteric; endotracheal tube with copious, thick, yellow secretions

Neck/Lymph Nodes

Trachea midline, no cervical lymphadenopathy or thyromegaly

CV

RRR; S$_1$, S$_2$ normal; no M/R/G

Lungs

Diffuse coarse rhonchi bilaterally, decrease air entry in right base. Right lateral chest tube site intact without crepitus. No air leak present.

Abd

Soft, non-distended, hypoactive bowel sounds

Genit/Rect

Normal external female anatomy; foley catheter in place draining clear yellow urine

MS/Ext

Capillary refill 3 seconds; no lower extremity edema; DP pulses 1+ bilaterally

Neuro

Agitated, not oriented, fluctuating mental status, inattentive, unable to answer yes/no questions, unable to follow commands; RASS +2; CPOT 6; no focal deficits

◼ Labs

Na 136 mEq/L	Glu 190 mg/dL	Bilirubin 1.1 mg/dL
K 4.5 mEq/L	Anion gap 19 mEq/L	AST 12 IU/L
Cl 99 mEq/L	Ca 8.9 mg/dL	ALT 40 IU/L
CO$_2$ 18 mEq/L	Protein total 7.1 g/dL	TSH 1.5 μIU/mL
BUN 45 mg/dL	Albumin 3.2 g/dL	
SCr 1.8 mg/dL (1 month prior 0.7 mg/dL)		Sputum gram stain: Gram-positive cocci in pairs and chains

◼ Chest Radiograph

1. Right lower lobe infiltrate, moderate right pneumothorax with midline trachea.
2. Endotracheal and nasogastric tubes in appropriate position. Left-sided central venous catheter well positioned with tip at the cavo-atrial junction. Right-sided chest tube in place with tip positioned apically. Trace residual apical pneumothorax.

◼ Assessment

A 72-year-old woman with a history of dyslipidemia and mild cognitive impairment admitted to ED, given emergent intubation, and diagnosed with right-sided moderate pneumothorax. She was admitted to the ICU to be managed for agitation associated with ICU delirium, pain, pneumonia, septic shock, and acute kidney injury.

QUESTIONS

Collect Information

1.a. What subjective and objective information indicates the presence of ICU delirium?

1.b. What additional information is needed to fully assess this patient's ICU delirium?

Assess the Information

2.a. Assess the severity of this patient's ICU delirium based on the subjective and objective information available.

2.b. Create a list of the patient's drug therapy problems and prioritize them. Include assessment of medication appropriateness, effectiveness, and safety.

Develop a Care Plan

3.a. What are the goals of pharmacotherapy for ICU delirium in this case?

3.b. What nondrug therapies for ICU delirium might be useful for this patient?

3.c. What feasible pharmacotherapeutic options are available for treating ICU delirium in this patient?

3.d. Create an individualized, patient-centered, team-based care plan to optimize medication therapy for this patient's ICU delirium and other drug therapy problems. Include specific drugs, dosage forms, doses, schedules, and durations of therapy.

Implement the Care Plan

4.a. What information should be provided to the patient/family to ensure successful therapy, and minimize adverse effects?

4.b. Describe how care should be coordinated with other healthcare providers.

Follow-Up: Monitor and Evaluate

5. Explain how to monitor and evaluate the care plan for medication appropriateness, effectiveness, safety, and patient adherence by using clinical and laboratory data, patient feedback, and other information.

◼ SELF-STUDY ASSIGNMENTS

1. Review treatment options for refractory ICU delirium. What is the quality of data supporting these alternate therapies and what are the safety considerations with their use?

2. Evaluate the clinical studies comparing propofol versus dexmedetomidine for routine ICU sedation. Considering the data available, develop a treatment algorithm to decide which drug to use in what scenario. Include goals of therapy and titration instructions.

3. Identify studies that have investigated transitions of care issues in patients receiving neuropsychiatric medications for ICU delirium (eg, antipsychotics, opioids). How would you recommend incorporating these therapies into practice without the risk of inadvertently continuing therapy beyond the ICU stay or hospitalization?

4. Consider how your choice of agents may change if encountering a patient with a history of polysubstance abuse (eg, alcohol, benzodiazepines, opioids, intravenous drugs, other illicit substances). Review the literature on this subject and determine how you would modify your approach for routine sedation in those patient scenarios.

CLINICAL PEARL

Delirium is a common occurrence in the ICU. It may be related to underlying conditions but may also be a risk associated with medications used to manage the agitated patient. In general, a strategy of no or light sedation should be incorporated along with the A-to-F bundle to optimize outcomes. Patients requiring pharmacologic management of ICU delirium and pain may be best treated with dexmedetomidine- or propofol-based sedation strategies and opioid-minimizing analgesia strategies.

REFERENCES

1. Devlin JW, Skrobik Y, Gélinas C, et al. Clinical practice guidelines for the prevention and management of pain, agitation/sedation, delirium, immobility, and sleep disruption in adult patients in the ICU. Crit Care Med. 2018;46(9):e825–e873.

2. Stollings JL, Kotfis K, Chanques G, Pun BT, Pandharipande PP, Ely EW. Delirium in critical illness: clinical manifestations, outcomes, and management. Intensive Care Med. 2021;47(10):1089–1103.

3. Khan BA, Perkins AJ, Gao S, et al. The confusion assessment method for the ICU-7 delirium severity scale: a novel delirium severity instrument for use in the ICU. Crit Care Med. 2017;45(5):851–857.

4. Reardon DP, Anger KE, Szumita PM. Pathophysiology, assessment, and management of pain in critically ill adults. Am J Health Syst Pharm. 2015;72(18):1531–1543.

5. Girard TD, Exline MC, Carson SS, et al; MIND-USA Investigators. Haloperidol and ziprasidone for treatment of delirium in critical illness. N Engl J Med. 2018;379(26):2506–2516.

6. Shehabi Y, Serpa Neto A, Howe BD, et al; SPICE III Study Investigators. Early sedation with dexmedetomidine in ventilated critically ill patients and heterogeneity of treatment effect in the SPICE III randomised controlled trial. Intensive Care Med. 2021;47(4):455–466.

7. Hughes CG, Mailloux PT, Devlin JW, et al; MENDS2 Study Investigators. Dexmedetomidine or propofol for sedation in mechanically ventilated adults with sepsis. N Engl J Med. 2021;384(15):1424–1436.

8. Corrado MJ, Kovacevic MP, Dube KM, Lupi KE, Szumita PM, DeGrado JR. The incidence of propofol-induced hypertriglyceridemia and identification of associated risk factors. Crit Care Explor. 2020;2(12):e0282.

9. Adams CD, Altshuler J, Barlow BL, et al. Analgesia and sedation strategies in mechanically ventilated adults with COVID-19. Pharmacotherapy 2020;40(12):1180–1191.

10. Witcraft EJ, Gonzales JP, Seung H, et al. Continuation of opioid therapy at transitions of care in critically ill patients. J Intensive Care Med. 2021;36(8):879–884.

73

MIGRAINE HEADACHE

It's Not Just a Headache! . . . . Level II

Susan R. Winkler, PharmD, BCPS, FCCP

Brittany Hoffmann-Eubanks, PharmD, MBA

LEARNING OBJECTIVES

After completing this case study, the reader should be able to:

• Develop pharmacotherapeutic goals for preventing and treating migraine headaches.

• Provide appropriate pharmacotherapeutic recommendations for an individual patient based on the patient's headache type and severity, medical history, previous drug therapy, concomitant problems, and pertinent laboratory data.

• Educate patients on the use of abortive and prophylactic agents for migraine headaches and menstrual migraines.

• Describe the appropriate use of a headache diary and how it may be used to refine headache treatment.

PATIENT PRESENTATION

■ Chief Complaint

"This new medication is not working for my migraines. My headaches are worse around my period, and I have gained 10 pounds!"

■ HPI

A 34-year-old woman presents to the neurology clinic for a follow-up of migraine headaches. She states that she used to get about two migraines every month; however, she recently went back to work full time and has two young children, ages 3 and 5, to care for. Since then, the frequency of her migraines has increased to about four to five per month. She states her migraines usually occur in the morning and are more frequent around her menses. Her typical headache evolves quickly (within 1 hour) and involves severe throbbing pain that is unilateral and temporal in distribution. Her headaches are preceded by an aura that consists of nausea and pastel lights flashing throughout her visual field. Photophobia occurs frequently, and vomiting may occur with an extreme headache. She reports experiencing severe migraine attacks that cause her to miss 1 day of work each month. She is unable to complete household chores and has a difficult time caring for her children on the days she has severe migraine attacks. She also complains of having mild migraine attacks lasting 3 days per month, during which her productivity at work and home is reduced by half. She typically has to retreat to a dark room and avoid any noise, or the severity of the migraine increases. She rates her migraines as 7–8 on a headache scale of 1–10, with 10 being the worst. At her previous visit to the neurology clinic 3 months ago, she was prescribed naratriptan 2.5 mg orally to be taken at the onset of headache. However, naratriptan has not been effective for half of her migraines in the past 3 months. During two of the attacks, she experienced partial pain relief, with the pain returning later in the day. She was prescribed naratriptan when Cafergot stopped working. She states she has taken her medications precisely as advised. She prefers to use medications that can be taken orally. She was also started on valproic acid at her last clinic visit for headache prophylaxis and has noticed a 10-lb weight gain. She inquires about switching from valproic acid to another medication.

■ PMH

Migraine with aura since age 29; previous medical workup, including an EEG and a head MRI, demonstrated no PVD, CVA, brain tumor, infection, cerebral aneurysm, or epileptic component; mild depression for 8 months

■ FH

Positive for migraines (both parents); hypertension and type 2 diabetes (mother)

■ SH

Secretary; recently changed jobs to a full-time position. Mother of two boys, ages 3 and 5. Denies alcohol use; started smoking cigarettes again 3 months ago due to stress, 1 ppd. Reports she also sometimes uses e-cigarettes as she would like to quit smoking. Occasional caffeine intake.

■ Meds

- Currently prescribed:
  - ✓ Naratriptan 2.5-mg tablets, one tablet PO at the onset of migraine, repeat dose of 2.5 mg PO in 4 hours if a partial response or if headache returns. Maximum dose 5 mg/24 hr.
  - ✓ Metoclopramide 10 mg PO at the onset of migraine
  - ✓ Valproic acid 500 mg PO at bedtime
  - ✓ Sertraline 50 mg PO at bedtime
- Past abortive migraine therapies:
  - ✓ Simple analgesics, NSAIDs, and Cafergot (good efficacy until 3 months ago)
  - ✓ Narcotics (good efficacy, but puts her "out of commission for days")
  - ✓ Midrin (no efficacy)
- Past prophylactic therapies prescribed:
  - ✓ Propranolol 20 mg BID (increased episodes of dizziness and lightheadedness; patient self-discontinued medication)
- Mild depression for 8 months, treated in the past with:
  - ✓ Bupropion SR 150 mg PO BID (minimal efficacy, self-discontinued 3 months ago)

■ All

NKDA

■ ROS

Complains of increased frequency of migraine headaches starting about 6 months ago; increased frequency around menses. Limited efficacy with naratriptan; no nausea, vomiting, diarrhea, or flashing lights at present.

■ Physical Examination

Gen

WDWN woman in mild distress

VS

BP 132/78 mm Hg, HR 76, RR 18, T 37.2°C; Wt 75 kg, Ht 5′3″

Skin

Normal skin turgor; no diaphoresis

HEENT

PERRLA; EOMI; no funduscopic exam performed

Neck

Supple; no masses, thyroid enlargement, adenopathy, bruits, or JVD

Chest

Good breath sounds bilaterally; clear to A&P

CV

RRR; S_1, S_2 normal; no murmurs, rubs, or gallops

Abd

Soft, NT/ND, no hepatosplenomegaly; (+) BS

Genit/Rect

Deferred

MS/Ext

UE/LE strength 5/5 with normal tone; radial and femoral pulses 3+ bilaterally; no edema; no evidence of thrombophlebitis; full ROM

Neuro

A&O × 3; no dysarthria or aphasia; memory intact; no nystagmus; no fasciculations, tremor, or ataxia; (–) Romberg; CN II–XII intact; sensory intact; DTRs: 2+ throughout; Babinski (–) bilaterally

■ Labs

Na 142 mEq/L	Hgb 13 g/dL	AST 23 IU/L
K 4.2 mEq/L	Hct 40%	ALT 25 IU/L
Cl 101 mEq/L	Plt 302 × 10³/mm³	Alk phos 35 IU/L
CO₂ 23 mEq/L	WBC 8 × 10³/mm³	Urine pregnancy test (–)
BUN 12 mg/dL	Differential WNL	
SCr 0.8 mg/dL		
Glu 95 mg/dL		

■ Assessment

A 34-year-old woman experiencing symptoms of migraine headache with increased frequency related to menses and increased stress, currently not optimally managed and not well prevented due to nonadherence.

QUESTIONS

Collect Information

1.a. What subjective and objective information indicates the presence of migraine headaches?

1.b. What additional information is needed to assess this patient's migraine headaches fully? (See Fig. 72-1 for MIDAS questionnaire.)

INSTRUCTIONS: Please answer the following questions about ALL the headaches you have had over the last 3 months. Write your answer in the box next to each question. Write zero if you did not do the activity in the last 3 months.

Days

1. How many days in the last 3 months did you miss work or school because of your headaches? ☐

2. How many days in the last 3 months was your productivity at work or school reduced by half or more because of headaches? *(Do not include days you counted in question 1 where you missed work or school.)* ☐

3. How many days in the last 3 months did you NOT do household work because of your headaches? ☐

4. How many days in the last 3 months was your productivity in household work reduced by half or more because of your headaches? *(Do not include days you counted in question 3 where you did not do household work.)* ☐

5. On how many days in the last 3 months did you miss family, social, or leisure activities because of your headaches? ☐

MIDAS Score: Add the total number of days from questions 1–5.   **Total** ☐

NOTE: Scores from A and B below are not included in the MIDAS score, but are used to assess frequency and intensity of pain.

A. How many days in the last 3 months did you have a headache? *(If a headache lasted more than 1 day, count each day.)* ☐

B. On a scale of 0–10, on average how painful were these headaches? *(0 = no pain, and 10 = pain as bad as it can be.)* ☐

Interpretation

The MIDAS questionnaire is scored in units of lost days. Depending on the MIDAS score, patients are assigned to I of IV grades:

MIDAS Grade	Definition	Score
I	Minimal or infrequent disability	0–5
II	Mild or infrequent disability	6–10
III	Moderate disability	11–20
IV	Severe disability	≥21

FIGURE 73-1. MIDAS questionnaire. (Reproduced with permission from Bigal ME, Lipton RB, Krymchantowski AV. The medical management of migraine. *Am J Ther.* 2004;11(2):130-140.)

Assess the Information

2.a. Assess the severity of the patient's migraine headaches based on the subjective and objective information available.

2.b. Create a list of the patient's drug therapy problems and prioritize them. Include an assessment of medication appropriateness, effectiveness, safety, and patient adherence.

Develop a Care Plan

3.a. What are the goals of pharmacotherapy in this case?

3.b. What non-drug therapies for migraine headaches might be useful for this patient?

3.c. What are feasible pharmacotherapeutic options available for (1) treating nausea associated with her migraine headaches, (2) acutely treating the migraine headaches, and (3) preventing migraine attacks?

3.d. Create an individualized, patient-centered, team-based care plan to optimize medication therapy for acute and preventive treatment of this patient's migraines and other drug therapy problems. Include specific drugs, dosage forms, doses, schedules, and duration of therapy.

Implement the Care Plan

4.a. What information should be provided to the patient to enhance adherence, ensure successful therapy, and minimize adverse effects?

4.b. Describe how care should be coordinated with other healthcare providers.

Follow-Up: Monitor and Evaluate

5. Explain how to monitor and evaluate the care plan for medication appropriateness, effectiveness, safety, and patient

adherence using clinical and laboratory data, patient feedback, and other information.

CLINICAL COURSE: ALTERNATIVE THERAPY

While discussing possible alternatives to her valproic acid therapy, the patient says a friend who also has migraines read about some herbal remedies used for migraine prevention. She asks whether any products like that could be used instead of or along with her prescription medications. The patient is very interested in a more "natural" therapy but only if it would reduce the number of migraines she experiences. For questions related to the use of butterbur and feverfew for the prevention of migraine headaches, see Section 19 (Complementary and Alternative Therapies) of this Casebook.

FOLLOW-UP QUESTION

1. Describe how a headache diary could help the treatment of this patient's migraine headaches. (See Fig. 72-2 for headache diary.)

SELF-STUDY ASSIGNMENTS

1. Evaluate the literature regarding the efficacy of IV agents (eg, dihydroergotamine, valproate sodium) for acute migraines.

2. Evaluate the literature on intranasal ketorolac and intranasal oxytocin for acute migraine.

3. Review the literature on the efficacy of the calcitonin gene-related peptide antagonists—erenumab (Aimovig), galcanezumab-gnlm (Emgality), and fremanezumab-vfrm (Ajovy)—for the prevention of migraine.

Name: _____ Month: _____ Year: _____

Date of Headache														
Headache Intensity														
Excruciating pain	10 9	10 9	10 9	10 9	10 9	10 9	10 9	10 9	10 9	10 9	10 9	10 9	10 9	10 9
Severe pain	8 7	8 7	8 7	8 7	8 7	8 7	8 7	8 7	8 7	8 7	8 7	8 7	8 7	8 7
Severe pain	6 5	6 5	6 5	6 5	6 5	6 5	6 5	6 5	6 5	6 5	6 5	6 5	6 5	6 5
Moderate pain	4 3	4 3	4 3	4 3	4 3	4 3	4 3	4 3	4 3	4 3	4 3	4 3	4 3	4 3
Mild pain	2	2	2	2	2	2	2	2	2	2	2	2	2	2
Aura only	1	1	1	1	1	1	1	1	1	1	1	1	1	1
Headache Duration (hours)														
Level of Disability														
Hospitalized														
Treatment by health care professional														
Bedrest required														
Decrease in activity by 50%														
Decrease in activity by 25%														
Normal activity														
Other (comment below)														
Associated Symptoms														
Nausea														
Vomiting														
Visual disturbances														
Menstrual period														
Neurological														
Other (comment below)														
Medications Taken														
1.														
2.														
3.														
4.														
5.														
Treatment Results														
Complete relief														
75% relief														
50% relief														
25% relief														
No relief														
Other (comment below)														
General Comments														

Note: A normal diary includes space to record a full month of headache activity. This form has been truncated for space purposes.

FIGURE 73-2. A headache diary.

4. Explain the role of onabotulinum toxin type A (Botox) for the prevention of chronic migraine.

CLINICAL PEARL

Migraines are three times more prevalent in women and are associated with estrogen levels. Sixty percent of women migraineurs report menstrually associated migraines, and 7–14% have migraines exclusively with menses.

REFERENCES

1. Patel PS, Minen MT. Complementary and integrative health treatments for migraine. J Neuroophthalmol. 2019;39(3):360–369. doi: 10.1097/WNO.0000000000000841.

2. Lipton RB. Risk factors for and management of medication-overuse headache. Continuum (Minneap Minn). 2015;21(4):1118–1131.

3. Banzi R, Cusi C, Randazzo C, Sterzi R, Tedesco D, Moja L. Selective serotonin reuptake inhibitors (SSRIs) and serotonin-norepinephrine reuptake inhibitors (SNRIs) for the prevention of migraine in adults. Cochrane Database Syst Rev. 2015. doi: 10.1002/14651858.CD011681.

4. Evans RW, Tepper SJ, Shapiro RE, Sun-Edelstein C, Tietjen GE. The FDA alert on serotonin syndrome with use of triptans combined with selective serotonin reuptake inhibitors or selective serotonin-norepinephrine reuptake inhibitors: American Headache Society position paper. Headache. 2010;50:1089–1099.

5. Marmura MJ, Silberstein SD, Schwedt TJ. The acute treatment of migraine in adults: the American Headache Society evidence assessment of migraine pharmacotherapies. Headache. 2015;55:3–20. doi: 10.1111/head.12499.

6. Thorlund K, Mills EJ, Wu P, et al. Comparative efficacy of triptans for the abortive treatment of migraine: a multiple treatment comparison meta-analysis. Cephalalgia. 2014;34(4):258–267.

7. Silberstein SD. Preventive migraine treatment. Continuum (Minneap Minn) 2015;21(4):973–989.

8. Sprenger T, Viana M, Tassorelli C. Current prophylactic medications for migraine and their potential mechanisms of action. Neurotherapeutics. 2018;15:313–323.

9. Nierenburg HC, Ailani J, Malloy M, Siavoshi S, Hu NN, Yusuf N. Systematic review of preventive and acute treatment of menstrual migraine. Headache. 2015;55:1052–1071.

10. Bucklan J, Ahmed Z. CGRP antagonists for decreasing migraine frequency: new options, long overdue. Cleve Clin J Med. 2020;87(4):211–218. doi: 10.3949/ccjm.87a.19048.

74

ATTENTION-DEFICIT HYPERACTIVITY DISORDER

He Is So Energized, He Keeps Going and Going and .... Level I

Jacob R. Peters, PharmD, BCPP, BCPS

LEARNING OBJECTIVES

After completing this case study, the reader should be able to:

- Determine the signs and symptoms of attention-deficit/hyperactivity disorder (ADHD) as defined by the *Diagnostic and Statistical Manual of Mental Disorders,* Edition 5 (DSM-5).

- Differentiate treatment options for ADHD with regard to effectiveness, tolerability, safety, monitoring parameters, and potential for drug interactions.

- Compare the advantages and disadvantages of once-daily stimulant preparations with short-acting stimulants.

- Develop strategies to enhance medication adherence for patients with ADHD.

- Perform patient assessment to determine efficacy with selected therapy and appropriate monitoring parameters.

PATIENT PRESENTATION

■ Chief Complaint

"My son has trouble focusing and sitting still while completing his afternoon homework."

■ HPI

A 10-year-old boy returns for a routine visit with his psychiatrist, accompanied by his mother, just after school dismissed for the day. He was diagnosed with ADHD 2 years ago and is currently being treated with Adderall XR 20 mg every morning. His mother states that during the last parent–teacher meeting, his teacher indicated that her son's behavior was well controlled during the day. Despite good behavior during the day, his mother reports difficulty getting her son to complete any afternoon tasks or assignments after school. The patient's mother established appropriate rules which include no playtime activities until he has completed his homework. Instead of focusing on homework, the patient insists on playing video games in his room and sometimes carelessly throws his controller. He also has exhibited impulsive and reckless behavior when interacting with

his younger brother. Initially, the patient's mother thought the medication was working. However, within the past year, his symptoms in the afternoon have progressively worsened. The mother finds it difficult to redirect him to his homework and is afraid his behavior at home will have repercussions on school performance. She asks, "What are my options?"

■ PMH

Asthma × 3 years
ADHD × 2 years
Tonsillectomy (1 year ago)
Broken wrist at age 8 (fell from tree)
Vaccinations up to date

■ FH

Both father and uncle have a history of ADHD and are currently receiving treatment as adults.

■ SH

Lives with both parents and younger brother in the suburbs

■ Meds

Adderall XR 20 mg daily (given every morning at 7:00 AM)
Albuterol inhaler two puffs Q 4–6 H PRN shortness of breath
Montelukast 5 mg PO daily

■ All

NKDA

■ ROS

Despite repeated requests, physical assessment was difficult to obtain as the patient could not sit still for more than 30 seconds and was jumping off the exam table. Asthma symptoms appear controlled with PRN inhaler use at bedtime only and daily montelukast.

■ PE

Gen

Well-nourished, healthy-appearing male child, normal physical development

VS

BP 110/72 mm Hg, P 82 bpm, RR 25, T 37.5°C; Wt 50 kg, Ht 5′2″

Skin

No signs of rash, skin irritation, or bruising noted. Scar noticed on left wrist from where he fell from tree. Minor cuts on knees from a recent fall while playing kickball at school.

HEENT

Unable to assess

Neck/Lymph Nodes
Unable to assess

Lungs/Thorax
No rales, rhonchi, or wheezing

CV
RRR

Abd
Deferred

Genit/Rect
Deferred

MS/Ext
Unable to assess

Neuro
A&O × 3; no underlying tics noted

■ Labs

Na 138 mEq/L   Hgb 14 g/dL   WBC 9 × 10³/mm³   Mag 1.8 mg/dL
K 3.8 mEq/L   Hct 44.5%   Neutros 66%   Serum iron 95 mcg/dL
Cl 106 mEq/L   RBC 4.6 × 10⁶/mm³   Bands 2%   TSH 3.6 mIU/L
CO₂ 23 mEq/L   Plt 278 × 10³/mm³   Eos 3%
BUN 18 mg/dL   MCV 85 μm³   Lymphs 24%
SCr 0.8 mg/dL   MCHC 33 g/dL   Monos 5%
Glu 110 mg/dL

■ ECG

NSR; changes not clinically significant

■ Assessment

A healthy, 10-year-old boy diagnosed with ADHD that is currently uncontrolled with 20 mg of dextroamphetamine and amphetamine extended-release capsules. His mild-persistent asthma is well controlled with PRN albuterol and daily montelukast.

QUESTIONS

Collect Information

1.a. What subjective and objective information indicates the presence or severity of ADHD?

1.b. What additional information is needed to fully assess this patient's ADHD?

Assess the Information

2.a. Assess the severity of ADHD based on the subjective and objective information available.

2.b. Create a list of the patient's drug therapy problems and prioritize them. Include assessment of medication appropriateness, effectiveness, safety, and patient adherence.

Develop a Care Plan

3.a. What are the goals of pharmacotherapy in this case?

3.b. What nondrug therapies might be beneficial for those diagnosed with ADHD?

3.c. What feasible pharmacotherapeutic options are available for the treatment of ADHD?

3.d. Create an individualized, patient-centered, team-based care plan to optimize medication therapy for this patient's ADHD and other drug problems. Include specific drugs, dosage forms, doses, schedules, and durations of therapy.

3.e. What alternatives would be appropriate if the initial care plan fails or cannot be used?

Implement the Care Plan

4.a. What information should be provided to the patient to enhance adherence, ensure successful therapy, and minimize adverse effects?

4.b. Describe how care should be coordinated with other healthcare providers.

Follow-Up: Monitor and Evaluate

5. Explain how to monitor and evaluate the care plan for medication appropriateness, effectiveness, safety, and patient adherence by using clinical and laboratory data, patient feedback, and other information.

■ SELF-STUDY ASSIGNMENTS

1. Many parents are apprehensive about starting stimulants in children because of abuse warnings in the prescribing information and media reports. After performing a literature search, prepare an educational brochure addressing the question, "What is the relationship between both untreated and treated ADHD and substance use disorders? Does stimulant treatment for ADHD increase the risk of substance use?"

2. Provide a summary that addresses the long-term effect stimulants have on growth and appetite, cardiovascular risks, sleep, and any psychiatric or behavioral effects.

3. ADHD is considered a chronic condition. Discuss various etiologies (including genetics) and population characteristics. Compare and contrast how symptoms and presentations change over the course of a lifetime. Include discussion of the different consequences from untreated ADHD spanning from childhood to adulthood.

4. Develop an appropriate recommendation for product conversion in a patient who is switching from oral methylphenidate (Concerta) 36 mg PO daily to methylphenidate (Daytrana) transdermal patch. Also, convert doses of mixed amphetamine salts (Adderall IR/Adderall XR) to lisdexamfetamine (Vyvanse).

5. Perform a literature search and defend or refute the role of modafinil, selective serotonin reuptake inhibitors, tricyclic antidepressants, and atypical antipsychotics in the treatment of ADHD.

CLINICAL PEARL

Because of well-established efficacy and tolerability, stimulant medications are considered first-line therapy in children with ADHD. The American Academy of Pediatrics reports at least an 80% response rate when these agents are used appropriately in the management of ADHD. If a patient does not respond adequately to initial stimulant therapy, a second or even third stimulant should be tried before initiating a nonstimulant medication. Most patients will be successfully treated by an alternative stimulant. Factors to consider when selecting a stimulant include age, tolerability, and dosage formulation preferences.

ACKNOWLEDGMENTS

This case is based on the patient case written for the 11th edition by Laura F. Ruekert, PharmD, BCPS, BCGP and Syed Khan, MD, MBA.

REFERENCES

1. American Psychiatric Association. Diagnostic and Statistical Manual of Mental Disorders. 5th ed. Washington, DC: American Psychiatric Association, 2013.
2. Wolraich ML, Hagan JF, Allan C, et al. Clinical practice guideline for the diagnosis, evaluation, and treatment of attention-deficit/hyperactivity disorder in children and adolescents. Pediatrics. 2019;144(4):e20192528.
3. The European Union. Attention Deficit Hyperactivity Disorder Drug Use Chronic Effect (ADDUCE) project, 2016. Available at: https://cordis.europa.eu/docs/results/260/260576/final1-public-final-report-all-sections.pdf. Accessed January 29, 2022.
4. The Medical Letter. Drugs for ADHD. Med Lett Drugs Ther. 2015;57(1464):37–40.
5. Sonuga-Barke EJ, Brandeis D, Cortese S, et al. Nonpharmacological interventions for ADHD: systematic review and meta-analyses of randomized controlled trials of dietary and psychological treatments. Am J Psychiatry. 2013;170:275–289.
6. Kollins SH, DeLoss DJ, Cañadas E, et al. A novel digital intervention for actively reducing severity of pediatric ADHD (STARS-ADHD): a randomised controlled trial. Lancet Digital Health. 2020;2:e168–e178.
7. Cortese S, Adamo N, Del Giovane C, et al. Comparative efficacy and tolerability of medications for attention-deficit hyperactivity disorder in children, adolescents, and adults: a systematic review and network meta-analysis. Lancet Psychiatry. 2018;5:727–738.
8. Pliszka S; AACAP Work Group on Quality Issues. Practice parameter for the assessment and treatment of children and adolescents with attention-deficit-hyperactivity disorder. J Am Acad Child Adolesc Psychiatry. 2007;46:894–921.
9. Stuhec M, Munda B, Svab V, et al. Comparative efficacy and acceptability of atomoxetine, lisdexamfetamine, bupropion and methylphenidate in treatment of attention deficit hyperactivity disorder in children and adolescents: a meta-analysis with focus on bupropion. J Affect Disord. 2015;178:149–159.
10. Henniseen L, Bakkar MJ, Banaschewski T, et al. Cardiovascular effects of stimulant and non-stimulant medication for children and adolescents with ADHD: a systematic review and meta-analysis of trials of methylphenidate, amphetamines, and atomoxetine. CNS Drugs. 2017;31:199–215.

75

BULIMIA NERVOSA

Self-Conscious Socialite........................ Level II

Laura F. Ruekert, PharmD, BCPP, BCGP

Cheen T. Lum, PharmD, BCPP

LEARNING OBJECTIVES

After completing this case study, the reader should be able to:

- Define bulimia nervosa according to the *Diagnostic and Statistical Manual of Mental Disorders*, Edition 5 (DSM-5) criteria.
- Assess signs and symptoms commonly associated with the presentation of bulimia nervosa.
- Recommend effective pharmacologic and nonpharcologic treatment options for the management of bulimia nervosa.
- Design a plan that includes monitoring, follow-up, and education for someone with an eating disorder, taking into account acute and long-term considerations.

PATIENT PRESENTATION

Chief Complaint

"I'm so unpopular, I just want to die!"

HPI

An 18-year-old female presented to the emergency department with her mom after multiple syncopal episodes while out shopping. After medical evaluation and treatment for hypomagnesemia and hypokalemia, she was medically cleared for a transfer to a behavioral health unit due to suicidal threats made while in the ED. Once in behavioral health, she reported worsening depressive symptoms after she was cut from the college dance team 6 months ago. She expressed anxious feelings of inadequacy and obsessions with her image after that incident and has been trying to lose weight to pursue other avenues of dance. She expresses frustration that no matter how long she goes without eating, she can't seem to lose enough weight. Subsequently, she is now purging up to eight times a week following the times when she eats anything unhealthy or fattening. She expressed self-hatred and losing control to impulsively binge on "a ton" of food. After eating, she becomes overwhelmed with guilt and anxiety leading to self-induced vomiting. In addition, she uses laxatives about three to four times a week. She tearfully stated that she is a failure and disappointment to her parents because she had to move back in with them after dropping out of school. She expresses guilty thoughts and not wanting to be a burden on her parents and said she wishes she didn't exist as "no one would miss me."

PMH

Bipolar disorder, type II (diagnosed 3 years ago by outpatient psychiatrist)

FH

Both parents living. Mother has a history of depression. Maternal aunt diagnosed with bipolar disorder. Maternal uncle and paternal aunt have a history of substance use.

SH

Completed almost 1 year of college as a dance major but dropped out 2 weeks ago. Recently moved from apartment into parents' home.

Meds

Ziprasidone 80 mg PO BID × 3 years
Bupropion SR 200 mg PO BID × 1 year

All

NKDA

Mental Status Exam

Patient is well-dressed and well-groomed; and her behavior is cooperative, although she exhibits poor eye contact and a dull affect.

She describes her mood as 'not good.' She is not experiencing hallucinations or delusions, and her thought processes are linear and associations, intact. The patient's speech is of normal content and articulation but is slowed at times. Her gait and station are normal and there are no tic, tremors, or EPS. Language/fund of knowledge is appropriate for level of education, but her insight and judgment are fair to poor.

■ ROS

Patient expresses feelings of hopelessness and frustration with her life in general. She states she rarely experiences relief from depressive symptoms. She endorses suicidal ideations with a plan of cutting her wrists or overdosing but denies any previous attempts. She reports high anxieties and obsessions with her image. She reports fatigue, weakness, dizziness, and low energy increasing in the past couple of weeks. Her LMP was 2 months ago, and her periods have been irregular.

■ PE

Gen

Tearful, thin, anxious-appearing female

VS

BP 98/72 mm Hg, P 52 bpm, RR 20, T 36.4°C; Wt 48 kg, Ht 5'4"

Skin

Abrasion on dorsum of right hand, numerous superficial scars, and cuts on the left forearm. No findings of lanugo on arms/upper body area.

HEENT

Atraumatic, normocephalic; PERRLA, no pallor or icterus; hearing grossly intact; no coryza or epistaxis; mucosal ulcerations in oral cavity

Neck/Lymph Nodes

Full ROM; bilateral parotid gland enlargement

Lungs/Thorax

Lungs CT A&P; no rales, rhonchi, wheezes

CV

RRR

Abd

Slightly distended, (–) BS

Genit/Rect

Deferred

MS/Ext

No cyanosis, clubbing; slight edema

Neuro

EOM intact; no facial weakness or asymmetry; cranial nerves II–XII intact
A&O × 3

■ Labs

Na 135 mEq/L	Hgb 14 g/dL	WBC 7.3 × 10³/mm³	AST 20 IU/L
K 3.3 mEq/L	Hct 39%	Neutros 60%	ALT 15 IU/L
Cl 100 mEq/L	RBC 5 × 10⁶/mm³	Bands 3%	Ca 8.6 mg/dL
HCO₃ 22 mEq/L	Plt 247 × 10³/mm³	Eos 2%	Mg 1.3 mg/dL
BUN 25 mg/dL	MCV 83 fL	Lymphs 31%	Serum iron
SCr 1.0 mg/dL	MCHC 34 g/dL	Monos 4%	96 mcg/dL
Glu 74 mg/dL	Albumin 3.4 g/dL		Folic acid
			9.3 ng/mL
			Ferritin
			110 ng/mL

Other:

UDS: negative   BAL <0.2   ECG shows QTc interval of 506 ms and bradycardia

HAM-D score 20   HCG (–)

■ Assessment

An 18-year-old woman being admitted to the inpatient psychiatric unit with a diagnosis of bulimia nervosa and also being treated for bipolar disorder type II, with currently depressed episodes.

QUESTIONS

Collect Information

1.a. What subjective and objective information indicates the presence of an eating disorder?

1.b. What additional information is needed to fully assess this patient's eating disorder?

Assess the Information

2.a. Assess the severity of bulimia nervosa, based on the subjective and objective information available.

2.b. Create a list of the patient's drug therapy problems and prioritize them. Include assessment of medication appropriateness, effectiveness, safety, and patient adherence.

Develop a Care Plan

3.a. What are the goals of pharmacotherapy for bulimia nervosa in this case?

3.b. What nondrug therapies for bulimia nervosa might be useful for this patient?

3.c. What feasible pharmacotherapeutic options are available for treating bulimia nervosa?

3.d. Create an individualized, patient-centered, team-based care plan to optimize medication therapy for this patient's eating disorder and other drug therapy problems. Include specific drugs, dosage forms, doses, schedules, and durations of therapy.

3.e. What alternatives would be appropriate if the initial care plan fails or cannot be used?

Implement the Care Plan

4.a. What information should be provided to the patient to enhance adherence, ensure successful therapy, and minimize adverse effects?

4.b. Describe how care should be coordinated with other healthcare providers.

Follow-Up: Monitor and Evaluate

5. Explain how to monitor and evaluate the care plan for medication appropriateness, effectiveness, safety, and patient adherence by using clinical and laboratory data, patient feedback, and other information.

■ SELF-STUDY ASSIGNMENTS

1. Compare and contrast etiologies and presentations of the eating disorders listed in the DSM-5.

2. Review the literature and discuss the incidence and types of psychiatric comorbidities with eating disorders and any pharmacotherapeutic treatment implications.

3. Prepare a table highlighting the different laboratory parameters seen in a patient presenting with acidosis secondary to laxative abuse versus a patient presenting with alkalosis secondary to excessive purging.

4. Review the literature and prepare a one-page paper describing the short- and long-term complications of eating disorders and the overall implications on long-term health.

CLINICAL PEARL

Fluoxetine at higher dosages is the only FDA-approved pharmacotherapy option for the treatment of bulimia nervosa.

ACKNOWLEDGMENT

Magdoline Daas, MD, assisted with the content and review of this case.

REFERENCES

1. Lock J, La Via MC, and the American Academy of Child and Adolescent Psychiatry (AACAP) Committee on Quality Issues (CQI). Practice parameters for the assessment and treatment of children and adolescent with eating disorders. J Am Acad Child Adolesc Psychiatry. 2015;54(5):412–425.

2. Campbell K, Peebles R. Eating disorders in children and adolescents: state of the art review. Pediatrics. 2014;134:582–592.

3. Hornberger LL, Lane MA, AAP The Committee On Adolescence. Identification and management of eating disorders in children and adolescents. Pediatrics. 2021;147(1):e2020040279. doi: 10.1542/peds.2020-040279.

4. Aigner M, Treasure J, Kaye W, Kasper S, WFSBP Task Force on Eating Disorders. World Federation of Societies of Biological Psychiatry (WFSBP) guidelines for the pharmacological treatment of eating disorders. World J Biol Psychiatry. 2011;12:400–443.

5. Hilbert A, Hoek HW, Schmidt R. Evidence-based clinical guidelines for eating disorders: international comparison. Curr Opin Psychiatry. 2017;30:423–437.

6. Bello NT, Yeomans BL. Safety of pharmacotherapy options for bulimia nervosa and binge-eating disorder. Expert Opinion on Drug Safety. 2018;17(1):17–23.

7. Tortorella A, Fabrazzo M, Monteleone AM, Steardo L, Monteleone P. The role of drug therapies in the treatment of anorexia and bulimia nervosa: a review of the literature. J Psychopathol. 2014;20:50–65.

8. Garner DM, Anderson ML, Keiper CD, Whynott R, Parker L. Psychotropic mediations in adult and adolescent eating disorders: clinical practice versus evidence-based recommendations. Eat Weight Disord. 2016;21:395–402.

9. Yager J, Devlin MJ, Halmi KA, et al. Guideline Watch (August 2012): practice guideline for the treatment of patients with eating disorders. 3rd ed. American Psychiatric Association, 2012. Available at: https://focus.psychiatryonline.org/doi/full/10.1176/appi.focus.120404. Accessed April 18, 2022.

10. Flament MF, Bissada H, Spettigue W. Evidence-based pharmacotherapy of eating disorders. Int J Neuropsychopharm. 2012;15:189–207.

76

OPIOID USE DISORDER

"Better on Bup" .... Level II

Tran H. Tran, PharmD, BCPS

Jenna Nikolaides, MD

LEARNING OBJECTIVES

After completing this case study, the reader should be able to:

- Identify the signs and symptoms of opioid use disorder (OUD).

- List the acute and chronic treatment goals for a patient with OUD.

- Devise an individualized treatment plan for successful buprenorphine induction, stabilization, and maintenance for OUD.

- Formulate monitoring and follow-up plans for a patient with OUD that includes recognizing, anticipating, and treating complications of buprenorphine and recovery.

PATIENT PRESENTATION

■ Chief Complaint

"I'm having trouble stopping my norco. I feel bad every time I try and am disappointed with myself when I can't."

■ HPI

A 34-year-old woman currently takes hydrocodone/acetaminophen daily. Two years ago, she had surgery for an ovarian cyst and has had trouble controlling pain in the weeks after the surgery. She ended up using 8–10 tablets per day, always ran out too soon, and started looking forward to taking them. She states, "I'm not addicted. I'm just crabby and sluggish at work if I don't take it. I just can't stand how I feel, so I take one. Then I take more to keep going. My husband is very supportive and put up with a lot while I was cutting my dose down, but I haven't told him I'm still using it. I don't have pain anymore although my back aches a little after my morning run. I stretch and the achiness goes away. I love my family and am happy with my life. Of course, I get tired since I have kids and a busy job. I notice that when I take norco, I feel more energy and I'm nicer. I was in therapy for a few years, but I don't need therapy. I just want to stop taking norco and feel normal. When I was drinking, I just decided to stop, and I did. I've been in AA ever since. I thought quitting norco would be like that, but it wasn't as simple. I heard that buprenorphine will help you get off pain medications. I don't need any more therapy since I was in therapy for years. I don't want to do urine tests; I'm not a junkie. I told you what I'm taking."

■ PMH

None

■ FH

Sister with alcohol use disorder, father had MI in his 50s.

■ SH

She is a schoolteacher and mother of three.

■ **Meds**

Hydrocodone/APAP 5-325 mg 1–2 tablets Q 6 H PRN pain

■ **All**

NKDA

■ **ROS**

Unremarkable

■ **PE**

Gen

Tall, slim, well-nourished appearing

VS

BP 120/72 mm Hg, P 88 bpm and regular, RR 20, T 38.2°C; Wt 66 kg, Ht 5′7″

Skin

Normal turgor; no obvious lesions, tumors, or moles

HEENT

Normocephalic, atraumatic, TMs clear, PERRLA

Neck/Lymph Nodes

Supple, without lymphadenopathy or thyromegaly

CV

RRR; S_1, S_2 normal; no MRG

Lungs

Clear to A&P

Abd

NTND

Genit/Rect

(–) occult blood in stool

MS/Ext

Normal ROM; pulses 2+ throughout

Neuro

A&O × 3

■ **Labs**

Na 138 mEq/L	Phos 2.8 mg/dL	AST 14 IU/L
K 4.0 mEq/L	Ca 9.4 mg/dL	ALT 38 IU/L
Cl 93 mEq/L	Bilirubin 0.8 mg/dL	GGT 33 IU/L
CO₂ 23 mEq/L	Protein total 8.1 g/dL	
BUN 11 mg/dL	Albumin 4.2 g/dL	
SCr 0.9 mg/dL		
Glu 97 mg/dL		

■ **Assessment**

A 34-year-old woman currently taking hydrocodone/acetaminophen daily with possible opioid use disorder (OUD) and depression.

QUESTIONS

Collect Information

1.a. What subjective and objective information indicates this patient has OUD and is a candidate for buprenorphine treatment?

1.b. What additional information is needed to fully assess the treatment for OUD in this patient?

Assess the Information

2.a. Assess the severity of this patient's OUD based on the subjective and objective information available.

2.b. Create a list of the patient's drug therapy problems and prioritize them. Include assessment of medication appropriateness, effectiveness, safety, and patient adherence.

Develop a Care Plan

3.a. What are the goals of therapy for this patient?

3.b. What nondrug therapies for OUD might be useful for this patient?

3.c. What feasible pharmacotherapeutic options are available for treating OUD?

3.d. Create an individualized, patient-centered, team-based care plan to optimize medication therapy for this patient's OUD. Include specific drugs, dosage forms, doses, schedules, and durations of therapy.

Implement the Care Plan

4.a. What information should be provided to the patient to enhance adherence, ensure successful therapy, and minimize adverse effects?

4.b. Describe how care should be coordinated with other healthcare providers.

Follow-Up: Monitor and Evaluate

5. Explain how to monitor and evaluate the care plan for medication appropriateness, effectiveness, safety, and patient adherence by using clinical and laboratory data, patient feedback, and other information.

■ SELF-STUDY ASSIGNMENTS

1. Methadone may be used to treat opioid withdrawal in the hospital; however, federal regulations restrict providers from prescribing methadone to patients after discharge from the hospital. Please review the legislation known as the 72-hour rule (Title 21, Code of Federal Regulation) that allows providers to prescribe methadone for opioid withdrawal in the hospital setting.

2. Despite the benefits of extended-release injectable naltrexone for patients with OUD studied in trials, discuss why it is difficult to initiate this medication.

CLINICAL PEARL

• The U.S. Food and Drug Administration now requires all opioids and medicines to treat OUD labeling include recommendations in their labeling that, as a routine part of prescribing these medicines, healthcare professionals should discuss the availability of naloxone with patients and caregivers.

- Historically, pharmacologic treatments for OUD were referred to as medication-assisted treatment (MAT), but more recently, it has been determined that the more appropriate term is medications for opioid use disorder (MOUD) to clearly convey that medications, in and of themselves, are treatments and not merely assisting abstinence or cognitive behavioral therapy.

- Buprenorphine has poor oral bioavailability due to extensive hepatic first-pass metabolism and is therefore formulated via nonoral routes of administration such as sublingual tablets and buccal films.

REFERENCES

1. Substance Abuse and Mental Health Services Administration. Medications for opioid use disorder: for healthcare and addiction professional, policymakers, patients, and families. Treatment Improvement Protocol (TIP) Series 63 Publication No. PEP21-02-01-002, July 2021. Available at: *https://store.samhsa.gov/sites/default/files/SAMHSA_Digital_Download/PEP21-02-01-002.pdf*. Accessed April 2, 2022.

2. Buprenorphine and naloxone sublingual film (Suboxone) prescribing information, 2015. Available at: *https://www.accessdata.fda.gov/drugsatfda_docs/label/2015/022410s020s022lbl.pdf*. Accessed April 2, 2022.

3. American College of Obstetricians and Gynecologists. Committee Opinion No. 711: opioid use and opioid use disorder in pregnancy. Obstet Gynecol. 2017;130(2):e81–e94. Available at: *https://www.acog.org/clinical/clinical-guidance/committee-opinion/articles/2017/08/opioid-use-and-opioid-use-disorder-in-pregnancy*. Accessed April 2, 2022.

4. Hasin DS, O'Brien CP, Auriacombe M, et al. DSM-5 criteria for substance use disorders: recommendations and rationale. Am J Psychiatry. 2013;170(8):834–851.

5. Department of Health and Human Services. Practice guidelines for the administration of buprenorphine for treating opioid use disorder. 2021. Available at: *https://www.federalregister.gov/documents/2021/04/28/2021-08961/practice-guidelines-for-the-administration-of-buprenorphine-for-treating-opioid-use-disorder*. Accessed April 2, 2022.

6. Falcon E, Browne C, Leon R, et al. Antidepressant-like effects of buprenorphine are mediated by kappa opioid receptors. Neuropsychopharmacology. 2016;41:2344–2351.

7. U.S. Food and Drug Administration. FDA requiring labeling changes for opioid pain medicines, opioid use disorder medicines regarding naloxone. Available at: *https://www.fda.gov/news-events/press-announcements/fda-requiring-labeling-changes-opioid-pain-medicines-opioid-use-disorder-medicines-regarding*. Accessed April 2, 2021.

8. Substance Abuse and Mental Health Services Administration. Frequently asked questions (FAQs) and fact sheets regarding the substance abuse confidentiality regulations. Available at: *https://www.samhsa.gov/about-us/who-we-are/laws-regulations/confidentiality-regulations-faqs*. Accessed April 2, 2022.

9. ADA National Network. The ADA, addiction, recovery, and employment. Available at: *https://adata.org/factsheet/ada-addiction-recovery-and-employment*. Accessed April 2, 2022.

77

ALCOHOL WITHDRAWAL

Cold Turkey Can Land You in Hot Water . . . . Level II

Kevin M. Tuohy, PharmD, BCPS

LEARNING OBJECTIVES

After completing this case study, the reader should be able to:

- Describe the signs and symptoms of acute alcohol withdrawal syndrome.

- Explain the common laboratory abnormalities seen in alcohol-dependent patients.

- Develop a treatment plan for acute alcohol withdrawal and alcohol-related seizures.

- Recommend an appropriate pharmacotherapeutic regimen for electrolyte replacement in an alcohol-dependent patient.

PATIENT PRESENTATION

■ Chief Complaint

"My husband has been acting strange, sweating, and shaking all day. I think he may have had a seizure about an hour ago."

■ HPI

A 54-year-old man who is brought to the ED by his wife. She states that her husband has abused alcohol since she met him while in college. She states that his typical daily consumption for the past 25 years has averaged about 14–18 alcoholic beverages. She reports that he has not been able to afford to drink as much over the past few months due to a recent job loss when his employer closed the restaurant where he worked. To save money, he has decided to quit drinking "cold turkey." He has not consumed any alcohol in the previous 48 hours.

■ PMH

Alcohol abuse and dependence
Alcohol withdrawal with seizure 4 years prior
Hypertension × 10 years
GERD × 4 years

■ SH

The patient is an unemployed restaurant worker. He has not worked for the past 6 months. He has been married for 22 years. He has been a heavy drinker for past 25 years. Drinks an average of 16 drinks (usually beer or whiskey-containing drinks) per day.

(+) Tobacco use: quit 5 years ago.
Denies any illicit drug use.

■ Meds

Hydrochlorothiazide 25 mg PO daily
Amlodipine 5 mg PO daily
OTC omeprazole 20 mg PO as needed for heartburn symptoms (usually requires a dose about four times a week)

■ **All**

NKDA

■ **ROS**

The patient exhibits overall confusion and is not responsive to questions. Wife states his mental status was normal until this afternoon when his confusion, sweating, and shakiness started.

■ **PE**

Gen

Tall, thin, undernourished-appearing man, in mild distress who is acutely confused and tremulous

VS

BP 150/85 mm Hg, P 107 bpm, RR 20, T 38.3°C; Wt 76 kg, Ht 6′6″

Skin

Moist, diaphoretic

HEENT

Head—atraumatic, icteric sclera, PERRLA, EOMI, mild AV nicking on funduscopic exam

Neck/Lymph Nodes

Supple, no thyromegaly or lymphadenopathy

Lungs/Thorax

Symmetric, lungs CTA

CV

RRR, no MRG

Abd

Soft, nontender; (+) bowel sounds; (+) hepatomegaly

Genit/Rect

(–) Occult blood in stool

MS/Ext

Confused, tremor in both hands

Neuro

A&O only to person, DTRs exaggerated

■ **Labs**

Na 139 mEq/L	Phos 2.8 mg/dL	PT 14.5 seconds
K 3.2 mEq/L	Ca 9.5 mg/dL	INR 1.30
Cl 88 mEq/L	GGT 310 units/L	EtOH (–)
CO_2 26 mEq/L	AST 250 units/L	
BUN 14 mg/dL	ALT 120 units/L	
SCr 1.1 mg/dL	T. bili 1.7 mg/dL	
Glu 99 mg/dL	D. bili 1.1 mg/dL	
Mg 1.6 mg/dL	Alb 2.1 g/dL	

■ **Assessment**

1. Acute alcohol withdrawal syndrome with possible witnessed alcohol withdrawal-related seizure

2. Alcohol use disorder

3. Hypertension

4. GERD

QUESTIONS

Collect Information

1.a. What subjective and objective information indicates the presence of acute alcohol withdrawal syndrome?

1.b. What additional information is needed to fully assess this patient's alcohol withdrawal syndrome?

Assess the Information

2.a. Assess the severity of acute alcohol withdrawal syndrome based on the subjective and objective information available.

2.b. Create a list of the patient's drug therapy problems and prioritize them. Include assessment of medication appropriateness, effectiveness, safety, and patient adherence.

Develop a Care Plan

3.a. What are the goals of pharmacotherapy in this case?

3.b. What nondrug therapies might be useful for this patient's acute alcohol withdrawal syndrome?

3.c. What feasible pharmacotherapeutic options are available for treating acute alcohol withdrawal syndrome?

3.d. Create an individualized, patient-centered, team-based care plan to optimize medication therapy for this patient. Include specific drugs, dosage forms, doses, schedules, and durations of therapy.

Implement the Care Plan

4.a. What information should be provided to the patient to enhance adherence, ensure successful therapy, and minimize adverse effects?

4.b. Describe how care should be coordinated with other healthcare providers.

Follow-Up: Monitor and Evaluate

5. Explain how to monitor and evaluate the care plan for medication appropriateness, effectiveness, safety, and patient adherence by using clinical and laboratory data, patient feedback, and other information.

■ SELF-STUDY ASSIGNMENTS

1. Research alcohol-related treatment on the Internet that can be recommended to patients with alcohol use disorder.

2. Discuss the pharmacologic options that are currently marketed in the United States (FDA-approved drugs) for the treatment of alcohol use disorder.

CLINICAL PEARLS

1. All benzodiazepines appear similarly efficacious in reducing signs and symptoms of alcohol withdrawal. The choice of the agent should be determined based on patient-specific factors and the pharmacokinetic profile of the drug.

2. Very high doses of benzodiazepines are often needed to control the symptoms of alcohol withdrawal. This is due to cross-tolerance between alcohol and benzodiazepines.

REFERENCES

1. The ASAM Clinical Practice Guideline on Alcohol Withdrawal Management. J Addict Med. 2020;14(3S Suppl 1):1–72.
2. Sullivan JT, Sykora K, Schneiderman J, Naranjo CA, Sellers EM. Assessment of alcohol withdrawal: the revised clinical institute withdrawal assessment for alcohol scale (CIWA-Ar). Br J Addict. 1989;84: 1353–1357. doi: 10.1111/j.1360-0443.1989.tb00737.x.
3. Schuckit MA. Recognition and management of withdrawal delirium (delirium tremens). N Engl J Med. 2014;371:2109–2113.
4. Muzyk AJ, Leung JG, Nelson S, Embury ER, Jones SR. The role of diazepam loading for the treatment of alcohol withdrawal syndrome in hospitalized patients. Am J Addict. 2013;22:113–118.
5. Martinotti G, diNicola M, Frustaci A, et al. Pregabalin, tiapride, and lorazepam in alcohol withdrawal syndrome: a multi-centre, randomized, single-blind comparison trial. Addiction. 2010;105:288–299.
6. Rosenson J, Clements C, Simon B. Phenobarbital for acute alcohol withdrawal: a prospective randomized double-blind placebo-controlled study. J Emerg Med. 2013;44:592–598.
7. Tidwell WP, Thomas TL, Pouliot JD, Canonico AE, Webber AJ. Treatment of alcohol withdrawal syndrome: phenobarbital vs CIWA-Ar protocol. Am J Crit Care. 2018 Nov;27(6):454–460.
8. Muzyk AJ, Fowler JA, Norwood DK, Chilipko A. Role of α2-agonists in the treatment of acute alcohol withdrawal. Ann Pharmacother. 2011;45:649–657.
9. Mueller SW, Preslaski CR, Kiser TH, et al. A randomized, double-blind, placebo-controlled dose range study of dexmedetomidine as adjunctive therapy for alcohol withdrawal. Crit Care Med. 2014;42:1131–1139.
10. National Institute on Alcohol Abuse and Alcoholism. Alcohol's effects on the body. U.S. Department of Health and Human Services. Available at: www.niaaa.nih.gov/alcohol-health/alcohols-effects-body. Accessed April 18, 2022.

78

NICOTINE DEPENDENCE

Gabriella A. Douglass, PharmD, BCACP, AAHIVP, BC-ADM

LEARNING OBJECTIVES

After completing this case study, the reader should be able to:

- Assess a patient's location in the stages of change process to develop a tailored intervention plan to promote smoking cessation and nicotine abstinence.

- Design a patient-specific plan for initiating lifestyle modifications and pharmacologic treatment to assist a patient in quitting smoking.

- Compare the side-effect profiles of individual nicotine replacement products.

- Develop appropriate educational information on the use of pharmacotherapy for treatment of nicotine dependence.

- Formulate monitoring and follow-up plans for a patient attempting to quit smoking based on patient-specific information and the prescribed regimen.

PATIENT PRESENTATION

■ Chief Complaint

"The machine at the pharmacy shows my blood pressure is running high, and I feel tired all the time. I think these cigarettes have something to do with how I'm feeling and I'm over it! I tried to quit once using nicotine gum for 2 days, but it made me sick to my stomach and made my jaw hurt; plus, I was still craving cigarettes. I have two kids and a wife, and I want to get better so I can take care of my family. I've seen commercials on what smoking can do to you and I'm scared that could happen to me!"

■ HPI

A 41-year-old man presents to the primary care clinic to review his most recent laboratory results. He wants to feel better because he wants to be able to continue to work and provide for his family.

■ PMH

Nicotine dependence × 18 years

■ FH

Father: 67 years old, prior myocardial infarction at age 45; hypertension
Mother: 64 years old; type 2 diabetes mellitus, ovarian cancer
Son: 12 years old; asthma
Daughter: 7 years old; ADHD

■ SH

Caffeine use: Daily cola consumption of 8+ cans a day
Tobacco use: Current everyday smoker for 18 years. Smokes a pack of cigarettes daily when he can afford to buy them. He wishes to stop smoking due to family pressure. He reports a previous unsuccessful attempt to stop smoking (see Table 78-1). He smokes his first cigarette within 5 minutes of waking. He finds it very difficult not to smoke while he is at work and that even if he sick and must be in bed most of the day he still smokes. He states his morning

TABLE 78-1	Stages of Change and Smoking Cessation Counseling	
Stage of Change	**Patient's Mindset**	**Response**
Precontemplation	Not interested in quitting, fails to recognize smoking as a problem	Provide concise and relevant statement about why the smoker should think about quitting smoking
Contemplation	Smoking is a problem and might consider quitting	State that there is good evidence that cigarette smoke and secondhand smoke are dangerous. Encourage smoker to quit
Preparation	Cigarette smoking is problematic and now ready to think about quitting	Discuss options for treatment—both pharmacotherapeutic and nonpharmacotherapeutic
Action	Motivated to quit, instituting a plan with an identified quit date and developing a plan to cope with stressors	Encourage quit attempt, offer to be a resource during the quit attempt, and praise former smokers' abstinent status
Maintenance	Former smokers who have not smoked for a period of time	Great job staying quit. Continued cessation is a positive move in becoming healthier

cigarette is the one he would hate to give up and that he smokes more frequently during the first hours after waking than during the rest of the day.

Alcohol use: One drink per day.

Habits: He sleeps on average 7 hours per day. He does not exercise.

Home environment: He lives with his spouse and two children. The living environment is secure and supportive.

Education: He has a high school diploma.

Work: He works full time at a local convenience store.

Financial: His income is marginal, enough to buy only necessities.

Language: Native language is English.

Marital Status: He is currently married. He is sexually active in a monogamous relationship.

■ Meds

None

■ All

NKDA

■ ROS

Systemic: No fever and no chills, feels tired
Head and neck: Discoloration of teeth to yellow
Gastrointestinal: No abdominal pain
Pulmonary: No dyspnea, no cough, no hemoptysis, and no wheezing
Cardiovascular: No chest pain or discomfort, and no palpitations

■ PE

Gen

Patient is alert and oriented and in no acute distress.

VS

BP 128/85, P 89, RR 20, T 37.0°C; Wt 125 kg, Ht 5'8"

Skin

No lesions noted, the skin showed no erythema, showed no ecchymosis, and the skin of the extremities was not cold. Yellow nail plates noted on his hands.

HEENT

Normocephalic with no lesions. Pupils are equal, round, and reactive to light and accommodation. The extraocular movements were normal. The pupils were normal. The conjunctiva exhibited no abnormalities. Visual fields normal. Nares appear normal. Mouth is well hydrated and without lesions. Mucous membranes are moist. Posterior pharynx is clear of any exudate or lesions. Canal and tympanic membranes are clear. Tympanic membrane was normal. No hearing abnormalities.

Neck/Lymph Nodes

No malformation or tenderness noted, no tenderness on palpation of the back, no muscle spasm of the back, and no costovertebral angle tenderness.

Lungs/Thorax

Clear to auscultation bilaterally with no rales, rhonchi, or wheezing. Respiration rhythm and depth was normal, the chest was normal to percussion, the lungs were clear to auscultation, and no decrease in breath sounds was heard. No rales/crackles were heard.

CV

JVP was normal. Heart rate and rhythm normal. Heart sounds normal, no S3 was heard, and no S4 was heard. No murmurs were heard. Arterial pulses were equal bilaterally and normal. Edema not present. Veins unremarkable.

Abd

Soft, nontender, and nondistended, with normal bowel sounds. No palpable masses or hepatosplenomegaly. The abdomen was normal on visual inspection. Abdominal auscultation revealed no abnormalities. Abdominal percussion was normal. Abdominal palpation revealed no abnormalities and no direct suprapubic tenderness. No rebound tenderness in the abdomen. The liver was normal to palpation and not enlarged. The spleen was normal to palpation.

Genit/Rect

Urinary system: Normal
Rectal exam: The prostate was normal

MS/Ext

No cyanosis, clubbing, lesions, or edema. Pulses normal bilaterally. Foot exam performed including visual inspection and sensory exam with monofilament and pulse exam. No abnormalities detected.

Neuro

Cranial nerves II–XII are grossly intact. No focal deficits and oriented to time, place, and person. The cranial nerves were normal. Gait and stance were normal. The reflexes were normal. No peripheral neuropathy was noted.

■ Labs

Na 142 mEq/L	Hgb 15.8 g/dL	T. chol 160 mg/dL
K 4.3 mEq/L	Hct 46.4%	Triglycerides 190 mg/dL
Cl 98 mEq/L	RBC 5.06 × 106/mm³	HDL-C 32 mg/dL
CO_2 21 mEq/L	MCV 92 μm³	VLDL-C 38 mg/dL
BUN 15 mg/dL	Plt 186 × 103/mm³	LDL-C 90 mg/dL
SCr 0.8 mg/dL	WBC 6.4 × 103/mm³	ALT (SGPT) 18 IU/L
Glu 86 mg/dL		AST (SGOT) 12 IU/L
HbA1c = 5.1%		Bilirubin, total 0.3 mg/dL
		Alk phos 40 IU/L

■ Assessment

A 41-year-old man with 18-year history of nicotine dependence, currently receiving no treatment but is desiring to quit smoking. He has risk factors for atherosclerotic cardiovascular disease (ASCVD) and need to discuss risk-reduction pharmacotherapy and lifestyle modifications.

QUESTIONS

Collect Information

1.a. What subjective and objective information indicates the presence of nicotine dependence?

1.b. What additional information is needed to fully assess this patient's nicotine dependence?

Assess the Information

2.a. Assess the severity of nicotine dependence based on the subjective and objective information available.

2.b. Create a list of the patient's drug therapy problems and prioritize them. Include assessment of medication appropriateness, effectiveness, safety, and patient adherence.

2.c. What economic, psychosocial, cultural, and ethical considerations are applicable to this patient?

Develop a Care Plan

3.a. What are the goals of pharmacotherapy for nicotine dependence in this case?

3.b. What nondrug therapies for nicotine dependence might be useful for this patient's nicotine dependence?

3.c. What feasible pharmacotherapeutic options are available for treating nicotine dependence?

3.d. Create an individualized, patient-centered, team-based care plan to optimize medication therapy for this patient's nicotine dependence and other drug therapy problems. Include specific drugs, dosage forms, doses, schedules, and durations of therapy.

3.e. What alternatives would be appropriate if the initial care plan fails or cannot be used?

Implement the Care Plan

4.a. What information should be provided to the patient to enhance adherence, ensure successful therapy, and minimize adverse effects?

4.b. Describe how care should be coordinated with other healthcare providers.

Follow-Up: Monitor and Evaluate

5. Explain how to monitor and evaluate the care plan for medication appropriateness, effectiveness, safety, and patient adherence by using clinical and laboratory data, patient feedback, and other information.

■ SELF-STUDY ASSIGNMENTS

1. Evaluate current literature concerning the use of quitlines to enhance quit-smoking attempts. What is the status of quitlines in your state? In a one-page paper, explain how you could educate your community about quitlines.

2. Describe the legal status (both federal and state) and explain the role of commercially used e-cigarettes.

CLINICAL PEARL

Patients with nicotine dependence who stop smoking and consume the same amount of caffeine as prior to their quit attempt are likely to feel the stimulant effects of caffeine much more. That is because nicotine doubles the rate at which the body depletes caffeine.

REFERENCES

1. Patnode CD, Henderson JT, Coppola EL, et al. interventions for tobacco cessation in adults, including pregnant persons: updated evidence report and systematic review for the US Preventive Services Task Force. JAMA. 2021;325:280. doi: 10.1001/jama.2020.23541.

2. Siu AL, U.S. Preventive Services Task Force. Behavioral and pharmacotherapy interventions for tobacco smoking cessation in adults, including pregnant women: U.S. Preventive Services Task Force recommendation statement. Ann Intern Med. 2015;163:622.

3. Boudreaux ED, Sullivan A, Abar B, et al. Motivation rulers for smoking cessation: a prospective observational examination of construct and predictive validity. Addict Sci Clin Pract. 2012;7(1):8. doi: 10.1186/1940-0640-7-8.

4. Heatherton TF, Kozlowski LT, Frecker RC, Fagerstrom K. Fagerström test for cigarette dependence (FTND). APA PsycTests 1991. doi: 10.1037/t03773-000.

5. Borland R, Yong HH, O'Connor RJ, Hyland A, Thompson ME. The reliability and predictive validity of the Heaviness of Smoking Index and its two components: findings from the International Tobacco Control Four Country study. Nicotine Tob Res. 2010;12 Suppl(Suppl 1):S45–S50. doi: 10.1093/ntr/ntq038.

6. Grundy SM, Stone NJ, Bailey AL, et al. 2018 AHA/ACC/AACVPR/AAPA/ABC/ACPM/ADA/AGS/APhA/ASPC/NLA/PCNA guideline on the management of blood cholesterol: a report of the American College of Cardiology/American Heart Association Task Force on clinical practice guidelines. Circulation. 2019;139:e1082. doi: 10.1161/CIR.0000000000000625.

7. U.S. Department of Health and Human Services. Smoking cessation: a report of the Surgeon General—executive summary. Atlanta, GA: U.S. Department of Health and Human Services, Centers for Disease Control and Prevention, National Center for Chronic Disease Prevention and Health Promotion, Office on Smoking and Health, 2020. Available at: https://www.hhs.gov/sites/default/files/2020-cessation-sgr-full-report.pdf. Accessed March 29, 2022.

8. Stead LF, Koilpillai P, Fanshawe TR, Lancaster T. Combined pharmacotherapy and behavioural interventions for smoking cessation. Cochrane Database Syst Rev. 2016;3:CD008286. doi: 10.1002/14651858.CD008286.pub3.

9. Baker TB, Piper ME, Stein JH, et al. Effects of nicotine patch vs varenicline vs combination nicotine replacement therapy on smoking cessation at 26 weeks: a randomized clinical trial. JAMA. 2016;315(4):371–379. doi: 10.1001/jama.2015.19284.

10. U.S. Department of Health and Human Services. Treating tobacco use and dependence: 2008 update. Available at: https://www.ncbi.nlm.nih.gov/books/NBK63952/. Accessed March 29, 2022.

79

SCHIZOPHRENIA

A Thousand Worms Inside My Body............ Level II

Leigh Anne Nelson, PharmD, BCPP

Benjamin Miskle, PharmD

LEARNING OBJECTIVES

After completing this case study, the reader should be able to:

- Describe the target symptoms of schizophrenia.

- Manage an acutely psychotic patient with appropriate pharmacotherapy.

- Identify and manage the adverse effects of antipsychotics.

- Discuss the role of second-generation antipsychotics in the treatment of schizophrenia.

PATIENT PRESENTATION

Chief Complaint

"I want to see my lawyer."

HPI

This is the first inpatient admission for a 32-year-old woman who was brought to the psychiatric hospital by the police. Earlier today, she was brought to the crisis center by a friend in her apartment building after the landlord threatened to call the police as she was creating a disturbance. At the crisis center, she became increasingly agitated and suspicious; the police were called; however, she left before being evaluated by staff. The patient apparently has been delusional and believes people sneak into her room at night when she is asleep and place a thousand worms inside her body. She also believes that she is being raped by passing men on the street. She is quite preoccupied about having massive wealth. She claims to have bought some gold and left it at the grocery store. She believes that her ideas have been given to a communist individual who has had plastic surgery to look like her and is using her identification to take possession of all her property. She states that she is having difficulty getting her property back.

Apparently, the precipitating event today that eventually resulted in her hospitalization was that she created a disturbance at a local fast-food restaurant, claiming that she owned it. Because of the disturbance, police were called, and she subsequently was sent here on an order of protective custody. According to the patient, she bought a hamburger and sat down to eat it, and for some reason, somebody called the police and charged her with illegal trespassing. She claims that 6 years ago, she was raped by a relative of a sister and broke her hip in the process. She states that her feet were cut off because she would not do what her impostors wanted her to do, and her feet were subsequently sent back to her and were reattached.

Her speech is quite rambling. She speaks of having been part of an experiment in which 38 eggs were taken from her body, and children were produced from them and then killed by the government. She claims that she has worms in her that are the type that kill dogs and horses and says that they have been put there by the government. She also claims that at one time, she had transmitters in her backbone and that it took 3 years to have them taken out by the government. She claims to have had surgery in the past, and the surgeon did not know what he was doing and took out her gallbladder and put it in the intestines where it exploded. The patient also states that on one occasion, a physician was removing snakes from her abdominal cavity, and the snakes killed the doctor and a nurse. She also claims that she worked as a surgeon herself before 1963.

Past Psychiatric History

Denies any prior hospitalization for mental health problems

PMH

Gallbladder surgery (cholecystectomy) 2 months ago.
Hypertension × 2 years.
No record of her ever being raped or having a broken hip is found.
No further medical history is known.

Family Psychiatric History

The patient claims that her alleged family is not really her family and that she is not sure who her family is.

SH

Divorced; heterosexual; lives in an apartment alone; employment history unknown
    Denies any smoking, illicit drug, or alcohol use

Meds

Lisinopril 20 mg PO once daily

All

Penicillin (rash)

Mental Status Examination

The patient is modestly dressed, with some disarray. She is morbidly obese. Her hair is unkept and unwashed. She is alert, oriented, and in no acute distress. Her speech is clear, constant, and pressured, with many grandiose delusions and illogical thoughts. She is quite tangential, going from one subject to the other without interruption. Her affect is mood-congruent, her mood is euphoric, and there is a marked degree of grandiosity. Her thought processes are quite illogical, with markedly delusional thinking. There is no current evidence of auditory hallucinations, and she denies visual hallucinations. She denies any suicidal or homicidal ideation, but she is quite verbal and pressured in her thought content, verbalizing a great deal about the things that have been taken away from her illegally by people impersonating her. She has marked delusional symptoms with paranoid ideation prominent. Her memory (immediate, recent, and remote) is fair. Her cognition and concentration are adequate. Her intellectual functioning is within the average range. Insight and judgment are markedly impaired.

ROS

Reports occasional GI upset; complains that worms are inside her stomach; otherwise negative

PE

VS

BP 140/85 mm Hg, P 80 bpm, RR 17, T 37.1°C; Wt 97 kg; Ht 5'3"

Skin

Scratches on both hands

HEENT

PERRLA; EOMI; fundi benign; throat and ears clear; TMs intact

Neck

Supple, no nodes; normal thyroid

Lungs

CTA & P

CV

RRR, normal S_1 and S_2

Abd

(+) BS, nontender

TABLE 79-1 Laboratory Values

Na 140 mEq/L	Hgb 14.6 g/dL	WBC $11.0 \times 10^3/mm^3$	AST 34 IU/L	Ca 9.6 mg/dL
K 3.9 mEq/L	Hct 45.7%	Neutros 66%	ALT 22 IU/L	Phos 5.1 mg/dL
Cl 104 mEq/L	RBC $4.7 \times 10^6/mm^3$	Lymphs 24%	Alk phos 89 IU/L	TSH 4.5 µIU/mL
CO_2 22 mEq/L	MCV 90.2 µm³	Monos 8%	GGT 38 IU/L	RPR negative
BUN 19 mg/dL	MCH 31 pg	Eos 1%	T. bili 0.9 mg/dL	Serum alcohol <10 mg/dL
SCr 1.1 mg/dL	MCHC 34.5 g/dL	Basos 1%	Alb 3.6 g/dL	Urine pregnancy (–)
Glu 100 mg/dL		Plt $232 \times 10^3/mm^3$	T. chol 208 mg/dL	

Urinalysis
Color yellow
Appearance slightly cloudy
Glucose (–)
Bilirubin (–)
Ketones, trace
SG 1.025
Blood (–)
pH 6.0
Protein (–)
Nitrites (–)
Leukocyte esterase (–)

Urine Drug Screen
Amphetamines (–)
Barbiturates (–)
Benzodiazepines (–)
Cannabinoids (–)
Cocaine (–)
Opiates (–)
PCP (–)
Oxycodone (–)

TABLE 79-2 Antipsychotic Treatment Recommendations

Recommendation	APA 2020	PORT 2009	NICE 2014
First episode	SGA, FGA	SGA (except clozapine and olanzapine), FGA	SGA, FGA (in combination with psychological interventions)
Second episode	SGA, FGA, clozapine	SGA, FGA	SGA, FGA (only if an SGA has already been tried)
Treatment refractory/ suicidal thoughts	Clozapine		
Poor adherence/ preference	LAI		

FGA = first-generation antipsychotics, SGA = second-generation antipsychotics, LAI = Long-acting injectable antipsychotics.

Ext

Full ROM, pulses 2+ bilaterally

Neuro

A&O × 3; reflexes symmetric; toes downgoing; normal gait; normal strength; sensation intact; CNs II–XII intact

■ Labs

See Table 79-1.

■ Assessment

A 32-year-old woman experiencing an acute episode of schizophrenia and needing evaluation and management of hypertension and obesity

QUESTIONS

Collect Information

1.a. What subjective and objective information indicates the presence of an acute episode of schizophrenia?

1.b. What additional information is needed to fully assess this patient's schizophrenia?

Assess the Information

2.a. Assess the severity of the acute episode of schizophrenia based on the subjective and objective information available.

2.b. Create a list of the patient's drug therapy problems and prioritize them. Include assessment of medication appropriateness, effectiveness, safety, and patient adherence.

Develop a Care Plan

3.a. What are the goals of pharmacotherapy in this case?

3.b. What nondrug therapies might be useful for this patient's schizophrenia?

TABLE 79-3 Recommended Monitoring Parameters for Patients Receiving SGA

Parameter	Baseline	4 Weeks	8 Weeks	12 Weeks	Quarterly	Annually
Personal/family history	X					
Weight (BMI)	X	X	X	X	X	
Blood pressure	X			X		X
Fasting plasma glucose	X			X		X
Fasting lipid profile	X			X		X
Waist circumference	X					X
Tardive dyskinesia evaluation	X					X
Hematologic profile[a]	X					X
CV status[b]	X					X

[a]Desirable for all SGA but required for clozapine according to a strict monitoring protocol.
[b]ECG if >40 years or h/o CV disease.

3.c. What feasible pharmacotherapeutic options are available for treating schizophrenia?

3.d. Create an individualized, patient-centered, team-based care plan to optimize medication therapy for this patient's schizophrenia and other drug therapy problems. Include specific drugs, dosage forms, doses, schedules, and durations of therapy.

3.e. What alternatives would be appropriate if the initial care plan fails or cannot be used?

Implement the Care Plan

4.a. What information should be provided to the patient to enhance medication adherence, ensure successful therapy, and minimize adverse effects?

4.b. Describe how care should be coordinated with other healthcare providers.

Follow-Up: Monitor and Evaluate

5. Explain how to monitor and evaluate the care plan for medication appropriateness, effectiveness, safety, and patient adherence by using clinical laboratory data, patient feedback, and other information.

■ SELF-STUDY ASSIGNMENTS

1. Perform a literature search regarding the metabolic side-effect risk associated with the second-generation antipsychotics. Which ones are more likely to cause weight gain, hyperglycemia, and hyperlipidemia? Which ones are less likely to cause weight gain, hyperglycemia, and hyperlipidemia?

2. Perform a literature search regarding QTc changes with both first- and second-generation antipsychotics. Which antipsychotics are more likely to alter the QTc interval?

3. Review the pharmacoeconomic literature for the second-generation antipsychotics. For your geographic area, compare costs for the average daily (monthly for long-acting injectable [LAI]) doses of haloperidol (oral and LAI formulation), chlorpromazine (oral formulation), clozapine (oral and orally disintegrating formulation), olanzapine (oral and orally disintegrating formulation), risperidone (oral, orally disintegrating, and LAI formulations), aripiprazole (oral, orally disintegrating, and LAI formulations), quetiapine and extended-release quetiapine (oral formulation), ziprasidone (oral formulation), paliperidone (oral and LAI formulation), asenapine (sublingual formulation), lurasidone (oral formulation), brexpiprazole (oral formulation), cariprazine (oral formulation), and lumateperone (oral formulation).

CLINICAL PEARL

A benzodiazepine (eg, lorazepam) may be used during the initiation of an antipsychotic to minimize anxiety, agitation, or aggression secondary to psychosis and allow time for the antipsychotic to take effect. For management of acute agitation or aggression, the addition of a benzodiazepine may also allow lower dosages of the antipsychotic to be used and help prevent antipsychotic-induced side effects such as extrapyramidal symptoms (eg, dystonia).

REFERENCES

1. American Psychiatric Association. Schizophrenia spectrum and other psychotic disorders. In: Diagnostic and Statistical Manual of Mental Disorders. 5th ed. Washington, DC: American Psychiatric Association; 2013:87–122.

2. Castle DJ, Buckley PF. Schizophrenia. 2nd ed. Oxford, UK: Oxford University Press; 2015.

3. Keepers GA, Fochtmann LJ, Anzia JM, et al. American Psychiatric Association Practice Guidelines; Work Group on Schizophrenia. Practice guideline for the treatment of patients with schizophrenia, 3rd ed. Am J Psychiatry. 2020;177(9):868–872.

4. Dixon LB, Perkins B, Calmas C. Guideline Watch (September 2009): practice guideline for the treatment of patients with schizophrenia. Psychiatry Online. Available at: *http://psychiatryonline.org/pb/assets/raw/sitewide/practice_guidelines/guidelines/schizophrenia-watch.pdf*. Accessed April 17, 2022.

5. Buchanan RW, Kreyenbuhl J, Kelly DL, et al. The 2009 schizophrenia PORT psychopharmacological treatment recommendations and summary statements. Schizophr Bull. 2010;36:71–93.

6. Hasan A, Falkai P, Wobrock T, et al. World Federation of Societies of Biological Psychiatry guidelines for biological treatment of schizophrenia, part 1: update on the acute treatment of schizophrenia and management of treatment resistance. World J Biol Psychiatry. 2012;13(14):2–44.

7. National Institute for Health and Care Excellence. Psychosis and schizophrenia in adults: prevention and management. Available at: *https://www.nice.org.uk/guidance/cg178*. Accessed April 17, 2022.

8. Lieberman JA, Stroup TS, McEvoy JP, et al., for the Clinical Antipsychotic Trials of Intervention Effectiveness (CATIE) Investigators. Effectiveness of antipsychotic drugs in patients with chronic schizophrenia. N Engl J Med. 2005;353:1209–1223.

9. American Diabetes Association, American Psychiatric Association, American Association of Clinical Endocrinologists, and North American Association for the Study of Obesity. Consensus development conference on antipsychotic drugs and obesity and diabetes. Diabetes Care. 2004;27:596–601.

80

MAJOR DEPRESSION

A Life Worth Living . . . . Level I

Katelynn Mayberry, PharmD

Brian L. Crabtree, PharmD

LEARNING OBJECTIVES

After completing this case study, the reader should be able to:

- Identify the signs and symptoms of depression.

- Develop a pharmacotherapy plan for a patient with depression.

- Compare adverse-effect profiles of various antidepressant drugs.

- Discuss pharmacoeconomic considerations when selecting antidepressant therapy.

PATIENT PRESENTATION

■ Chief Complaint

"I don't know if I can handle this anymore."

■ HPI

A 41-year-old woman was referred by her family physician to an outpatient mental health clinic. She complains of feeling down and sad, with crying spells, trouble sleeping, increased eating, impaired concentration, and fatigue. She has not worked in over 2 months and has used up her vacation and sick leave from work. She went through treatment for alcohol use disorder over 1 year ago. Things were going fairly well for her after her treatment, and she remarried approximately 8 months ago. Arguments with her teenage sons about family issues and past incidents have made her increasingly depressed over the past few months. Her older son, 17, moved out to live with his father. Her younger son, 12, moved to live with his paternal grandparents. She divorced the boys' father after approximately 10 years of marriage when she discovered that he was having an affair with another woman. She left her second husband after approximately 2 years because of problems involving his children that caused increasing conflict with her then-husband. Without a second income in the household, she accumulated large credit card debts. She began drinking and soon developed a pattern of using alcohol to relieve stress. Just before entering alcoholism treatment, there was a sexual fondling incident involving one of her son's friends while the friend was visiting her son at her house, but she was amnestic for the incident the next day. Her present husband, her third, has been supportive of her, but she feels guilty about her failed previous marriages and her sons, worries about her debt, and has become more despondent. She has taken a leave of absence from her job as an administrative assistant at an elementary school. The patient sought treatment for depression 3 months ago from her family physician, who prescribed mirtazapine. Her spirits have not improved, and she says the medication made her gain weight. Because of vague references that the physician believed could possibly indicate suicidal ideas, she has been referred for psychiatric evaluation.

■ PMH

Childhood illnesses: she has had all the usual childhood illnesses. She was hospitalized at age 3 for bacterial meningitis but knows of no residual effects.

Adult illnesses: no current nonpsychiatric adult illnesses; no previous psychiatric treatment.

Trauma: fractured arm due to bicycle accident at age 9, otherwise unremarkable.

Surgeries: hx childbirth by C-section; tonsillectomy at age 6.

Travel: no significant travel history.

Diet: no dietary restrictions. Despite not having much of an appetite, reports eating more since taking mirtazapine.

Exercise: no regular exercise program.

Immunizations: no personal records of childhood vaccinations; had tetanus booster 9 years ago; does not remember when she had most recent influenza immunization.

■ FH

Father is deceased, had coronary artery disease, but ultimately died of colon cancer. Mother has well-controlled HTN. A sister has depression and anxiety and takes antidepressant medication (patient does not know its name). A second sister died by suicide.

■ SH

High school graduate; works as an administrative assistant but on leave for approximately 2 months. Married approximately 8 months, two previous divorces. Lived with husband and sons until sons moved out in the past few weeks. Health insurance is through the school district where she is employed; includes adjusted copay on prescriptions. Reports heavy credit card debt. Attended church regularly in the past (Protestant), but not recently. Attends AA weekly.

Denies drinking alcohol since substance use disorder treatment. Denies smoking. Drinks three to four cups of caffeinated coffee per day; usually drinks iced tea with evening meal; drinks colas as leisure beverage. Used marijuana a few times after high school, denies use in more than 10 years; denies present or past use of other illicit substances.

■ Meds

Mirtazapine 30 mg PO QHS (started on mirtazapine 15 mg PO QHS approximately 3 months ago)

St. John's wort 300 mg PO TID for the past 2 weeks at suggestion of husband (purchased at health food store)

OTC antihistamines and decongestants for colds or allergies; none in recent months

■ All

NKDA

■ ROS

General appearance: pt c/o feeling tired much of the time

HEENT: wears contact lenses; no tinnitus, ear pain, or discharge; no c/o nasal congestion; hx of dental repair for caries

Chest: no hx of asthma or other lung disease

CV: reports occasional feelings of "pounding heart"; no hx of heart disease

GI: reports infrequent constipation; takes MOM PRN; has gained 9 lb in last 2 months

GU: has regular menses; LMP ended a week ago

Neuromuscular: occasional headaches, worse over the past few months; no syncope, vertigo, weakness or paralysis, numbness or tingling

Skin: no complaints

■ PE

Performed by nurse practitioner

Gen

Overweight WF, slightly unkempt

VS

BP 132/78 mm Hg, P 88 bpm, RR 22, T 36.9°C; Wt 187 lb, Ht 5′8″

Skin

Normal skin, hair, and nails

HEENT

PERRLA; EOM intact, no nystagmus. Fundus—disks sharp, no retinopathy; no nasal discharge or nasal polyps; TMs gray and shiny bilaterally; minor accumulation of cerumen.

Neck/Lymph Nodes

Supple without thyromegaly or lymphadenopathy

Chest/Lungs

Frequent sighing during examination, but no tachypnea or SOB; chest CTA

Breasts

No masses, tenderness, or discharge

Heart

RRR without murmur

Abd

Soft, nontender; (+) BS; no organomegaly

Genit/Rect

Deferred

MS/Ext

Unremarkable

Neuro

CN: EOM intact, no nystagmus, no weakness of facial or tongue muscles. Casual gait normal. Finger-to-nose normal.
Motor: normal symmetric grip strength. DTRs 2+ and equal.
Sensory: intact bilaterally.

Mental Status

When seen in the clinic, the patient is pale and appears moderately overweight, dressed in casual slacks and sweater. Grooming is fair and without makeup. She speaks slowly, often not responding to questions for approximately 30 seconds before beginning answers. She describes depressed mood and lack of energy and says she feels no pleasure in life. Her husband is good to her, but she feels everyone else she loves has left her. She has no social contacts other than occasional visits by her parents. She spends most of her time in bed. She feels worthless and blames herself for her problems. She feels particularly anguished about the incident with her son's friend even though she does not remember it. She is often anxious and worries about the future. She wonders if her sons love her and if they will ever return. She worries how she will repay her financial debts. Her speech is logical, coherent, and goal-oriented. She denies suicidal intent but says the future seems dim to her, and she wonders sometimes if life is worth living. She admits she sometimes wishes she could just go to sleep and not wake up. She denies hallucinations. Paranoid delusions, FOI, IOR, and LOA are absent. There is no dysarthria or anomia.

■ Labs (Collected 11:45 AM)

Na 139 mEq/L	Hgb 14.0 g/dL	AST 34 IU/L
K 4.2 mEq/L	Hct 46.2%	ALT 42 IU/L
Cl 102 mEq/L	MCV 92 μm³	GGT 38 IU/L
CO₂ 24 mEq/L	MCH 29 pg	T. bili 0.8 mg/dL
BUN 12 mg/dL	Plt 234 × 10³/mm³	T. prot 7.0 g/dL
SCr 0.9 mg/dL	WBC 7.3 × 10³/mm³	Alb 4.4 g/dL
Glu 98 mg/dL	Segs 49%	CK 57 IU/L
Ca 9.5 mg/dL	Bands 1%	T₄ 8.6 mcg/dL
Mg 1.7 mEq/L	Lymphs 42%	T₃ uptake 29%
Uric acid 4.0 mg/dL	Monos 2%	TSH 2.8 mIU/L
	Eos 6%	

■ UA

Glucose (–); ketones (–); pH 5.8; SG 1.016; bilirubin (–); WBC 1/hpf, protein (–), amorphous—rare, epithelial cells 1/hpf; color yellow; blood (–), RBC 0/hpf; mucus—rare; bacteria—rare; casts 0/lpf; appearance clear

■ Assessment

A 41-year-old woman requiring change in therapy for major depressive disorder, single episode, with melancholic features, and potential drug-drug interactions with St. John's wort.

Collect Information

1.a. What subjective and objective information indicates the presence of depression?

1.b. What additional information is needed to fully assess this patient's depression?

Assess the Information

2.a. Assess the severity of depression based on the subjective and objective information available.

2.b. Create a list of the patient's drug therapy problems and prioritize them. Include assessment of medication appropriateness, effectiveness, safety, and patient adherence.

2.c. What economic, psychosocial, cultural, racial, and ethical considerations are applicable to this patient?

Develop a Care Plan

3.a. What are the goals of pharmacotherapy for depression in this case?

3.b. What nondrug therapies might be useful for this patient's depression?

3.c. What feasible pharmacotherapeutic options are available to treat this patient's depression?

3.d. Create an individualized, patient-centered, team-based care plan to optimize medication therapy for this patient's depression and other drug therapy problems. Include specific drugs, dosage forms, doses, schedules, and durations of therapy.

3.e. What alternatives would be appropriate if the initial care plan fails or cannot be used?

Implement the Care Plan

4.a. What information should be provided to the patient to enhance adherence, ensure successful therapy, and minimize adverse effects?

4.b. Describe how care should be coordinated with other healthcare providers.

Follow-Up: Monitor and Evaluate

5. Explain how to monitor and evaluate the care plan for medication appropriateness, effectiveness, safety, and patient adherence by using clinical and laboratory data, patient feedback, and other information.

■ CLINICAL COURSE: ALTERNATIVE THERAPY

The patient understands that she must stop the St. John's wort she has been taking because of an interaction with her prescribed mirtazapine, but she wonders if it would have been helpful if she had started it when she first began feeling depressed. See Section 19 in this Casebook for questions about the use of St. John's wort for treatment of depression.

■ SELF-STUDY ASSIGNMENTS

1. The selective serotonin reuptake inhibitor (SSRI) antidepressants are commonly used and have the same serotonin reuptake pharmacology; contrast the agents in this class, considering relative side effects, dosing, and drug interactions.

2. Compare other antidepressants with SSRIs with regard to adverse effects and relative advantages and disadvantages.

3. Discuss the role of combination drug therapy in the treatment of depression, including the use of drugs not usually classified as antidepressants.

4. Review the medical literature and evaluate the scientific evidence for the efficacy of St. John's wort in the treatment of depression.

CLINICAL PEARL

Although SSRIs are of one pharmacologic class, they are not of one chemical class. Therefore, failure to respond to one SSRI does not reliably predict failure to respond to others.

REFERENCES

1. American Psychiatric Association. Depressive disorders. In: Diagnostic and Statistical Manual of Mental Disorders, 5th ed. Washington, DC: American Psychiatric Association; 2013:155–188.

2. VandenBerg AM. Major depressive disorder. In: DiPiro JT, Yee GC, Posey L, Haines ST, Nolin TD, Ellingrod V, eds. Pharmacotherapy: A Pathophysiologic Approach, 11e. McGraw Hill; 2020.

3. Cuijpers P, Noma H, Karyotaki E, Vinkers CH, Cipriani A, Furukawa TA. A network meta-analysis of the effects of psychotherapies, pharmacotherapies and their combination in the treatment of adult depression. World Psychiatry 2020;19(1):92–107. doi: 10.1002/wps.20701.

4. Linde K, Kriston L, Rucker G, et al. Efficacy and acceptability of pharmacological treatments for depressive disorders in primary care: systematic review and network meta-analysis. Ann Fam Med. 2015;13:69–79.

5. Hoffelt C, Gross T. A review of significant pharmacokinetic drug interactions with antidepressants and their management. Ment Health Clin. 2016;6:35–41.

6. Perry PJ. Pharmacotherapy for major depression with melancholic features: relative efficacy of tricyclic versus selective serotonin reuptake inhibitor antidepressants. J Affect Disord. 1996;39:1–6.

7. Bishop JR, Stevenson JM, Burghardt KJ. Pharmacogenetics in mental health. In: Johnson JA, Ellingrod VL, Kroetz DL, Kuo GM, eds. Pharmacogenomics: Application to Patient Care. 3rd ed. Lenexa, KS: American College of Clinical Pharmacy; 2015:115–134.

81

BIPOLAR DISORDER

Up All Night . . . . Level II

Jason M. Noel, PharmD, BCPP

LEARNING OBJECTIVES

After completing this case study, the reader should be able to:

- Given a description of a patient case, assess the symptoms of an acute episode of bipolar disorder.

- Recommend appropriate pharmacotherapy for patients with acute mania.

- Generate parameters for monitoring anticonvulsant therapy for bipolar disorder.

- Identify the pharmacotherapeutic options for treating the subtypes of bipolar disorder.

PATIENT PRESENTATION

■ Chief Complaint

"I am trying to keep the evil spirits away!"

■ HPI

A 28-year-old man was brought by the police to the Crisis Center for an emergency evaluation. According to neighbors who called the police, the patient has been acting increasingly strange. The lights in the house are left on all night, and loud music is played at all hours. Last evening, he dug a trench around his front yard with an electric lawn edger and filled it with various herbal plants. This evening, he hung wreaths and horseshoes on his front door and threw many of his belongings into his yard and the street. When approached by neighbors, he apparently began screaming and preaching at them. When the police arrived, they found the patient standing naked on the dining room table in his front yard preaching. When the police approached, he began throwing garlic cloves at them and screaming, "I refuse to let you all curse me in my own home." He became increasingly hostile during the arrest shouting, "You can't do this—I have rights!" He then tried to bite one of the officers.

■ PMH

Manic episodes first occurred while he was in college, leading to psychiatric admissions at ages 21 and 23 for acute mania. Patient was treated with haloperidol and lithium, with adequate response and discharged on both occasions after about a month. Adherence to outpatient treatment has been inconsistent, with several documented missed appointments and prescription refills.

He also receives outpatient treatment for migraine headaches and shift work disorder.

■ Patient Interview

Patient is disheveled with pungent body odor. He is pacing the room, waving his hands in the air, and preaching in an elated, loud, sing-songy voice. He is wearing a dirty T-shirt and jeans. When asked how he felt, he stated, "Playful, with intense clarity, sharp, spiffy, and clean." He then became hostile and angry, insisting that he be discharged before sunrise, or he would "be tormented by the demons forever." He claims to have witnessed spirits that attached themselves to various people and that now control their thoughts and actions. He spoke in long run-on sentences with many political, religious, and sexual references. He was very difficult to interrupt. For example, at one point, he stated, "Can't you see, or are you an idiot?! I am being persecuted by the evil spirits I must stop them now and if you don't get that, you're an idiot."

When asked about his sleep, he angrily replied, "Would you sleep at a time like this? If I sleep, this whole town will be taken over! I cannot allow that to happen." The patient stated that he has not been eating and has not taken his lithium in several days because, "Lithium is of the ground, the underworld. The Lord will sustain me." When his interviewers challenged him on these beliefs, he suspected them of being part of plot to undermine his mission. When told that he might need to be in the hospital so we can help him with his problems, he screamed, "You can't help me! You're nonbelievers."

■ Abnormal Involuntary Movements

Excessive eye blinking and mild grimacing; unclear whether abnormal (patient states this is the "demon blood trying to take over my body"). He is bothered by it in that to him, it represents his "sinful nature."

■ FH

Father has a history of depression; paternal grandmother was placed in an "asylum" for hysteria secondary to childbirth. Mother and brother have type 2 diabetes.

■ SH

Recently fired from his job as a nursing assistant at a local hospital, where he worked the night shift on a "7 on/7 off" schedule. Patient states that he drinks "only occasionally," but he was noted to be intoxicated, with a BAC 0.14%, on a previous admission.

■ Meds

Haloperidol 5 mg PO daily
Lithium carbonate 600 mg PO twice daily
Acetaminophen/butalbital/caffeine two tablets PO as needed for headaches
Modafinil 200 mg PO at 9 PM for shift work disorder

■ All

NKDA

■ ROS

Migraine headaches about twice a month, no aura, (+) nausea and photophobia. Occasional GI upset with no clear relationship to meals or time of day, frequent loose stools.

■ Physical Examination

VS

BP 118/73 mm Hg, P 83 bpm, RR 16, T 37.1°C; Wt 94 kg, Ht 5'11"

HEENT

PERRLA; EOMI; fundi benign; throat and ears clear; TMs intact; rapid eye blinking and facial grimacing (may indicate early tardive dyskinesia)

Skin

Psoriatic plaques evident on both elbows

Neck

Supple, bite mark, no nodes

Lungs

CTA & P

CV

RRR; S_1, S_2 normal; no MRG

Abd

(+) BS, nontender

Ext

Full ROM, pulses 2+ bilaterally

Neuro

A & O × 3; reflexes symmetric; toes downgoing; normal gait; normal strength; sensation intact; CNs II–XII intact

■ Labs

Na 141 mEq/L	Hgb 14.6 g/dL	WBC 12.0 ×	AST 32 IU/L
K 3.8 mEq/L	Hct 45.7%	10^3/mm³	ALT 21 IU/L
Cl 103 mEq/L	RBC 4.73 ×	Neutros 67%	Alk phos 87 IU/L
CO_2 24 mEq/L	10^6/mm³	Lymphs 23%	GGT 46 IU/L
BUN 19 mg/dL	MCV 90.2 μm³	Monos 7%	T. bili 0.9 mg/dL
SCr 1.1 mg/dL	MCH 31 pg	Eos 2%	T. chol
Glu 89 mg/dL	MCHC 34.4 g/dL	Basos 1%	218 mg/dL
Ca 9.7 mg/dL	Plt 256 × 10^3/mm³	TSH 4.1 μIU/mL	Alb 3.7 g/dL
Phos 5.3 mg/dL			RPR: neg
			Lithium
			0.1 mEq/L

■ UA

Color yellow; appearance slightly cloudy; glucose (–), bili (–), ketones trace; SG 1.025, blood (–), pH 6.0, protein (–), nitrites (–), leukocyte esterase (–)

■ Assessment

A 28-year-old man with bipolar I disorder having a manic episode with psychotic features, migraine headaches, shift work disorder, and possible medication-related problems.

QUESTIONS

Collect Information

1.a. What subjective and objective information indicates the presence of a manic episode?

1.b. What additional information is needed to fully assess this patient's bipolar disorder?

Assess the Information

2.a. Assess the severity of the current manic episode based on the subjective and objective information available.

2.b. Create a list of the patient's drug therapy problems and prioritize them. Include assessment of medication appropriateness, effectiveness, safety, and patient adherence.

Develop a Care Plan

3.a. What are the goals of pharmacotherapy in this case?

3.b. What nondrug therapies might be useful for this patient's bipolar disorder?

3.c. What feasible pharmacotherapeutic options are available for treating of bipolar disorder?

3.d. Create an individualized, patient-centered, team-based care plan to optimize medication therapy for this patient. Include specific drugs, dosage forms, doses, schedules, and durations of therapy.

3.e. What alternatives would be appropriate if the initial care plan fails or cannot be used?

Implement the Care Plan

4.a. What information should be provided to the patient to enhance compliance, ensure successful therapy, and minimize adverse effects?

4.b. Describe how care should be coordinated with other healthcare providers.

Follow-Up: Monitor and Evaluate

5. Explain how to monitor and evaluate the care plan for medication appropriateness, effectiveness, safety, and patient adherence by using clinical and laboratory data, patient feedback, and other information.

■ SELF-STUDY ASSIGNMENTS

1. Perform a literature search and explore the anticonvulsants that are not specifically approved for use in bipolar disorder (eg, gabapentin, oxcarbazepine, and topiramate) in the treatment of bipolar disorder.

2. Standardized rating scales are often used in clinical trials and occasionally in clinical practice to quantify the presence of symptoms in people with psychiatric disorders and drug-induced movement disorders. Perform a Web search for each of the following rating scales. For each scale, determine the symptom domains measured, the overall score ranges, and severity score cutoff ranges (e.g., mild, moderate, and severe).

   Mania:

   Young Mania Rating Scale (YMRS)

   Depression:

   Hamilton Depression Rating Scale (HAM-D)

   Montgomery–Åsberg Depression Rating Scale (MADRS)

   Movement Disorders:

   Abnormal Involuntary Movement Scale (AIMS)

   Dyskinesia Identification System: Condensed User Scale (DISCUS)

CLINICAL PEARL

When a patient admitted with acute mania is taking activating drugs such as antidepressants or stimulants, those drugs should be tapered and withdrawn. In some patients, antidepressants and stimulants may activate mania or increase the rate of cycling, and potentially delay response to antimanic/mood stabilizers.

REFERENCES

1. National Institute for Health and Care Excellence (NICE). Clinical Guideline CG185. Bipolar disorder: assessment and management. Available at: *https://www.nice.org.uk/guidance/cg185/resources/bipolar-disorder-assessment-and-management-pdf-35109814379461*. Accessed March 15, 2022.

2. Yatham LN, Kennedy SH, Parikh SV, et al. Canadian Network for Mood and Anxiety Treatments (CANMAT) and International Society for Bipolar Disorders (ISBD) 2018 guidelines for the management of patients with bipolar disorder. Bipolar Disord. 2018;20:97–170.

3. Grunze EV, Goodwin GM, Bowden C, et al. The World Federation of Societies of Biological Psychiatry (WFSBP) guidelines for the biological treatment of bipolar disorders: update 2009 on the treatment of acute mania. World J Biol Psychiatry. 2009;10:85–116.

4. Goodwin G, Haddad P, Ferrier I, et al. Evidence-based guidelines for treating bipolar disorder: Revised third edition recommendations from the British Association for Psychopharmacology. J Psychopharmacol. 2016;30(6):495–553.

5. Bowden CL, Perlis RH, Thase ME, et al. Aims and results of the NIMH Systematic Treatment Enhancement Program for Bipolar Disorder (STEP-BD). CNS Neurosci Ther. 2012;118:243–249.

6. Cipriani A, Reid K, Young AH, et al. Valproic acid, valproate and divalproex in the maintenance treatment of bipolar disorder. Cochrane Database Syst Rev. 2013. doi: 10.1002/14651858.CD003196.pub2.

82

GENERALIZED ANXIETY DISORDER

Bundle of Nerves .... Level I

Sarah T. Melton, PharmD, BCPP, BCACP, FASCP

Cynthia K. Kirkwood, PharmD, BCPP

LEARNING OBJECTIVES

After completing this case study, the reader should be able to:

- Identify target symptoms associated with generalized anxiety disorder (GAD).

- Construct pharmacotherapeutic goals for GAD.

- Recommend appropriate pharmacotherapy and duration of treatment for the acute, continuation, and maintenance phases of GAD.

- Develop a care plan and coordinate care with other healthcare providers.

- Develop a monitoring plan for a patient treated for GAD based on the treatment regimen.

PATIENT PRESENTATION

■ Chief Complaint

"I am so worried all the time that I can't do anything else. I need some serious help."

■ HPI

A 55-year-old man presents to his family physician with complaints of severe irritability, feelings of "being on edge," and inability to fall asleep at night. He states that he always feels tense and exhausted with constant muscle tension and body aches. He was laid off from his job as a manager at a building supply store 9 months ago. Over the past year, he has had difficulty concentrating when filling out job application forms, and his mind often "goes blank" when talking with people. His irritability has impacted his relationship with his wife, and he is worried that she will leave him. He has developed frequent abdominal pain and occasional episodes of diarrhea. He constantly worries about the lack of financial resources, his wife losing her job, and his relationship with his wife. He is afraid that he and his wife will lose their house and cars. He states that he cannot control his constant worry and that his anxiety has increased in intensity over the past 6 months. He denies having obsessive–compulsive thoughts or behaviors or symptoms of panic disorder or social anxiety disorder. He recently went to the emergency department (ED) because he was so worried about multiple issues in his life that he could not eat or sleep for 2 days. He was given an IM injection of hydroxyzine and sent home with a prescription for hydroxyzine 25-mg capsules orally four times daily as needed for anxiety. He stopped this medication last week secondary to constipation. He tried kava kava from an herbal store a few months ago. It was not effective, and he discontinued it after 2 weeks because of severe abdominal pain.

PMH

Records from the family physician indicate frequent visits over the past 9 months for insomnia, headaches, abdominal pain, and diarrhea. He has been treated with buspirone for anxiety for the past 6 months. He has a history of peptic ulcer disease treated with ranitidine 6 years ago. He currently takes famotidine 1–2 times per week as needed for dyspepsia.

After a recent visit to the ED, he was prescribed hydroxyzine to be taken up four times daily as needed for anxiety.

Past psychiatric history is significant for episode of depression and alcohol use disorder when he was 33 years old, which were treated with fluoxetine. He took the fluoxetine for 2 weeks and discontinued it secondary to insomnia.

FH

Father, 80 year old, on "nerve medication" for several years. Mother deceased at age 73 from breast cancer with history of major depression and alcohol use disorder. Patient has one sister who was treated with multiple medications in the past for anxiety and depression, and was treated for sedative, hypnotic, or anxiolytic use disorder 5 years ago.

SH

Married for 25 years; no children; high school graduate; past nicotine use disorder (quit 5 years ago with 40 pack-year history); alcohol use disorder (has been sober for 10 years and attends Alcoholics Anonymous on a weekly basis); little exercise because of time constraints; drinks four to five cups of coffee per day and three to four Mountain Dew soft drinks throughout the day. He admits to occasional cannabis use when his anxiety is "out of control." (*Note*: cannabis is not legal for medical or recreational use in his state.) He does not have any prescription drug coverage at this time.

Meds

Buspirone 30 mg PO BID for anxiety
Phenylephrine 10 mg PO QID PRN for nasal congestion
Loperamide 2 mg PO Q 6 H PRN for diarrhea
Famotidine 20 mg PO daily PRN for dyspepsia

All

Sulfa (hives); codeine (nausea)

ROS

Positive for paresthesia, headaches, and mild diaphoresis; negative for dizziness, palpitations, SOB, chest pain

PE

Gen

Anxious, well-groomed man sitting on examination table; cooperative; oriented × 3

VS

BP 125/85 mm Hg, P 98 bpm, RR 18, T 36.5°C; Wt 90 kg, Ht 5′11″

Skin

Clammy; no rashes, lesions, or track marks

HEENT

EOMI; PERRLA; fundi benign; ear and nose clear; dentition intact; tonsils 1+

Neck/Lymph Nodes

Supple, no lymphadenopathy; thyroid symmetric and of normal size

Lungs/Chest

Symmetric chest wall movement; BS equal bilaterally; no rub; clear to A&P

CV

RRR, normal S_1 and S_2, no MRG

Abd

Symmetric; NTND; normal BS; no organomegaly or masses

Genit/Rect

Deferred

MS/Ext

Average frame; normal bones, joints, and muscles

Neuro

CNs II–XII intact; motor and sensory grossly normal; coordination intact

MSE

Appearance and behavior: well groomed, fair eye contact, wringing hands, and bouncing legs
Speech: well spoken and coherent with normal rate and rhythm
Mood: anxious, worried about everything in his life, and concerned that he is very sick
Affect: full
Thought processes: linear, logical, and goal-directed
Thought content: negative for suicidal or homicidal ideations, obsessions/compulsions, delusions, or hallucinations
Memory: 3/3 at 0 minutes, 2/3 at 5 minutes; spelled "world" backward
Abstractions: good
Judgment: good by testing
Insight: fair
Score on Hamilton Anxiety Scale = 34 points (see Figure 82-1)

Labs

Na 142 mEq/L	Hgb 14.0 g/dL
K 4.3 mEq/L	Hct 38%
Cl 105 mEq/L	TSH 4.1 mIU/L
CO_2 28 mEq/L	AST 29 IU/L
BUN 15 mg/dL	ALT 28 IU/L
SCr 1.0 mg/dL	Alk phos 23 IU/L
Glu 80 mg/dL	Vit D 25-OH 51 ng/mL

ECG

NSR; rate 88 bpm

Urine Toxicology Screen

Positive for 9-carboxy-THC

Assessment

1. GAD treated and uncontrolled with buspirone

2. Substance use disorder

Mark and score as follows: 0, not present; 1, mild; 2, moderate; 3, severe; 4, very severe

Anxious mood

_4_ Worries, anticipation of the worst, fearful anticipation, irritability

Tension

_3_ Feelings of tension, fatigability, startle response, moved to tears easily, trembling, feelings of restlessness, inability to relax

Fears

_1_ Of dark, of strangers, of being left alone, of animals, of traffic, of crowds

Insomnia

_4_ Difficulty in falling asleep, broken sleep, unsatisfying sleep and fatigue on waking, dreams, nightmares, night terrors

Intellectual

_3_ Difficulty in concentration, poor memory

Depressed mood

_1_ Loss of interest, lack of pleasure in hobbies, depression, early waking, diurnal swing

Somatic (muscular)

_3_ Pains and aches, twitchings, stiffness, myoclonic jerks, grinding of teeth, unsteady voice, increased muscular tone

Somatic (sensory)

_1_ Tinnitus, blurring of vision, hot and cold flushes, feelings of weakness, pricking sensation

Cardiovascular symptoms

_2_ Tachycardia, palpitations, pain in chest, throbbing of vessels, fainting feelings, sighing, dyspnea

Respiratory symptoms

_1_ Pressure or constriction in chest, choking feelings, sighing, dyspnea

Gastrointestinal symptoms

_3_ Difficulty in swallowing, wind, abdominal pain, burning sensations, abdominal fullness, nausea, vomiting, borborygmi, looseness of bowels, loss of weight, constipation

Genitourinary symptoms

_2_ Frequency of micturition, urgency of micturition, amenorrhea, menorrhagia, development of frigidity, premature ejaculation, loss of libido, impotence

Autonomic symptoms

_3_ Dry mouth, flushing, pallor, tendency to sweat, giddiness, tension, headache, raising of hair

Behavior at interview

_3_ Fidgeting, restlessness or pacing, tremor of hands, furrowed brow, strained face, sighing or rapid respiration, facial pallor, swallowing, etc.

Total score: _34_

FIGURE 82-1. Score on Hamilton Anxiety Rating Scale (HAM-A)

QUESTIONS

Collect Information

1.a. What subjective and objective information indicates the presence or severity of GAD?

1.b. What additional information is needed to fully assess this patient's GAD?

Assess the Information

2.a. Assess the severity of GAD based on the subjective and objective information available.

2.b. Create a list of the patient's drug therapy problems and prioritize them. Include assessment of medication appropriateness, effectiveness, safety, and patient adherence.

Develop a Care Plan

3.a. What are the goals of pharmacotherapy in this case?

3.b. What nondrug therapies for GAD might be useful for this patient?

3.c. What feasible pharmacotherapeutic options are available for treating GAD?

3.d. Create an individualized, patient-centered, team-based care plan to optimize medication therapy for the GAD. Include specific drugs, dosage forms, doses, schedules, and durations of therapy.

3.e. What alternatives would be appropriate if the optimal plan fails or cannot be used?

Implement the Care Plan

4.a. What information should be provided to the patient to enhance adherence, ensure successful therapy, and minimize adverse effects?

4.b. Describe how care should be coordinated with other healthcare providers.

Follow-Up: Monitor and Evaluate

5. Explain how to monitor and evaluate the care plan for medication appropriateness, effectiveness, safety, and patient adherence by using clinical and laboratory data, patient feedback, and other information.

■ CLINICAL COURSE: ALTERNATIVE THERAPY

The patient is still worried about the adverse effects of prescription drugs to treat his anxiety and whether he will be able to afford them. He states that he has read a lot of information about kava that "it really works for anxiety." The patient says, "Maybe I was just using a bad product last time I tried it and that's why it didn't help much and hurt my stomach. Should I get a better product and try it again?" Please see Section 19 of this Casebook for questions about the use of kava kava for the treatment of GAD.

■ SELF-STUDY ASSIGNMENTS

1. Perform a literature search to review the role of pregabalin in the treatment of GAD. Write a summary of the controlled trials that evaluated the use of pregabalin in GAD as monotherapy.

2. Individuals with GAD may misuse alcohol, cannabis, or other substances in an effort to ameliorate their anxiety. Review and summarize the recommendations put forth by the International Psychopharmacology Algorithm Project on treating patients with GAD and a history of or current substance use disorder.

3. Many patients with mental illness do not have prescription drug insurance coverage, and this impacts the choice of pharmacotherapy. Using this case example, go to a Web-based pharmacy discount site or patient assistance program and document how you would go about helping this patient obtain a first-line agent that he otherwise would not be able to afford (eg, escitalopram, duloxetine, venlafaxine extended-release capsules).

CLINICAL PEARL

With effective pharmacotherapy available for the acute and long-term therapy of GAD, the treatment goal for anxiety is remission. Many patients exhibit treatment response but still have anxiety symptoms and social and functional impairment. Remission is a more rigorous treatment goal that requires a HAM-A score of ≤7 or reduction of at least 70% in baseline levels of symptoms.

REFERENCES

1. Hamilton M. Hamilton Anxiety Scale. In: Guy W, ed. ECDEU Assessment Manual for Psychopharmacology. Rockville, MD: U.S. Department of Health, Education, and Welfare; 1976:193–198.

2. Baldwin DS, Anderson IM, Nutt DJ, et al. Evidence-based pharmacological treatment of anxiety disorders, post-traumatic stress disorder and obsessive-compulsive disorder: a revision of the 2005 guidelines from the British Association for Pharmacology. J Psychopharmacol. 2014;28:403–439.

3. Davidson JR, Zhang W, Connor KM, et al. A psychopharmacological treatment algorithm for generalized anxiety disorder (GAD). J Psychopharmacol. 2010;24:3–26.

4. Zhang Y, Huang G, Yang S, Liang W, Zhang L, Wang C. Duloxetine in treating generalized anxiety disorder in adults: a meta-analysis of published randomized, double-blind, placebo-controlled trials. Asia Pac Psychiatry. 2016;8(3):215–225.

5. Bandelow B, Sher L, Bunevicius R, et al. Guidelines for the pharmacological treatment of anxiety disorders, obsessive-compulsive disorder and posttraumatic stress disorder in primary care. Int J Psychiatry Clin Pract. 2012;16:77–84.

6. Frampton JE. Pregabalin: a review of its use in adults with generalized anxiety disorder. CNS Drugs. 2014;28:835–854.

7. Evoy KE, Morrison MD, Saklad SR. Abuse and misuse of pregabalin and gabapentin. Drugs. 2017;77(4):403–426.

8. Maneeton N, Maneeton B, Woottiluk P, et al. Quetiapine monotherapy in acute treatment of generalized anxiety disorder: a systematic review and meta-analysis of randomized controlled trials. Drug Des Devel Ther. 2016;10:259–276.

9. Sarris J, LaPorte E, Schweitzer I. Kava: a comprehensive review of efficacy, safety, and psychopharmacology. Aust N Z J Psychiatry. 2011;45:27–35.

83

OBSESSIVE–COMPULSIVE DISORDER

Don't Use That, It's Poison! . . . . Level I

Lindsey Miller, PharmD, BCPP

Chris Paxos, PharmD, BCPP, BCPS, BCGP

LEARNING OBJECTIVES

After completing this case study, the reader should be able to:

- Identify target symptoms associated with obsessive–compulsive disorder (OCD).

- Determine goals of pharmacotherapy for OCD.

- Develop an appropriate plan and duration of therapy for the management of OCD.

- Educate patients and consult with providers about the pharmacotherapy used for OCD.

- Develop a monitoring plan for a patient treated for OCD based on the treatment regimen.

PATIENT PRESENTATION

■ Chief Complaint

"I can't take it anymore!"

■ HPI

A 24-year-old woman presents to her primary care provider. Her roommate has become increasingly alarmed with the patient's behaviors, prompting this visit with the provider. The patient is unable to leave a room without turning the light on and off three times. She believes that by not completing this task, she will be involved in a horrible car accident. She rarely leaves her apartment. She states, "I know this is absurd, but I can't help it! If I don't do it, I know I will get hurt. I just know it!" The patient has been experiencing a great deal of anxiety over the past several months. She is currently treated for obsessive–compulsive disorder; however, her anxiety has become more notable as the deadline to her master's thesis approaches. More recently, the patient will not allow her roommate to eat anything that is not pre-packaged for fear of poisoning. She continually checks the food in the kitchen to make sure it is all pre-packaged. The patient states that her anxiety has risen to a level that she has never experienced before, and she no longer knows what to do. When asked about suicidal ideation, she reports fleeting thoughts of suicide but does not have a plan. She understands that these thoughts are irrational and wants them to go away. She is concerned because her thoughts and rituals consume 6 or more hours each day and have impeded her ability to complete her coursework and be "present" at school. She reports that her checking behaviors have begun to cause tension at home but also says that she needs relief from the overwhelming anxiety that develops throughout the day from her intrusive thoughts. She has tried to hide her compulsions from her roommate, but it has become so time-consuming and distressful that it is nearly impossible to ignore. This has only added to her anxiety. The patient has been treated with sertraline 200 mg daily for approximately 1 year with minimal improvement in her Yale–Brown Obsessive Compulsive Scale score (decreased from 35 to 31). Her provider has tried to increase the dose of sertraline beyond 200 mg daily, but the patient experienced restlessness and could not tolerate the dose increase.

■ PMH

Obsessive–compulsive disorder × 8 years
Menorrhagia × 4 years
Surgeries: none
Trauma: none
Immunizations: current with all vaccinations

■ FH

Mother has a history of major depressive disorder and atrial fibrillation. Father has a history of generalized anxiety disorder and hypertension. Older brother is a "perfectionist" and has to have everything "just right."

■ SH

Single, with no children; working toward her master's degree in business administration; bachelor's degree in accounting and currently works as an intern for a human resource firm; denies tobacco use but admits to alcohol use 1–2 times per week. Currently lives with roommate; has one cat and one dog. She has commercial insurance coverage.

■ Meds

Sertraline 200 mg PO daily
Levonorgestrel intrauterine system

■ All

Amoxicillin (hives)

■ ROS

Reports anxiety throughout the day that is temporarily relieved by counting and checking behaviors. Denies fatigue, headaches, abdominal pain, or changes in sleep.

■ Physical Examination

Gen

Patient displaying severe anxiety

VS

BP 120/74 mm Hg, P 85 bpm, RR 18, T 37°C; Wt 76 kg, Ht 6'1"

Skin

Normal skin turgor; hair and nails are normal

HEENT

PERRLA; EOMI; fundi benign

Neck/Lymph Nodes

No lymphadenopathy or thyromegaly

Lungs/Chest

CTA bilaterally

CV

Heart sounds normal; no MRG

Abd

Normal BS; no organomegaly or masses

Genit/Rect

Deferred

MS/Ext

No CCE; pulses intact

Neuro

A&O × 3; CN II-XII intact; normal gait

Mental Status Examination

Patient is a 24-year-old woman who appears her stated age. She is well groomed and appropriately dressed for the weather with good attention to overall hygiene. She is wearing a significant amount of jewelry as per her usual baseline. She has appropriate psychomotor activity. Her mood is anxious, and affect is congruent. Speech is clear, soft, regular rate and tone. Thoughts are positive for obsessions. Compulsions include counting rituals and checking behaviors. Continues to have suicidal ideation chronically. No homicidal ideation detected or elicited. No auditory or visual hallucinations. She is alert and oriented to the context of the examination. Attention is good; concentration is impaired. Insight and judgment are good.

Yale–Brown Obsessive Compulsive Scale score = 31

■ Labs

Na 140 mEq/L	Hgb 13.2 g/dL
K 3.8 mEq/L	Hct 40.5%
Cl 103 mEq/L	WBC 5.2×10^3/mm³
CO_2 25 mEq/L	AST 20 IU/L
BUN 15 mg/dL	ALT 30 IU/L
SCr 0.8 mg/dL	Alk phos 44 IU/L
Glu 77 mg/dL	Albumin 4.2 g/dL
HCG negative	TSH 1.4 mIU/L

■ ECG

NSR; QTc—420 milliseconds

■ Urine Toxicology Screen

Negative

■ Assessment

A 24-year-old women with obsessive-compulsive disorder, currently uncontrolled with sertraline, and menorrhagia managed with pharmacologic therapy.

QUESTIONS

Collect Information

1.a. What subjective and objective information indicates the presence of OCD?

1.b. What additional information is needed to fully assess this patient's OCD?

Assess the Information

2.a. Assess the severity of OCD based on the subjective and objective information available.

2.b. Create a list of the patient's drug therapy problems and prioritize them. Include assessment of medication appropriateness, effectiveness, safety, and patient adherence.

Develop a Care Plan

3.a. What are the goals of pharmacotherapy for OCD in this case?

3.b. What nondrug therapies for OCD might be useful for this patient?

3.c. What feasible pharmacotherapeutic options are available for treating OCD?

3.d. Create an individualized, patient-centered, team-based care plan to optimize medication therapy for the OCD and other drug therapy problems identified. Include specific drugs, dosage forms, doses, schedules, and durations of therapy.

3.e. What alternatives would be appropriate if the initial care plan fails or cannot be used?

Implement the Care Plan

4.a. What information should be provided to the patient to enhance adherence, ensure successful therapy, and minimize adverse effects?

4.b. Describe how care should be coordinated with other healthcare providers.

Follow-Up: Monitor and Evaluate

5. Explain how to monitor and evaluate the care plan for medication appropriateness, effectiveness, safety, and patient adherence by using clinical and laboratory data, patient feedback, and other information.

■ ADDITIONAL CASE QUESTIONS

1. When is a decrease in the Yale–Brown Obsessive Compulsive Scale score considered clinically significant?

2. If this patient had presented to the prescriber desiring to become pregnant after 6 months of pharmacotherapy, what would your recommendations be regarding pharmacotherapy?

3. When is a patient with OCD considered to be "treatment-refractory?" What other pharmacologic alternatives are available if this patient is determined to be refractory to standard pharmacotherapy?

■ SELF-STUDY ASSIGNMENTS

1. Prepare a grid contrasting the pros and cons of each SSRI in the management of OCD.

2. Perform a literature search and write a short paper on the treatment options used to augment antidepressant monotherapy in patients with OCD who have a partial response or are resistant to treatment.

3. Visit the National Institute of Mental Health website and review the brochure "PANDAS—Questions and Answers," to learn about PANDAS–related obsessive–compulsive symptoms.

CLINICAL PEARL

Antidepressant doses used to treat OCD are often higher than doses used to treat major depressive disorder. Guidelines recommend occasional off-label use of high-dose antidepressant therapy for patients with minimal response after 8 weeks of maximum dosing.

Examples of occasional maximum doses include sertraline 400 mg daily and fluoxetine 120 mg daily. Occasional high-dose antidepressant therapy should be considered only when patients are tolerating the antidepressant with minimal or no adverse effects.

REFERENCES

1. Fineberg NA, Reghunandanan S, Simpson HB, et al. Obsessive-compulsive disorder (OCD): practical strategies for pharmacological and somatic treatment in adults. Psychiatry Res. 2015;227:114–125.
2. Rush AJ, First MB, Blacker D, eds. Handbook of Psychiatric Measures. 2nd ed. Washington, DC: American Psychiatric Publishing; 2008:547–549.
3. Koran LM, Simpson HB. Guideline watch (March 2013): Practice guideline for the treatment of patients with obsessive-compulsive disorder. Available at: *http://psychiatryonline.org/pb/assets/raw/sitewide/practice_guidelines/guidelines/ocd-watch.pdf*. Accessed April 15, 2022.
4. American Psychiatric Association. Diagnostic and Statistical Manual of Mental Disorders. 5th ed. Washington, DC: American Psychiatric Publishing; 2013. doi: 10.1176/appi.books.9780890425596.
5. American Psychiatric Association. Practice guideline for the treatment of patients with obsessive–compulsive disorder. Arlington, VA: American Psychiatric Association; 2007. Available at: *http://psychiatryonline.org/pb/assets/raw/sitewide/practice_guidelines/guidelines/ocd.pdf*. Accessed April 15, 2022.
6. Katzman MA, Bleau P, Blier P, et al. Canadian clinical practice guidelines for the management of anxiety, posttraumatic stress and obsessive-compulsive disorders. BMC Psychiatry. 2014;14(Suppl 1):S1.
7. Fonseka TM, Richter MA, Müller DJ. Second generation antipsychotic-induced obsessive-compulsive symptoms in schizophrenia: a review of the experimental literature. Curr Psychiatry Rep. 2014;16(11):510.
8. Alwan S, Friedman JM, Chambers C. Safety of selective serotonin reuptake inhibitors in pregnancy: review of current evidence. CNS Drugs. 2016;30:499–515.
9. Orsolini L, Bellantuaono C. Serotonin reuptake inhibitors and breastfeeding: a systematic review. Hum Psychopharmacol Clin Exp. 2015;30:4–20.
10. Baldwin DS, Anderson IM, Nutt DJ, et al. Evidence-based pharmacological treatment of anxiety disorders, post-traumatic stress disorder, and obsessive–compulsive disorder: a revision of the 2005 guidelines from the British Association for Psychopharmacology. J Psychopharmacol. 2014;28:403–439.

84

INSOMNIA

Restless Nights and the Blue Moon . . . . Level II

Suzanne C. Harris, PharmD, BCPP, CPP

Rachel Marie E. Salas, MD, MEd, FAAN, FANA

LEARNING OBJECTIVES

After completing this case study, the reader should be able to:

- Identify the psychosocial, disease-related, and drug-induced causes of insomnia.

- Explain the impact of poor medication adherence on chronic illnesses.

- Design a therapeutic plan for the treatment of insomnia.
- Educate a patient regarding nonpharmacologic treatments for insomnia.

PATIENT PRESENTATION

■ Chief Complaint

"I can't sleep."

■ HPI

A 55-year-old woman is referred by her family medicine physician to a pharmacotherapy clinic for medication therapy management for insomnia. She receives help paying for her medications from medication assistance programs. She has been experiencing long-standing insomnia for approximately 9 months. Specifically, she is having difficulty falling and staying asleep at least four to five times during the week, and then sleeps all day on Sunday. The patient is currently taking temazepam 30 mg daily at bedtime that was recently increased from 15 mg. She said that she started taking valerian root 600 mg 6 weeks ago based on a friend's recommendation but does not feel any benefit. Additionally, she has been experiencing vivid dreams that she attributes to the valerian root. When she had health insurance, she started cognitive behavioral therapy for insomnia (CBT-I); however, when she lost her insurance, she was only able to complete six out of eight sessions, with last session over 4 weeks ago. She endorsed moderate benefit from CBT-I but still complained of residual symptoms. She is also experiencing depression due to not having any employment and a stress of a partner who recently moved in with her because he could not pay his apartment rent. Her most recent Patient Health Questionnaire-9 (PHQ-9) result was 20. She admits to being intermittently nonadherent and missing doses of scheduled inhaled medications for COPD and sertraline, olanzapine/fluoxetine, and valerian root one to two times per week. She reports that she is no longer able to see her psychiatrist due to cost of the visits.

■ PMH

Insomnia for many years
COPD
Depression
Allergic rhinitis

■ FH

Mother is alive and well and lives nearby. Father died of MI at age 65.

■ SH

She is in a new relationship with her partner who recently moved in due to his own financial difficulties. Unemployed, leading to stress at home to pay bills but receives some money from her mother. She smokes approximately five cigarettes per day now but has smoked up to two ppd in the past. She does not drink alcohol. She sees a deacon at her church for counseling regularly. She receives medication assistance for several of her medications from a local agency.

■ Medications

Temazepam 30 mg PO QHS PRN sleep
Fluticasone/salmeterol DPI 250/50 one inhalation twice daily
Albuterol MDI two puffs Q 6 H PRN SOB
Tiotropium Handihaler one inhalation daily
Sertraline 200 mg PO Q AM
Olanzapine 3 mg/fluoxetine 25 mg PO Q PM
Pseudoephedrine 30 mg PO Q 6 H PRN allergies
Valerian root supplement 600 mg PO QHS

■ All

NKDA

■ ROS

Patient reports that she does not sleep at all during the week and only sleeps on Sunday. She also reports some improvement in sleep hygiene based on previous recommendations, such as avoiding eating too close to bedtime and long naps, but she continues to exercise in late evenings and reads and watches television in bed. She has cut back to three cups of coffee throughout the day, reduced from six to eight cups of coffee throughout the day. She continues to experience difficulty going to sleep and staying asleep and reports having had this problem for several years. Additionally, the temazepam does not seem to help much. Due to reports of awakening during the night and risk factors for obstructive sleep apnea (ie, postmenopausal, increased BMI), her primary care provider ordered a sleep study that was normal other than some minimal snoring. She has a long history of depression but has never been hospitalized. She currently is not experiencing a "blue mood" or any thoughts of suicide, and her PHQ-9 score today is 20. She has been prescribed sertraline, which she tolerates well, and the combination of olanzapine and fluoxetine to help with her depressive symptoms. Her COPD is secondary to a long history of smoking but is currently controlled on tiotropium, fluticasone/salmeterol, and albuterol PRN. She has runny nose, congestion, and itchy eyes in the spring.

■ Physical Examination (from the last visit with her PCP)

Gen

Obese (per BMI criteria), woman in NAD who looks her stated age

VS

BP 125/80 mm Hg, P 76 BPM, RR 16, T 37°C; Wt 105 kg; Ht 5′6″

Skin

Normal skin color and turgor, no lesions noted

HEENT

Normocephalic, PERRLA, EOMI

Neck/Lymph Nodes

Supple with normal size thyroid, (–) adenopathy

Lungs

CTA bilaterally

CV

Normal S_1, S_2; no MRG

Abd

NTND, no HSM

Genit/Rect

Deferred. Last PAP smear was WNL 6 months ago.

Ext

No C/C/E; normal muscle bulk and tone; muscle strength 5/5 and equal in all extremities; normal pulses

Neuro

Oriented to person, place, and time; CN II–XII intact; Mini-Mental State Examination results: 30/30

■ Labs

Na 141 mEq/L	Hgb 13 g/dL	AST 36 IU/L	Lipid panel
K 3.9 mEq/L	Hct 38%	ALT 32 IU/L	T. chol 215 mg/dL
Cl 105 mEq/L	RBC $4.4 \times 10^6/mm^3$	LDH 112 IU/L	LDL 100 mg/dL
CO_2 26 mEq/L	Plt $236 \times 10^3/mm^3$	GGT 47 IU/L	HDL 45 mg/dL
BUN 12 mg/dL	WBC $6.8 \times 10^3/mm^3$	T. bili 0.6 mg/dL	TG 160 mg/dL
SCr 0.7 mg/dL	TSH 3.9 mIU/L	T. prot 7.1 g/dL	
Glu 85 mg/dL	Free T_4 4.0 ng/dL	Alb 4.0 g/dL	

■ Assessment

1. Insomnia, with poor sleep hygiene and sleep environment, that is inadequately managed with long-term use of benzodiazepine
2. Depression evidenced by PHQ-9 score of 20
3. Allergic rhinitis and pseudoephedrine use
4. Health maintenance and nonadherence to medication
5. Multiple stressors and poor access to healthcare

QUESTIONS

Collect Information

1.a. What subjective and objective information indicates the presence of insomnia?

1.b. What additional information is needed to fully assess this patient's insomnia?

Assess the Information

2.a. Assess the severity of insomnia based on the subjective and objective information available.

2.b. Create a list of the patient's drug therapy problems and prioritize them. Include assessment of medication appropriateness, effectiveness, safety, and patient adherence.

2.c. What economic, psychosocial, cultural, and ethical considerations are applicable to this patient?

Develop a Care Plan

3.a. What are the goals of pharmacotherapy for this patient?

3.b. What nonpharmacologic therapies might be useful for this patient's insomnia?

3.c. What feasible pharmacotherapeutic options are available to treat this patient's insomnia?

3.d. Create an individualized, patient-centered, team-based care plan to optimize medication therapy for this patient's insomnia and other drug therapy problems. Include specific drugs, dosage form, dose, schedule, and durations of therapy.

3.e. What alternatives would be appropriate if the initial therapy fails or cannot be used?

Implement the Care Plan

4.a. What information should be provided to the patient to enhance adherence, ensure successful therapy, and minimize adverse effects?

4.b. Describe how care should be coordinated with other healthcare providers.

Follow-Up: Monitor and Evaluate

5. Explain how to monitor and evaluate the care plan for medication appropriateness, effectiveness, safety, and patient adherence by using clinical laboratory data, patient feedback, and other information.

■ CLINICAL COURSE: ALTERNATIVE THERAPY

The patient states that her neighbor had suggested using a melatonin product to help her stay asleep. She would like to know whether that is a good option to help keep her from waking up after she has fallen asleep. See Section 19 of this Casebook for questions about the use of melatonin to help manage insomnia.

■ SELF-STUDY ASSIGNMENTS

1. Discuss clinician's interventions that can improve medication adherence.
2. Explain important monitoring parameters for patients receiving atypical antipsychotics.

CLINICAL PEARL

Patients with underlying depression frequently have insomnia, and poor medication adherence to antidepressants can exacerbate sleep disorders.

REFERENCES

1. Qaseem A, Kansagara D, Forciea MA, et al. Management of chronic insomnia disorder in adults: a clinical practice guideline from the American College of Physicians. Ann Intern Med. 2016;165(2):125–133.
2. Edinger JD, Arnedt JT, Bertisch SM, et al. Behavioral and psychological treatments for chronic insomnia disorder in adults: an American Academy of Sleep Medicine clinical practice guideline. J Clin Sleep Med. 2021;17(2):255–262.
3. Perez MN, Salas RME. Insomnia. Continuum (Minneap Minn) 2020;26(4):1003–1015.
4. Sateia MJ, Buysse DJ, Krystal AD, et al. Clinical practice guideline for the pharmacologic treatment of chronic insomnia in adults: an American Academy of Sleep Medicine Clinical Practice Guideline. J Clin Sleep Med. 2017;13(2):307–349.
5. 2019 American Geriatrics Society Beers Criteria Update Expert Panel. American Geriatrics Society 2019 updated AGS beers criteria for potentially inappropriate medication use in older adults. J Am Geriatr Soc. 2019;67(4):674–694.
6. U.S. Food and Drug Administration. FDA Drug Safety Communication: Risk of next-morning impairment after use of insomnia drugs; FDA requires lower recommended doses for certain drugs containing zolpidem (Ambien, Ambien CR, Edluar, and Zolpimist). Available at: *http://wayback.archive-it.org/7993/20170111080036/http://www.fda.gov/Drugs/DrugSafety/ucm334033.htm.* Accessed April 15, 2022.
7. U.S. Food and Drug Administration. FDA Drug Safety Communication: FDA warns of next-day impairment with sleep aid Lunesta (eszopiclone) and lowers recommended dose. Available at: *https://www.fda.gov/drugs/drug-safety-and-availability/fda-drug-safety-communication-fda-warns-next-day-impairment-sleep-aid-lunesta-eszopiclone-and-lowers.* Accessed April 15, 2022.
8. Schroeck JL, Ford J, Conway EL, et al. Review of safety and efficacy of sleep medicines in older adults. Clin Ther. 2016;38(11):2340–2372.
9. Cleare A, Pariante CM, Young AH, et al. Evidence-based guidelines for treating depressive disorders with antidepressants: a revision of the 2008 British Association for Psychopharmacology guidelines. J Psychopharmacol. 2015;29(5):459–525.
10. Finan PH, Richards JM, Gamaldo CE, et al. Validation of a wireless, self-application, ambulatory electroencephalographic sleep monitoring device in healthy volunteers. J Clin Sleep Med. 2016;12(11):1443–1451.

85

TYPE 1 DIABETES MELLITUS AND KETOACIDOSIS

Disconnected .... Level II

Holly S. Divine, PharmD, BCACP, BCGP, CDCES, FAPhA

Carrie L. Isaacs, PharmD, CDCES, MLDE

Rachel C. Minrath, PharmD

LEARNING OBJECTIVES

After completing this case study, the reader should be able to:

- Recognize signs and symptoms of diabetic ketoacidosis (DKA).

- Determine laboratory parameters for the diagnosis and monitoring of DKA.

- Identify anticipated fluid and electrolyte abnormalities associated with DKA and their treatment.

- Recommend appropriate insulin therapy for treating DKA.

- Identify therapeutic decision points in DKA treatment and provide parameters for altering therapy at those points.

PATIENT PRESENTATION

■ Chief Complaint

"I felt weak and nauseated during softball practice. I checked my blood glucose and it read 'HI' (blood glucose >600 mg/dL)."

■ HPI

A 21-year-old woman with a history of type 1 diabetes diagnosed 3 years ago is a college senior at the local university where she also plays softball. She started using an insulin pump approximately 6 months ago.

She noticed she was unusually tired and short of breath at the beginning of her practice and then began feeling weak and nauseated. She was also very thirsty during practice. Her softball coach said she seemed "a little confused." He advised her to check her blood glucose, and it read "HI". She checked her insulin pump and noticed the pump had become disconnected. She is unsure how long she has been without insulin. She vomited two times since shortly thereafter and was transported via EMS to the ED.

■ PMH

Type 1 DM diagnosed 3 years ago. No prior hospitalizations for DKA or prior surgeries.

■ FH

Parents are alive and healthy. One twin sister who also has type 1 DM.

■ SH

College student; no tobacco, alcohol, or illicit drug use. Sexually active; in a monogamous relationship.

■ Meds

NovoLog 100 U/mL, per insulin pump
Basal rates:
    0.6 U/hr 0000–0300
    0.9 U/hr 0300–0700
    0.8 U/hr 0700–1100
    0.7 U/hr 1100–1730
    0.8 U/hr 1730–0000
Correction factor: 1 U:40 mg/dL >120 mg/dL
Insulin:carbohydrate ratios:
    1:10 insulin:carbohydrate before breakfast
    1:15 insulin:carbohydrate before lunch and dinner
Glucagon injection kit, as needed
Sprintec (35 mcg ethinyl estradiol/0.25 mg norgestimate) one tablet PO once daily × 3 years

■ All

NKDA

■ ROS

Complains of blurry vision, lethargy, shortness of breath, nausea, polyuria, and polydipsia. Denies constipation, diarrhea, and headache.

■ Physical Examination

Gen

WDWN woman appearing her stated age, with deep respirations, ketones on her breath, and slurred speech; slightly confused, but responds appropriately to questions

VS

BP 101/72 mm Hg, P 123 bpm, RR 32, T 37.0°C; Wt 56 kg, Ht 5′6″; BMI 19.9 kg/m²

Skin

Unremarkable

HEENT

PERRLA, EOMI; mucous membranes are dry

Neck/Lymph Nodes

Supple without lymphadenopathy or thyromegaly

Lungs

CTA, Kussmaul respirations

CV

S_1 and S_2 are normal without S_3, S_4, murmur or rub; RRR

Abd

NT/ND

Genit/Rect

Deferred

MS/Ext

No edema, pulses 2+ throughout, mild calluses

Neuro

A&O × 3; DTRs 2+ throughout; feet with normal sensation and vibration

■ Labs

Na 136 mEq/L	WBC $15.0 \times 10^3/mm^3$
K 4.8 mEq/L	RBC $4.61 \times 10^6/mm^3$
Cl 101 mEq/L	Hgb 14.2 g/dL
CO_2 10 mEq/L	Hct 40.7%
BUN 23 mg/dL	Platelets $239 \times 10^3/mm^3$
SCr 1.4 mg/dL	Ketones positive
Glu 479 mg/dL	hCG negative

■ ABG

pH 7.26; $PaCO_2$ 21 mm Hg; PaO_2 128 mm Hg; HCO_3 7.1 mEq/L; O_2 sat 97%

■ UA

(+) Ketones; (+) glucose

■ Chest X-Ray

Normal

■ ECG

Sinus tachycardia

■ Assessment

DKA precipitated by insulin deficiency

QUESTIONS

Collect Information

1.a. What subjective and objective information indicates the presence and severity of DKA?

1.b. What are the precipitating risk factors for DKA, and which of those risk factors are present in this patient?

1.c. What are the diagnostic criteria for DKA?

Assess the Information

2.a. What problems need to be addressed in DKA besides hyperglycemia?

2.b. Create a list of the patient's drug therapy problems and prioritize them. Include assessment of medication appropriateness, effectiveness, safety, and patient adherence.

Develop a Care Plan

3.a. What are the goals of pharmacotherapy for DKA in this case?

3.b. What therapeutic options are available to correct the metabolic derangements of DKA?

3.c. Create an individualized, patient-centered, team-based care plan to optimize medication therapy for this patient's DKA and other drug therapy problems. Include specific drugs, dosage forms, doses, schedules, and durations of therapy.

Implement the Care Plan

4.a. What information should be provided to the patient regarding prevention of future DKA?

4.b. Describe how care should be coordinated with other healthcare providers.

Follow-up: Monitor and Evaluate

5. Explain how to monitor and evaluate the care plan for medication appropriateness, effectiveness, safety, and patient adherence by using clinical and laboratory data, patient feedback, and other information.

■ SELF-STUDY ASSIGNMENTS

1. What does the ADA state about DKA and hyperosmolar hyperglycemic state (HHS) in patients with type 2 DM? Compare these two disorders with respect to prevention, precipitating causes, signs and symptoms, pathophysiology, and treatment.

2. Investigate other causes of DKA, such as illness, and write a sick day management plan for this patient.

3. How might the use of continuous glucose monitors (CGMs) be beneficial in patients with type 1 DM?

4. Review euglycemic DKA and its relationship to the sodium-glucose cotransporter-2 (SGLT2) inhibitor drug class.

CLINICAL PEARL

Sodium-glucose cotransporter-2 (SGLT2) inhibitors increase the risk for diabetic ketoacidosis, particularly in patients with type 1 diabetes or latent autoimmune diabetes in adulthood (LADA) and those with type 2 diabetes with certain high-risk conditions. Over a third of patients with ketoacidosis associated with SGLT2 inhibitor use have normal or only mildly elevated blood glucose levels (<250 mg/dL) which can delay diagnosis.

REFERENCES

1. Kitabchi AE, Umpierrez GE, Miles JM, Fisher JN. Hyperglycemic crises in adult patients with diabetes. Diabetes Care. 2009;32:1335–1343.

2. Umpierrez G, Korytkowski M. Diabetic emergencies-ketoacidosis, hyperglycaemic hyperosmolar state and hypoglycemia. Nat Rev Endocrinol. 2016;12:222–232.

3. Dingle HE, Slovis C. Diabetic ketoacidosis and hyperosmolar hyperglycemic syndrome management. Emerg Med. 2018;50(8):161–171.

4. American Diabetes Association. Standards of Medical Care in Diabetes—2022. Diabetes Care. 2022;45(Suppl 1):S1–S2.

5. American Association of Clinical Endocrinologists and American College of Endocrinology. Clinical practice guidelines for developing a diabetes mellitus comprehensive care plan—2015. Endocr Pract. 2015;21(Suppl 1):1–87.

6. The management of type 1 diabetes in adults: a consensus report by the American Diabetes Association (ADA) and the European Association for the Study of Diabetes (EASD). Diabetes Care. 2021;44:2589–2625.

7. Andrade-Castellanos CA, Colunga-Lozano LE, Delgado-Figueroa N, Gonzalez-Padilla DA. Subcutaneous rapid-acting insulin analogues for diabetic ketoacidosis. Cochrane Database Syst. Rev. 2016:1. doi: 10.1002/14651858.CD011281.pub2.

8. Duhon B, Attridge RL, Franco-Martinez AC, Maxwell PR, Hughes DW. Intravenous sodium bicarbonate therapy in severely acidotic diabetic ketoacidosis. Ann Pharmacother. 2013;47:970–975.

9. American Association of Diabetes Educators AADE practice paper: continuous subcutaneous insulin infusion (CSII) without and with sensor integration. Available at: *www.diabeteseducator.org/docs/default-source/default-document-library/continuous-subcutaneous-insulin-infusion-2018-v2.pdf?sfvrsn=0*. Accessed January 11, 2022.

10. Beck J. Greenwood DA, Blanton L, et al; 2017 Standards Revision Task Force. 2017 national standards for diabetes self-management education and support. Diabetes Care. 2017;40:1409–1419.

86

TYPE 2 DIABETES MELLITUS: NEW ONSET

The Candy Man. . . . . Level II

Nicole C. Pezzino, PharmD, BCACP, CDCES

Deanne L. Hall, PharmD, BCACP, CDCES

LEARNING OBJECTIVES

After completing this case study, the reader should be able to:

- Recognize the signs, symptoms, and risk factors associated with type 2 diabetes mellitus (DM).

- Identify the comorbidities in type 2 DM associated with insulin resistance (metabolic syndrome).

- Compare the pharmacotherapeutic options in the management of type 2 DM including mechanism of action, contraindications, and adverse effects.

- Develop appropriate educational information for a patient regarding blood glucose monitoring (BGM).

- Design a patient-specific pharmacotherapeutic plan for the treatment and monitoring of type 2 DM.

PATIENT PRESENTATION

■ Chief Complaint

"My vision has been blurred lately and it seems to be getting worse."

■ HPI

A 68-year-old man presents to his family physician's office complaining of periodic blurred vision for the past month. He further complains of fatigue and lack of energy that prohibits him from working in his garden and participating in physical activity.

■ PMH

HTN × 18 years
Dyslipidemia × 8 years
Hypothyroidism × 15 years
Overweight × 25 years

■ FH

Diabetes present in mother. Immigrated to the United States with his mother and sister after their father died suddenly from unknown causes at age 45. One younger sibling died of breast cancer at age 48.

■ SH

Retired candy salesman, married × 46 years with three children and two grandchildren. No tobacco use. Drinks one to two glasses of homemade wine with meals. He reports adherence with his medications.

■ Meds

Lisinopril 20 mg PO once daily
Levothyroxine 0.088 mg PO once daily

■ All

NKDA

■ ROS

Occasional polydipsia, polyphagia, fatigue, weakness, and blurred vision. Denies chest pain, dyspnea, tachycardia, dizziness or light-headedness on standing, tingling or numbness in extremities, leg cramps, peripheral edema, changes in bowel movements, GI bloating or pain, nausea or vomiting, urinary incontinence, or presence of skin lesions.

■ Physical Examination

Gen

The patient is a centrally obese, Caucasian man who appears to be restless and in mild distress.

VS

BP 124/76 mm Hg without orthostasis, P 80 bpm, RR 18, T 37.2°C; Wt 77 kg, Ht 66″; BMI 27.4 kg/m²

Skin

Dry with poor skin turgor; no ulcers or rash

HEENT

PERRLA; EOMI; TMs intact; no hemorrhages or exudates on funduscopic examination; mucous membranes normal; nose and throat clear w/o exudates or lesions

Neck/Lymph Nodes

Supple; without lymphadenopathy, thyromegaly, or JVD

Lungs/Thorax

CTA

CV

RRR; normal S_1 and S_2; no S_3, S_4, rubs, murmurs, or bruits

Abd

Soft, NT, central obesity; normal BS; no organomegaly or distention

Genit/Rect

Normal external male genitalia

MS/Ext

Normal ROM and sensation; peripheral pulses 2+ throughout; no lesions, ulcers, or edema

Neuro

A&O × 3, CN II–XII intact; DTRs 2+ throughout; feet with normal vibratory and pinprick sensation (5.07/10 g monofilament)

■ Labs

Na 141 mEq/L	Ca 9.9 mg/dL	A1C 7.8%
K 4.0 mEq/L	Phos 3.2 mg/dL	*Fasting lipid profile*
Cl 96 mEq/L	AST 21 IU/L	T. chol 280 mg/dL
CO_2 22 mEq/L	ALT 15 IU/L	HDL 27 mg/dL
BUN 24 mg/dL	Alk phos 45 IU/L	LDL 193 mg/dL
SCr 1.1 mg/dL	T. bili 0.9 mg/dL	Trig 302 mg/dL
Random glu 202 mg/dL		

■ UA

(–) Ketones, (–) protein, (–) microalbuminuria

■ Assessment

68-year-old overweight man with new onset type 2 DM.

■ Clinical Course

The patient returned to clinic 3 days later for lab work, which revealed: TSH 1.8 mIU/L, free T_4 1.2 ng/dL, and a FBG of 157 mg/dL. Additionally, updated immunization status was provided, which revealed up-to-date on all childhood vaccines, annual influenza, COVID-19 first and second dose (Pfizer series), and pneumococcal polysaccharide (PPSV 23) administered at 65 years old.

QUESTIONS

Collect Information

1.a. What risk factors for type 2 DM are present in this patient?

1.b. What subjective and objective information indicates the presence of new-onset type 2 DM?

1.c. What information indicates the presence of insulin resistance?

1.d. What additional information is needed to fully assess this patient's type 2 DM?

Assess the Information

2.a. Create a list of this patient's drug therapy problems and prioritize them. Include assessment of medication appropriateness, effectiveness, safety, and patient adherence.

Develop a Care Plan

3.a. What are the goals of pharmacotherapy for type 2 DM in this case?

3.b. Considering his other medical problems, what other treatment goals should be established?

3.c. What nondrug therapies might be useful for this patient's type 2 DM?

3.d. What feasible pharmacotherapeutic options are available for treating this patient's type 2 DM?

3.e. Create an individualized, patient-centered, team-based care plan to optimize medication therapy for this patient's type 2 DM and other drug therapy problems. Include specific drugs, dosage forms, doses, schedules, and durations of therapy.

3.f. What alternatives would be appropriate if the initial care plan fails or cannot be used?

Implement the Care Plan

4.a. What information should be provided to the patient about diabetes and its treatment to enhance adherence, ensure successful therapy, minimize adverse effects, and prevent future complications?

4.b. How would you educate the patient regarding how and when to check his blood glucose?

4.c. Describe how care should be coordinated with other healthcare providers.

Follow-up: Monitor and Evaluate

5.a. Explain how to monitor and evaluate the care plan for medication appropriateness, effectiveness, safety, and patient adherence by using clinical and laboratory data, patient feedback, and other information.

5.b. The patient's physician suggested that he obtain a blood glucose meter for BGM. What evidence supports BGM, and what are the healthcare provider's responsibilities with respect to patients and BGM?

5.c. Identify at least four potential situations in which the information provided by BGM would be useful to patients and healthcare providers.

5.d. What factors should be considered in the selection of an appropriate blood glucose meter?

■ CLINICAL COURSE: ALTERNATIVE THERAPY

While discussing the patient's diagnosis with him, he states that his neighbor with diabetes told him that she just follows her diabetic diet and takes cinnamon and something called "alip acid" and does not have to take any prescriptions for her blood sugar. He also says that he has read about fish oil being used for diabetes. The patient asks if he should start any of those to help get his blood sugar under control. See Section 19 in this Casebook for questions about the use of fish oil, cinnamon, and alpha-lipoic acid for treatment of diabetes.

■ FOLLOW-UP QUESTIONS

1. What nonprescription products could be recommended for patients to use in treating hypoglycemic episodes?

2. List several potential sources of error in BGM.

3. When starting patients on insulin, the use of combination oral antihyperglycemic agents and insulin offers several advantages over switching entirely to insulin:

   (a) What are the advantages of adding insulin to existing therapies with oral agents?

   (b) List an appropriate method of starting insulin therapy to adequately control fasting hyperglycemia in patients on combination oral agents.

SELF-STUDY ASSIGNMENTS

1. Describe how you would evaluate and monitor this patient's quality of life.

2. Characterize the relationship between insulin resistance and the risk for ASCVD.

3. Prepare a list of medications that have been associated with increasing blood glucose. Provide literature evidence on the strength of the association with each medication.

4. Review the literature and conduct a comparative review of the efficacy of inhaled insulin therapy relative to the insulin products commercially available for subcutaneous injection.

CLINICAL PEARL

The leading cause of morbidity and mortality for individuals with diabetes is atherosclerotic cardiovascular disease (ASCVD). ADA 2022 guidelines support reducing cardiovascular risk and choosing first-line therapy based on ASCVD/indicators of high risk, HF, and CKD. Utilizing agents that reduce the risk of cardiovascular events, such as metformin and/or certain GLP-1 receptor agonists and SGLT-2 inhibitors, is preferred considering many common conditions that coexist with diabetes are also risk factors for ASCVD.[1]

REFERENCES

1. American Diabetes Association. Standards of medical care in diabetes—2022. Diabetes Care. 2022;45(1 Suppl):S1–S264.

2. Bloomgarden ZT. Insulin resistance: current concepts. Clin Ther. 1998;20:216–231.

3. American College of Endocrinology and American Association of Clinical Endocrinologists. Clinical practice guidelines for developing a diabetes mellitus comprehensive care plan—2015. Endocr Pract. 2015;21(Suppl 1):1–87.

4. American College of Endocrinology and American Association of Clinical Endocrinologists. Consensus statement by the American Association of Clinical Endocrinologists and American College of Endocrinology on the comprehensive type 2 diabetes management algorithm—2020 executive summary. Endocr Pract. 2020;26(1):107–139.

5. Grundy SM, Stone NJ, Bailey AL, et al. 2018 AHA/ACC/AACVPR/AAPA/ABC/ACPM/ADA/AGS/APhA/ASPC/NLA/PCNA guideline on the management of blood cholesterol: a report of the American College of Cardiology/American Heart Association Task Force on clinical practice guidelines. J Am Coll Cardiol. 2018 November. doi: 10.1016/j.jacc.2018.11.003.

6. Whelton PK, Carey RM, Aronow WS, et al. 2017 ACC/AHA/AAPA/ABC/ACPM/AGS/APhA/ASH/ASPC/NMA/PCNA guideline for the prevention, detection, evaluation, and management of high blood pressure in adults: executive summary: a report of the American College of Cardiology/American Heart Association Task Force on clinical practice guidelines. Circulation. 2018;138(17):e426–e483.

7. Davies MJ, D'Alessio DA, Fradkin J, et al. Management of hyperglycemia in type 2 diabetes, 2018: a consensus report by the American Diabetes Association (ADA) and the European Association for the Study of Diabetes (EASD). Diabetes Care. 2018;41(12):2669–2701.

8. Cho TM, Wideman RD, Kieffer TJ. Clinical application of glucagon-like peptide 1 receptor agonists for the treatment of type 2 diabetes mellitus. Endocrinol Metab. 2013;28:262–274.

9. Centers for Disease Control and Prevention. Pneumococcal vaccination: Summary of who and when to vaccinate. Available at: https://www.cdc.gov/vaccines/vpd/pneumo/hcp/who-when-to-vaccinate.html. Updated January 24, 2022. Accessed April 8, 2022.

87

TYPE 2 DIABETES MELLITUS: EXISTING DISEASE

Establishing Optimal Control . . . . Level II

Sharon S. Gatewood, PharmD, BCACP, FAPhA

Margaret A. Landis, PharmD

LEARNING OBJECTIVES

After completing this case study, the reader should be able to:

- Identify the goals of therapy for the treatment of type 2 diabetes mellitus (DM).

- Discuss the risk factors and comorbidities associated with type 2 DM.

- Compare options for drug therapy management of type 2 DM, including mechanisms of action, combination therapies, comorbidities, and patient-friendly treatment plans.

- Develop an individualized drug therapy management plan, including dosage regimens, therapeutic endpoints, and monitoring parameters.

- Provide patient education regarding medications and the importance of adhering to the treatment plan, monitoring the disease state, maintaining blood glucose control, and seeking advice from healthcare providers when necessary.

PATIENT PRESENTATION

Chief Complaint

"I have had diabetes for about six months and would like to have my blood sugar tested. I think that my blood sugar is running low, because I have a terrible headache."

HPI

A 45-year-old woman who comes to the pharmacy for a diabetes education class taught by the pharmacist. She would like for the pharmacist to check her blood sugar before the class begins. She was diagnosed with type 2 DM about 6 months ago. She had been attempting to control her disease with diet and exercise, but had no success. Her physician started her on metformin 1000 mg twice daily with food about 3 months ago. She has gained 10 lb over the past year. She monitors her blood sugar once a day, and her results have ranged from 200 to 230 mg/dL. Her fasting blood sugars have averaged 200 mg/dL.

PMH

Type 2 DM × 6 months
HTN × 17 years
Bipolar disorder × 25 years
Dyslipidemia × 12 years
Morbid obesity × 20 years

FH

Father has a history of HTN, dyslipidemia, and bipolar disorder. Mother has a history of dyslipidemia and hypothyroidism. Brother has DM thought to be secondary to alcoholism.

SH

Has been married for 23 years. She has two children who are teenagers and one child in college. She works as a sales associate in the electronics department of a local mass merchandiser. She denies any use of tobacco products after stopping smoking 10 years ago, but does drink alcohol occasionally (three beers or glasses of wine per week).

Meds

Metformin 1000 mg PO BID with food
Lisinopril 20 mg PO once daily
Olanzapine 5 mg PO QHS
Carbamazepine ER 200 mg PO BID
Lorazepam 1 mg PO TID PRN (takes once a month)
Fluoxetine 20 mg PO Q AM
Pravastatin 40 mg PO once daily

All

Penicillin—hives

ROS

Complains of nocturia, polyuria, and polydipsia on a daily basis. Denies nausea, constipation, diarrhea, signs or symptoms of hypoglycemia, paresthesias, and dyspnea.

Physical Examination

Gen

WDWN severely obese, white woman in NAD

VS

BP 154/90 mm Hg, P 98 bpm, RR 18, T 37.0°C; Wt 109 kg, Ht 5′8″, waist circ 38″

HEENT

PERRLA, EOMI, R&L fundus exam without retinopathy

Neck/Lymph Nodes

No LAN

Lungs

CTA & P

CV

RRR, no m/r/g

Abd

NT/ND

Genit/Rect

Deferred

MS/Ext

Carotids, femorals, popliteals, and right dorsalis pedis pulses 2+ throughout; left dorsalis pedis 1+; feet show mild calluses on MTPs

Neuro

DTRs 2+ throughout, feet with normal sensation (5.07 monofilament) and vibration

Labs

Na 138 mEq/L	Ca 9.4 mg/dL	*Fasting lipid profile*
K 3.7 mEq/L	Phos 3.3 mg/dL	T. chol 244 mg/dL
Cl 103 mEq/L	AST 16 IU/L	LDL 141 mg/dL
CO$_2$ 31 mEq/L	ALT 19 IU/L	HDL 58 mg/dL
BUN 16 mg/dL	Alk phos 62 IU/L	Trig 225 mg/dL
SCr 0.9 mg/dL	T. bili 0.4 mg/dL	TC/HDL ratio 4.2
Glu (random) 223 mg/dL	A1C 9.0%	

UA

1+ protein, (+) microalbuminuria

Assessment

The patient reports that she exercises at most once a week and her diet is difficult to maintain due to being busy with her children's schedules and having an erratic eating schedule at both work and home. Her glycemic control has worsened from an A1C of 8% 6 months ago. She has had a moderate weight gain of 10 lb over the past year. Her blood pressure and cholesterol are not at goal on the current drug therapy. Her bipolar disorder is controlled on the current drug therapy. When the patient is in a depression or manic phase, she tends to use food to "treat" the symptoms.

QUESTIONS

Collect Information

1.a. What subjective and objective information indicates the presence of uncontrolled diabetes?

1.b. What additional information is needed to fully assess this patient's diabetes?

Assess the Information

2.a. Assess the severity of the diabetes based on the subjective and objective information available.

2.b. Create a list of the patient's drug therapy problems and prioritize them. Include assessment of medication appropriateness, effectiveness, safety, and patient adherence.

Develop a Care Plan

3.a. What are the goals of pharmacotherapy for diabetes in this case?

3.b. What nondrug therapies might be useful for this patient's diabetes?

3.c. What feasible pharmacotherapeutic options are available for treating this patient's diabetes?

3.d. Create an individualized, patient-centered, team-based care plan to optimize medication therapy for this patient's diabetes and other drug therapy problems. Include specific drugs, dosage forms, doses, schedules, and durations of therapy.

3.e. What alternatives would be appropriate if the initial care plan fails or cannot be used?

Implement the Care Plan

4.a. What information should be provided to the patient to enhance adherence, ensure successful therapy, and minimize adverse effects?

4.b. Describe how care should be coordinated with other healthcare providers.

Follow-up: Monitor and Evaluate

5. Explain how to monitor and evaluate the care plan for medication appropriateness, effectiveness, safety, and patient adherence by using clinical and laboratory data, patient feedback, and other information.

■ SELF-STUDY ASSIGNMENTS

1. Discuss the phenomenon known as the metabolic syndrome and the role that insulin resistance is postulated to play in its sequelae.

2. Explore and discuss the importance of monitoring postprandial blood glucose levels and its impact on overall glucose control, A1C levels, and progression of diabetes complications.

3. Research the various blood glucose monitors available, and compare, among available monitors, the features that meet the needs of individual patients and improve adherence to testing regimens.

4. Research new therapies for diabetes and discuss their potential role in the management of patients with type 2 DM.

5. Keep a food diary, including carbohydrate counting for each meal, and exercise log for 1 week. Evaluate and discuss your experience from the viewpoint of a patient with type 2 DM.

6. Investigate continuous blood glucose monitoring systems (CGMS) technology, and discuss the role of CGMS in a patient with type 2 DM.

7. Research and compare current insulin pumps in the market. Discuss the role of insulin pump therapy in a patient with type 2 DM and what patient characteristics make or eliminate the patient as an insulin pump candidate.

CLINICAL PEARL

Although metformin is considered the first-line therapy for a patient with type 2 DM, not all patients with type 2 DM are appropriate candidates for metformin as it has several contraindications. After a thorough assessment of comorbid conditions, patients generally must have good renal, hepatic, cardiac, and respiratory function to be considered a candidate for metformin therapy.

REFERENCES

1. American Diabetes Association. Standards of medical care in diabetes—2022. Diabetes Care. 2022;45(1 Suppl):S1–S255.

2. Grundy SM, Stone NJ, Bailey AL, et al. AHA/ACC/AACVPR/AAPA/ABC/ACPM/ADA/AGS/APhA/ASPC/NLA/PCNA guideline on the management of blood cholesterol: executive summary: a report of the American College of Cardiology/American Heart Association Task Force on clinical practice Guidelines. J Am Coll Cardiol. 2018 November. doi: 10.1016/j.jacc.2018.11.003.

3. Whelton PK, Carey RM, Aronow WS, et al. 2017 ACC/AHA/AAPA/ABC/ACPM/AGS/APhA/ASH/ASPC/NMA/PCNA guideline for the prevention, detection, evaluation, and management of high blood pressure in adults: executive summary. J Am Coll Cardiol. 2018 May; 71(19):e127–e248.

4. U.S. Department of Agriculture and U.S. Department of Health and Human Services. Dietary Guidelines for Americans, 2020–2025. 9th ed. December 2020:1–149.

5. Burghardt KJ, Seyoum B, Mallisho A, et al. Atypical antipsychotics, insulin resistance and weight; a meta-analysis of healthy volunteer studies. Prog Neuropsychopharmacol Biol Psychiatry. 2018 April 20;83:55–63.

6. Koski RR. Practical review of oral antihyperglycemic agents for type 2 diabetes mellitus. Diabetes Educ. 2006;32(2):869–876.

7. Inzucchi SE, Bergenstal RM, Buse JB, et al. Management of hyperglycemia in type 2 diabetes, 2015: a patient-centered approach. Update to a position statement of the American Diabetes Association and the European Association for the Study of Diabetes. Diabetes Care 2015;38:140–149.

8. Jamerson K, Weber MA, Bakris GL, et al. Benazepril plus amlodipine or hydrochlorothiazide for hypertension in high-risk patients. N Engl J Med. 2008;359:2417–2428.

9. Pepine CJ, Handberg EM, Cooper-DeHoff RM. A calcium antagonist vs a noncalcium antagonist hypertension treatment strategy for patients with coronary artery disease: the International Verapamil-Trandolapril Study (INVEST): a randomized control trial. JAMA. 2003;290:2805–2816.

10. Edwards SJ, Smith CJ. Tolerability of atypical antipsychotics in the treatment of adults with schizophrenia or bipolar disorder: a mixed treatment comparison of randomized controlled trials. Clin Ther. 2009;31:1345–1359.

88

HYPERTHYROIDISM: GRAVES DISEASE

Gland Central................................. Level II

Kristine S. Schonder, PharmD

LEARNING OBJECTIVES

After completing this case study, the reader should be able to:

• Describe the signs, symptoms, and laboratory parameters associated with hyperthyroidism, and relate them to the pathophysiology of the disease.

• Select and justify appropriate patient-specific initial and follow-up pharmacotherapy for patients with hyperthyroidism.

• Develop a plan for monitoring the pharmacotherapy for hyperthyroidism.

• Provide appropriate education to patients receiving drug therapy for hyperthyroidism.

PATIENT PRESENTATION

■ Chief Complaint

"My heart feels like it is racing, and I feel jittery."

■ HPI

A 23-year-old woman presents to her PCP with complaints of palpitations and a fine tremor. The palpitations started a few months ago and would come and go until the past week when they began occurring more frequently, almost daily. She denies CP. She reports that she began noticing a fine tremor approximately 3 weeks ago. She also reports loose stools and a 5-kg weight loss over the past 6 months, despite a good appetite and food intake. She feels hot all of the time and sweats a lot. She further states that she has been losing her hair recently and that she is more irritable than usual.

TABLE 88-1	Lab Values			
Na 140 mEq/L	Hgb 12.8 g/dL	RDW 10.2%	AST 14 IU/L	Total T$_4$ 24 mcg/dL
K 4.1 mEq/L	Hct 38.4%	WBC 4.8 × 10^3/mm^3	ALT 16 IU/L	Free T$_4$ 4 ng/dL
Cl 98 mEq/L	RBC 3.08 × 10^6/mm^3	Polys 72%	T. bili 0.2 mg/dL	TSH 0.02 mIU/L
CO$_2$ 23 mEq/L	Plt 298 × 10^3/mm^3	Lymphs 27%	Amylase <30 IU/L	T$_3$ resin uptake 35%
BUN 9 mg/dL	MCV 86.4 μm^3	Monos 1%	Ca 9.5 mg/dL	Total T$_3$ 550 ng/dL
SCr 0.6 mg/dL	MCH 27.1 pg	Basos 2%	Mg 2.0 mEq/L	Free thyroxine index 28.7
Glu 78 mg/dL	MCHC 31.8 g/dL		Phos 3.7 mg/dL	Thyrotropin receptor antibody 1.8 IU/L (≤1.75 IU/L)

■ PMH

She has been healthy up to this point with no medical conditions. She reports having had "the flu" last November but states that she did not seek medical attention at that time.

■ FH

Father has HTN; mother had a history of Graves disease and passed away 1 year ago from breast CA at age 53. Her oldest sister is 32 years of age and has breast CA; she has two other sisters, ages 29 and 25, and one brother, age 27, all of whom are healthy. Her aunt (mother's sister) and grandmother both had Graves disease.

■ SH

She smokes 1.5 ppd × 5 years and drinks alcohol socially on the weekends ("a few drinks on Fridays and Saturdays").

■ Meds

Drospirenone 3 mg/ethinyl estradiol 20 mcg PO daily

■ All

None

■ ROS

She reports mild diplopia occasionally; denies CP or dyspnea. She has occasional N/V/D.

■ Physical Examination

Gen

Patient is a thin, tanned woman in NAD. She appears anxious and has a fine motor tremor in her hands.

VS

BP 136/80 mm Hg, P 120 bpm, RR 18, T 38.1°C; Wt 48 kg, Ht 5′6″

Skin

Hair is fine and sparse in the temporal area.

HEENT

PERRLA, EOMI, (+) lid lag, (+) proptosis, mild periorbital edema

Neck/Lymph Nodes

Supple, (+) smooth, symmetrically enlarged thyroid (approximately 1.5 times the normal size), prominent pulsations in neck vessels

Lungs

CTA bilaterally, no wheezes or rales

Breasts

Nontender, no discharges, no palpable masses or nodes

CV

Regular rhythm, tachycardic without murmurs; (–) bruits

Abd

Soft, NT/ND; (+) hyperactive BS; no HSM or masses. Aortic pulsations palpable.

Genit/Rect

Denies frequency, urgency, hematuria, vaginal discharge, or lesions; pelvic exam normal; guaiac (–) stool

Ext

Normal pulses bilaterally, no calf tenderness. No cyanosis. Fingernails and toenails are flaking. Thumbnails have prominent ridges.

Neuro

A&O × 3; fine tremor with outstretched hands; no asterixis; hyperreflexia at knees; no proximal muscle weakness

■ Labs

See Table 88-1.

■ ECG

NSR, with HR of 120 bpm

■ Assessment

A 23-year-old woman with small goiter, probable hyperthyroidism. Most likely cause is Graves disease.

QUESTIONS

Collect Information

1. What subjective and objective information indicates the presence of hyperthyroidism?

Assess the Information

2.a. Assess the severity of hyperthyroidism based on the subjective and objective information available.

2.b. Create a list of the patient's drug therapy problems and prioritize them. Include assessment of medication appropriateness, effectiveness, safety, and patient adherence.

Develop a Care Plan

3.a. What are the goals of pharmacotherapy for hyperthyroidism in this case?

3.b. What nondrug therapies might be useful for this patient's hyperthyroidism?

3.c. What feasible pharmacotherapeutic options are available for treating hyperthyroidism?

3.d. Create an individualized, patient-centered, team-based care plan to optimize medication therapy for this patient's hyperthyroidism and other drug therapy problems. Include specific drugs, dosage forms, doses, schedules, and durations of therapy.

3.e. What alternatives would be appropriate if the initial care plan fails or cannot be used?

Implement the Care Plan

4.a. What information should be provided to the patient to enhance adherence, ensure successful therapy, and minimize adverse effects?

4.b. Describe how care should be coordinated with other healthcare providers.

Follow-Up: Monitor and Evaluate

5. Explain how to monitor and evaluate the care plan for medication appropriateness, effectiveness, safety, and patient adherence by using clinical and laboratory data, patient feedback, and other information.

■ CLINICAL COURSE

The patient is started on the treatment you recommended and returns for a 6-month follow-up visit. She reports that she has noticed marked improvement in her symptoms. The palpitations and tremor have both resolved, and she is no longer experiencing diplopia. Periorbital edema and proptosis have also resolved on physical exam. She states that she missed her last menses and is concerned that she may be pregnant. The following vital signs and laboratory results are obtained:

VS: BP 124/70 mm Hg, P 88 bpm, RR 16, T 37.2°C

Hgb 12.5 g/dL	WBC 5.8 ×10³/mm³	AST 18 IU/L
Hct 37.5%	Polys 65%	ALT 16 IU/L
MCV 85.6 μm³	Lymphs 30%	T. bili 0.2 mg/dL
MCH 26.5 pg	Monos 2%	Total T$_4$ 14.2 mcg/dL
MCHC 30.9 g/dL	Basos 2%	TSH <0.17 mIU/L
RDW 9.4%	Basos 1%	hCG 2637 mIU/mL

■ FOLLOW-UP QUESTIONS

1. What changes to the patient's treatment for Graves disease, if any, would you suggest at this point?

2. What other interventions would you recommend for this patient?

■ SELF-STUDY ASSIGNMENTS

1. Develop a monitoring protocol for the pharmacotherapy of hyperthyroidism.

2. Design a systematic approach for a patient counseling technique for the drug therapy of hyperthyroidism.

3. Formulate a plan for the pharmacotherapy of moderate to severe thyroid eye disease (TED).

CLINICAL PEARL

Thyroid eye disease (TED) associated with Graves disease can produce significant morbidity in patients and can cause blindness in severe cases that affect the optic nerve or cornea. Graves TED is thought to be an autoimmune disorder mediated by autoreactive T lymphocytes and cytokine release. The most common symptoms include diplopia, photophobia, tearing, and pain. Correction of the underlying hyperthyroidism can improve symptoms of Graves TED in most cases. However, symptoms can temporarily worsen with radioactive iodine treatment, until the hyperthyroidism is corrected. Severe cases of Graves TED should be treated with systemic corticosteroids or teprotumumab. Alternative therapies include other immunomodulating drugs, such as azathioprine, cyclosporine, methotrexate, and rituximab. Surgery is reserved for the most severe cases that threaten vision or those refractory to steroids and immunomodulating therapies. Surgery is also used as rehabilitation therapy to reverse sequelae of inflammation and lid lag.

REFERENCES

1. Ross DS, Burch HB, Cooper DA, et al. 2016 American Thyroid Association guidelines for diagnosis and management of hyperthyroidism and other causes of thyrotoxicosis. Thyroid. 2016;26(10):1343–1421.

2. Roos CP, Murthy R. Update on the clinical assessment and management of thyroid eye disease. Curr Opin Ophthalmol. 2019;30:401–406.

3. De Leo S, Lee SY, Braverman LE. Hyperthyroidism. Lancet. 2016; 388(10047):906–918.

4. Alexander EK, Pearce EN, Brent GA, et al. 2017 guidelines of the American Thyroid Association for the diagnosis and management of thyroid disease during pregnancy and the postpartum. Thyroid. 2017;27(3):315–389.

5. Kumari R and Saha BC. Advances in the management of thyroid eye diseases: an overview. Int Ophthalmol. 2018;38:2247–2255.

6. Johnson BT, Jameyfield E, Aakalu VK. Optic neuropathy and diplopia from thyroid eye disease: update on pathophysiology and treatment. Curr Opin Neurol. 2021;34(1):116–121.

7. Wiersinga WM. Smoking and thyroid. Clin Endocrinol. 2013;79:145–151.

8. Committee on Underserved Women, Committee on Obstetric Practice. Committee opinion no. 721: smoking cessation during pregnancy. Obstet Gynecol. 2017;130(4):e200–e204.

89

HYPOTHYROIDISM

Trying to Have a Baby Is Making Me Tired!....... Level II

Michael D. Katz, PharmD

LEARNING OBJECTIVES

After completing this case study, the reader should be able to:

• Recognize the signs, symptoms, and associated complications of mild and overt hypothyroidism.

• Identify the goals of therapy for hypothyroidism.

• Develop an appropriate treatment and monitoring plan for thyroid replacement based on individual patient characteristics.

• Select an appropriate product for thyroid replacement therapy.

• Properly educate a patient taking thyroid replacement therapy.

PATIENT PRESENTATION

■ Chief Complaint

"We are trying so hard to have a baby. Maybe that's why I'm so tired all the time … too much pressure."

■ HPI

A 31-year-old woman who presents with her husband (age 33) to the endocrinology clinic after being referred by her OB-GYN based on the results of some recent blood work. They have been trying to have a baby for almost 2 years but have been unable to conceive. The infertility workup done by the OB-GYN showed that he had a normal sperm count and sperm motility, and that she had no anatomical abnormalities of her reproductive tract and no evidence of endometriosis. Her serum sex hormone and gonadotropin levels were all normal. The couple is contemplating in vitro fertilization but wants to make sure that there are no hormone-related causes of her infertility. She says that for the past few months, she has felt increasingly fatigued, which she attributes to the stress of her unsuccessful attempts to become pregnant. She wonders if she is becoming depressed. She also notes that for the past few months, she has had more difficulty concentrating at work, and she has "gained a few pounds." Over the past 6 months, she has noticed that her periods are a little heavier than normal and are somewhat more irregular. Two years ago, she attended a local health fair that provided a variety of laboratory tests. The result of her TSH at that time was 4.2 mIU/L. Her PCP at that time felt that the TSH value was within the normal range and required no follow-up.

■ PMH

Infertility × 2 years
Iron deficiency anemia as a teenager

■ FH

Father, age 55, has mild COPD; mother, age 54, has type 2 DM, HTN; she has one sister, age 32, who has hypothyroidism.

■ SH

Married × 6 years, first marriage for both. No history of STDs. Works as an immigration attorney for a private firm. Social drinker in past but has not used alcohol since attempting to become pregnant; (–) tobacco or illicit drug use.

■ Meds

MiraLAX PO daily PRN constipation
Seasonique one PO daily (stopped 2 years ago)
$FeSO_4$ 300 mg PO daily
Calcium carbonate 500 mg PO twice daily
Acetaminophen 325–650 mg PO PRN headache, body aches

■ All

Skin rash from sulfa drug many years ago

■ ROS

(+) Fatigue that she attributes to stress, (+) occasional insomnia, (+) constipation relieved with MiraLAX; (+) occasional headaches relieved with non-aspirin pain reliever; (–) tinnitus, vertigo, or infections; (–) urinary symptoms; (+) dry skin

■ Physical Examination

Gen

Well-appearing woman in NAD

VS

BP 112/74 mm Hg, P 64 bpm, RR 12, T 36.8°C; Wt 62 kg, Ht 5'7"

Skin

Slightly dry-appearing skin; (–) rashes or lesions

HEENT

PERRLA, EOMI; (–) sinus tenderness; TMs appear normal

Neck/Lymph Nodes

(–) Thyroid nodules, possible slight thyroid enlargement to palpation; (–) lymphadenopathy, (–) carotid bruits

Lungs/Thorax

CTA

Breasts

(–) Lumps/masses

CV

RRR, normal S_1, S_2; (–) S_3 or S_4

Abd

NT/ND, (–) organomegaly

Neuro

A&O × 3; DTRs 2+, symmetric

GU

Deferred given recent extensive w/u by OB-GYN

■ Labs (Fasting)

Na 138 mEq/L	Hgb 13.1 g/dL	Anti-TPO antibody +
K 4.2 mEq/L	Hct 39.2%	TSHRAbs –
Cl 98 mEq/L	WBC 6.8 ×10³/mm³	TSH 9.8 mIU/L
CO_2 25 mEq/L	MCV 89 μm³	Free T_4 0.72 ng/dL
BUN 8 mg/dL	Ca 9.6 mg/dL	T. chol 212 mg/dL
SCr 0.7 mg/dL	Mg 2.0 mEq/L	LDL chol 142 mg/dL
Glu 98 mg/dL	PO_4 3.8 mg/dL	HDL chol 45 mg/dL
	Albumin 4.0 g/dL	TG 125 mg/dL
	AST 22 IU/L	
	ALT 19 IU/L	
	T. bili 0.4 mg/dL	
	Alk phos 54 IU/L	

■ Assessment

A 31-year-old woman with infertility, fatigue, other nonspecific symptoms, and an elevated TSH level, suggestive of hypothyroidism

QUESTIONS

Collect Information

1.a. What subjective and objective information indicates the presence of hypothyroidism?

1.b. What additional information is needed to fully assess this patient's hypothyroidism?

Assess the Information

2.a. Assess the severity of this patient's hypothyroidism based on the subjective and objective information available.

2.b. Create a list of the patient's drug therapy problems and prioritize them. Include assessment of medication appropriateness, effectiveness, safety, and patient adherence.

Develop a Care Plan

3.a. What are the goals of pharmacotherapy for hypothyroidism in this case?

3.b. What nondrug therapies might be useful for this patient's hypothyroidism?

3.c. What feasible pharmacotherapeutic options are available for treating this patient's hypothyroidism?

3.d. Create an individualized, patient-centered, team-based care plan to optimize the medication therapy for this patient's hypothyroidism and other drug therapy problems. Include specific drugs, dosage forms, doses, schedules, and durations of therapy.

Implement the Care Plan

4.a. What information should be provided to the patient to enhance adherence, ensure successful therapy, and minimize adverse effects?

4.b. Describe how care should be coordinated with other healthcare providers.

Follow-Up: Monitor and Evaluate

5. Explain how to monitor and evaluate the care plan for medication appropriateness, effectiveness, safety, and patient adherence by using clinical and laboratory data, patient feedback, and other information.

■ ADDITIONAL CASE QUESTION

1. What changes in her thyroid therapy might be necessary if she does become pregnant?

■ SELF-STUDY ASSIGNMENTS

1. Review the effects of untreated hypothyroidism during pregnancy on both mother and baby.

2. Research information on the US bioequivalence testing of levothyroxine (LT_4) products. How does US bioequivalence testing of LT_4 products differ from that of other oral products? Does LT_4 bioequivalence ensure therapeutic equivalence? Is there a consensus regarding the substitution of LT_4 products?

3. Review the factors that may alter LT_4 dose requirements, including drug interactions.

CLINICAL PEARL

Pregnant women who are receiving LT_4 replacement must undergo monthly monitoring of the TSH level to ensure adequate replacement. The majority of such women will require an increase of their LT_4 dose during pregnancy to ensure adequate replacement for both mother and fetus.

REFERENCES

1. Taylor PN, Albrecht D, Scholz D, et al. Global epidemiology of hyperthyroidism and hypothyroidism. Nature Rev Endocrinol. 2018 May;14:301–316.

2. Canaris GJ, Manowitz NR, Mayor G, Ridgway EC. The Colorado thyroid disease prevalence study. Arch Intern Med. 2000;160:526–534.

3. Alexander EK, Pearce EN, Brent GA, et al. 2017 guidelines of the American Thyroid Association for the diagnosis and management of thyroid disease during pregnancy and the postpartum. Thyroid. 2017;27:315–389.

4. Jonklaas J, Bianco AC, Bauer AJ, et al. Guidelines for the treatment of hypothyroidism: prepared by the American Thyroid Association Task Force on thyroid hormone replacement. Thyroid. 2014;24:1670–1751.

5. Biondi B, Cappola AR, Cooper DS. Subclinical hypothyroidism. A review. JAMA. 2019 July 9;322:153–160.

6. Benvenga S, Carle A. Levothyroxine formulations: pharmacological and clinical implications of generic substitution. Adv Ther. 2019 September 4; 36:S59–S71.

7. Dong BJ, Hauck WW, Gambertoglio JG, et al. Bioequivalence of generic and brand-name levothyroxine products in the treatment of hypothyroidism. JAMA. 1997;277:1205–1213.

8. Mayor GH, Orlando T, Kurtz NM. Limitations of levothyroxine bioequivalence evaluation: an analysis of an attempted study. Am J Ther. 1995;2:417–432.

9. Mateo RC, Hennessey JV. Thyroxine and treatment of hypothyroidism: seven decades of experience. Endocrine. 2019 July 18;66:10–17.

10. Shan Z, Teng W. Thyroid hormone therapy of hypothyroidism in pregnancy. Endocrine. 2019 January;66:35–42.

90

CUSHING SYNDROME

A Tale of Two Glands.............................. Level II

Christie R. Monahan, PharmD

Steven M. Smith, PharmD, MPH, FCCP

John G. Gums, PharmD, FCCP

LEARNING OBJECTIVES

After completing this case study, the reader should be able to:

- Recognize and differentiate the signs, symptoms, and laboratory changes associated with the various forms of Cushing syndrome.

- Recognize the biochemical, anatomic, and emotional changes that can occur with Cushing syndrome.

- Recommend appropriate treatment regimens for patients with Cushing syndrome.

- Provide patient counseling on proper dosing, administration, and adverse effects of treatment for Cushing disease.

PATIENT PRESENTATION

■ Chief Complaint

"I have been tired and weak lately, and I've noticed some swelling in my legs recently."

HPI

A 31-year-old woman presents to her family physician complaining of fatigue, weakness, and edema. She also reports weight gain (50 lb over 2 years) and depression with insomnia.

PMH

Patient has been healthy with no other major medical illnesses, except seasonal allergic rhinitis. She had two healthy children by uncomplicated vaginal deliveries.

FH

Mother is alive at age 54 with type 2 DM; father is living at age 56 with HTN. She has two sisters: one is healthy and the other has depression.

SH

Patient does not smoke and drinks occasionally. She is a photographer. Children are 6 years and 3 years old.

Meds

Seasonique one tablet PO once daily as directed
Nasonex two sprays in each nostril once daily PRN allergic symptoms
Unisom SleepTabs 25 mg PO QHS PRN sleep
Advil 200 mg one to two tablets PO Q6H PRN headache

All

Sulfa—rash

ROS

(+) For fatigue, weakness, occasional back pain, and weight gain; also reports episodes of sadness, depressed mood, and insomnia; skin bruises easily; occasional headache, blurred vision, and heartburn; no CP, wheezing, or SOB. Normal menstruation with regular periods. LMP 7 weeks ago.

Physical Examination

Gen

WDWN obese, cushingoid-appearing woman in NAD

VS

BP 165/86 mm Hg, HR 85 bpm, RR 14/min, T 37.0°C, Wt 82.1 kg, Ht 5′3″

Skin

Thin skin with some bruising and scratches; purple striae visible on abdomen

HEENT

Rounded face; moderate facial hair; PERRLA; EOMI; funduscopic exam shows normal retinal background, optic cup-to-disc ratios 0.4; visual fields appear to be grossly intact; OP moist and pink

Neck/Lymph Nodes

Supple; (+) JVD at 30° (7 cm); (–) bruits, adenopathy, or thyromegaly

Chest

CTA bilaterally

Breasts

No lumps or masses

CV

RRR, no MRG

Abd

Obese, soft, NT, (–) masses or organomegaly

Genit/Rect

Guaiac (–); normal external genitalia; no masses

MS/Ext

Appears to have decreased strength bilaterally; DTR 1–2+ and symmetric throughout all four extremities; 2+ pitting pedal edema bilaterally; pedal pulses palpable with moderate intensity

Neuro

Oriented × 3; flat affect; CNs II–XII intact

Labs

Na 138 mEq/L	Hgb 13.4 g/dL	AST 9 IU/L	TSH 2.33 mIU/L
K 3.3 mEq/L	Hct 38.5%	ALT 7 IU/L	A1C 7.1%
Cl 105 mEq/L	RBC 4.0 × 10⁶/mm³	Alk phos	*Fasting lipid profile*
CO_2 25 mEq/L	Plt 264 × 10³/mm³	180 IU/L	T. chol 261 mg/dL
BUN 12 mg/dL	WBC 14.5 × 10³/mm³	T. bili	HDL 62 mg/dL
SCr 0.9 mg/dL		0.5 mg/dL	LDL 120 mg/dL
Glu 160 mg/dL		Alb 4.5 g/dL	Trig 396 mg/dL
		UA 5.6 mg/dL	

Assessment

Probable Cushing syndrome of unknown etiology requiring further evaluation by an endocrinologist

Clinical Course

The patient was seen by an endocrinologist for further evaluation. Baseline 24-hour UFC was 356 and 362 mcg on separate days. A midnight salivary cortisol concentration was 0.54 mcg/dL. An overnight 1-mg DST showed a plasma cortisol concentration of 9.2 mcg/dL. Plasma ACTH concentrations on 2 consecutive days at 1:00 PM were 103 and 110 pg/mL. A CRH stimulation test revealed a baseline plasma cortisol of 10.4 mcg/dL and ACTH of 108 pg/mL, with an increase to a plasma cortisol of 13.5 mcg/dL and ACTH of 187 pg/mL following CRH administration. An MRI revealed an enlarged pituitary gland; the same finding was seen on a focused repeat MRI. There was no focal inhomogeneity that would suggest an isolated adenoma (ie, the tumor cannot be localized).

The risks and benefits of all the treatments were explained to the patient. She preferred to undergo radiation treatments rather than exploratory-type surgery. She indicated that she would like to have more children and would prefer to try other treatments prior to surgery.

QUESTIONS

Collect Information

1.a. What information (signs, symptoms, laboratory values) indicates the presence of Cushing syndrome?

1.b. What information (presentation, history, laboratory values, imaging) can be used to identify the most likely etiology of Cushing syndrome?

Assess the Information

2.a. Assess the severity of the Cushing syndrome based on the subjective and objective information available.

2.b. Create a list of this patient's drug therapy problems and prioritize them. Include assessment of medication appropriateness, effectiveness, safety, and patient adherence.

2.c. What psychosocial and ethical considerations are applicable to this patient?

Develop a Care Plan

3.a. What are the goals of pharmacotherapy for Cushing syndrome in this case?

3.b. What nondrug therapies might be useful for this patient's Cushing syndrome?

3.c. What feasible pharmacotherapeutic options are available for the treatment of Cushing syndrome?

3.d. Create an individualized, patient-centered, team-based care plan to optimize medication therapy for this patient's Cushing syndrome and other drug therapy problems. Include specific drugs, dosage forms, doses, schedules, and durations of therapy.

3.e. What adjunctive pharmacotherapy may be required if the therapy identified in 3.d. above is successful?

3.f. What alternatives would be appropriate if the initial care plan fails or cannot be used?

Implement the Care Plan

4.a. What information should be provided to the patient to enhance adherence, ensure successful therapy, and minimize adverse events?

4.b. Describe how care should be coordinated with other healthcare providers.

Follow-Up: Monitor and Evaluate

5. Explain how to monitor and evaluate the care plan for medication appropriateness, effectiveness, safety, and patient adherence by using clinical and laboratory data, patient feedback, and other information.

■ FOLLOW-UP QUESTION

1. What are the advantages of measuring late-night salivary cortisol over measuring late-night serum cortisol concentrations?

■ CLINICAL COURSE

The patient received radiation therapy with adjuvant pharmacotherapy to reduce cortisol levels. Given that it may take several months for therapy to normalize cortisol, several other interventions were initiated to ameliorate the complications of Cushing disease. She received hydrochlorothiazide 25 mg daily for hypertension, pioglitazone 30 mg daily for elevated blood glucose, rosuvastatin 5 mg daily for dyslipidemia, and escitalopram 10 mg daily for depression. A DXA scan revealed a Z-score of −2.4 standard deviations at the hip and −2.6 vertebrally. Accordingly, she received a diagnosis of steroid-induced osteoporosis. One month following initiation of the above agents, she presented to her physician for follow-up. She reported increased weakness, leg cramps, and palpitations. Lab work revealed a serum potassium concentration of 2.7 mEq/L.

2. What pharmacologic therapy would you recommend to reduce her risk of fracture?

3. What medication changes would you suggest at this time?

■ SELF-STUDY ASSIGNMENTS

1. Many of the tests used in the differential diagnosis of Cushing syndrome require drug therapy (eg, DST, CRH). Create a table to assist healthcare providers in performing these tests correctly (include possible adverse events, timing, critical values, and evaluation of the results).

2. Compare the retail costs in your area for each of the pharmacotherapeutic alternatives for the treatment of Cushing syndrome. Write a brief summary of your findings, and describe whether this information would cause you to change your recommendation for the initial drug therapy for this patient.

3. Describe methods that may be used to minimize drug-induced Cushing syndrome.

CLINICAL PEARL

Most patients with Cushing disease are treated with transsphenoidal surgery because of its high cure rate (80–90%). Pharmacotherapy is usually used as adjunctive therapy and has proven an effective option for those unable to have surgery. Combination therapy can be considered for those experiencing adverse effects or minimal benefit with monotherapy.

REFERENCES

1. Newell-Price J, Bertagna X, Grossman AB, Nierman LK. Cushing syndrome. Lancet. 2006;367:1605–1617.
2. Sharma ST, Nieman LK, Feelders RA. Cushing syndrome: epidemiology and developments in disease management. Clin Epidemiol. 2015;7:281–293.
3. Nieman LK, Biller BMK, Findling JW, et al. Treatment of Cushing syndrome: an Endocrine Society Clinical Practice Guideline. J Clin Endocrinol Metab. 2015;100:2807–2831.
4. Lacroix A, Feelders RA, Stratakis CA, Nieman LK. Cushing syndrome. Lancet. 2015;386(9996):913–927.
5. Broersen LHA, Jha M, Biermasz NR, Pereira AM, Dekkers OM. Effectiveness of medical treatment for Cushing's syndrome: a systematic review and meta-analysis. Pituitary. 2018;21(6):631–641.
6. Dougherty JA, Desai DS, Herrera JB. Osilodrostat: a novel steroidogenesis inhibitor to treat Cushing's disease. Ann Pharmacother. 2021;55(8):1050–1060.

91

ADDISON DISEASE

I May Look Great, but I Don't Feel Well. . . . . Level II

Zachary A. Weber, PharmD, BCPS, BCACP, CDCES, FASHP

LEARNING OBJECTIVES

After completing this case study, the reader should be able to:

- Recognize the clinical presentation, symptoms, and laboratory changes associated with Addison disease.

- Optimize pharmacologic and nonpharmacologic therapy for patients with Addison disease and comorbid conditions.

- Provide education and counseling to patients and family members about Addison disease and the proper administration, side effects, and adverse effects of corticosteroids and mineralocorticoids, and the importance of adherence to therapy.

- Provide counseling and education about common side effects associated with high and low serum cortisol concentrations.

- Compare corticosteroids with respect to relative glucocorticoid and mineralocorticoid potencies.

PATIENT PRESENTATION

■ Chief Complaint

"I've noticed that over the past six months, my son's skin is getting darker, and he has been more lethargic, somewhat withdrawn, and sleeping more. I have also noticed that he has been making some poor choices, in terms of friends and activities."

■ HPI

A 19-year-old man is brought to the emergency department (ED) by his mother after she found him crying, confused, and disoriented. His mother states that she has recently noticed that he has not had the same level of energy, and has been complaining about not being able to run and play basketball with his friends at the park. She has also noticed he has been hanging out with a different group of friends, and she is concerned he may be involved in some abhorrent activities and has not been taking his medications appropriately.

■ PMH

Type 1 DM × 7 years
Hypothyroidism × 3 years

■ FH

Mother, 52 years old, has HTN; father, 54 years old, has hypothyroidism; sister, 24 years old, has both HTN and type 1 DM.

■ SH

Denies use of alcohol, tobacco, or illicit drugs; lives with his mother.

■ Meds

Lantus 24 units subcutaneously at bedtime
NovoLog 1:15 scale carbohydrate counting ratio, subcutaneously with meals
Levothyroxine 100 mcg PO daily

■ All

NKDA

■ ROS

Increased tanning of the skin noted over the past 6 months. Increased fatigue, nausea, and a 2.5-kg weight loss over the past month.

■ Physical Examination

Gen

Alert, somewhat disoriented and confused

VS

BP 84/47 mm Hg, HR 91 bpm, RR 16/min, T 36.2°C; Wt 62.5 kg, Ht 5'4"

Skin

Warm, dry, and intact; slightly tanned color.

HEENT

Normocephalic; oral mucosa moist; PERRL; EOMI

Neck

No JVD. Nontender. No thyroid nodularity

Lungs

CTA; respirations are nonlabored

CV

Normal rate and rhythm; no murmurs; normal perfusion; no edema

Abd

Soft, NT/ND; normal BS

MS/Ext

No CCE; normal ROM

Neuro

Alert, somewhat disoriented

Psych

Somnolent, but cooperative

■ Labs (Fasting, Drawn at 10:15 AM)

Na 116 mEq/L	Hgb 14.2 g/dL	AST 111 IU/L	T. chol 168 mg/dL
K 4.9 mEq/L	Hct 43.8%	ALT 59 IU/L	Trig 120 mg/dL
Cl 99 mEq/L	RBC 4.88 × 10⁶/mm³	Alk phos	Fe 93 mcg/dL
CO_2 26 mEq/L	Plt 244 × 10³/mm³	75 IU/L	TSH 25.8 mIU/L
BUN 14 mg/dL	WBC 3.6 × 10³/mm³	GGT 63 IU/L	Free T_4 0.41 ng/dL
SCr 0.9 mg/dL	Neutros 41%	LDH 173 IU/L	Cortisol 0.4 mcg/dL
Glu 140 mg/dL	Lymphos 43%	T. bili 1.1 mg/dL	ACTH 2003 pg/mL
Ca 9.2 mg/dL	Monos 13%	D. bili 0.5 mg/dL	A1C 8.2%
Phos 5.1 mg/dL	Eos 2%	T. prot 7.3 g/dL	
Uric acid	Basos 1%	Alb 4.1 g/dL	
4.1 mg/dL			

Reference range for cortisol: AM 8–25 mcg/dL, PM 4–20 mcg/dL; ACTH 0–130 pg/mL

■ UA

Clear, pale yellow, SG 1.020, pH 6.8

■ Other

CT scan negative; ECG normal

■ Assessment

1. Primary adrenal insufficiency, most likely due to an autoimmune disease

2. Hypothyroidism with an elevated TSH, likely secondary to nonadherence to prescribed levothyroxine regimen

3. Type 1 DM with an elevated A1C, likely secondary to nonadherence to prescribed insulin regimen

QUESTIONS

Collect Information

1.a. What subjective and objective information indicates the presence of Addison disease?

1.b. What additional information is needed to fully assess this patient's Addison disease?

Assess the Information

2.a. Assess the severity of Addison disease based on the subjective and objective information available.

2.b. Create a list of the patient's drug therapy problems and prioritize them. Include assessment of medication appropriateness, effectiveness, safety, and patient adherence.

2.c. What psychosocial considerations are applicable to this patient?

Develop a Care Plan

3.a. What are the goals of pharmacotherapy for Addison disease in this case?

3.b. What nondrug therapies might be useful for this patient's Addison disease?

3.c. What feasible pharmacotherapeutic options are available for treating Addison disease?

3.d. Create an individualzed, patient-centered, team-based care plan to optimize medication therapy for this patient's Addison disease and other drug therapy problems. Include specific drugs, dosage forms, doses, schedules, and durations of therapy.

3.e. What alternatives would be appropriate if the initial care plan fails or cannot be used?

Implement the Care Plan

4.a. What information should be provided to the patient to enhance adherence, ensure successful therapy, and minimize adverse effects?

4.b. Describe how care should be coordinated with other healthcare providers.

Follow-Up: Monitor and Evaluate

5. Explain how to monitor and evaluate the care plan for medication appropriateness, effectiveness, safety, and patient adherence by using clinical and laboratory data, patient feedback, and other information.

■ SELF-STUDY ASSIGNMENTS

1. Review the signs and symptoms of an acute adrenal crisis, and describe the treatment.

2. Differentiate the glucocorticoids with respect to duration of activity, glucocorticoid potency, and mineralocorticoid potency.

3. Differentiate the biologic functions of cortisol and aldosterone.

CLINICAL PEARL

Although rare, a decrease in insulin requirements and unexplained hypoglycemia in patients with type 1 DM may be initial signs of Addison's disease.

REFERENCES

1. Bornstein SR, Allolio B, Arlt W, et al. Diagnosis and treatment of primary adrenal insufficiency: an Endocrine Society clinical practice guideline. J Clin Endocrinol Metab. 2016;101(2):364–389.
2. Griffing GT. Addison Disease. Available at: *https://emedicine.medscape.com/article/116467-overview*. Accessed September 30, 2021.
3. Addison's Disease Self-Help Group. Diagnosing Addison's: A Guide for GPs. Available at: *https://www.addisonsdisease.org.uk/Handlers/Download.ashx?IDMF=ce8a8a9d-f063-4604-b5ec-46a7d30f5798*. Accessed February 28, 2022.
4. Michels A, Michels N. Addison disease: early detection and treatment principles. Am Fam Phys. 2014;89(7):563–568.
5. Abdel-Motleb M. The neuropsychiatric aspect of Addison's disease: a case report. Innov Clin Neurosci. 2012 Oct;9(10):34–36. Available at: *http://www.ncbi.nlm.nih.gov/pmc/articles/PMC3508960/*. Accessed September 30, 2021.
6. Kordonouri O, Maguire AM, Knip M, et al. Other complications and associated conditions with diabetes in children and adolescents. Ped Diab. 2009;10(Suppl 12):204–210.
7. Barker JM, Fain PR, Eisenbarth GS. Addison's disease and type 1 diabetes. Curr Opin Endocr Diabetes. 2005;12(4):280–284.
8. Reisch N, Arlt W. Fine tuning for quality of life: 21st century approach to treatment of Addison's disease. Endocrinol Metab Clin N Am. 2009;38:407–418.
9. Arlt W. The approach to the adult with newly diagnosed adrenal insufficiency. J Clin Endocrinol Metab. 2009;94(4):1059–1067.
10. Elbelt U, Hahner S, Allolio B. Altered insulin requirement in patient with type 1 diabetes and primary adrenal insufficiency receiving standard glucocorticoid replacement therapy. Eur J Endocrinol. 2009;160:919–924.

92

HYPERPROLACTINEMIA

The Missing Period . . . . Level I

Amy Heck Sheehan, PharmD

LEARNING OBJECTIVES

After completing this case study, the reader should be able to:

• Recognize the signs and symptoms of hyperprolactinemia.

• Recommend appropriate treatment options for hyperprolactinemia.

• Design a plan to monitor the response to the pharmacologic treatment of hyperprolactinemia.

PATIENT PRESENTATION

■ Chief Complaint

"I haven't had my period for almost a year."

■ HPI

A 31-year-old woman with a history of oligomenorrhea (menstrual cycle every 2–6 months) since menarche at age 14 presents to her gynecologist after 11 months of amenorrhea and a small amount of milky discharge from her left breast, which she first noticed 1–2 months ago.

The patient and her husband would like to have a baby, but she is concerned that she may be unable to have children. The patient states that she and her husband have not used birth control for more than 1 year, and she has had several negative home pregnancy tests.

■ **PMH**

GERD
Seasonal allergies
Depression

■ **FH**

Father died at age 58 from an AMI; mother (age 62) has type 2 DM and HTN. Patient has two brothers (ages 33 and 35) who are alive and well.

■ **SH**

The patient is employed as an administrative assistant. She does not smoke and has less than one drink of alcohol per month. She has been married for 5 years and lives with her husband and two stepdaughters (ages 7 and 9).

■ **Meds**

Omeprazole 20 mg PO daily
Desloratadine 5 mg PO daily
Fluoxetine 20 mg PO daily
Prenatal vitamin one PO daily
Acetaminophen 500 mg PO PRN

■ **All**

Codeine (hives)

■ **ROS**

Galactorrhea of the left breast and amenorrhea for 11 months as described in the HPI. No active GERD.

■ **Physical Examination**

Gen

The patient is a WDWN woman in NAD.

VS

BP 124/71 mm Hg, P 72 bpm, RR 13, T 37.1°C; Wt 72 kg, Ht 5′8″

Skin

Normal, intact, warm, and dry

HEENT

PERRLA, EOMI, normal funduscopic exam, normal visual fields

Neck/Lymph Nodes

Normal thyroid, no lymphadenopathy

Lungs/Chest

CTA & P

Breasts

Galactorrhea of left breast, no masses

CV

RRR, S_1 and S_2 normal, no MRG

Abd

Soft, nontender, no organomegaly, (+) bowel sounds

GU

LMP 11 months ago, normal pelvic exam and Pap smear

MS/Ext

Normal ROM, no edema, pulses 2+ throughout

Neuro

A&O × 3, bilateral reflexes intact, normal gait

■ **Labs**

Na 138 mEq/L	AST 23 IU/L	TSH 2.1 mIU/L
K 4.0 mEq/L	ALT 31 IU/L	T_3 111 ng/dL
Cl 101 mEq/L	Alk phos 110 IU/L	Total T_4 7.5 mcg/dL
CO_2 25 mEq/L	T. bili 0.5 mg/dL	Free T_4 1.3 ng/dL
BUN 13 mg/dL		Serum β-hCG negative
SCr 0.8 mg/dL		FSH 12 IU/L
Glu 89 mg/dL		

Serum prolactin on 3 separate days: 133, 159, and 142 mcg/L

■ **Other Test Results**

DXA T-score –0.90 at the lumbar spine (no previous DXA results). MRI of the pituitary gland revealed an 8-mm pituitary adenoma.

■ **Assessment**

Hyperprolactinemia due to a microprolactinoma

QUESTIONS

Collect Information

1.a. What signs, symptoms, and laboratory values indicate the presence of hyperprolactinemia?

1.b. What additional information is needed to fully assess this patient's hyperprolactinemia?

Assess the Information

2.a. Assess the severity of hyperprolactinemia based on the subjective and objective information available.

2.b. Create a list of this patient's drug therapy problems and prioritize them. Include assessment of medication appropriateness, effectiveness, safety, and patient adherence.

Develop a Care Plan

3.a. What are the goals of pharmacotherapy for hyperprolactinemia in this case?

3.b. What nondrug therapies might be useful for the treatment of hyperprolactinemia?

3.c. What pharmacotherapeutic options are available for treating this patient's hyperprolactinemia?

3.d. Create an individualized, patient-centered, team-based care plan to optimize medication therapy for this patient's hyperprolactinemia and other drug therapy problems. Include specific drugs, dosage forms, doses, schedules, and durations of therapy.

Implement the Care Plan

4.a. What information should be provided to the patient to enhance adherence, ensure successful therapy, and minimize adverse effects?

4.b. Describe how care should be coordinated with other healthcare providers.

Follow-Up: Monitor and Evaluate

5. Explain how to monitor and evaluate the care plan for medication appropriateness, effectiveness, safety, and patient adherence by using clinical and laboratory data, patient feedback, and other information.

■ CLINICAL COURSE

The patient was started on the regimen you recommended, and she returned to the clinic 4 weeks later complaining of significant nausea and abdominal pain that was temporally associated with medication administration. Serum prolactin concentrations measured 10 minutes apart were 140, 151, and 137 mcg/L. Galactorrhea and amenorrhea were unchanged.

■ FOLLOW-UP QUESTIONS

1. Identify the possible reasons for the patient's poor initial response to therapy.

2. Given the new patient information, what alternative therapies should be considered?

3. How long will this patient require drug treatment for the prolactinoma?

■ SELF-STUDY ASSIGNMENTS

1. Review the available information on the safety of dopamine agonist pharmacotherapy in pregnant women. If this patient eventually becomes pregnant, should a dopamine agonist be continued throughout the pregnancy?

2. Research information on the use of hormone replacement therapy in patients with hyperprolactinemia. Is this patient a candidate for hormone replacement therapy? Why or why not?

3. Describe the treatment of hyperprolactinemia in the presence of a macroadenoma. How would the management of hyperprolactinemia be different if the patient were diagnosed with a macroprolactinoma instead of a microprolactinoma?

CLINICAL PEARL

Although dopamine agonists are the mainstay of therapy for hyperprolactinemia, approximately 5–10% of patients do not respond to these agents because of poor adherence, suboptimal dosing, or the presence of a treatment-resistant prolactinoma.

REFERENCES

1. Melmed S, Casanueva FF, Hoffman AR, et al. Diagnosis and treatment of hyperprolactinemia: an Endocrine Society clinical practice guideline. J Clin Endocrinol Metab. 2011;96:273–288.

2. Chanson P, Maiter D. The epidemiology, diagnosis, and treatment of prolactinomas: the old and the new. Best Pract Res Clin Endocrinol Metab. 2019;33:101290.

3. Auriemma RS, Pirchio R, De Alcublerre D, Pivoneilo R, Colao A. Dopamine agonists: from the 1970s to today. Neuroendocrinology. 2019;109:34–41.

4. dos Santos Nunes V, El Dib R, Boquszewski CL, Noqueira CR. Cabergoline versus bromocriptine in the treatment of hyperprolactinemia: a systematic review of randomized controlled trials and meta-analysis. Pituitary. 2011;14(3):259–265.

5. Glezer A, Bronstein MD. Prolactinomas in pregnancy: considerations before conception and during pregnancy. Pituitary. 2020;23:65–69.

93

PREGNANCY AND LACTATION

Nauseous and Cautious.......................... Level II

Sneha Baxi Srivastava, PharmD, BCACP, CDCES, DipACLM, CDE

Ziemowit Mazur, PhD, EdM, MS, PA-C, DFAAPA

LEARNING OBJECTIVES

After completing this case study, the reader should be able to:

- Describe each FDA pregnancy category using the US Food and Drug Administration Drug Classification System and the Pregnancy and Lactation Labeling Rule (PLLR).

- Determine the factors (clinical vs pharmacologic) that should be considered when treating a patient who is pregnant or lactating.

- List the risks and benefits associated with pharmacologic interventions during pregnancy for a patient with hyperthyroidism, depression, mechanical heart valve requiring chronic anticoagulation for thromboembolism prophylaxis, and gestational diabetes.

- Design a pharmacotherapeutic plan for a pregnant patient with depression, hypertension, and a mechanical heart valve including treatment options, appropriate monitoring, and therapeutic goals.

- Apply shared decision-making when it comes to the treatment options, benefits, risks, and monitoring of antidepressants, antihypertensives, and anticoagulants during pregnancy.

PATIENT PRESENTATION

Chief Complaint

"I have been nauseated and vomiting for the past week. I took a pregnancy test yesterday, and it was positive! I am taking a lot of different medications. Could I have harmed my baby?"

HPI

A 34-year-old female reports experiencing two to three episodes of nausea per day with occasional vomiting mostly in the mornings and evenings. She typically wakes up feeling nauseous every day and vomits one to two times a week. These symptoms began about 2 weeks ago and have remained consistent, preventing her from going to work consistently or being able to work effectively. She states that she feels "run down" all the time and needs to start feeling better soon, or she will lose her job. She took a pregnancy test today, and it is positive. She is very concerned about her "blood thinner"

medication, remembering that she could not take it with her previous pregnancy. Additionally, she reports being diagnosed with depression 2 years ago and has not had any depressive symptoms in the last year. She states she stopped taking the paroxetine a year ago, with her health care provider's oversight, because she was no longer having any symptoms and wanted to see how she would feel without the medication. She has noted that since she incorporated exercise, she has also seen an improvement in her mood. Overall, she lives a healthy lifestyle, eating well (follows a plant-based diet) and exercising three to four times a week.

PMH

Depression
History of multiple, unprovoked, lower extremity DVTs
Hyperthyroidism (diagnosed 9 months ago)
S/P gestational diabetes

FH

Mother alive with DM2 and HTN, father alive with celiac disease. A patient has one twin sister who is alive and well.

SH

Married, mother to one daughter. She is a physician assistant at an outpatient clinic. She runs and does strength training three to four times a week and follows a plant-based diet. She currently tobacco-free for the last 5 years with a previous history of smoking half a pack per day × 5 years, and occasionally drinks a glass of wine with dinner on the weekends.

Meds

Self-discontinued paroxetine 20 mg PO once daily (discontinued 1 year ago)
Methimazole 10 mg PO once daily
Warfarin 5 mg PO MWF, 7.5 mg rest of the week
Acetaminophen 375 mg PO PRN (takes once a month for a rare headache)

All

NKDA

ROS

Fatigue

PE

Gen

WDWN concerned woman

VS

BP 120/62 mm Hg, P 72 bpm, RR 18, T 36.3°C; Wt 50 kg, Ht 5'3"

Skin

Warm, dry, no eruptions, boils, or lesions

HEENT

WNL

Neck/Lymph Nodes

No adenopathy, no thyromegaly, supple

Lungs

CTA bilaterally

Breasts

Tender to palpation; no masses

CV

Mechanical click systolic murmur, grade 2/4

Abd

Soft, NT, (+) BS; no masses, no bruits

Genit/Rect

Pelvic exam confirms pregnancy; stool heme/guaiac (–)
Urine (–) for protein/glucose

Ext

(–) CCE; pulses intact

Neuro

Normal sensory and motor levels

■ Labs

Ultrasound: confirmed pregnancy

Na 138 mEq/L	Hgb 13 g/dL	Blood type: O–
K 4 mEq/L	Hct 40%	PT/INR 10.0 sec/3.0
Cl 102 mEq/L	WBC 8.0×10^3/mm^3	Fasting glucose 80 mg/dL
CO$_2$ 27 mEq/L	Plt 345×10^3/mm^3	A1c 5.4%
BUN 10 mg/dL	TSH 1.45 mIU/L	Serum HCG 42,000 IU/L
SCr 0.9 mg/dL		Stool heme/guaiac (–)
		Urine (–) for protein/glucose

■ Assessment

A 34-year-old female experiencing nausea and emesis due to pregnancy, requiring pharmacologic and nonpharmacologic management. She also needs careful evaluation and management related to hyperthyroidism diagnosed 9 months ago, depression, gestational diabetes, and her history of multiple, unprovoked, lower extremity DVTs.

QUESTIONS

Collect Information

1.a. What subjective and objective information indicates the presence of nausea and vomiting secondary to pregnancy?

1.b. What additional information is needed to fully assess this patient's nausea and vomiting secondary to pregnancy?

Assess the Information

2.a. Assess the severity of nausea and vomiting based on the subjective and objective information available.

2.b. Create a list of the patient's drug therapy problems and prioritize them. Include an assessment of medication appropriateness, effectiveness, safety, and patient adherence.

2.c. What economic, psychosocial, cultural, racial, and ethical considerations are applicable to this patient?

Develop a Care Plan

3.a. What are the goals of pharmacotherapy in this case?

3.b. What non-drug therapies for nausea and vomiting secondary to pregnancy might be useful for this patient?

3.c. What feasible pharmacotherapeutic options are available to treat this patient's nausea and vomiting?

3.d. Create an individualized, patient-centered, team-based care plan to optimize medication therapy for this patient's nausea and vomiting and other drug therapy problems. Include specific drugs, dosage forms, doses, schedules, and duration of therapy.

3.e. What alternatives would be appropriate if the initial care plan fails or cannot be used?

Implement the Care Plan

4.a. What information should be provided to the patient to enhance adherence, ensure successful therapy, and minimize adverse effects?

4.b. Describe how care should be coordinated with other healthcare providers.

Follow-Up: Monitor and Evaluate

5. Explain how to monitor and evaluate the care plan for medication appropriateness, effectiveness, safety, and patient adherence by using clinical and laboratory data, patient feedback, and other information.

■ CLINICAL COURSE

The patient's nausea and vomiting improved by week 15 and progressed through the pregnancy, having a healthy baby girl. The patient returns to your office 4 weeks, reporting that her clinical symptoms of depression have intensified postpartum and would like to know if she should reinitiate her antidepressant, and if so, at what dose.

■ FOLLOW-UP QUESTIONS

1. Based on the American College of Obstetricians and Gynecologists (ACOG) guidelines, what would you recommend to the patient for postpartum depression?

2. What is the Pregnancy and Lactation Labeling Rule?

CLINICAL PEARLS

Electronic resources for information related to fetal and neonatal effects in pregnancy and lactation include Reprotox (*www.reprotox.org*) and TERIS (*http://depts.washington.edu/terisweb*). There are also post-marketing pregnancy exposure registries available through the US Food and Drug Administration Pregnancy Labeling Task Force. Alternatively, there is General Practice Research Database (GPRD) that can be utilized as the data source for investigating drug exposure during pregnancy.

REFERENCES

1. American College of Obstetricians and Gynecologists. Committee on Practice Bulletins-Obstetrics. ACOG Practice Bulletin No. 189: nausea and vomiting of pregnancy. Obstet Gynecol. 2018;131(1):e15–e30.

2. Bates SM, Greer IA, Middeldorp S, Veenstra DL, Prabulos AM, Vandvik PO. VTE, thrombophilia, antithrombotic therapy, and pregnancy: antithrombotic therapy and prevention of thrombosis, 9th ed. American College of Chest Physicians evidence-based clinical practice guidelines. Chest. 2012;141(2 Suppl):e691S–e736S.

3. Alexander EK, Pearce EN, Brent GA, et al. 2017 Guidelines of the American Thyroid Association for the diagnosis and management of thyroid disease during pregnancy and the postpartum. Thyroid. 2017;27(3):315–389.

4. De Groot L, Abalovich M, Alexander EK, et al. Management of thyroid dysfunction during pregnancy and postpartum: an Endocrine Society clinical practice guideline. J Clin Endocrinol Metab. 2012;97(8):2543–2565.

5. Peleg D, Cada S, Peleg A, Ben-Ami M. The relationship between maternal serum thyroid-stimulating immunoglobulin and fetal and neonatal thyrotoxicosis. Obstet Gynecol. 2002;99(6):1040–1043.

6. Nguyen CT, Sasso EB, Barton L, Mestman JH. Graves' hyperthyroidism in pregnancy: a clinical review. Clin Diabetes Endocrinol. 2018;4:4.

7. Morales DR, Slattery J, Evans S, Kurz X. Antidepressant use during pregnancy and risk of autism spectrum disorder and attention deficit hyperactivity disorder: systematic review of observational studies and methodological considerations. BMC Med. 2018;6(1):6.

8. Yonkers KA, Wisner KL, Stewart DE, et al. The management of depression during pregnancy: a report from the American Psychiatric Association and the American College of Obstetricians and Gynecologists. Gen Hosp Psychiatry. 2009;31(5):403–413.

9. American Diabetes Association. 14. Management of Diabetes in Pregnancy: Standards of Medical Care in Diabetes—2021. Diabetes Care. 2021;44(Suppl 1):S200–S210.

10. U.S. Food and Drug Administration. Pregnancy and lactation labeling (drug) final rule. Available at: https://www.fda.gov/drugs/labeling-information-drug-products/pregnancy-and-lactation-labeling-drugs-final-rule. Accessed April 15, 2022.

11. U.S. Food and Drug Administration. Pregnancy, lactation, and reproductive potential: Labeling for human prescription drug and biological products—content and format guidance for industry. Available at: www.fda.gov/media/90160/download. Accessed April 15, 2022.

94

CONTRACEPTION

Stork Landing Prohibited .... Level II

Julia M. Koehler, PharmD, FCCP

Jennifer R. Guthrie, MPAS, PA-C

LEARNING OBJECTIVES

After completing this case study, the reader should be able to:

- Discuss the absolute and relative contraindications to the use of hormonal contraceptives.
- Discuss the advantages and disadvantages of the various forms of contraceptives, including both oral and nonoral hormonal formulations as well as intrauterine devices.
- Compare and contrast the marketed contraceptive options and select the best product for an individual patient.
- Develop strategies for managing the possible side effects of oral contraceptives (OCs) and prepare appropriate alternative treatment plans.
- Provide specific patient education on the administration and expected side effects of selected hormonal contraceptives.

PATIENT PRESENTATION

■ Chief Complaint

"My fiancé and I are getting married soon, and we're not ready for kids just yet."

■ HPI

A 24-year-old female graduate student presents to the women's health clinic for her annual exam and contraceptive counseling. She and her fiancé are planning to be married in approximately 4 months. The patient states that she and her partner have been in a monogamous sexual relationship for the past 3 years and that their primary method of contraception has been via the inconsistent use of male condoms. She is here today to be evaluated for the use of hormonal contraceptives. The patient states she began menses at age 14 years, with irregular cycles occurring every 25–36 days and 8–10 days in length. Her last menses was 2 weeks ago and described as "normal." The patient denies having had sexual intercourse since the start of her last menses. The patient states she has heard about contraceptive options that "decrease your number of periods" and wants to know more about those options and if they would be okay for her to try.

■ PMH

Nulligravida; migraine headaches without aura or focal neurologic symptoms, well-controlled for the past 12 months on prophylactic therapy; no history of HTN, dyslipidemia, or heart disease.

■ FH

Mother, age 53 years, has HTN and osteoporosis and went through natural menopause at age 50 years. Maternal grandmother, age 74 years, has a history of breast cancer which was diagnosed at age 60 years. Father, age 55 years, has osteoarthritis, HTN, and dyslipidemia. Paternal grandfather, age 76, has coronary artery disease and a history of MI at age 60 years.

■ SH

Currently lives in a house on campus, which she rents with three other graduate students. Once she and her fiancé are married, they plan to rent an apartment together until she finishes graduate school. She admits to occasional social use of alcohol ("a few drinks at parties on the weekends"). Otherwise, she denies regular alcohol use during the week. Denies tobacco and illicit drug use.

■ Meds

Propranolol LA 160 mg PO once daily for migraine prophylaxis
Naproxen 220 mg, 1–2 tablets PO Q 8 H PRN mild menstrual cramps

■ All

NKDA

■ ROS

Nulligravida and nulliparous with no history of abnormal Pap smears. Last Pap smear was normal at age 21 years. Denies missed periods, excessive vaginal bleeding, abnormal vaginal discharge, dyspareunia, or significant pelvic pain with menses. Menstrual periods are the most irregular during midterm and final exam times. No history of STIs. She has mild acne on her forehead and nose, which are treated with facial wash. Denies weight change, recent skin changes, breast tenderness, nausea, or vomiting. Migraine headaches are not accompanied by aura or focal neurologic symptoms and have been well controlled on prophylactic medication—patient states she has not had a migraine for more than 12 months; however, prior to being placed on propranolol for migraine prophylaxis, she reported experiencing menstrual-related headaches in addition to frequent migraines. No history or current symptoms of depression or anxiety. Immunizations are up to date, including HPV and hepatitis B vaccinations.

■ PE

VS

BP 110/72 mm Hg, P 68 bpm, RR 14, T 37°C; Wt 59 kg, Ht 5′7″, BMI 20.4 kg/m^2

Gen

Thin, well-developed woman in NAD

Skin

Warm, dry, and without rashes; mild noninflammatory facial acne limited to forehead and nose; normal pigmentation

HEENT

Deferred

Neck/Lymph Nodes

Supple without lymphadenopathy or masses. No thyroid tenderness or thyromegaly.

Lungs

CTA, no wheezing

CV

RRR; no MRG

Breasts

Symmetric in size without nodularity or masses, nontender; nipples appear normal, everted, and without discharge

Abd

Soft, nontender, no masses or organomegaly

Genit/Rect

Normal-appearing external genitalia without lesions; no cervical discharge or motion tenderness; uterus anteverted, mobile, and without masses or tenderness; ovaries palpable, of normal size, and without tenderness; rectal exam not performed. Pap test collected.

MS/Ext

Normal ROM and strength of bilateral extremities; no peripheral edema

Neuro/Psych

A&O × 3; normal mood and affect

■ Labs

Negative UPT

■ Assessment

1. Contraception management, initial encounter
2. Irregular menses and menstrual headaches
3. Migraine headache
4. Acne vulgaris, mild

QUESTIONS

Collect Information

1.a. What subjective and objective information indicates consideration for hormonal contraception for this patient?

1.b. What additional information is needed to fully assess this patient's request for hormonal contraception?

Assess the Information

2.a. Assess the urgency for provision of pharmacologic contraception based on the subjective and objective information available.

2.b. Create a list of the patient's drug therapy problems and prioritize them. Include assessment of medication appropriateness, effectiveness, safety, and patient adherence.

Develop a Care Plan

3.a. What are the goals of pharmacotherapy in this case?

3.b. What nondrug contraceptive options might be useful for this patient?

3.c. What feasible pharmacotherapeutic options are available for prevention of pregnancy?

3.d. Create an individualized, patient-centered, team-based care plan to optimize medication therapy for this patient's contraceptive needs and other drug therapy problems. Include specific drugs, dosage forms, doses, schedules, and durations of therapy.

Implement the Care Plan

4.a. What information should be provided to the patient to enhance adherence, ensure successful therapy, and minimize adverse effects?

4.b. Describe how care should be coordinated with other healthcare providers.

Follow-Up: Monitor and Evaluate

5. Explain how to monitor and evaluate the care plan for medication appropriateness, effectiveness, safety, and patient adherence by using clinical and laboratory data, patient feedback, and other information.

■ CLINICAL COURSE

The patient returns to the clinic in 2 months complaining of worsening acne and breakthrough bleeding.

■ FOLLOW-UP QUESTIONS

1. What medical conditions can be the cause of breakthrough bleeding?

2. If breakthrough bleeding is not caused by an underlying medical condition, how can it be managed?

3. What recommendations can be made to address this patient's complaint of worsening acne?

■ SELF-STUDY ASSIGNMENTS

1. Compare the costs of each method of contraception and prepare a report that contains your conclusions as to which method provides the best efficacy at the most reasonable cost.

2. Visit a pharmacy and review the various home pregnancy tests; determine how you would counsel a patient to use each one and evaluate them for ease of use.

3. Review the US Medical Eligibility Criteria for Contraceptive Use and create a list of "Category 4" conditions that pose unacceptable health risks to patients who might use combined oral contraceptives.

CLINICAL PEARL

Except for latex and synthetic condoms, most contraceptives do not protect against the acquisition of STIs. Thus, it is important to properly educate patients who are sexually active about the importance of taking necessary precautions to minimize their risk for acquiring an STI, regardless of the type of hormonal contraceptive used.

REFERENCES

1. Hatcher RA, Nelson AL, Trussel J, et al. Contraceptive Technology. 21st ed. New York: Ayer Company Publishers, Inc., 2018.

2. U.S. Preventive Services Task Force. USPSTF A and B recommendations, 2021. Available at: *http://www.uspreventiveservicestaskforce.org/Page/Name/uspstf-a-and-b-recommendations/*. Accessed April 15, 2022.

3. Curtis KM, Tepper NK, Jatlaoui TC, et al. U.S. medical eligibility criteria for contraceptive use, 2016. MMWR Recomm Rep. 2016;65(No. RR-3):1–104. Available at: *https://www.cdc.gov/mmwr/volumes/65/rr/rr6503a1.htm*. Accessed April 15, 2022.

4. Tepper NK, Whiteman MK, Zapata LB, Marchbanks PA, Curtis KM. Safety of hormonal contraceptives among women with migraine: a systematic review. Contraception 2016;94(6):630–640. doi: 10.1016/j.contraception.2016.04.016.

5. Curtis KM, Jatlaoui TC, Tepper NK, et al. U.S. selected practice recommendations for contraceptive use, 2016. MMWR Recomm Rep. 2016;65(No. RR-4):1–66. Available at: *https://www.cdc.gov/mmwr/volumes/65/rr/rr6504a1.htm*. Accessed April 15, 2022.

6. Vinogradova Y, Coupland C, Hippisley-Cox J. Use of combined oral contraceptives and risk of venous thromboembolism: nested case-control studies using the QResearch and CPRD databases. BMJ. 2015;350:h2135. doi: 10.1136/bmj.h2135. Accessed January 28, 2022.

7. Oedingen C, Scholz S, Razum O. Systematic review and meta-analysis of the association of combined oral contraceptives on the risk of venous thromboembolism: the role of the progestogen type and estrogen dose. Thromb Res. 2018;165:68–78.

8. Machado RB, Pereira AP, Coelho GP, Neri L, Martins L, Luminoso D. Epidemiological and clinical aspects of migraine in users of combined oral contraceptives. Contraception. 2010;81:202–208.

9. American College of Obstetricians and Gynecologists. Updated Cervical Cancer Screening Guidelines Practice Advisory, April 2021. Available at: *https://www.acog.org/clinical/clinical-guidance/practice-advisory/articles/2021/04/updated-cervical-cancer-screening-guidelines*. Accessed April 15, 2022.

10. Committee on Practice Bulletins—Gynecology. Practice Bulletin No. 179: breast cancer risk assessment and screening in average-risk women. Obstet Gynecol. 2017;130:e1–e16. doi: 10.1097/AOG.0000000000002158. Accessed April 15, 2022.

95

EMERGENCY CONTRACEPTION

More Than Just Plan B .... Level II

Rebecca H. Stone, PharmD, BCPS, BCACP, FCCP

LEARNING OBJECTIVES

After completing this case study, the reader should be able to:

• Describe the advantages and disadvantages of the various options for emergency contraception.

• Describe the efficacy of each emergency contraception method and factors that may influence the efficacy.

• Discuss the possible adverse effects and contraindications of the various forms of emergency contraceptives, including both oral and nonoral options.

• Educate patient regarding the use of emergency contraception.

PATIENT PRESENTATION

■ Chief Complaint

"I forgot to restart my birth control pill pack 3 days ago. I have gone 10 days without a pill. I'm not ready to be pregnant yet!"

■ HPI

A 19-year-old woman presents to the family medicine clinic in a panic. She states that she typically throws out the last week of pills in her pack, "since they are not 'real' pills anyway," and she forgot to start her new oral contraceptive pack on time. She had intercourse with her partner 2 days ago and wants to know what she should do to avoid pregnancy.

■ PMH

Seasonal allergies
Menorrhagia

■ SH

Denies smoking
Enjoys an occasional glass of wine
Married × 1 year—reports mutually monogamous relationship

■ Meds

Cetirizine 10 mg PO once daily × 5 years
Ethinyl estradiol 20 mcg/ levonorgestrel 0.1 mg (Aviane) 1 tablet PO once daily × 2 years

■ **All**

NKDA

■ **ROS**

Patient is a nulligravida woman, she takes a combined oral contraceptive (OC) to regulate her menstrual cycle and reduce menorrhagia. She denies any heavy bleeding or breakthrough bleeding or spotting with routine use. She is tolerating the OC well.

■ **PE**

Gen

WDWN woman appearing anxious

VS

BP 106/70 mm Hg, P 60 bpm, RR 13, T 37°C; Wt 53.5 kg, Ht 5'5", BMI 19.6 kg/m²

Exam

Deferred; she had a complete examination 3 months ago that was normal

■ **Labs**

3 months ago

Negative Pap smear

1 year ago

Tests negative for chlamydia, gonorrhea, syphilis, and HIV

■ **Assessment**

A 19-year-old woman with seasonal allergy and contraception, currently in need of emergency contraception and a reliable contraception method for adherence

QUESTIONS

Collect Information

1.a. What subjective and objective information indicates that this patient is appropriate for emergency contraception?

1.b. What additional information is needed to fully assess this patient's need for emergency contraception?

Assess the Information

2.a. Assess the urgency of emergency contraception access based on the subjective and objective information available.

2.b. Create a list of the patient's drug therapy problems and prioritize them. Include assessment of medication appropriateness, effectiveness, safety, and patient adherence.

2.c. What economic, psychosocial, cultural, racial, and ethical considerations are applicable to this patient?

Develop a Care Plan

3.a. What are the goals of pharmacotherapy in this case?

3.b. What nondrug therapies might be useful for this patient?

3.c. What feasible pharmacotherapeutic options are available for addressing this patient's risk of unintended pregnancy?

3.d. Create an individualized, patient-centered, team-based care plan to optimize medication therapy for this patient. Include specific drugs, dosage forms, doses, schedules, and durations of therapy.

3.e. What alternatives would be appropriate if the initial care plan fails or cannot be used?

Implement the Care Plan

4.a. What information should be provided to the patent to enhance adherence, ensure successful therapy, and minimize adverse effects?

4.b. Describe how care should be coordinated with other healthcare providers.

Follow-Up: Monitor and Evaluate

5. Explain how to monitor and evaluate the care plan for medication appropriateness, effectiveness, safety, and patient adherence by using clinical and laboratory data, patient feedback, and other information.

■ CLINICAL COURSE

A few weeks later, the patient calls into the clinic to report that she started her period and is not pregnant. She states that she is thankful for the advice provided to her.

■ SELF-STUDY ASSIGNMENTS

1. For other forms of hormonal contraception, such as the patch, the ring, progestin-only OCs, and injectables, create a table identifying when emergency contraception may be needed if these methods are not used appropriately.

2. For patients not using hormonal contraception, identify additional scenarios for which emergency contraception may be utilized.

3. Explain how BMI or body weight may influence efficacy of emergency contraceptive products.

CLINICAL PEARL

Although not FDA-approved for this purpose, a copper IUD may also be used as emergency contraception within the first 120 hours after inadequately protected intercourse.

REFERENCES

1. Curtis KM, Jatlaoui TC, Tepper NK, et al. U.S. Selected practice recommendations for contraceptive use, 2016. MMWR Recomm Rep. 2016;65(4):1–66.

2. American College of Obstetricians and Gynecologists. Practice Bulletin No. 152: Emergency contraception. Obstet Gynecol. 2015;126(3):e1–e11.

3. Curtis KM, Tepper NK, Jatlaoui TC, et al. U.S. Medical eligibility criteria for contraceptive use, 2016. MMWR Recomm Rep. 2016;65(3):1–103.

4. Haeger KO, Lamme J, Cleland K. State of emergency contraception in the U.S., 2018. Contracept Reprod Med. 2018;3:20.

5. Gemzell-Danielsson K, Berger C. Emergency contraception—mechanisms of action. Contraception. 2013;87(3):300–308.

6. American College of Obstetricians and Gynecologists. Practice Bulletin No. 186: Long-acting reversible contraception: implants and intrauterine devices. Obstet Gynecol. 2017;130(5):e251–e269.

7. Turok DK, Gero A, Simmons RG, et al. Levonorgestrel vs. copper intrauterine devices for emergency contraception. N Engl J Med. 2021;384(4):335–344. doi: 10.1056/NEJMoa2022141.

8. Berger C, Boggavarapu NR, Menezes J, Lalitkumar PG, Gemzell-Danielsson K. Effects of ulipristal acetate on human embryo attachment and endometrial cell gene expression in an in vitro co-culture system. Hum Reprod. 2015;30(4):800–811.

9. Banh C, Rautenberg T, Duijkers I, et al. The effects on ovarian activity of delaying versus immediately restarting combined oral contraception after missing three pills and taking ulipristal acetate 30 mg. Contraception. 2020;102(3):145–151.

10. Glasier A, Cameron ST, Blithe D, et al. Can we identify women at risk of pregnancy despite using emergency contraception? Data from randomized trials of ulipristal acetate and levonorgestrel. Contraception. 2011;84(4):363–367.

96

PREMENSTRUAL DYSPHORIC DISORDER

Miserable Menses .... Level II

Autumn Stewart-Lynch, PharmD, BCACP

Sea-oh McConville, DO

LEARNING OBJECTIVES

After completing this case study, the reader should be able to:

- Differentiate between the clinical presentation and diagnosis of premenstrual syndrome (PMS) and premenstrual dysphoric disorder (PMDD).

- Identify the desired therapeutic outcomes for patients with PMDD.

- Design an appropriate therapeutic plan for a patient with PMDD.

- Design an appropriate monitoring plan for a patient with PMDD, considering patient-specific factors.

- Educate patients and other healthcare professionals about PMDD and therapeutic options.

PATIENT PRESENTATION

Chief Complaint

"My partner and I want to get pregnant, but we keep fighting."

HPI

A 32-year-old female presents to her family medicine clinic for help regarding preconception counseling. She and her partner have been unsuccessful in becoming pregnant after trying for 9 months and she worries her family goals are suffering because of conflict in their relationship. She attributes these conflicts to her emotional state and an inability to engage in emotional and physical intimacy due to fatigue, irritability, and "feeling down." Although she feels love and attraction toward her partner, she is less interested in sexual intercourse and worries he will become less understanding and supportive if she continues to push him away. She describes episodes of interpersonal conflict at home and work brought on by feeling out of control of labile emotions (eg, anger, irritability, sadness, frustration) and has at times yelled at her partner. She has kept a diary of her symptoms for the past 3 months, and these episodes appear to follow a trend of monthly occurrences during the last week of her menstrual cycle (the week prior to onset of menses) and are accompanied by symptoms of bloating, breast tenderness, and headaches. She has tried over-the-counter ibuprofen and acetaminophen with minimal relief. She noted better control of these symptoms when she was on an oral contraceptive which she stopped approximately 12 months ago when they decided to start trying to conceive.

ROS

Denies SI/HI. Negative except for listed in the HPI.

PMH

Migraines without aura
Mild intermittent asthma

FH

Mother has dyslipidemia. Father has irritable bowel syndrome.

SH

Married to male partner for 4 years. No children.
Tobacco use: ½ ppd for 5 years, quit 10 years ago.
Alcohol: drinks 2–3 glasses of wine once a week (at weekly book club).
She works full time as a professor at a small community college.
Negative IPV screening; feels safe at home.

Meds

Albuterol HFA inhaler, two inhalations as needed for SOB
Fluticasone/salmeterol 100 mcg/50 mcg dry powder inhaler, one inhalation twice daily
Sumatriptan 100 mg PO PRN migraine headache, may repeat × 1 dose
Women's multivitamin gummies, takes two daily

All

NKDA

PE

Gen

Tearful, petite woman

VS

BP 108/66 mm Hg, P 55 bpm, RR 17, T 98.3°F; Wt 112 lb (50.8 kg), Ht 5'3", BMI 19.8 kg/m²

Skin

Normal; intact; warm and dry

HEENT

PERRLA; EOMI; moist mucous membranes; TMs intact

Neck/Lymph Nodes

Supple without evidence of JVD, lymphadenopathy, or thyromegaly

Lungs/Thorax

CTA, no wheezes, rhonchi, rales

Breasts

Symmetric; no lumps or masses; nipples without discharge; bilaterally diffusely tender to touch

CV

RRR without MRG

Abd

Soft, NT/ND; +BS; no masses

Genit/Rect

Normal pelvic exam

Ext

Normal ROM; pulses 2+; No cyanosis, clubbing, or edema

Neuro

A&O × 3; CN II–XII intact; DTRs +2/4 throughout

■ Labs

Na 141 mEq/L	Ca 9.2 mg/dL	*Fasting lipid profile*	WBC 6 × 10³/mm³
K 3.5 mEq/L	AST 20 IU/L	T. chol 190 mg/dL	Hgb 13 g/dL
Cl 104 mEq/L	ALT 17 IU/L	TG 120 mg/dL	Hct 39%
CO_2 27 mEq/L	Alb 3.9 g/dL	LDL 95 mg/dL	MCV 92.8 μm³
Glu 81 mg/dL	TSH 0.74 mIU/L	HDL 71 mg/dL	MCH 31.7 pg
BUN 14 mg/dL			MCHC 34.2 g/dL
SCr 0.9 mg/dL			Plt 249 × 10³/mm³
			Urine Hcg: Negative

■ Assessment

1. PMDD
2. Preconception care
3. Migraines without aura
4. Mild intermittent asthma

QUESTIONS

Collect Information

1.a. What subjective and objective information indicates the presence of PMDD versus PMS?

1.b. What additional information is needed to fully assess this patient's PMDD?

Assess the Information

2.a. Assess the severity of PMDD based on the subjective and objective information available.

2.b. Create a list of the patient's drug therapy problems and prioritize them. Include assessment of medication appropriateness, effectiveness, safety, and patient adherence.

Develop a Care Plan

3.a. What are the goals of pharmacotherapy in this case?

3.b. What nondrug therapies for PMDD might be useful for this patient?

3.c. What feasible pharmacotherapeutic alternatives are available to treat this patient's PMDD?

3.d. Create an individualized, patient-centered, team-based care plan to optimize medication therapy for this patient's PMDD and other drug therapy problems. Include specific drugs, dosage forms, doses, schedules, and durations of therapy.

Implement the Care Plan

4.a. What information should be provided to the patient to enhance adherence, ensure successful therapy, and minimize adverse effects?

4.b. Describe how care should be coordinated with other healthcare providers.

Follow-Up: Monitor and Evaluate

5. Explain how to monitor and evaluate the care plan for medication appropriateness, effectiveness, safety, and patient adherence by using clinical and laboratory data, patient feedback, and other information.

■ SELF-STUDY ASSIGNMENTS

1. Develop a patient educational handout that outlines the differences between PMS and PMDD and provides resources for patients to get more information on PMDD.

2. List the preconception prevention and management options to ensure optimal maternal health and improve pregnancy outcomes.

3. Discuss how the treatment options might differ if the patient was not trying to become pregnant or trying to prevent pregnancy.

CLINICAL PEARL

Symptoms of PMDD and PMS overlap, but the severity of symptoms is generally worse in PMDD. Selective serotonin reuptake inhibitors, dosed continuously or during the luteal phase only, are first-line therapy. Combined hormonal contraceptives (CHC) can improve physical symptoms in PMS and a 20 mcg ethinyl estradiol CHC containing drospirenone is FDA-approved for the treatment of premenstrual symptoms in PMDD.

ACKNOWLEDGMENT

This case is based on the patient case written for the 11th edition by Larissa N.H. Bossaer, PharmD, BCPS.

REFERENCES

1. American Psychiatric Association: Diagnostic and Statistical Manual of Mental Disorders, 5th edition. Arlington, VA, American Psychiatric Association, 2013.

2. Futterman LA, Rapkin AJ. Diagnosis of premenstrual disorders. J Reprod Med. 2006;51:349–358.

3. Appleton, S. Premenstrual syndrome: evidence-based evaluation and treatment. Clin Obstet and Gynecol. 2018;61(1):52–61.

4. Endicott J, Nee J, Harrison W. Daily record of severity of problems (DRSP): reliability and validity. Arch Women Ment Health 2006;9:41–49.

5. Yonkers KA, Simoni MK. Premenstrual disorders. Am J Obstet Gynecol. 2018;218(1):68–74.

6. Maharaj S, Trevino K. A comprehensive review of treatment options for premenstrual syndrome and premenstrual dysphoric disorder. J Psychiatr Pract. 2015;21(5):334–350.

7. Marjoribanks J, Brown J, O'Brien PM, Wyatt K. Selective serotonin reuptake inhibitors for premenstrual syndrome. Cochrane Database Syst Rev. 2013;6:CD001396.

8. Global Initiative for Asthma. Global Strategy for Asthma Management and Prevention, 2021. Available at: www.ginasthma.org. Accessed January 10, 2022.

9. Institute of Medicine. Dietary Reference Intakes for Calcium and Vitamin D. Washington, DC: The National Academies Press, 2011. Available at: https://doi.org/10.17226/13050.

10. American College of Obstetricians and Gynecologists (ACOG) Committee on Practice Bulletins-Obstetrics. Practice Bulletin No. 187: Neural Tube Defects. Obstet Gynecol. 2017;130(6):e279–e290.

97

ENDOMETRIOSIS

Persistent Pelvic Pain...........................Level I

Erin C. Raney, PharmD, FCCP, BCPS, BC-ADM

LEARNING OBJECTIVES

After completing this case study, the reader should be able to:

- Identify the signs and symptoms associated with endometriosis.
- Compare and contrast the benefits and risks associated with various hormonal medications used for the treatment of endometriosis-associated pelvic pain.
- Determine a treatment approach for this case taking into account other health issues and potential health benefits.
- Discuss possible side effects associated with treatment for endometriosis.

PATIENT PRESENTATION

Chief Complaint
"I am not getting relief from my endometriosis pain with Tylenol, and I would like to see what other options I have."

HPI
A 36-year-old woman presents to the clinic today to establish care and evaluate continued endometriosis-related pain. She was diagnosed with endometriosis at age 30 by a previous provider based on a history of dysmenorrhea and dyspareunia. She does not find relief despite treatment with acetaminophen which she has been using when the pain is most severe during her menstrual period. During these times, the acetaminophen reduces her pain from a 6 on a 10-point scale to a 5. When first diagnosed with endometriosis, she was treated with combined oral contraceptives for 2 years. Pain relief was limited by poor adherence with daily dosing. The oral contraceptive was discontinued when she resumed cigarette use.

PMH
Endometriosis
G0P0A0

FH
Mother (aged 60 years) has a history of endometriosis, no other health conditions; father (aged 62 years) has hypertension; one male sibling (aged 34 years) has asthma.

SH
Patient is an information technology specialist. She has no children and states no desire for conceiving in the future. She is unmarried and currently sexually active with one partner. She uses male condoms for contraception. She smokes ½ pack of cigarettes per day, decreased from 1 pack per day 1 year ago. She reports cigarette use from age 16 to 24, at which time she quit "cold turkey." She resumed smoking at age 32 due to stress from a divorce and career change. She is not interested in quitting tobacco use at this time. She consumes no more than two alcohol-containing beverages per week. She exercises 30 minutes one to two times per week.

Meds
Acetaminophen 1000 mg PO four times daily as needed for menstrual pain
Multivitamin one tablet PO daily

All
Ibuprofen (hives, anaphylaxis)

ROS
(+) For moderate pain in pelvic region, (–) for constipation, menstrual periods occur at regular intervals of 28 days. Experiences mild pain during sexual intercourse, approximately 2–3 on a 10-point pain scale (with 10 being the worst possible pain).

PE
Gen
WDWN woman in NAD

VS
BP 120/72 mm Hg, P 65 bpm, RR 15, T 37°C; Wt 60 kg, Ht 5'6"; patient has maintained same weight for the last 4 years

Skin
No lesions

HEENT
WNL, normal nasal mucosa, no rhinorrhea

Neck/Lymph Nodes
Supple, no bruits, no adenopathy, no thyromegaly

Lungs/Thorax
CTA bilaterally; no wheezes

Breasts
Supple; no masses

CV

RRR, normal S_1 and S_2

Abd

Soft; patient states, at baseline, she experiences pain that averages a 2–3 on a 10-point pain scale, this worsens to a 6 during the first 2–3 days of her menstrual period. (+) BS; no masses noted.

Genit/Rect

Pelvic exam: (+) adnexal pain elicited and rated at 5 on a 10-point pain scale, no masses

MS/Ext

Pulses intact

Neuro

Normal sensory and motor levels

■ Labs

Na 135 mEq/L	*Fasting lipid profile*
K 4.3 mEq/L	T. chol 149 mg/dL
Cl 104 mEq/L	LDL 60 mg/dL
CO_2 25 mEq/L	HDL 65 mg/dL
BUN 10 mg/dL	Trig 120 mg/dL
SCr 0.8 mg/dL	
Fasting glu 84 mg/dL	

■ Other

PAP test: Normal
HPV/chlamydia/gonorrhea: Negative
Urine pregnancy test: Negative
Vaginal ultrasound (from previous medical records): Normal

■ Assessment

1. Endometriosis
2. Tobacco use

QUESTIONS

Collect Information

1.a. What subjective and objective information indicates the presence of endometriosis?

1.b. What additional information is needed to fully assess this patient's endometriosis?

Assess the Information

2.a. Assess the severity of endometriosis based on the subjective and objective information available.

2.b. Create a list of the patient's drug therapy problems and prioritize them. Include assessment of medication appropriateness, effectiveness, safety, and patient adherence.

Develop a Care Plan

3.a. What are the goals of pharmacotherapy for endometriosis in this case?

3.b. What nondrug therapies might be useful for the treatment of pain associated with this patient's endometriosis?

3.c. What pharmacotherapeutic options are available for treating pain associated with endometriosis?

3.d. Create an individualized, patient-centered, team-based care plan to optimize medication therapy for endometriosis and other drug therapy problems identified. Include specific drugs, dosage forms, doses, schedules, and durations of therapy.

Implement the Care Plan

4.a. What information should be provided to the patient to enhance adherence, ensure successful therapy, and minimize adverse effects?

4.b. Describe how care should be coordinated with other healthcare providers.

Follow-Up: Monitor and Evaluate

5. Explain how to monitor and evaluate the care plan for medication appropriateness, effectiveness, safety, and patient adherence by using clinical and laboratory data, patient feedback, and other information.

■ CLINICAL COURSE

The patient returns to her primary care provider 6 months after starting medroxyprogesterone acetate 150 mg intramuscular injections every 3 months. She reports that her pelvic pain is better controlled with an overall average pain rating of 1 on the 10-point scale. She states that she had intermittent spotting initially but now has no menstrual periods. She continues to smoke cigarettes but has further reduced her use to 5–10 cigarettes per day. Her weight is 62 kg, and she denies changes in mood.

■ FOLLOW-UP QUESTIONS

1. What is the optimal length of time for a patient to continue medroxyprogesterone acetate injections for the treatment of endometriosis-related chronic pelvic pain?

2. Would your recommendation change if this patient had risk factors for osteopenia or osteoporosis?

3. Would your recommendation change if this patient had indicated an interest in having a child in the next 1–2 years?

4. Would your recommendation change if this patient quit tobacco use?

■ SELF-STUDY ASSIGNMENTS

1. Review the contraindications of the various contraceptive agents used for the treatment of endometriosis.

2. Research the strategies used to treat infertility associated with endometriosis.

CLINICAL PEARL

The use of combined hormonal contraceptives for endometriosis-related pelvic pain can be associated with pain recurrence during the hormone-free interval of the cyclical pattern of these contraceptive agents. Using the products in a continuous pattern without a hormone-free interval can address this complaint, although an erratic breakthrough bleeding pattern is common and may be treatment limiting. Progestogens also cause breakthrough bleeding, but many patients experience eventual amenorrhea after longer intervals of use, which further alleviates pain associated with menstrual bleeding.

REFERENCES

1. European Society of Human Reproduction and Embryology. Endometriosis: Guideline of European Society of Human Reproduction and Embryology, 2022. Available at: *https://www.eshre.eu/Guidelines-and-Legal/Guidelines/Endometriosis-guideline.aspx.* Accessed April 1, 2022.

2. Practice Committee of the American Society for Reproductive Medicine. Treatment of pelvic pain associated with endometriosis: a committee opinion. Fertil Steril. 2014;101:927–935.

3. Centers for Disease Control and Prevention. U.S. medical eligibility criteria for contraceptive use, 2016. Available at: *https://www.cdc.gov/mmwr/volumes/65/rr/rr6503a1.htm.* Accessed April 1, 2022.

4. Mira, RAA, Buen MM, Borges MG, Yela D, Benetti-Pinto CL. Systematic review and meta-analysis of complementary treatments for women with symptomatic endometriosis. Int J Gynecol Obstet. 2018;143:2–9.

5. Ferrero S, Barra F, Maggiore ULR. Current and emerging therapeutics for the management of endometriosis. Drugs. 2018;78:995–1012.

6. Vercellini P, Buggio L, Berlanda N, Barbara G, Somigliana E, Bosari S. Estrogen-progestins and progestins for the management of endometriosis. Fertil Steril. 2016;106:1552–1571.

7. Hatcher RA, Nelson AL, Trussell J, et al. Contraceptive Technology, 21st ed. New York: Ayer Company Publishers, 2018.

8. Leyland N, Estes SJ, Lessey BA, Advincula AP, Taylor HS. A clinician's guide to the treatment of endometriosis with elagolix. J Womens Health. 2021;30:569–578.

9. American College of Obstetricians and Gynecologists. Committee opinion: depot medroxyprogesterone acetate and bone effects. Obstet Gynecol. 2014;123:1398–1402.

98

MANAGING MENOPAUSAL SYMPTOMS

Too Hot to Handle............................ Level II

Veronica P. Vernon, PharmD, BCPS, BCACP, NCMP

LEARNING OBJECTIVES

After completing this case study, the reader should be able to:

- Identify the signs and symptoms associated with menopause.

- List the risks and benefits associated with hormone therapy (HT), and identify appropriate candidates for HT.

- Describe differences between transdermal, vaginal, and oral forms of HT and their place in therapy.

- Recommend nonpharmacologic therapy for managing menopausal symptoms.

- Identify alternative, nonhormonal therapies for managing menopausal symptoms.

- Design a comprehensive pharmacotherapeutic plan for a patient on HT including treatment options, monitoring, and duration of therapy.

- Determine the desired therapeutic outcomes for a patient taking HT.

- Educate patients on the treatment options, benefits, risks, and monitoring of HT.

PATIENT PRESENTATION

■ Chief Complaint

"I have been having hot flashes for a several months. They are getting worse and interfering with my life at home and work."

■ HPI

A 52-year-old G2P2 woman reports experiencing at least twelve hot flashes per day. She also states she is awakened from sleep about four times per week feeling hot and "drenched with sweat." She has trouble falling back asleep after these episodes and it leaves her feeling exhausted the next day. She also finds it embarrassing when she spends the night with her new partner. Her symptoms began about 8 months ago, and over that time, they have increased in frequency and severity, and they are interfering with her daily function. When she is doing presentations or participating in important meetings at work, it seems to trigger a hot flash. She also complains of vaginal dryness and painful intercourse. She states that her older sister was prescribed a medication for similar symptoms, but she is hesitant to take the same thing because she heard on the news and from friends that the medication may not be safe. She states she does not want to "start having periods again." Her anxiety is currently controlled with paroxetine. She exercises three times a week and tries to follow a healthy diet with lean protein and lots of fruits and vegetables. She admits to "stress eating" and eating unhealthy foods when she travels for work.

■ PMH

Generalized anxiety disorder

■ FH

Mother, age 74, has HTN; father died of MI at age 72. Patient has one sister, age 54, who is in good health but has HTN.

■ SH

Divorced 10 years ago, lives with two teenage sons. Started dating a man 3 months ago. She is a financial executive for a large company and often travels for important meetings and presentations. She walks on her local greenway two times a week, does yoga once a week, and is trying to follow a healthy diet although inconsistently. She does not smoke. She drinks one glass of red wine each night with dinner and has two cups of black coffee every morning.

■ Meds

Paroxetine 20 mg PO once daily at bedtime

■ All

NKDA

■ ROS

(+) Hot flashes, night sweats, vaginal dryness/dyspareunia. (−) weight gain, constipation. LMP 14 months ago.

■ PE

Gen

WDWN woman in NAD

VS

BP 118/76 mm Hg, P 78 bpm, RR 15, T 36.4°C; Wt 76.2 kg, Ht 5'6"

Skin

Warm, dry, no lesions

HEENT

WNL

Neck/LN

Supple, no bruits, no adenopathy, no thyromegaly

Lungs/Thorax

CTA bilaterally

Breasts

Supple; no masses

CV

RRR, normal S_1 and S_2; no MRG

Abd

Soft, NT/ND, (+) BS; no masses

Genit/Rect

Pelvic exam normal except (+) mucosal atrophy; stool guaiac (−)

Ext

(−) CCE; pulses intact

Neuro

Normal sensory and motor levels

■ Labs

Na 136 mEq/L	Hgb 12.7 g/dL	Ca 9.3 mg/dL	*Fasting lipid profile*
K 3.9 mEq/L	Hct 39.3%	AST 32 IU/L	T. chol 190 mg/dL
Cl 104 mEq/L	WBC 6.5 × 10³/mm³	ALT 30 IU/L	LDL 132 mg/dL
CO₂ 25 mEq/L	Plt 208 × 10³/mm³	TSH 2.46 mIU/L	HDL 50 mg/dL
BUN 10 mg/dL		FSH 70.8 mIU/mL	Trig 180 mg/dL
SCr 0.7 mg/dL		Estradiol 5.6 pg/mL	
Random glu 98 mg/dL		UPT (−)	

■ Other

Pap smear and mammogram: Normal

■ Assessment

A 52-year-old woman experiencing multiple symptoms of menopause, currently affecting her daily living. Her symptoms of generalized anxiety disorder are controlled with therapy.

QUESTIONS

Collect Information

1.a. What subjective and objective information indicates the presence of menopausal symptoms?

1.b. What additional information is needed to fully assess this patient's menopausal symptoms?

Assess the Information

2.a. Assess the severity of menopausal symptoms based on the subjective and objective information available.

2.b. Create a prioritized list of the patient's drug therapy problems, including assessment of medication appropriateness, effectiveness, safety, and patient adherence.

2.c. What economic, psychosocial, cultural, racial, and ethical considerations are applicable to this patient?

Develop a Care Plan

3.a. What are the goals of pharmacotherapy for menopausal symptoms in this case?

3.b. What nondrug therapies might be useful for this patient's menopausal symptoms?

3.c. What feasible pharmacotherapeutic options are available for treating menopausal symptoms?

3.d. Create an individualized, patient-centered, team-based care plan to optimize medication therapy for this patient's menopausal symptoms and other drug therapy problems identified. Include specific drugs, dosage forms, doses, schedules, and durations of therapy.

3.e. What alternatives would be appropriate if the initial care plan fails or cannot be used?

Implement the Care Plan

4.a. What information should be provided to the patient to enhance adherence to the medication, ensure successful therapy, and minimize adverse effects?

4.b. Describe how care should be coordinated with other healthcare providers.

Follow-Up: Monitor and Evaluate

5. Explain how to monitor and evaluate the care plan for medication appropriateness, effectiveness, safety, and patient adherence by using clinical and laboratory data, patient feedback, and other information.

■ CLINICAL COURSE

The patient returns to her provider after 1 year of HT. She reports that her hot flashes and night sweats have decreased in number and intensity, and her vaginal dryness is not bothering her. She is wondering if she should continue her HT regimen, and if so, for how long?

■ FOLLOW-UP QUESTIONS

1. What is the optimal dose and length of time for a patient to continue on HT?

2. How should HT be discontinued after successful treatment?

3. Would your recommendation for HT change if the patient had been complaining of genital symptoms only? Why or why not?

4. Would your recommendation for HT change if this patient were to have had significant risk factors for CHD or a personal history of breast cancer? Why or why not?

5. How would you respond to the patient if she asked you about taking compounded bioidentical HT?

■ CLINICAL COURSE: ALTERNATIVE THERAPY

The patient is considering stopping her HT because her cousin was recently diagnosed with breast cancer. She still desires relief from hot flashes and asks for additional information on other alternatives. She has heard that black cohosh should not be used in women with breast cancer, but she has a friend who also has a family history of breast cancer who has been on black cohosh for about 9 months on the recommendation of her physician. Her friend has a checkup with lab tests every 6 months. The patient asks if black cohosh or soy would be an appropriate option to help keep her hot flushes under control. See Section 19 in this Casebook for questions about the use of black cohosh for managing menopausal symptoms.

■ SELF-STUDY ASSIGNMENTS

1. Research nonhormonal therapies that have been studied for the relief of menopausal symptoms and compare the scientific evidence of their efficacy to traditional hormonal medications.

2. Review the results of the Women's Health Initiative (WHI) study from 2002 and the 2007 reanalysis of the WHI results regarding the impact of HT on cardiovascular disease related to age and duration of HT use. Provide a summary of the overall findings regarding HT and cardiovascular and breast cancer risk.

3. Develop a recommendation based on the available evidence for the use of herbal therapies to treat menopausal symptoms. What agents, if any, are preferred? Would you recommend an herbal therapy for a patient with breast cancer?

4. Research the evidence surrounding the use of calcium and vitamin D supplementation for osteoporosis prevention in community-dwelling postmenopausal patients.

CLINICAL PEARL

The most effective treatment for vasomotor symptoms is systemic hormone therapy. Transdermal estradiol and micronized progesterone may be the preferred types of systemic HT, given the lower incidence of adverse effects.

ACKNOWLEDGMENT

This case is based on the patient cases written for the 11th edition by Andrea Franks, PharmD and Julie Jeter, MD.

REFERENCES

1. Stuenkel CA, Davis SR, Gompel A, et al. Treatment of symptoms of the menopause: an Endocrine Society clinical practice guideline. J Clin Endocrinol Metab. 2015;100(11):3975–4011.

2. Faubion SS, Crandall CJ, Davis L, et al. The 2022 hormone therapy position statement of The North American Menopause Society. Menopause. 2022;29(7):767–794.

3. North American Menopause Society. Nonhormonal management of menopause-associated vasomotor symptoms: 2015 position statement of The North American Menopause Society. Menopause. 2015;22:1155–1172.

4. Grundy SM, Stone NJ, Bailey AL, et al. 2018 AHA/ACC/AACVPR/AAPA/ABC/ACPM/ADA/AGS/APhA/ASPC/NLA/PCNA guideline on the management of blood cholesterol: a report of the American College of Cardiology/American Heart Association Task Force on clinical practice guidelines. Circulation 2019;139(25):e1082–e1143. doi: 10.1161/CIR.0000000000000625.

5. North American Menopause Society. Management of osteoporosis in postmenopausal women: The 2021 position statement of The North American Menopause Society. Menopause 2021;28(9):973–997.

6. The 2020 genitourinary syndrome of menopause position statement of The North American Menopause Society. Menopause. 2020;27(9):976–992. doi: 10.1097/GME.0000000000001609.

7. Liu JH, Pinkerton JV. Prescription therapies. In: Crandall CJ, ed. Menopause Practice: A Clinician's Guide, 6th edition. The North American Menopause Society; 2019:277–309.

8. Vinogradova Y, Coupland C, Hippisley-Cox J. Use of hormone replacement therapy and risk of venous thromboembolism: nested case-control studies using the QResearch and CPRD databases. BMJ. 2019;364:k4810. doi: 10.1136/bmj.k4810.

9. National Academies of Sciences, Engineering, and Medicine; Health and Medicine Division; Board on Health Sciences Policy; Committee on the Clinical Utility of Treating Patients with Compounded Bioidentical Hormone Replacement Therapy, Jackson LM, Parker RM, Mattison DR, eds. The Clinical Utility of Compounded Bioidentical Hormone Therapy: A Review of Safety, Effectiveness, and Use. Washington, DC: National Academies Press; 2020. doi: 10.17226/25791.

10. Franco OH, Chowdhury R, Troup J, et al. Use of plant-based therapies and menopausal symptoms: a systematic review and meta-analysis. JAMA. 2016;315(23):2554–2563.

99

ERECTILE DYSFUNCTION

Where There's a Pill, There's a Way . . . . Level III

Cara Liday, PharmD, CDCES

LEARNING OBJECTIVES

After completing this case study, the reader should be able to:

- Recognize risk factors associated with development of erectile dysfunction (ED).

- Provide brief descriptions of the advantages and disadvantages of the common therapies available for treating ED.

- Recommend appropriate first- and second-line therapy for treatment of ED.

- Provide appropriate patient education on administration and expected adverse effects of selected treatment modalities for ED.

PATIENT PRESENTATION

Chief Complaint

"I'm having trouble in the bedroom lately…."

HPI

A 63-year-old man presents to his PCP with the above complaint. On questioning, he states that for the past year, he has been able to achieve only partial erections that are insufficient for intercourse. He notices occasional nocturnal penile tumescence. He feels that the problem is leading to a strained relationship with his wife. He has tried a couple of herbal products or "natural supplements" that he ordered over the Internet, but they did not help.

PMH

Type 2 DM × 14 years
HTN
Dyslipidemia
CKD stage 3

FH

Father deceased at age 72 secondary to MI; mother alive with HTN

SH

Married for 38 years; no history of marital problems; 20 pack-year smoking history; does not drink alcohol; walks for 30 minutes 3 days per week

Meds

Insulin glargine U-100 60 units SC at bedtime
Metformin 1000 mg PO BID
Dulaglutide 1.5 mg SQ once weekly
Lisinopril 40 mg PO once daily
Hydrochlorothiazide 25 mg PO once daily
Atorvastatin 80 mg PO once daily
ASA 81 mg PO once daily

All

NKDA

ROS

Denies significant life stressors, fatigue, urgency, or symptoms of prostatitis. Complains of occasional nocturia and difficulty achieving and maintaining erections.

Physical Examination

Gen

Centrally obese, alert, well-developed, cooperative man in NAD

VS

BP 131/78 mm Hg, P 60 bpm, RR 18, T 37.2°C; Wt 120 kg, Ht 5′10″

HEENT

NC/AT; EOMI; PERRLA

Lungs/Chest

Clear to A&P bilaterally

CV

RRR; normal S_1 and S_2; no MRG

Abd

Soft, obese; NTND; normal bowel sounds; no masses or organomegaly

Genit/Rect

Normal scrotum, testes descended; NT w/o masses; penis without discharge or curvature

MS/Ext

Muscle strength 5/5 throughout; full ROM in all extremities; pulses 2+ throughout; no edema present; multiple toenails with yellow discoloration and thickening

Neuro

CNs II–XII intact; DTRs 2+ and equal bilaterally. No motor deficits; feet with reduced sensation (monofilament) and vibration; normal pain sensation with sharp pinprick bilaterally.

■ Labs

			Fasting lipid profile
Na 139 mEq/L	Hgb 16.0 g/dL	Ca 9.5 mg/dL	
K 3.9 mEq/L	Hct 50%	Mg 1.8 mEq/L	T. chol 192 mg/dL
Cl 102 mEq/L	AST 35 IU/L	A1C 8.5%	HDL 41 mg/dL
CO_2 24 mEq/L	ALT 18 IU/L	Testosterone 700 ng/dL	LDL 94 mg/dL
BUN 27 mg/dL		TSH 1.54 mIU/L	TG 167 mg/dL
SCr 1.8 mg/dL			VLDL
Glu (fasting)			19 mg/dL
166 mg/dL			

■ UA

SG 1.00; pH 5.1; leukocyte esterase (–); nitrite (–); protein 100 mg/dL; glucose 2+; ketones (–); urobilinogen normal; bilirubin (–); blood (–); albumin/Cr ratio 28 mg/g

■ IIEF-5 (International Index of Erectile Function-5)

Score 8/25

■ Assessment

A 63-year-old man with ED, hypertension, chronic kidney disease, dyslipidemia, poor long-term control of type 2 diabetes, and probable diagnosis of onychomycosis

QUESTIONS

Collect Information

1.a. What subjective and objective information indicates the presence of ED?

1.b. What risk factors for ED are present in this patient?

1.c. What additional information is needed to fully assess this patient's ED?

Assess the Information

2.a. Assess the severity of ED based on the information available.

2.b. Create a list of the patient's drug therapy problems and prioritize them. Include assessment of medication appropriateness, effectiveness, safety, and patient adherence.

Develop a Care Plan

3.a. What are the goals of therapy for ED in this case?

3.b. What nondrug therapies might be useful for treating ED in this patient?

3.c. What feasible pharmacotherapeutic alternatives are available for treating ED?

3.d. Create an individualized, patient-centered, team-based care plan to optimize initial therapy for this patient's ED and other drug therapy problems. Include specific drugs, dosage forms, doses, schedules, and durations of therapy.

Implement the Care Plan

4.a. What information should be provided to the patient to enhance adherence, ensure successful therapy, and minimize adverse effects with ED therapy?

4.b. Describe how care should be coordinated with other healthcare providers.

Follow-Up: Monitor and Evaluate

5. Explain how to monitor and evaluate the care plan for medication appropriateness, effectiveness, safety, and patient adherence by using clinical and laboratory data, patient feedback, and other information.

■ SELF-STUDY ASSIGNMENTS

1. If therapy for onychomycosis is desired, what medication would be optimal, and how would the addition of this agent change your treatment of the patient's ED?

2. β-Blockers are typically associated with an increased incidence of ED. Determine why nebivolol may have a lower incidence of ED and may possibly improve erectile function.

3. Discuss the possible benefits of using a PDE-5 inhibitor in patients with symptomatic benign prostatic hyperplasia (BPH).

4. Determine a treatment plan for a patient presenting with ED with a documented low testosterone concentration.

CLINICAL PEARL

The relationship between testosterone and erectile function is complicated. Testosterone plays a significant role in libido and a secondary role in erectile function by increasing nitric oxide, which leads to intracavernosal vasodilation and an erection. In men with a reduced libido and ED, testosterone supplementation may improve erectile function although additional therapies are frequently needed.

REFERENCES

1. Gandaglia G, Briganti A, Jackson G, et al. A systematic review of the association between erectile dysfunction and cardiovascular disease. Eur Urol. 2014;65(5):968–978.

2. Rosen RC, Cappelleri JC, Smith MD, Lipsky J, Pena BM. Development and evaluation of an abridged, 5-item version of the International Index of Erectile Function (IIEF-5) as a diagnostic tool for erectile dysfunction. Int J Impot Res. 1999;11(6):319–326.

3. Razdan S, Greer AB, Patel A, Alameddine M, Jue JS, Ramasamy R. Effect of prescription medications on erectile dysfunction. Postgrad Med J. 2018;94(1109):171–178.

4. Salonia A, Bettocchi C, Carvalho J, et al. European Association of Urology guidelines on sexual and reproductive health—2021 update. Available at: *https://uroweb.org/guideline/sexual-and-reproductive-health*. Accessed December 20, 2021.

5. Burnett AL, Nehra A, Breau RH, et al. Erectile dysfunction: AUA guideline. J Urol. 2018;200(3):633–641.

6. Nehra A, Jackson G, Miner M, et al. The Princeton III Consensus recommendations for the management of erectile dysfunction and cardiovascular disease. Mayo Clin Proc. 2012;87:766–778.

7. Cui T, Kovell RC, Brooks DC, Terlecki RP. A urologist's guide to ingredients found in top-selling nutraceuticals for men's sexual health. J Sex Med. 2015;12(11):2105–2117.

8. U.S. Food and Drug Administration. Consumer updates. "All natural" alternatives for erectile dysfunction: a risky proposition. Available at: *https://www.fda.gov/ForConsumers/ConsumerUpdates/ucm465024.htm*. Accessed November 14, 2021.

9. Diehm N, Borm AK, Keo HH, Wyler S. Interdisciplinary options for diagnosis and treatment of organic erectile dysfunction. Swiss Med Wkly 2015;145:1–12.

100

BENIGN PROSTATIC HYPERPLASIA

Trouble with Dribbles.......................... Level II

Kathryn Eroschenko, PharmD

Michael A. Biddle Jr., PharmD, BCPS

LEARNING OBJECTIVES

After completing this case study, the reader should be able to:

- Recognize the clinical manifestations of benign prostatic hyperplasia (BPH) and lower urinary tract symptoms (LUTS) secondary to BPH.

- Differentiate between obstructive and irritative symptoms in patients with BPH.

- Recommend appropriate pharmacotherapeutic treatment for BPH.

- Identify and manage a drug interaction associated with BPH pharmacotherapy.

- Recognize when surgical therapies should be considered for patients with BPH.

- Understand how some drugs can exacerbate BPH symptoms.

PATIENT PRESENTATION

■ Chief Complaint

"I'm up four to five times a night feeling that I have to urinate, and then when I get to the bathroom all I do is dribble. I have a girlfriend now, but I am finding it difficult to be intimate with her."

■ HPI

A 65-year-old man is being evaluated in an outpatient clinic for complaints of worsening urinary hesitancy, nocturia, and dribbling. He also has a new complaint of ED. He would like information on prescription medications to treat his urinary symptoms but is also asking about use of natural products.

■ PMH

HTN
BPH
Type 2 DM
ED
Obesity
Cat allergy (new onset)

■ FH

Educated through the 12th grade. Father died of massive MI at age 78; mother died of natural causes at age 91.

■ SH

Worked for 35 years in a grocery store; retired 7 years ago. Married once. Wife deceased 6 months ago (stroke); one daughter, two granddaughters. Lives alone but is starting to become more socially active. He recently joined a senior dating website and has started dating a 60-year-old woman. He also just adopted a 3-year-old cat from the humane society. Although he reports being allergic to cat dander, he feels that she has added happiness back into his life and uses medications to keep his allergies under control because he doesn't want to give up the cat. Used smokeless tobacco × 35 years (quit 10 years ago); heavy ETOH in the past, occasional glass of wine now.

■ ROS

In conversation, he is alert, friendly, and courteous. He has no c/o dyspepsia, dysphagia, abdominal pain, hematemesis, urinary incontinence, or visible blood in the stool.

■ Meds

Metformin 1000 mg PO BID
Rosuvastatin 20 mg PO once daily
Lisinopril 20 mg PO once daily
Claritin-D 24-hour one tablet PO daily (allergy to cats)

■ All

NKDA; allergic to cat dander

■ Physical Examination

Gen

NAD; well-kept appearance; A&O × 3

VS

BP 120/80 mm Hg, P 70 bpm, RR 18, T 37°C; Wt 254 lb, Ht 6′0″

Skin

Warm, dry with good turgor

HEENT

PERRLA; EOMI; TMs intact; nose and throat clear w/o exudate or lesions

Neck/Lymph Nodes

Supple w/o LAD or masses; thyroid in midline

Lungs/Thorax

CTA, distant sounds

CV

RRR w/o murmurs

Abd

Soft, NTND w/o masses or scars; (+) BS

Genit/Rect

Testes ↓↓, penis circumcised w/o DC; guaiac (–) stool

MS/Ext

No erythema, pain, or edema; pulses 2+

Neuro

DTRs 2+; CNs II–XII grossly intact

TABLE 100-1 | Laboratory Values

Na 136 mEq/L	Hgb 12.6 g/dL	WBC 5.6 × 10³/mm³	AST 12 IU/L	Ca 8.5 mg/dL
K 4.1 mEq/L	Hct 37.9%	Neutros 75%	ALT 16 IU/L	Phos 3.5 mg/dL
Cl 103 mEq/L	MCV 78 μm³	Lymphs 16%	Alk phos 55 IU/L	Uric acid 3.5 mg/dL
CO_2 41 mEq/L	MCH 29 pg	Monos 5%	LDH 121 IU/L	T_4 7.3 mcg/dL
BUN 9 mg/dL	MCHC 33.0 g/dL	Eos 3%	T. bili 0.6 mg/dL	TSH 1.04 mIU/L
SCr 0.7 mg/dL	Plt 191 × 10³/mm³	Basos 1%	T. prot 6.1 g/dL	A1C 7%
Glu 120 mg/dL			T. chol 146 mg/dL	PSA 4.5 ng/mL

■ Labs

See Table 100-1.

■ UA

Color straw; appearance clear; SG 1.010; pH 6.5; glucose (–); bilirubin (–); ketones (–); blood (–); urobilinogen 0.2 mg/dL; nitrite (–); leukocyte esterases (–); epithelial cells—occasional per hpf; WBC—occasional per hpf; RBC—none seen; bacteria—trace; amorphous—none seen; crystals—1+ calcium oxalate; mucus—none seen. Culture not indicated.

■ GU Consult

Urine clear; negative for glucose. Bladder examination with ultrasound revealed postvoid residual estimate of 300 mL. Prostate approximately 35 g, benign. AUA Symptom Score = 20. Uroflowmetry (Qmax) = 8 mL/sec. A 3-day urine frequency volume chart was completed and showed no polyuria.

■ Assessment

BPH
ED
HTN

Type 2 DM
Obesity
Cat allergy (recent onset with adoption of new cat)

QUESTIONS

Collect Information

1.a. What subjective and objective information is consistent with the presence of BPH?

1.b. What additional information is needed to fully assess this patient's BPH (Figure 100-1)?

Assess the Information

2.a. Assess the severity of BPH based on the subjective and objective information available.

2.b. Create a list of the patient's drug therapy problems and prioritize them. Include assessment of medication appropriateness, effectiveness, safety, and patient adherence.

Patient Name: _____ DOB: _____ ID: _____ Date of assessment: _____

Initial Assessment ( ) Monitor during: _____ Therapy ( ) after: _____ Therapy/surgery ( ) _____

AUA BPH Symptom Score

	Not at all	Less than 1 time in 5	Less than half the time	About half the time	More than half the time	Almost always	
1. Over the past month, how often have you had a sensation of not emptying your bladder completely after you finished urinating?	0	1	2	3	4	5	
2. Over the past month, how often have you had to urinate again less than two hours after you finished urinating?	0	1	2	3	4	5	
3. Over the past month, how often have you found you stopped and started again several times when you urinated?	0	1	2	3	4	5	
4. Over the past month, how often have you found it difficult to postpone urination?	0	1	2	3	4	5	
5. Over the past month, how often have you had a weak urinary stream?	0	1	2	3	4	5	
6. Over the past month, how often have you had to push or strain to begin urination?	0	1	2	3	4	5	
	None	1 time	2 times	3 times	4 times	5 or more times	
7. Over the past month, how many times did you most typically get up to urinate from the time you went to bed at night until the time you got up in the morning?	0	1	2	3	4	5	
						Total Symptom Score	

FIGURE 100-1. The American Urologic Association (AUA) symptom index for benign prostatic hyperplasia (BPH). (Reproduced with permission from Barry MJ, Fowler FJ Jr, O'Leary MP, et al. The American Urological Association symptom index for benign prostatic hyperplasia. The Measurement Committee of the American Urological Association. *J Urol.* 1992;148(5):1549-1564.)

Develop a Care Plan

3.a. What are the goals of pharmacotherapy for BPH in this case?

3.b. What nondrug therapies might be useful for this patient's BPH?

3.c. What feasible pharmacotherapeutic options are available for treating BPH?

3.d. Create an individualized, patient-centered, team-based care plan to optimize medication therapy for BPH and other drug therapy problems. Include specific drugs, dosage forms, doses, schedules, and durations of therapy.

Implement the Care Plan

4.a. What information should be provided to the patient to enhance adherence, ensure successful therapy, and minimize adverse effects?

4.b. Describe how care should be coordinated with other healthcare providers.

Follow-Up: Monitor and Evaluate

5. Explain how to monitor and evaluate the care plan for medication appropriateness, effectiveness, safety, and patient adherence by using clinical and laboratory data, patient feedback, and other information.

■ CLINICAL COURSE: ALTERNATIVE THERAPY

You perform a literature search on the use of saw palmetto for BPH. You discover that there are reports of the dietary supplement both improving and worsening symptoms of ED. In addition, your readings indicate that saw palmetto should really only be used by patients with mild to moderate BPH. Based on this information, you do not recommend use of saw palmetto for the patient's BPH symptoms. However, because the patient is requesting information on natural products, you search for alternative dietary supplements that may provide some benefit for this patient's BPH without contributing to ED. Would *Pygeum africanum* be a reasonable option to consider? For questions related to the use of *P. africanum* for the treatment of BPH, please see Section 19 of this Casebook.

■ CLINICAL COURSE

After your recommendations were implemented, the patient's BPH and ED symptoms improved remarkably. Over the ensuing weeks, he continued to experience occasional urgency and hesitancy. After 6 months of watchful waiting, he opted for laser prostatectomy. This procedure was successful in alleviating his symptoms.

■ SELF-STUDY ASSIGNMENTS

1. Compare the efficacy of saw palmetto (*Serenoa repens*) to finasteride and α1-antagonists for the treatment of BPH.

2. Compare treatment options for ED in patients with BPH. Identify the risks and potential benefits of using α1-antagonists and 5α-reductase inhibitors in treating comorbid ED and BPH.

3. Identify the BPH patient subpopulation that would benefit most from finasteride/dutasteride therapy.

4. Perform a literature search for evidence that supports use of phosphodiesterase type 5 inhibitors and α1-antagonists as combination therapy for BPH/ED.

5. Perform a literature search for the use of phosphodiesterase type 5 inhibitors as monotherapy for LUTS secondary to BPH.

CLINICAL PEARL

Shared decision-making between patient and provider is encouraged to determine the best pharmacotherapy plan for each patient. Watchful waiting is also an option if patients are hesitant to start drug therapy when symptoms are minimal and do not affect the quality of their daily lives.

REFERENCES

1. McVary KT, Roehrborn CG, Avins AL, et al. Update on AUA guideline on the management of benign prostatic hyperplasia. J Urol. 2011;185(5):1793–1803.

2. Miner M, Rosenberg MT, Perelman MA. Treatment of lower urinary tract symptoms in benign prostatic hyperplasia and its impact on sexual function. Clin Ther. 2006;28:13–25.

3. Kaminetsky JC. Comorbid LUTS and erectile dysfunction: optimizing their management. Curr Med Res Opin. 2006;22:2407–2506.

4. Hollingsworth J, Wilt T. Lower urinary tract symptoms in men. BMJ 2014;349:g4474. doi:10.1136/bmj.g4474.

5. Narayan P, Evans CP, Moon T. Long-term safety and efficacy of tamsulosin for the treatment of lower urinary tract symptoms associated with benign prostatic hyperplasia. J Urol. 2003;170(Pt 1):498–502.

6. Sarma AV, Wei JT. Clinical practice. Benign prostatic hyperplasia and lower urinary tract symptoms. N Engl J Med. 2012;19:367(3):248–257.

7. Greco KA, McVary KT. The role of combination medical therapy in benign prostatic hyperplasia. Int J Impot Res. 2008;20(Suppl 3):S33–S43.

8. Van Asseldonk B, Barkin J, Elterman D. Medical therapy for benign prostatic hyperplasia: a review. Can J Urol. 2015;22(Suppl 1):7–17.

9. Donatucci CF, Brock GB, Goldfischer ER, et al. Tadalafil administered once daily for lower urinary tract symptoms secondary to benign prostatic hyperplasia: a 1-year, open-label extension study. BJU Int. 2011;107(7):1110–1116.

10. Tacklind J, MacDonald R, Rutks I, Stanke JU, Wilt TJ. *Serenoa repens* for benign prostatic hyperplasia. Cochrane Database Syst Rev. 2012 (Dec 12);12:CD001423.

101

URINARY INCONTINENCE

Getting In and Out of Bed .... Level II

Mary W. L. Lee, PharmD, BCPS, FCCP

Roohollah R. Sharifi, MD, FACS

LEARNING OBJECTIVES

After completing this case study, the reader should be able to:

• Distinguish the symptoms of overactive bladder syndrome from those of stress urinary incontinence.

• Recommend appropriate nondrug therapy for managing overactive bladder syndrome.

• Explain how concomitant medications may exacerbate symptoms of overactive bladder syndrome.

• Compare and contrast the efficacy and adverse effects of antimuscarinic medications and β3-adrenergic agonists when used for overactive bladder syndrome.

- Compare and contrast muscarinic receptor selectivity, lipophilicity, and pharmacokinetic properties of commonly used antimuscarinic agents for managing overactive bladder syndrome and discuss the clinical implications of these properties.

PATIENT PRESENTATION

■ Chief Complaint

"I can't seem to control my urine. I feel like I have to urinate all the time. However, when I do go to the bathroom, I pass only a small amount of urine. Sometimes I wet myself. I was started on a medication for my leaking a few weeks ago, but it doesn't seem to be working. I also can't seem to remember anything. It is a wonder that I remembered to come to the clinic today. My daughter seems to spend more and more time taking care of me because I am too forgetful."

■ HPI

A 65-year-old woman with urinary urgency, frequency, and incontinence presents to the urology clinic for a follow-up visit. She reports soiling her underwear at least two to three times during the day and night and has resorted to wearing panty liners or disposable underwear. Urinary leakage is not worsened by laughing, coughing, sneezing, carrying heavy objects, or walking up and down stairs. She does not report wetting herself without warning. She has been taking oxybutynin extended-release 15 mg PO BID for the past month with no improvement in her voiding symptoms, and she complains of new-onset confusion and difficulty remembering routine tasks.

The patient is accompanied by her daughter, who confirms that the patient's confusion seems to have started shortly after oxybutynin was started. The patient cannot remember what day it is and can no longer tell time. Also, the patient gets out of bed at night many times to void, and the family is worried that she will fall and hurt herself. The daughter implores the clinician to initiate a more effective treatment for her mother.

■ PMH

HTN for many years, treated with medications for 10 years
Dyslipidemia for 5 years, controlled with a low-cholesterol diet, weight control, regular exercise, and medication
Postmenopausal; stopped ovulating at age 52
Mild Parkinson disease for the past 5 years treated with amantadine without adverse effects
Has difficulty falling asleep and often has sleepless nights; takes a sedative most nights
No history of spinal or pelvic surgery

■ FH

Noncontributory

■ SH

Nonsmoker; social drinker; married, but husband is not involved with her care

■ Meds

Hydrochlorothiazide 25 mg PO once daily with supper
Irbesartan 300 mg PO daily
Pravastatin 40 mg PO at bedtime
Oxybutynin extended-release 15 mg PO BID
Diphenhydramine 25–50 mg PO at bedtime as needed, usually about five times a week
Amantadine extended-release 274 mg PO once daily at bedtime

■ All

NKDA

■ Physical Examination

Gen
WDWN woman

VS
BP 170/94 mm Hg, P 90 bpm, RR 16, T 37°C; Wt 70 kg, Ht 5'2"

Skin
No rashes, wounds, or open sores

HEENT
PERRLA; EOMI; no AV nicking or hemorrhages

Neck/Lymph Nodes
No palpable thyroid masses; no lymphadenopathy

Pulm
Clear to A&P

Breasts
Normal; no lumps

CV
Regular S_1, S_2; (+) S_4; (−) S_3, murmurs, or rubs

Abd
Soft, NTND, (+) bowel sounds

Genit/Rect
Genital examination shows atrophic vaginitis consistent with postmenopausal status. Perineal sensation and anal sphincter tone are normal.
Pelvic examination shows no uterine prolapse and a mild degree of cystocele. Cervix is normal. No pelvic, adnexal, or uterine masses found.
External hemorrhoids; heme (−) stool.

Ext
Normal; equal motor strength in both arms and legs

Neuro
Although alert, the patient is not oriented to correct month, day, or year. CNs II–XII grossly intact; DTRs 3/5 bilaterally; negative Babinski. When asked to recall a series of five objects after 5 minutes, the patient had difficulty and could only recall one object.

■ Labs

Na 140 mEq/L	Hgb 12 g/dL
K 4.2 mEq/L	Hct 37%
Cl 105 mEq/L	Plt 400 × 10³/mm³
CO_2 28 mEq/L	WBC 5.0 × 10³/mm³
BUN 17 mg/dL	
SCr 1.2 mg/dL	
Glu 100 mg/dL	

▪ UA

No bacteria; no WBC

▪ Other

Using an ultrasonic bladder scan, a residual urine volume was measured after the patient voided. No residual urine was found. The bladder was then filled with 300 mL saline. The patient felt the first desire to void at 100 mL. The catheter was removed. The patient was asked to cough in different positions. No stress urinary incontinence was demonstrated. The patient voided the entire volume of saline that was instilled.

▪ Assessment

Overactive bladder with symptoms of urinary urgency, frequency, and incontinence, which has not responded to oxybutynin extended-release 15 mg PO BID for 1 month. Patient is also having new-onset confusion and forgetfulness, temporally related to starting oxybutynin. The central nervous system adverse effects of oxybutynin are worsened by concomitant use of diphenhydramine, but probably not amantadine. Will evaluate carefully and consider alternative medication options.

QUESTIONS

Collect Information

1.a. What subjective and objective information indicates the presence of urge incontinence?

1.b. What additional information is needed to fully assess this patient?

Assess the Information

2.a. Assess the severity of incontinence based on the subjective and objective information available.

2.b. Create a list of the patient's drug therapy problems and prioritize them. Include assessment of medication appropriateness, effectiveness, safety, and patient adherence.

Develop a Care Plan

3.a. What are the goals of pharmacotherapy in this case?

3.b. What nondrug therapies might be useful for this patient?

3.c. What oral pharmacotherapeutic options are available for treating overactive bladder?

3.d. Create an individualized, patient-centered, team-based care plan to optimize medication therapy for this patient's urinary incontinence and other drug therapy problems. Include specific drugs, dosage forms, doses, schedules, and durations of therapy.

▪ CLINICAL COURSE

The physician stopped oxybutynin and started solifenacin 5 mg PO daily, and the patient returned to the clinic 3 weeks later. Although her confusion and forgetfulness are somewhat improved, the daughter states that her mother's memory is still poor and her symptoms of overactive bladder syndrome seem to have worsened. The patient complains of multiple episodes of nocturia that disturb her sleep. She says that she cannot tolerate this and wants different drug treatment.

Implement the Care Plan

4.a. What information should be provided to the patient to enhance adherence, ensure successful therapy, and minimize adverse effects of solifenacin?

4.b. Describe how care should be coordinated with other healthcare providers.

Follow-Up: Monitor and Evaluate

5. Explain how to monitor and evaluate the care plan for medication appropriateness, effectiveness, safety, and patient adherence by using clinical and laboratory data, patient feedback, and other information.

▪ FOLLOW-UP QUESTION

1. The clinician discontinued solifenacin and started mirabegron. Discuss the potential benefits and risks of mirabegron for this patient.

▪ SELF-STUDY ASSIGNMENTS

1. Patients have been classified as extensive versus poor metabolizers of tolterodine. Describe the characteristics of these patients and the clinical implications of this patient classification.

2. Mirabegron and antimuscarinic agents have been used in combination to treat overactive bladder syndrome. What are the advantages and disadvantages of combination therapy?

3. Mirabegron and vibegron are considered to have comparable effectiveness for management of overactive bladder syndrome. When might vibegron be preferred over mirabegron?

CLINICAL PEARL

A uroselective antimuscarinic agent generally exerts systemic clinical effects. Although inhibition of M_3 receptors will cause bladder relaxation and decrease involuntary detrusor contractions, M_3 receptors are also located in the colon and salivary glands. Therefore, antagonism of M_3 receptors may relieve overactive bladder symptoms but may also produce dose-related antimuscarinic adverse effects such as constipation and dry mouth.

REFERENCES

1. Raju R, Linder BJ. Evaluation and treatment of overactive bladder in women. Mayo Clin Proc. 2020;95(2):370–377.

2. Nambiar AK, Bosch R, Cruz F, et al. EAU guidelines on assessment and nonsurgical management of urinary incontinence. Eur Urol. 2018;73(4):596–609.

3. Shaw C, Wagg A. Overactive bladder in frail adults. Drugs Aging. 2020;37(8):559–565.

4. Yamada S, Ito Y, Nishijima S, Kadekawa K, Sugaya K. Basic and clinical aspects of antimuscarinic agents used to treat overactive bladder. Pharmacol Ther. 2018;189:130–148.

5. Mostafaei H, Shariat SF, Salehi-Pourmehr H, et al. The clinical pharmacology of the medical treatment for overactive bladder in adults. Expert Rev Clin Pharmacol. 2020;13(7):707–720.

6. Araklitis G, Robinson D, Cardozo L. Cognitive effects of anticholinergic load in women with overactive bladder. Clin Interv Aging. 2020;15:1493–1503.

7. Deeks ED. Mirabegron: a review in overactive bladder syndrome. Drugs. 2018;78(8):833–844.

8. Wani MS, Sheikh MI, Bhat T, Bhat Z, Bhat A. Comparison of antimuscarinic drugs to beta adrenergic agonists in overactive bladder: a literary review. Curr Urol. 2021;15(3):153–160.

9. Lightner DJ, Gomelsky A, Souter L, Vasavada SP. Diagnosis and treatment of overactive bladder (non-neurogenic) in adults: AUA/SUFU Guideline Amendment 2019. J Urol. 2019;202(3):558–563.

10. Sahai A, Belal M, Hamid R, Tooz-Hobson P, Granitsiotis P, Robinson D. Shifting the treatment paradigm in idiopathic overactive bladder. Int J Clin Pract. 2021;75(14):e13847. doi: 10.1111/ijcp.13847. Epub Jan 21, 2021.

102

SYSTEMIC LUPUS ERYTHEMATOSUS

Sometimes, It's Lupus......................... Level II

Nicole Paolini Albanese, PharmD, CDE, BCACP

LEARNING OBJECTIVES

After completing this case study, the reader should be able to:

- Discuss the clinical presentation of SLE, including its complications.

- Design appropriate therapy for the treatment of SLE and the complications of antiphospholipid syndrome (APS) and iron deficiency anemia.

- Construct a monitoring plan for SLE, including disease activity, drug efficacy, and drug toxicity.

- Recommend appropriate therapy for the treatment of SLE during pregnancy.

PATIENT PRESENTATION

■ Chief Complaint

"My knees are killing me, I'm tired all the time, and I've got horrible pain in my stomach."

■ HPI

A 32-year-old woman reports having knee pain on and off for about 2 years. She has been to the doctor a few times since then with the same complaint. Workups showed no radiologic changes to the knees, and the doctor settled on a diagnosis of early arthritis. She was not evaluated by a rheumatologist. Despite scheduled APAP and ibuprofen throughout the day, the pain has not decreased much. The pain seems to be cyclical; it is very bad for a period of weeks, and then it wanes over time. It is also worse in the summer. She reports this pain in both knees as well as occasional swelling. No matter how much sleep she gets, it does not seem to be enough; a couple of sleep medications later, she is no better than before she tried them. She has also noticed a darkening of her stool over the past couple of months.

■ PMH

Knee pain × 2 years
HTN × 1 year
Fatigue × 1 year

■ FH

Father alive in his mid-60s; has HTN and dyslipidemia. Mother alive in her mid-60s; has asthma and seasonal allergies.

■ SH

Employed as a travel agent; married 5 years; occasional EtOH use and no current or past tobacco use. On inquiry, patient reports that she and her husband are trying to conceive.

■ Meds

Hydrochlorothiazide 12.5 mg PO once daily
Amlodipine 5 mg PO once daily
Ibuprofen 800 mg PO four times daily
Acetaminophen 500 mg PO three times daily
Past meds: Zolpidem 10 mg PO at bedtime and ramelteon 8 mg PO at bedtime (stopped using both after inefficacy)

■ All

NKDA

■ ROS

(+) Fatigue; (−) rash, fever, chills, peripheral edema, or alopecia

■ Physical Examination

Gen

Tired-looking woman in moderate pain.
Pain scale: Presently 6/10; per patient, her worst pain is 10/10; her best score is 0/10.

VS

BP 136/82 mm Hg, P 74 bpm, RR 17, T 38°C, Wt 59 kg, Ht 5′4″

Skin

Warm; moist to touch

HEENT

PERRLA; EOMI

Neck/Lymph Nodes

Supple without adenopathy

Lungs/Thorax

CTA; no rales/rhonchi

CV

RRR; S$_1$ and S$_2$ normal

Abd

Tender, nondistended; (+) bowel sounds; (+) stool guaiac

Ext

Peripheral pulses intact; no edema

Joint examination: (+) synovitis of the knees bilaterally; (−) bony proliferation, crepitus, muscle atrophy, or deformities; no limitations on range of motion

Neuro

A&O × 3; CN II–XII intact; Babinski negative

■ Labs

Na 136 mEq/L	RBC 3.2 10^6/mm³	ESR 66 mm/hr
K 4.7 mEq/L	Hgb 11.0 g/dL	RF titer 1:40
Cl 105 mEq/L	Hct 25%	Anti-CCP antibody (−)
CO_2 25 mEq/L	MCV 78 fL	ANA titer 1:320 (rim pattern)
BUN 13 mg/dL	WBC 7.2 × 10³/mm³	C3 50 mg/dL
SCr 0.8 mg/dL	Plt 250 × 10³/mm³	C4 10 mg/dL
Uric acid 5.5 mg/dL	Fe 35 mcg/dL	Lupus anticoagulant (+)
Glucose 82 mg/dL	TIBC 455 mcg/dL	Anticardiolipin Ab (+)
	Ferritin 8 ng/mL	dsDNA Ab (+)

■ UA

(−) WBC, RBC, RBC casts; (+) microalbuminuria; (−) protein

■ Radiologic Joint Evaluation

(−) Patellar or tibial fracture, (−) displacement, (−) fragments, (−) ligament damage, no evident soft tissue damage

■ Assessment

Mild SLE with biomarkers for APS; iron deficiency anemia possibly secondary to NSAID use.

QUESTIONS

Collect Information

1.a. What subjective and objective information indicates the presence of SLE?

1.b. What additional information is needed to fully assess this patient's SLE?

Assess the Information

2.a. Assess the severity of SLE based on the subjective and objective information available.

2.b. Create a list of the patient's drug therapy problems and prioritize them. Include assessment of medication appropriateness, effectiveness, safety, and patient adherence.

Develop a Care Plan

3.a. What are the goals of pharmacotherapy for SLE with APS in this patient?

3.b. What nondrug therapies might be useful for treating SLE?

3.c. What feasible pharmacotherapeutic options are available for treating SLE in this patient?

3.d. Create an individualized, patient-centered, team-based care plan to optimize medication therapy for this patient's SLE and other drug therapy problems. Include specific drugs, dosage forms, doses, schedules, and durations of therapy.

Implement the Care Plan

4.a. What information should be provided to the patient to enhance adherence, minimize relapses, ensure successful therapy, and minimize adverse effects?

4.b. Describe how care should be coordinated with other healthcare providers.

Follow-Up: Monitor and Evaluate

5. Explain how to monitor and evaluate the care plan for medication appropriateness, effectiveness, safety, and patient adherence by using clinical and laboratory data, patient feedback, and other information.

■ FOLLOW-UP QUESTIONS

1. What can this patient do to increase the chances of having a successful pregnancy?

■ SELF-STUDY ASSIGNMENTS

1. How do B-lymphocyte stimulator antagonists work, and what is their role in the pharmacotherapy of SLE?

CLINICAL PEARL

Because UV light exacerbates SLE, drugs that induce photosensitivity should be avoided in patients with the disease.

REFERENCES

1. Lam NC, Ghetu MV, Bieniek ML. Systemic lupus erythematosus: primary care approach to diagnosis and management. Am Fam Physician. 2016;94(4):284–294.

2. Lewis MJ, Jawad AS. The effect of ethnicity and genetic ancestry on the epidemiology, clinical features and outcome of systemic lupus erythematosus. Rheumatology 2017;56(Suppl 1):i67–i77.

3. Kiriakidou, M, Ching, CL. Systemic lupus erythematosus. Ann Intern Med. 2020;172(11):ITC81–ITC96.

4. Petri M, Orbai AM, Alarcón GS, et al. Derivation and validation of the Systemic Lupus International Collaborating Clinics classification criteria for systemic lupus erythematosus. Arthritis Rheum. 2012;64(8):2677–2686.

5. Thong B, Olsen NJ. Systemic lupus erythematosus diagnosis and management. Rheumatology (Oxford) 2017;56(Suppl 1):i3–i13.

6. DeLoughery, TG, Iron deficiency anemia. Med Clin North Am. 2017;101(2):319–332.

7. Vreede AP, Bockenstedt PL, Knight JS. Antiphospholipid syndrome: an update for clinicians and scientists. Curr Opin Rheumatol. 2017;29(5):458–466.

8. Schreiber K, Hunt BJ. Managing antiphospholipid syndrome in pregnancy. Thromb Res. 2019;181(Suppl 1):S41–S46.

9. Resman-Targoff BH. Systemic lupus erythematosus. In: DiPiro JT, Yee GC, Posey L, eds. Pharmacotherapy: A Pathophysiologic Approach, 11th edition. McGraw Hill; 2020. Available at: *http://www.accesspharmacy.com*. Accessed October 28, 2021.

10. Whelton PK, Carey RM, Aronow WS, et al. 2017 ACC/AHA/AAPA/ABC/ACPM/AGS/APhA/ASH/ASPC/NMA/PCNA guideline for the prevention, detection, evaluation, and management of high blood pressure in adults. A Report of the American College of Cardiology/American Heart Association Task Force on Clinical Practice Guidelines. Hypertension. 2018;71(6):1269–1324.

103

ALLERGIC DRUG REACTION

Return of the 3-Day Itch .... Level II

Sheila K. Wang, PharmD, BCPS, BCIDP

LEARNING OBJECTIVES

After completing this case study, the reader should be able to:

- Interpret drug allergy information (eg, timing of the reaction, signs, and symptoms) to identify the likelihood of an IgE-mediated reaction.

- Assess the potential for cross-reactivity between penicillins and carbapenems.

- Differentiate desensitization from graded challenge dosing procedures and identify patients who are appropriate candidates for each procedure.

- Select appropriate antibiotic therapy for a patient with multiple antibiotic allergies.

PATIENT PRESENTATION

■ Chief Complaint

"My cough is back and I feel like I did when I was admitted three weeks ago."

■ HPI

A 55-year-old man with a history of COPD who is an inpatient on the general medicine service at an academic medical center presented nearly 3 weeks ago to the ED complaining of a 3-day history of tiredness and cough productive of greenish sputum. He has had four admissions this year for COPD and pneumonia. Sputum cultures at that time revealed *Pseudomonas aeruginosa* susceptible to amikacin, aztreonam, cefepime, and meropenem; intermediate to piperacillin–tazobactam, gentamicin, tobramycin, and ciprofloxacin; and resistant to levofloxacin. Due to his multiple antibiotic allergies, the patient underwent desensitization to cefepime. He was subsequently treated as an inpatient for 7 days with IV cefepime without incident. He has remained an inpatient for continued COPD management. Received prednisone 40 mg PO once daily × 5 days starting on admission.

■ PMH

COPD × 17 years
Received pneumococcal vaccine (PPSV23) and annual influenza vaccine
Chronic empyema secondary to bronchial pleural fistulae with chest tube placement 7 months ago
HTN × 10 years
S/P MI 15 years ago

■ SH

Lives with his mother; he is unemployed. He has a 40 pack-year smoking history. Admits to occasional alcohol use; denies use of recreational drugs.

■ Meds

Albuterol MDI two puffs Q 6 H PRN
Ipratropium MDI two puffs Q 6 H
Aspirin 81 mg PO once daily
Amlodipine 10 mg PO once daily
Atorvastatin 40 mg PO once daily (FLP 1 year ago: TC 142, LDL 67, HDL 46, TG 145)

■ All

Ampicillin–sulbactam: facial edema, tongue swelling, and periorbital edema
Ceftazidime: urticarial rash on chest and face with shortness of breath
Codeine: nausea, pruritus

■ ROS

(+) Fatigue, fever, sore throat, shortness of breath, and cough with thick sputum; (–) nausea, vomiting, diarrhea, chills, or chest pain

■ Physical Examination

Gen

A 55-year-old man appearing older than his stated age in moderate respiratory distress. He is lethargic and hard of hearing.

VS

BP 100/60 mm Hg, P 85 bpm, RR 16, T 39°C; Wt 52 kg, Ht 5′5″

Skin

Dry scaly skin; no tenting

HEENT

PERRLA, EOM intact, dry mucous membranes, difficulty hearing L > R

Neck/Lymph Nodes

(–) Bruits, (–) lymphadenopathy

Lungs/Thorax

(+) Diffuse crackles at the left base; wheezes throughout with poor breath sounds

CV

Normal S_1 and S_2, RRR, (–) MRG

Abd

Distended with (+) bowel sounds; (–) hepatosplenomegaly

Ext

(+) Clubbing; (–) cyanosis or edema; poor muscle tone

Neuro

Alert, oriented, and cooperative. CNs II–XII are intact. Tone and strength are 4/5 in both arms, and 4/5 in both legs. Sensory exam is normal. Reflexes are 2+ in UE and 3+ in LEs.

■ Labs

Na 137 mEq/L	Hgb 14.8 g/dL	WBC 17 × 10³/mm³
K 3.7 mEq/L	Hct 44.6%	Neutros 72%
Cl 96 mEq/L	RBC 5.36 × 10⁶/mm³	Bands 5%
CO₂ 29 mEq/L	Plt 244 × 10³/mm³	Eos 4%
BUN 22 mg/dL	MCV 83.2 μm³	Lymphs 11%
SCr 1.0 mg/dL	MCHC 33.2 g/dL	Monos 8%
Glu 119 mg/dL		Basos 0%

■ **ABG**

pH 7.44, PaO$_2$ 55 mm Hg, PaCO$_2$ 38 mm Hg, O$_2$ sat 90%

■ **Chest X-Ray**

Haziness in the left lower lobe

■ **Sputum Gram Stain**

Pending

■ **Sputum Cultures**

Pending

■ **Blood Cultures**

Pending

■ **Assessment**

1. HAP
2. COPD
3. HTN
4. S/P MI

QUESTIONS

Collect Information

1.a. What subjective and objective information indicates the presence of an allergic drug reaction?

1.b. What additional information would be helpful to fully assess the patient's risk of hypersensitivity reactions to β-lactam antibiotics?

1.c. What additional information would be helpful to assess whether the patient experiences true hypersensitivity versus pseudo allergy to codeine?

Assess the Information

2.a. Based on the patient's allergy history, how should his allergies to ampicillin–sulbactam and ceftazidime be categorized—as low-risk, medium-risk, or high-risk reactions?

2.b. Create a list of the patient's drug therapy problems and prioritize them. Include assessment of medication appropriateness, effectiveness, safety, and patient adherence.

Develop a Care Plan

3.a. What are the goals for treating pneumonia in this case?

■ CLINICAL COURSE

The patient is started on standing DuoNeb (albuterol 3 mg/3 mL and ipratropium 0.5 mg/3 mL) by nebulizer 3 mL Q 2 H, guaifenesin with codeine (100 mg/10 mg/5 mL) PO Q 4 H PRN, and

TABLE 103-2	Initial Empiric Treatment for HAP in Patients with Risk Factors for Drug-Resistant Pathogens and Receipt of Intravenous Antibiotics During the Previous 90 Days[a]

Two of the following, avoiding two β-lactams:

β-Lactam/β-lactamase inhibitor
   Piperacillin-tazobactam 4.5 g IV Q 6 H
Or antipseudomonal cephalosporin
   Cefepime 2 g IV Q 8 H
   Ceftazidime 2 g IV Q 8 H
Or antipseudomonal fluoroquinolone
   Levofloxacin 750 mg IV daily
   Ciprofloxacin 400 mg IV Q 8 H
Or antipseudomonal carbapenem
   Imipenem 500 mg IV Q 6 H
   Meropenem 1 g IV Q 8 H
Or aminoglycoside
   Amikacin 15–20 mg/kg IV daily
   Gentamicin 5–7 mg/kg IV daily
   Tobramycin 5–7 mg/kg IV daily
Or monocyclic β-lactam (monobactam)
   Aztreonam 2 g Q 8 H[b]
PLUS
Vancomycin 15 mg/kg IV Q 8–12 H with target trough level of 15–20 mcg/mL
Or
Linezolid 600 mg IV Q 12 H

HAP, hospital-acquired pneumonia.
[a]Kalil AC, Metersky ML, Klompas M, et al. Management of adults with hospital-acquired and ventilator-associated pneumonia: 2016 Clinical Practice Guidelines by the Infectious Diseases Society of American and the American Thoracic Society. Clin Infect Dis. 2016;63(5):e61–e111.
[b]If patient has severe penicillin allergy and aztreonam will be used instead of any β-lactam antibiotic, include coverage for methicillin-sensitive Staphylococcus aureus (MSSA).

acetaminophen 325–650 mg PO Q 4 H PRN. While cultures are pending, the team reviews the hospital course to date, the culture and susceptibilities obtained 3 weeks ago, the facility-wide antibiogram (Table 103-1), and the hospital guideline for treating HAP. As a result, empiric therapy is initiated with meropenem 1 g IV Q 8 H, amikacin 15 mg/kg IV daily, and vancomycin 1 g IV Q 12 H. The medical team discusses the appropriateness of starting meropenem in this patient.

3.b. The initial empiric regimens recommended for hospital-acquired pneumonia (HAP) are summarized in Table 103-2. Both cefepime and aztreonam are alternatives to meropenem in these multidrug regimens. Based on this patient's history, are cefepime and aztreonam safe alternatives to meropenem for empiric therapy of HAP? (See Fig. 103-1 for the chemical structures of cefepime and ceftazidime.)

3.c. If a multidrug regimen including cefepime was chosen for empiric therapy, would this patient require another course of desensitization prior to initiating full-dose cefepime therapy?

3.d. Assess the risk of a hypersensitivity cross-reaction to meropenem in this patient. Based on your review of the literature, determine which of the following courses of action is best: (a) initiation of full-dose meropenem therapy; (b) desensitization to meropenem prior to initiating full treatment doses; or (c) graded challenge dosing of meropenem prior to initiating full treatment

TABLE 103-1	Facility-wide Antibiogram with Percentage of Isolates Susceptible to Associated Pathogens

Organism	Amik	Aztr	Cefe	Cipr	Mero	Oxac	Pip-Taz	Tobr	Vanc
E.coli	99	88	88	74	100		93	89	
K. pneumoniae	99	87	87	90	98		90	90	
P. aeruginosa	97	76	91	86	90		88	96	
S. aureus						66			100

Amik, amikacin; Aztr, aztreonam; Cefe, cefepime; Cipr, ciprofloxacin; Mero, meropenem, Oxac, oxacillin, Pip-Taz, piperacillin-tazobactam; Tobr, tobramycin; Vanc, vancomycin

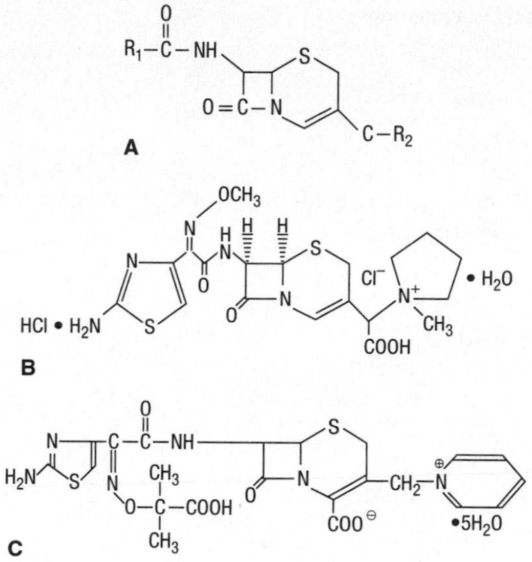

FIGURE 103-1. Chemical structures of cefepime and ceftazidime. *A.* Basic cephalosporin structure. *B.* Cefepime. *C.* Ceftazidime.

doses. Substantiate your position on the most appropriate course of action based on evidence from the literature.

Implement the Care Plan

4.a. What information should be provided to the patient about his drug allergies to minimize allergic events in the future?

4.b. Describe how care should be coordinated with other healthcare providers.

Follow-Up: Monitor and Evaluate

5. Explain how to monitor and evaluate the care plan for medication appropriateness, effectiveness, safety, and patient adherence by using clinical and laboratory data, patient feedback, and other information.

■ SELF-STUDY ASSIGNMENTS

1. Define the following terms: CAP, HAP, and VAP. Differentiate the initial empiric regimens for each of these types of pneumonia.

2. Develop a care map for patients allergic to penicillin for whom a carbapenem is ordered. Outline the process by which the clinician would determine the most appropriate course of action for these patients. Be specific as to the type of allergy to the penicillin (ie, maculopapular rash vs Stevens–Johnson syndrome vs anaphylactic reaction).

3. Apply the concepts of graded challenge dosing and desensitization (see the section "Clinical Pearl") to the issue of β-lactam hypersensitivity. Develop criteria describing those patients with history of β-lactam hypersensitivity who would be appropriate candidates for graded challenge dosing versus desensitization to structurally related antibiotics.

CLINICAL PEARL

A graded challenge dose (test dosing) involves the cautious administration of a medication to a patient. Graded challenge doses are often recommended for patients who have history of hypersensitivity to a structurally-related medication and the risk of a cross-reaction is

deemed unlikely. Unlike desensitization, graded challenge dosing is higher and typically limited to two or three steps in the dosing process (starting dose 1/10th to 1/100th of final treatment dose) and does not temporarily alter the body's immune response to an antigenic medication. Therefore, tolerance of the drug after a graded challenge procedure indicates the patient is not allergic to it.

ACKNOWLEDGMENT

This case is based on the patient case written for the 11th edition by Lynne M. Sylvia, PharmD.

REFERENCES

1. Shenoy ES, Macy E, Rowe T, Blumenthal KG. Evaluation and management of penicillin allergy: a review. JAMA. 2019;321(2):188–199.
2. Solensky R, Khan DA. Drug allergy: an updated practice parameter. Ann Allergy Asthma Immunol. 2010;105:273.e1–e78.
3. Bland CM, Brookstaver PB, Griffith NC, et al. A practical guide for pharmacists to successfully implement penicillin allergy skin testing. Am J Health-Syst Pharm. 2019;76(3):136–147.
4. Macy E, Blumenthal KG. Are cephalosporins safe for use in penicillin allergy without prior allergy evaluation? J Allergy Clin Immunol Pract. 2018;6(1):82–89.
5. Romano A, Gaeta F, Arribas Poves MF, Valluzzi RL. Cross-reactivity among beta-lactams. Curr Allergy Asthma Rep. 2016;16:24.
6. Lieberman P, Nicklas RA, Randolph C, et al. Anaphylaxis—a practice parameter update 2015. Ann Allergy Asthma Immunol. 2015;115:341–384.
7. Picard M, Robitaille G, Karam F, et al. Cross-reactivity to cephalosporins and carbapenems in penicillin-allergic patients: two systematic reviews and meta-analyses. J Allergy Clin Immunol Pract. 2019;7(8):2722–2738.
8. Caruso C, Valluzzi RL, Colantuono S, Gaeta F, Romano A. β-lactam allergy and cross-reactivity: a clinician's guide to selecting an alternative antibiotic. J Asthma Allergy. 2021;14:31–46.
9. Gaeta F, Valluzzi RL, Alonzi C, Maggioletti M, Caruso C, Romano A. Tolerability of aztreonam and carbapenems in patients with IgE-mediated hypersensitivity to penicillins. J Allergy Clin Immunol. 2015;135:972–976.
10. Wilson DL, Owens RC, Zuckerman JB. Successful meropenem desensitization in a patient with cystic fibrosis. Ann Pharmacother. 2003;37:1424–1428.

104

SOLID ORGAN TRANSPLANTATION

Kidney—Don't Fail Me Now! . . . . Level III

Kristine S. Schonder, PharmD

LEARNING OBJECTIVES

After completing this case study, the reader should be able to:

• Develop a patient-specific care plan for acute cellular rejection following solid organ transplantation.

- Assess a transplant medication regimen for potential drug interactions and develop a plan to resolve any identified interactions.
- Describe possible adverse effects of immunosuppressive medications and prophylactic medications for solid organ transplant recipients and develop a plan to resolve these effects.
- Counsel a transplant recipient on the importance of medication adherence and implement strategies to enhance adherence.

PATIENT PRESENTATION

■ Chief Complaint
"I have pain over my kidney transplant, my legs are swollen, and my urine output is decreased."

■ HPI
A 48-year-old woman presents to the renal transplant clinic for evaluation of the above complaints. She states the symptoms began about 1 week ago and have gotten progressively worse.

■ PMH
Five months S/P living kidney transplant from her sister-in-law. She is CMV seronegative; her donor was CMV seropositive.
ESRD secondary to non-recovery after viral infection
Atypical hemolytic uremic syndrome
Hyperlipidemia
HTN
Recurrent vaginal candidiasis—most recent infection occurred 1 month ago, for which she was prescribed itraconazole for 14 days

■ FH
No history of kidney disease in her family. Father is alive with hypertension. Mother is alive and healthy.

■ SH
Drinks alcohol rarely. She used to smoke 0.5 ppd for 20 years but quit when she was diagnosed with kidney disease. Denies IVDA.

■ Meds
Tacrolimus 1 mg PO BID (last dose taken last night at 8:00 PM)
Mycophenolic acid 360 mg PO BID
Atovaquone 1500 mg PO daily
Valganciclovir 900 mg PO daily
Carvedilol 25 mg PO BID
Magnesium chloride 64 mg PO BID
Atorvastatin 40 mg PO daily
Itraconazole 200 mg PO daily for 14 days (finished course 2 weeks ago)

■ All
Sulfa (rash)

■ ROS
She has pain in the left lower quadrant of the abdomen (at the site of the kidney transplant) and bilateral lower extremity edema. She also notes that her total daily urine output has decreased over the past week; she estimates that she is now producing about 1.5 L of urine/day, compared to more than 2 L/day 2 weeks ago, despite drinking the same amount of liquid every day.

■ Physical Examination

Gen
WDWN woman in NAD

VS
BP 142/92 mm Hg, P 66 reg, RR 14, T 37.4°C; Wt 58 kg (previous Wt 56 kg 2 weeks ago), Ht 5'1"

Skin
Warm and dry

HEENT
PERRLA; EOMI

Chest
CTA & P

CV
Normal S_1 and S_2; no MRG

Abd
Tenderness in LLQ (over kidney allograft); incisional wound healed; liver size normal

GU
Negative; no evidence of yeast or infection

Ext
3+ pitting edema in ankles, extending to the knee; 2+ DP pulses bilaterally. No cyanosis.

Neuro
A&O × 3; CN II–XII intact; DTRs 2+ throughout; decreased sensation to filament test

■ Labs
At 8:00 AM today (fasting):

Na 136 mEq/L	Hgb 11.4 g/dL	Ca 9.1 mg/dL
K 5.3 mEq/L	Hct 31.4%	Phos 2.2 mg/dL
Cl 99 mEq/L	RBC 3.68 × 10⁶/mm³	Mg 1.5 mg/dL
CO₂ 21 mEq/L	Plt 223 × 10³/mm³	TAC <2 ng/mL*
FBG 78 mg/dL	WBC 1.9 × 10³/mm³	
BUN 28 mg/dL	Polys 68%	
SCr 1.8 mg/dL	Lymphs 27%	
	Monos 2%	
	Eos 1%	
	Basos 2%	

*Tacrolimus (TAC) whole blood concentration (therapeutic range, 5–20 ng/mL).

■ Renal Biopsy
Moderate acute T-cell mediated rejection (TMCR) Grade IIB; moderate inflammation (i2); moderate tubulitis (t2); moderate intimal arteritis (v2); no glomerulitis (g0).

■ Assessment
1. Acute rejection of kidney allograft (last BUN 20 mg/dL, SCr 1.1 mg/dL 4 weeks ago)
2. Hyperkalemia (serum potassium 4.9 mEq/L 4 weeks ago)

QUESTIONS

Collect Information

1. What subjective and objective information indicates rejection of the kidney allograft?

Assess the Information

2.a. Assess the severity of kidney transplant rejection based on the subjective and objective information available.

2.b. Create a list of the patient's drug therapy problems and prioritize them. Include assessment of medication appropriateness, effectiveness, safety, and patient adherence.

Develop a Care Plan

3.a. What are the goals of pharmacotherapy for rejection of the kidney allograft?

3.b. What nondrug therapies might be useful for treating this patient's kidney allograft rejection?

3.c. What feasible pharmacotherapeutic alternatives are available for treating kidney allograft rejection?

3.d. Create an individualized, patient-centered, team-based care plan to optimize medication therapy for the patient's kidney allograft rejection and other drug therapy problems. Include specific drugs, dosage forms, doses, schedules, and durations of therapy.

3.e. What alternatives would be appropriate if the initial therapy for acute rejection fails or cannot be used?

Implement the Care Plan

4.a. What information should be provided to the patient to enhance adherence, ensure successful therapy, and minimize adverse effects?

4.b. Describe how care should be coordinated with other healthcare providers.

Follow-Up: Monitor and Evaluate

5. Explain how to monitor and evaluate the care plan for medication appropriateness, effectiveness, safety, and patient adherence by using clinical and laboratory data, patient feedback, and other information.

■ CLINICAL COURSE

The patient received the treatment you recommended for acute cellular rejection. Tacrolimus dose was gradually increased to 3 mg PO BID based on blood concentrations. Valganciclovir was discontinued 6 months post-transplant as per the usual protocol. The rejection episode resolved, and renal function returned to baseline levels.

CLINICAL PEARL

Acute rejection can occur in up to 20% of kidney transplant recipients within the first 6 months after transplant. Although an abrupt rise in serum creatinine ≥30% over baseline can signal an acute rejection episode, a renal biopsy must be performed for a definitive diagnosis. The greatest risk factor for acute cellular rejection is a decrease in the level of immunosuppression. Treatment of acute rejection is typically based on the severity of the rejection episode.

REFERENCES

1. Whelton PK, Carey RM, Aronow WS, et al. 2017 ACC/AHA/AAPA/ABC/ACPM/AGS/APhA/ASH/ASPC/NMA/PCNA guideline for the prevention, detection, evaluation, and management of high blood pressure in adults: executive summary. J Am Coll Cardiol. (2017). doi: 10.1016/j.jacc.2017.11.005.

2. Weir MR, Burgess ED, Cooper JE, et al. Assessment and management of hypertension in transplant patients. J Am Soc Nephrol. 2015;26(6):1248–1260.

3. Baker RJ, Mark PB, Patel RK, Stevens KK, Palmer N. Renal association clinical practice guideline in post-operative care in the kidney transplant recipient. BMC Nephrol. 2017;18:174.

4. van der Zwan M, Clahsen-Van Groningen MC, Roodnat JI, et al. The efficacy of rabbit anti-thymocyte globulin for acute kidney transplant rejection in patients using calcineurin inhibitor and mycophenolate-based immunosuppressive therapy. Ann Transplant. 2018;23:577–590.

5. Baia LC, Heilberg IP, Navi G, de Borst MH. Phosphate and FGF-23 homeostasis after kidney transplantation. Nat Rev Nephrol. 2015;11:656–666.

105

OSTEOARTHRITIS

Dealing with Wear and Tear . . . . Level II

Christopher M. Degenkolb, PharmD, BCPS

LEARNING OBJECTIVES

After completing this case study, the reader should be able to:

- Describe the most common signs and symptoms of osteoarthritis (OA).

- Design an appropriate pharmacotherapeutic regimen for treating OA considering the patient's other medical problems and drug therapy.

- Incorporate potential adjunctive therapies (pharmacologic, nonpharmacologic, and alternative) into the regimen of a patient with OA.

- Assess and evaluate the efficacy of an analgesic regimen for a patient with OA and formulate an alternative plan if the regimen is inadequate or causes unacceptable toxicity.

PATIENT PRESENTATION

■ Chief Complaint

"What can I take to help this pain? This new medication has only made me feel worse!"

■ HPI

The patient is a 74-year-old man who comes in to see his PCP today complaining of right knee and right hip pain for the past 10 years since he retired from an assembly plant. He often did very heavy lifting in his job and put a lot of strain on his back and legs; now the patient feels he is paying the price for his hard work. The patient wakes up every morning very stiff, and his right knee cracks when he gets up out of bed. The cracking in the joint goes away after he finishes his breakfast, but the aching in his knee and hip persists and chronically bothers him. For several months the patient has been taking scheduled doses of Tylenol Extra Strength. He visited his PCP 3 weeks ago with similar complaints and was prescribed Norco for additional pain management. He reports being given a month supply and taking this new medication three to four times per day. He reports good adherence to prescribed medications; however, he is not sure what medications he has tried in the past; all he knows is that whatever he is taking is not helping. He reports some vague abdominal cramping and intermittent nausea. Additionally, patient complains of lack of energy due to sleepiness during the day and has been unable to do any exercise. He states he is very depressed because he can't enjoy time with family and his two grandchildren. His PCP wants more aggressive pain management and asking for your dosing recommendation on converting his Norco to a long-acting opioid given his past medical history and limited treatment options.

■ PMH

OA × 10 years
HTN × 20 years
Obesity × 15 years
Seizure disorder × 12 years (last seizure was 5 years ago)
CKD × 5 years

■ PSH

Appendectomy 35 years ago

■ FH

Father died at age 68 due to myocardial infarction
Mother died at age 81 of CVA
Lives at home with wife and two grandchildren

■ SH

Retired and lives on small pension from his company
Lives in small rural area and must travel a long way for appointments
Denies tobacco use
Occasional EtOH (two to three beers on weekends)

■ Meds

Amlodipine 10 mg PO daily in AM
Lisinopril 10 mg PO daily in AM
Metoprolol 50 mg PO BID
Hydrocodone/acetaminophen 5 mg/325 mg two tablets PO Q 6 H PRN pain
Acetaminophen 500 mg one tablet PO Q 6 H PRN pain
Levetiracetam 1000 mg PO BID

■ All

NKDA; reports allergy to egg products

■ ROS

Positive for pain and stiffness in the right knee and right hip; has low back pain with occasional shooting and aching pains radiating to the buttocks and groin area; negative for headache, neck stiffness, joint swelling, or erythema; no SOB or palpitations; reports some vague abdominal cramping, intermittent nausea; and no bowel movement in the past 5 days

■ Physical Examination

Gen

Well-developed, obese, Caucasian man with moderate pain, otherwise in NAD

VS

BP 148/89 mm Hg, P 68 bpm, RR 18, T 37.1°C; Ht 5'9", Wt 225 lb (102.1 kg), pain 6/10. No orthostatic changes.

Skin

Warm, dry, intact

HEENT

NC/AT; PERRLA; funduscopic exam reveals sharp disks; mild AV nicking, but no hemorrhages or exudates; no scleral icterus; TMs intact; mucous membranes moist; poor dentition with gingival erythema; no lateral deviation of tongue; no pharyngeal edema or erythema

Neck/Lymph Nodes

Supple; no thyromegaly or lymphadenopathy; no carotid bruits

Lungs

CTA

CV

Distant heart sounds, normal S_1 and S_2; PMI at fifth ICS/MCL; RRR; no MRG; no JVD or HJR

Abd

Obese, soft, mild tenderness on palpation; no guarding; diminished BS; unable to assess liver size on palpation

Genit/Rect

Prostate gland normal; normal sphincter tone; guaiac (–) stool in rectal vault

MS/Ext

Back pain radiating to right buttock with straight leg raising at 60°; right hip pain with flexion >90° and with internal and external rotation >45°; right hip tender to palpation; right knee (+) crepitus; no swelling or edema; good pedal pulses

Neuro

Oriented × 3; normal affect; appears at times to alternate between apathy and anger/frustration; CN II–XII intact; DTRs equal bilaterally except for slightly diminished Achilles reflexes bilaterally; no focal deficits; gait impaired secondary to hip and knee pain; Babinski downgoing

■ Labs

Na 135 mEq/L	Hgb 11.8 g/dL	AST 38 IU/L
K 4.7 mEq/L	Hct 34.5%	Alk phos 96 IU/L
Cl 98 mEq/L	WBC 6.5 × 10³/mm³	T. prot 7.4 g/dL
CO₂ 26 mEq/L	Plt 286 × 10³/mm³	Alb 4.2 g/dL
BUN 18 mg/dL	MCV 85.3 μm³	Phos 4.5 mg/dL
SCr 1.8 mg/dL	MCH 28.4 pg	ESR 18 mm/hr
Glu 99 mg/dL	MCHC 34.5 g/dL	Ca 11.2 mg/dL

■ UA

SG 1.011; pH 6.5; WBC (–), RBC (–), leukocyte esterase (–), nitrite (–), 2+ protein; microscopic examination reveals two to five epithelial cells/hpf and no bacteria

■ X-Rays

Lumbar spine: advanced degenerative changes at L3–4 and at L4–5
Right hip: moderate degenerative changes with some spurring of the femoral head and slight decrease in joint space
Right knee: moderate degenerative changes; no effusion

■ Assessment

A 74-year-old man with pain in his right knee, hip, and back, secondary to a long-standing history of OA—his current medications are inadequate to control his pain. He also needs pharmacotherapy management for uncontrolled hypertension, obesity, CKD, and seizure disorder.

QUESTIONS

Collect Information

1.a. What subjective and objective information indicates the presence of osteoarthritis?

1.b. What additional information is needed to fully assess this patient's osteoarthritis?

Assess the Information

2.a. Assess the severity of OA based on the subjective and objective information available.

2.b. Create a list of the patient's drug therapy problems and prioritize them. Include assessment of medication appropriateness, effectiveness, safety, and patient adherence.

2.c. What economic, psychosocial, cultural, racial, and ethical considerations are applicable to this patient?

Develop a Care Plan

3.a. What are the goals of pharmacotherapy for osteoarthritis in this case?

3.b. What nondrug therapies might be useful for this patient's osteoarthritis?

3.c. What feasible pharmacotherapeutic options are available for treating this patient's osteoarthritis?

3.d. Create an individualized, patient-centered, team-based care plan to optimize medication therapy for this patient's osteoarthritis and other drug therapy problems. Include specific drugs, dosing forms, doses, schedules, and durations of therapy.

3.e. What alternatives would be appropriate if the initial care plan fails or cannot be used?

Implement the Care Plan

4.a. What information should be provided to the patient to enhance adherence, ensure successful therapy, and minimize adverse effects?

4.b. Describe how care should be coordinated with other healthcare providers.

Follow-Up: Monitor and Evaluate

5. Explain how to monitor and evaluate the care plan for medication appropriateness, effectiveness, safety, and patient adherence by using clinical and laboratory data, patient feedback, and other information.

■ CLINICAL COURSE: ALTERNATIVE THERAPY

While discussing multiple treatment options, he says, "This may seem silly, but I have a neighbor a couple years older than me who was getting some pretty bad arthritis in both knees a few years ago. He says he hardly has any pain anymore because he's taking these glucosamine and chondroitin pills. He even started back to golfing! Is there any way those could help me with my pain?" See Section 19 in this Casebook for questions and answers about the use of glucosamine and chondroitin for osteoarthritis.

■ SELF-STUDY ASSIGNMENTS

1. Many patients who deal with pain and osteoarthritis often turn to unproven methods to control their pain. Research some of these unproven methods online and try to find active ingredients to determine if these are unsafe to recommend for patients with complex medication regimens.

2. Evaluate this patient's CKD. What stage of CRI does this patient have, and what is the most likely etiology of his renal disease? Prepare a paper describing some of the complications of long-standing kidney disease and how such complications should be managed.

CLINICAL PEARLS

At least one in ten older adults have symptomatic OA but there are no treatment options that provide disease-state modifications. Therefore, treatment recommendations and current guidelines provide an array of pharmacologic and non-pharmacologic options to provide symptomatic relief in combination with one another. It is important to take a patient-centric approach prioritizing safety and preventing harm with treatment interventions. There are many unproven and unsubstantiated treatment options that are imperative for the clinician to recognize and utilize a shared decision-making approach when treating the most prevalent chronic joint disease in adults.

REFERENCES

1. Kolasinski SL, Neogi T, Hochberg MC, et al. 2019 American College of Rheumatology/Arthritis Foundation guideline for the management of osteoarthritis of the hand, hip, and knee. Arthritis Care Res. (Hoboken) 2020;72:149–162.

2. Dowell D, Haegerich TM, Chou R. CDC guideline for prescribing opioids for chronic pain—United States, 2016. MMWR Recomm Rep. 2016;65:1. Available at: https://www.cdc.gov/mmwr/volumes/65/rr/rr6501e1.htm. Accessed February 28, 2022.

3. Busse JW, Wang L, Kamaledin M, et al. Opioids for chronic noncancer pain: a systematic review and meta-analysis. JAMA. 2018;320:2448–2460.

4. American Academy of Orthopaedic Surgeons (AAOS). American Academy of Orthopaedic Surgeons clinical practice guideline on treatment of osteoarthritis of the knee. 2nd ed. Available at: https://aaos.org/quality/quality-programs/lower-extremity-programs/osteoarthritis-of-the-knee/. Accessed February 28, 2022.

5. Bannuru RR, Osani MC, Vaysbrot EE, et al. Osteoarthritis Research Society International (OARSI) guidelines for the non-surgical management of knee, hip, and polyarticular osteoarthritis. Osteoarthritis Cartilage. 2019;27(11):1578–1589.

6. Ebell MH. Osteoarthritis: rapid evidence review. Am Fam Physician. 2018;97(8):523–526.

7. Machado GC, Maher CG, Ferreira PH, et al. Efficacy and safety of paracetamol for spinal pain and osteoarthritis: systematic review and meta-analysis of randomized placebo controlled trials. BMJ. 2015;350:h1225. doi: 10.1136/bmj.h1225.

8. Osani MC, Bannuru RR. Efficacy and safety of duloxetine in osteoarthritis: a systematic review and meta-analysis. Korean J Intern Med. 2019;34:966–973.

106

RHEUMATOID ARTHRITIS

Not Responding to Therapy. Level II

Brett E. Glasheen, PharmD

Kami Roake, PharmD

LEARNING OBJECTIVES

After completing this case study, the reader should be able to:

• Identify signs and symptoms of rheumatoid arthritis (RA) and assess disease severity.

• Recommend appropriate nonpharmacologic therapy for adjunctive management of RA.

• Recommend evidence-based, patient-specific analgesic, anti-inflammatory, and disease-modifying drug therapy for patients with RA.

• Develop an evidence-based, patient-specific monitoring plan to assess disease progress and evaluate the safety and efficacy of medication therapy.

• Educate patients and their families about the medications used to treat RA.

PATIENT PRESENTATION

■ Chief Complaint

"I don't feel like my methotrexate is working anymore. My joints are sore, and I am tired all the time."

■ HPI

A 51-year-old woman presents to rheumatology clinic with complaints of generalized arthralgias, fatigue, and morning stiffness. She has a 17-year history of RA currently treated with methotrexate. She reports worsening in her symptoms over the past 6 months.

■ PMH

RA × 17 years
Hypertension × 4 years

■ FH

Father is alive and being treated for hypertension. Mother is alive and being treated for severe RA. Two siblings with no major health concerns.

■ SH

Hypnotherapist; married for 25 years; heterosexual, sexually active, monogamous. Past smoker, 5 pack-year history. Drinks one to two glasses of wine per week.

■ Meds

Methotrexate 50 mg/2 mL, 1.0 mL (25 mg) subcutaneously once a week
Folic acid 1 mg PO once daily

Hydrochlorothiazide 25 mg daily

Diclofenac 1% transdermal gel as needed

Patient receives medications at a local community pharmacy. Medication profile indicates that she refills her medications on time on the first of each month.

■ All

NKDA

■ ROS

Complains of swelling and pain in both hands; reports decreased ROM in hands and wrists; has morning stiffness every day for about 2 hours and fatigue daily during the afternoon hours; denies HA, chest pain, bleeding episodes, or syncope; no nausea, vomiting, diarrhea, loss of appetite, or weight loss.

■ Physical Examination

Gen

Women in distress because of pain, swelling, and fatigue related to arthritis

VS

BP 110/72 mm Hg, P 61 bpm, RR 15, T 37.1°C; Wt 65 kg, Ht 5′6″

Skin

No rashes; normal turgor; no breakdown or ulcers; no subcutaneous nodules

HEENT

Normocephalic, atraumatic; moist mucous membranes; PERRLA; EOMI; pale conjunctiva bilaterally; TMs intact; no oral mucositis

Neck/Lymph Nodes

Neck supple, no JVD or thyromegaly; no thyroid bruit; no lymphadenopathy

Chest

CTA

Breasts

Deferred

CV

RRR; normal S_1, S_2; no MRG

Abd

Soft, NT/ND; (+) BS

Genit/Rect

Deferred

MS/Ext

Total of 16 tender and 16 swollen joints bilaterally

Hands: swelling and tenderness on palpation of second, third, fourth, and fifth PIP and MTP joints bilaterally; decreased grip strength, L > R (patient is left-handed)

Wrists: decreased ROM

Elbows: good ROM

Shoulders: decreased ROM (especially abduction) bilaterally

Hips: good ROM

Knees: good ROM, no pain bilaterally

Feet: no obvious swelling of MTP joints; full plantar flexion; reduced dorsiflexion; 2+ pedal pulses

Neuro

CN II–XII intact; muscle strength 4/5 UE, 4/5 LE, DTRs 2+ throughout

■ Labs

Na 136 mEq/L	Hgb 11.4 g/dL	AST 18 IU/L	CK <20 IU/L
K 4.1 mEq/L	Hct 33%	ALT 14 IU/L	ANA negative
Cl 102 mEq/L	WBC 5.2 × 10³/mm³	Alk phos 56 IU/L	Wes ESR
CO₂ 21 mEq/L	Plt 372 × 10³/mm³	T. bili 0.8 mg/dL	60 mm/hr
BUN 14 mg/dL	Ca 9.1 mg/dL	Alb 4.2 g/dL	RF (+) 50 U/mL
SCr 0.8 mg/dL	Urate 5.1 mg/dL	HbsAb (+)	Anti-CCP 70 EU
Glu 92 mg/dL	TSH 0.74 mIU/L	HbsAg (−)	aPTT 31 seconds
		HepB core Ab (−)	INR 1.0
		Anti-HCV (−)	

■ UA

Normal

■ Chest X-Ray

No fluid, masses, or infection; no cardiomegaly

■ Hand X-Ray

Multiple erosions of MCP and PIP joints bilaterally; measurable joint space narrowing from previous X-ray 1 year ago

■ DAS 28

6.2 today; 3.0 one year ago

■ Assessment

A 51-year-old woman experiencing worsening symptoms of RA for the past 6 months, not responding to current treatment

QUESTIONS

Collect Information

1.a. What subjective and objective information indicates the presence of rheumatoid arthritis?

1.b. What additional information is needed to fully assess this patient's rheumatoid arthritis?

Assess the Information

2.a. Assess the severity of rheumatoid arthritis based on the subjective and objective information available.

2.b. Create a list of the patient's drug therapy problems and prioritize them. Include assessment of medication appropriateness, effectiveness, safety, and patient adherence.

2.c. What economic, psychosocial, cultural, racial, and ethical considerations are applicable to this patient?

Develop a Care Plan

3.a. What are the goals of pharmacotherapy in this case?

3.b. What nondrug therapies for rheumatoid arthritis might be useful for this patient?

3.c. What feasible pharmacotherapeutic options are available for treating rheumatoid arthritis?

3.d. Create an individualized, patient-centered, team-based care plan to optimize medication therapy for this patient's rheumatoid arthritis and other drug therapy problems. Include specific drugs, dosage forms, doses, schedules, and durations of therapy.

3.e. What alternatives would be appropriate if the initial therapy for rheumatoid arthritis fails or cannot be used?

Implement the Care Plan

4.a. What information should be provided to the patient to enhance adherence, ensure successful therapy, and minimize adverse effects?

4.b. Describe how care should be coordinated with other healthcare providers.

Follow-Up: Monitor and Evaluate

5. Explain how to monitor and evaluate the care plan for medication appropriateness, effectiveness, safety, and patient adherence by using clinical and laboratory data, patient feedback, and other information.

■ SELF-STUDY ASSIGNMENTS

1. Create a list of clinically significant drug interactions for NSAIDs and DMARDs, including methotrexate.

2. Compare the biologic agents used to treat RA with respect to drug class, route of administration, efficacy, contraindications, and adverse effects.

CLINICAL PEARL

Patients receiving immunosuppressant therapy are at increased risk of TB and hepatitis B reactivation. Reactivation of latent tuberculosis and hepatitis B is a concern with all immunosuppressant therapy but has been specifically associated with corticosteroid use, all biologic agents (TNF-α antagonists, IL-1 and IL-6 receptor inhibitors, B-cell–depleting agents, T-cell costimulation inhibitors), and some nonbiological agents (JAK-inhibitors and leflunomide).

ACKNOWLEDGMENT

This case is based on the patient cases written for the 11th edition by Andrea Franks, PharmD and Julie Jeter, MD.

REFERENCES

1. U.S. Food and Drug Administration. FDA requires warnings about increased risk of serious heart-related events, cancer, blood clots, and death for JAK inhibitors that treat certain chronic inflammatory conditions. Available at: *https://www.fda.gov/drugs/drug-safety-and-availability/fda-requires-warnings-about-increased-risk-serious-heart-related-events-cancer-blood-clots-and-death*. Accessed April 3, 2022.

2. Niewold TB, Harrison MJ, Paget SA. Anti-CCP antibody testing as a diagnostic and prognostic tool in rheumatoid arthritis. QJM. 2007;100(4):193–201.

3. Aletaha D, Neogi T, Silman A, et al. 2010 Rheumatoid arthritis classification criteria. Arthritis Rheum. 2012;62:2569–2581.

4. Fransen J, van Riel PLCM. The disease activity score and the EULAR response criteria. Rheum Dis Clin North Am. 2009;35:745–757.

5. Fraenkel L, Bathon JM, England BR, et al. 2021 American College of Rheumatology guideline for the treatment of rheumatoid arthritis. Arthritis Care Res. (Hoboken) 2021;73(7):924–939. doi: 10.1002/acr.24596.

6. Marmor MF, Kellner U, Lai TY, Melles RB, Mieler WF; American Academy of Ophthalmology. Recommendations on screening for chloroquine and hydroxychloroquine retinopathy (2016 revision). Ophthalmology. 2016;123(6):1386–1394. doi: 10.1016/j.ophtha.2016.01.058.

7. Singh JA, Christensen R, Wells GA, et al. Biologics for rheumatoid arthritis: an overview of Cochrane reviews (Protocol). Cochrane Database Syst Rev. 2009;2:CD007848. doi: 10.1002/14651858.CD007848.

8. Curtis JR, Patkar N, Xie A, et al. Risk of serious bacterial infections among rheumatoid arthritis patients exposed to tumor necrosis factor alpha antagonists. Arthritis Rheum. 2007;56:1125–1133.

9. Saag KG, Teng GG, Patkar NM, et al. American College of Rheumatology 2008 recommendations for the use of nonbiologic and biologic disease-modifying antirheumatic drugs in rheumatoid arthritis. Arthritis Care Res. 2008;59:762–784.

10. Ramiro S, Gaujoux-Viala C, Nam JL, et al. Safety of synthetic and biological DMARDs: a systematic literature review informing the 2013 update of the EULAR recommendations for management of rheumatoid arthritis. Ann Rheum Dis. 2014;73(3):529–535. doi: 10.1136/annrheumdis-2013-204575.

107

OSTEOPOROSIS

No Bones About It: Osteoporotic Fractures Warrant Treatment . . . . Level II

Mollie Ashe Scott, PharmD, BCACP, CPP, FASHP

Lisa LaVallee, MD

LEARNING OBJECTIVES

After completing this case study, the reader should be able to:

• Identify the risk factors for the development of osteoporosis and use the Fracture Risk Assessment Tool (FRAX) to assess risk of an osteoporotic fracture.

• Recommend appropriate nonpharmacologic measures for the prevention and treatment of osteoporosis.

• Recommend appropriate calcium and vitamin D supplementation required for the prevention and treatment of osteoporosis.

• Design an appropriate pharmacologic treatment regimen for the treatment of osteoporosis in postmenopausal women.

• Provide patient education regarding osteoporosis and its therapy.

• Discuss the role that the fracture liaison service plays in coordinating care and preventing additional fractures.

PATIENT PRESENTATION

■ Chief Complaint

"I recently fell while walking my dog, and my lower back is sore. I would also like to get the results of my DXA scan. My mother is still undergoing rehabilitation in the nursing home after her hip fracture three weeks ago. I've heard osteoporosis can run in families, and I don't want to experience what she is going through."

HPI

Patient is a 65-year-old woman with a history of hypertension. She presents to the family medicine clinic for her yearly physical and to discuss the results of her recent labs and DXA scan.

In an effort to become more active, she recently started walking around her neighborhood every day but fell 3 days ago and injured her back. She admits that she has a hard time remembering to take her medications faithfully. She states she takes her medicines "most of the time." She states that she was prescribed alendronate 2 years ago but that she is "afraid of its side effects" and did not start it.

PMH

Hypertension
Menopause at age 51
GERD with history of esophageal stricture

FH

Paternal history (+) for hypertension; father died in his sleep at age 80
Maternal history (+) for stroke; hip fracture

SH

Married; G_2P_2; drinks occasionally, retired real estate agent, lives independently with her husband and dog, manages her own medicines, completed college, does not have a Medicare Part D plan, nonsmoker

Meds

Omeprazole 20 mg PO once daily × 1 year
Hydrochlorothiazide 25 mg PO once daily

All

NKDA

ROS

Reports vaginal dryness; has noticed that her height has decreased by 2″ since she was "in her prime;" denies headache, chest pain, GI pain, or heartburn

Physical Examination

Gen

WDWN woman in NAD, ambulating with a cane

VS

Today

BP initially 133/88 mm Hg sitting, repeated at end of office visit 100/64 mm Hg standing, P 70 bpm sitting 90 standing, RR 18, T 37°C, Wt 53.5 kg, Ht 5′3″
Timed Up and Go (TUG) test: 15 seconds

1 Month Ago

BP 130/82 mm Hg, P 66 bpm, RR 20, T 37°C; Wt 53.5 kg, Ht 5′3″

Skin

No lesions noted

HEENT

PERRLA; EOMI; eyes and throat clear; poor dentition

Neck/Lymph Nodes

Supple, without obvious nodes; no JVD, no thyromegaly

Chest

Clear to auscultation; no rales or rhonchi

Breasts

Normal

CV

RRR; no MRG

Abd

Soft, NT/ND, (+) BS, no mass, no hepatosplenomegaly

Genit/Rect

Deferred

MS/Ext

Good pulses bilaterally, spine straight without scoliosis, moderate kyphosis, tender midthoracic tenderness to palpation, no stigmata of Cushing disease

Neuro

CN II–XII intact; DTRs 2+; sensory and motor levels intact

Labs

Na 145 mEq/L	SCr 1.1 mg/dL	25-OH vitamin D 15 ng/mL
K 4.0 mEq/L	Glu 97 mg/dL	ALP 52 IU/L
Cl 104 mEq/L	AST 32 IU/L	
CO_2 25 mEq/L	ALT 27 IU/L	
BUN 18 mg/dL	Corrected Ca 9.1 mg/dL	

Other

DXA scan results from Hologic machine 2 weeks prior:
Lumbar spine 2 weeks ago reveals: L2–4 = 0.780 g/cm^2 (T score: –3.2 SD); right femoral neck = 0.52 g/cm^2 (T score: –2.8 SD)
X-ray of the spine today shows a compression fracture in T10
Patient is referred to fracture liaison service for coordination of care

Assessment

A 65-year-old woman with a recent fall, untreated osteoporosis, vertebral compression fracture, and vitamin D deficiency, currently being treated for hypertension and GERD

QUESTIONS

Collect Information

1.a. What subjective and objective information indicates the presence of osteoporosis?

1.b. What additional information is needed to fully assess this patient's osteoporosis?

Assess the Information

2.a. Assess the severity of osteoporosis based on the subjective and objective information available.

2.b. Create a list of the patient's drug therapy problems and prioritize them. Include assessment of medication appropriateness, effectiveness, safety, and patient adherence.

2.c. What economic, psychosocial, cultural, racial, and ethical considerations are applicable to this patient?

Develop a Care Plan

3.a. What are the goals of pharmacotherapy in this case?

3.b. What nondrug therapies might be useful for this patient?

3.c. What feasible pharmacotherapeutic options are available for treating osteoporosis?

3.d. Create an individualized, patient-centered, team-based care plan to optimize medication therapy for this patient's osteoporosis and other drug therapy problems. Include specific drugs, dosage forms, doses, schedules, and durations of therapy.

3.e. What alternatives would be appropriate if the initial care plan fails or cannot be used?

Implement the Care Plan

4.a. What information should be provided to the patient to enhance adherence, ensure successful therapy, and minimize adverse effects?

4.b. Describe how care should be coordinated with other healthcare providers.

Follow-Up: Monitor and Evaluate

5. Explain how to monitor and evaluate the care plan for medication appropriateness, effectiveness, safety, and patient adherence by using clinical and laboratory data, patient feedback, and other information.

■ SELF-STUDY ASSIGNMENTS

1. Create a list of medications and disease states that are associated with an increased risk for developing osteoporosis.

2. Investigate the sclerostin inhibitor, romosozumab, and its role in the treatment of osteoporosis.

3. Discuss the role of the fracture liaison service and the different responsibilities of the members of the interprofessional team in the clinical care of patients with fracture.

CLINICAL PEARL

Patients with osteoporosis who are prescribed bisphosphonates should be evaluated for a drug holiday after 3–5 years of therapy.

REFERENCES

1. Eastell R, Rosen CJ, Black DM, et al. Pharmacologic management of osteoporosis in postmenopausal women: an Endocrine Society clinical practice guideline. J Clin Endo Metab. 2019;104(5):1595–1622.

2. Cosman F, de Beur SJ, LeBoff MS, et al. Clinician's guide to prevention and treatment of osteoporosis. Osteoporosis Int. 2014;25:2359–2381.

3. The North American Menopause Society. Management of osteoporosis in postmenopausal women: the 2021 position statement of The North American Menopause Society. Menopause. 2021;28(9):973–997.

4. Wu CH, Tu ST, Chang YF, Chan DC, Chien JT, et al. Fracture liaison services improve outcomes for patients with osteoporosis-related fracture: a systematic literature review and meta-analysis. Bone. 2018;111:92–100.

5. American Geriatrics Society. 2019 updated AGS Beers Criteria for potentially inappropriate medication use in older adults. J Am Geriatr Soc. 2019;67(4):674–694.

6. Centers for Disease Control and Prevention. STEADI: stopping elderly accidents, deaths, and injuries. Available at: https://www.cdc.gov/steadi/index.html. Accessed April 19, 2022.

7. Zhou B, Huang Y, Li H, Sun W, Liu J. Proton-pump inhibitors and risk of fractures: an update meta-analysis. Osteopor Int. 2016;27:339–347.

8. American Association of Clinical Endocrinologists and American College of Endocrinologists. Vitamin D deficiency. 2019. Available at: https://pro.aace.com/sites/default/files/2019-02/Vitamin_D_Deficiency_formatted.pdf. Accessed April 19, 2022.

9. Miller PD, Hattersley G, Riis JR, et al. Effect of abaloparatide vs placebo on new vertebral fractures on postmenopausal women with osteoporosis. A randomized clinical trial. JAMA. 2016;316:722–733.

10. Cummings SR, Ferrari S, Eastell R, et al. Vertebral fractures after discontinuation of denosumab: a post hoc analysis of the randomized placebo-controlled FREEDOM trial and its extension. J Bone Miner Res. 2018;33(2):190–198.

108

GOUT AND HYPERURICEMIA

The King of Oktoberfest . . . . Level II

Erik D. Maki, PharmD, BCPS

LEARNING OBJECTIVES

After completing this case study, the reader should be able to:

- Identify major risk factors for developing gout, including drugs that may contribute to or cause this disorder.

- Develop a pharmacotherapeutic plan for a patient with acute gouty arthritis that includes individualized drug selection and assessment of the treatment for efficacy or toxicity.

- Identify patients in whom maintenance therapy for gout and hyperuricemia is warranted.

- Identify medications not used primarily for gout that may have a beneficial effect on serum uric acid (SUA) levels.

PATIENT PRESENTATION

■ Chief Complaint

"My toe is on fire."

■ HPI

A 78-year-old patient presents to the ED complaining of significant toe pain. The patient states, "I think I'm paying the price for my fun at Oktoberfest." The patient reports having spent the weekend indulging on beer and sausage at the local Oktoberfest festival. In the early hours of Monday morning (approximately 3 hours ago), he awoke to sudden excruciating pain in the right big toe. Over the past hour, this toe has become red, swollen, and so painful that ambulating is difficult. The patient has not experienced any trauma or injuries and denies having experienced these symptoms previously.

■ PMH

HTN × 28 years
Obesity × 40 years

■ SH

The patient typically drinks "a can of beer or two" daily but drank significantly on Friday, Saturday, and Sunday. Does not smoke or use illicit drugs.

■ Meds

Chlorthalidone 25 mg PO daily, started 1 month ago

■ All

NKDA

■ ROS

Other than feeling somewhat dehydrated from attendance at the festival, the patient has no major complaints prior to this ED visit. No chest pain, nausea/vomiting, or respiratory symptoms. Bowel habits are normal. No prior history of arthritic symptoms or joint problems.

■ Physical Examination

Gen

A healthy-appearing, obese, patient in acute distress

VS

BP 135/70 mm Hg, P 105 bpm, RR 17, T 37.5°C; Wt 88 kg, Ht 5′6″

Skin

Poor skin turgor. No rashes or other dermatologic abnormalities.

HEENT

PERRLA, dry mucous membranes, throat/ears clear of redness or inflammation

Neck/Lymph Nodes

Negative for lymph node swelling or masses

Lungs/Thorax

Clear to auscultation bilaterally, symmetric movement with inspiration

CV

Tachycardic, normal rhythm, normal S_1 and S_2

Abd

Obese, but soft, nontender; positive bowel sounds in all quadrants

Genit/Rect

Deferred

MS/Ext

Erythematous, edematous right first metatarsophalangeal joint, which is very warm to touch; joint is exquisitely painful with patient relating the pain as currently a 10/10 (on a 1–10 scale with 0 being no pain and 10 being the worse pain the patient has ever suffered); no swelling of any other joints. No signs of tophi present.

Neuro

A&O × 3; CN II–XII grossly intact, no focal neurologic deficits

■ Labs

Ankle and foot radiographs: negative for fracture
Aspirated fluid from first metatarsophalangeal joint tap: >50 WBC/hpf, containing negatively birefringent monosodium urate crystals

Na 143 mEq/L	Hgb 15 g/dL	WBC 12.9 × 10³/mm³
K 3.7 mEq/L	Hct 44%	Neutros 88%
Cl 99 mEq/L	RBC 4.9 × 10⁶/mm³	Bands 0%
CO₂ 22 mEq/L	Plt 225 × 10³/mm³	Eos 1%
BUN 63 mg/dL	MCV 84 μm³	Lymphs 10%
SCr 3.0 mg/dL	MCHC 37 g/dL	Monos 1%
Glu 101 mg/dL	ESR 47 mm/hr	RF negative
SUA 11.6 mg/dL		

■ Assessment

1. Primary presentation of acute gouty arthritis
2. Acute kidney injury
3. Hypertension

QUESTIONS

Collect Information

1.a. What subjective and objective information indicates the presence of gout?

1.b. What additional information is needed to fully assess this patient's gout?

Assess the Information

2.a. Assess the severity of gout based on the subjective and objective information available.

2.b. Create a list of the patient's drug therapy problems and prioritize them. Include assessment of medication appropriateness, effectiveness, safety, and patient adherence.

Develop a Care Plan

3.a. What are the goals of pharmacotherapy in this case?

3.b. What nondrug therapies for gout might be useful for this patient?

3.c. What feasible pharmacotherapeutic options are available for treating gout?

3.d. Create an individualized, patient-centered, team-based care plan to optimize medication therapy for this patient's gout and other drug therapy problems. Include specific drugs, dosage forms, doses, schedules, and durations of therapy.

3.e. What alternatives would be appropriate if the initial care plan fails or cannot be used?

Implement the Care Plan

4.a. What information should be provided to the patient to enhance adherence, ensure successful therapy, and minimize adverse effects?

4.b. Describe how care should be coordinated with other healthcare providers.

Follow-Up: Monitor and Evaluate

5. Explain how to monitor and evaluate the care plan for medication appropriateness, effectiveness, safety, and patient adherence by using clinical and laboratory data, patient feedback, and other information.

■ CLINICAL COURSE

The patient responded to the therapy you recommended, and within 96 hours, the pain has subsided significantly. Toe redness and swelling have decreased to near normal. Additionally, with fluids, the SCr has returned to baseline (0.8 mg/dL). After consultation with you, the patient's physician decides against maintenance therapy to decrease SUA levels. The patient, remembering the severe pain this episode caused, follows your recommended lifestyle changes and is adherent to the new medication you recommended for hypertension. At the 6-month follow-up appointment, the patient reports no additional gout flares. Additionally, the patient has lost 20 lb. and no longer drinks ethanol. Measured SUA level has decreased to 6.9 mg/dL, and BP is 130/80 mm Hg.

■ ADDITIONAL CASE QUESTIONS

1. Should chronic treatment to decrease the patient's SUA level be initiated at this time? Why or why not?

2. If at some point maintenance therapy to decrease SUA is begun, what additional therapy is needed to prevent acute flares?

■ SELF-STUDY ASSIGNMENTS

1. List antihyperuricemic agents that are available in the United States and their relative advantages and disadvantages. Describe new agents that are being studied for this indication and what clinical data support their use.

2. List medications that can either increase or decrease serum uric acid concentrations.

CLINICAL PEARL

Historically, colchicine was used for treating acute gout flares at doses of 0.6 mg Q 1–2 H until symptoms resolved or adverse GI symptoms developed (6 mg maximum). GI side effects were employed as a clinical endpoint for discontinuing the drug because these side effects tended to occur prior to the more severe adverse effects of colchicine-induced myopathy and myelosuppression. However, current recommendations are to use low-dose colchicine at a dose of 1.2 mg, followed in 1 hour with a single dose of 0.6 mg. For patients receiving prophylactic colchicine prior to the flare, it is recommended to wait 12 hours after treatment dosing before resuming prophylactic dosing.

REFERENCES

1. Richette P, Doherty M, Pascual E, et al. 2018 updated European League against rheumatism evidence-based recommendations for the diagnosis of gout. Ann Rheum Dis. 2020;79(1):31–38.

2. FitzGerald JD, Dalbeth N, Mikuls T, et al. 2020 American College of Rheumatology guideline for the management of gout. Arthritis Rheumatol. 2020;72(6):879–895. doi: 10.1002/art.41247.

3. Richette P, Doherty M, Pascual E, et al. 2016 updated EULAR evidence-based recommendations for the management of gout. Ann Rheum Dis. 2017;76(1):29–42.

4. Hui M, Carr A, Cameron S, et al. The British Society for Rheumatology guideline for the management of gout. Rheumatology. 2017;56(7): e1–e20. doi: 10.1093/rheumatology/kex156.

5. Khanna D, Khanna PP, Fitzgerald JD, et al. 2012 American College of Rheumatology guidelines for management of gout. Part 2: therapy and antiinflammatory prophylaxis of acute gouty arthritis. Arthritis Care Res. (Hoboken) 2012;64:1447–1461.

6. Abhishek A, Doherty M. Education and non-pharmacological approaches for gout. Rheumatology. 2018;57:i51–i58.

7. Wilson L, Nair KV, Saseen JJ. Comparison of new-onset gout in adults prescribed chlorthalidone vs hydrochlorothiazide for hypertension. J Clin Hypertens. (Greenwich) 2014;16:864–868.

8. Wolff ML, Cruz JL, Vanderman AJ, Brown JN. The effect of angiotensin II receptor blockers on hyperuricemia. Ther Adv Chronic Dis. 2015;6:339–346.

9. Choi H, Soriano L, Zhang Y, et al. Antihypertensive drugs and risk of incident gout among patients with hypertension: population-based case-control study. BMJ. 2012;344:d8190. doi: 10.1136/bmj.d8190.

10. Dalbeth N, Merriman TR, Stamp LK. Gout. Lancet. 2016;388:2039–2052.

109

GLAUCOMA

Silent Blindness.................................Level III

Brian McMillan, MD

Ashlee McMillan, PharmD, BCACP

LEARNING OBJECTIVES

After completing this case study, the reader should be able to:

- Identify the importance of regular eye examinations and the early diagnosis of glaucoma.

- List the risk factors for developing open-angle glaucoma.

- Select and recommend agents from different pharmacologic classes when indicated and provide the rationale for drug selection, including combination products to increase adherence.

- Recommend conventional glaucoma therapy as well as other options in glaucoma management when indicated.

- Formulate basic ophthalmologic monitoring parameters used in glaucoma therapy.

- Counsel patients on medication regimens and proper ophthalmic administration technique.

- Discuss potential adverse drug reactions with patients to increase therapy adherence.

PATIENT PRESENTATION

■ Chief Complaint

"My vision is closing down and I am having difficulty seeing cars at intersections while driving."

■ HPI

A 75-year-old woman presents for follow-up of advanced primary open-angle glaucoma (POAG). She reports adherence with latanoprost nightly and timolol/brimonidine (Combigan) two times daily in the right eye and dorzolamide three times daily in the left eye. She feels that her vision in the left eye is beginning to blur, and she is having more difficulty seeing objects in the top part of her vision. She finds that she has to move her head more to see objects in her periphery. She denies eye pain, flashes, or floaters. She is feeling more tired recently.

She was first diagnosed with POAG 20 years ago during a routine eye exam to update her eyeglass prescription. She had no visual disturbances at that time, and her best-corrected vision was 20/20 OU. She was started on pilocarpine 1% three times daily in both eyes and developed brow ache and blurred vision. This was discontinued and she was started on timolol 0.5% twice daily in both eyes. Her highest IOP prior to treatment was 30 mm Hg, which improved to 25 mm Hg on timolol. Her eye pressure gradually increased requiring the addition of brimonidine three times daily and latanoprost nightly in both eyes. She underwent cataract surgery 2 years ago and experienced an IOP spike to 55 mm Hg and was given acetazolamide 250 mg PO four times daily for 5 days after surgery until her pressure improved. Three months after surgery, her IOP control had improved, and therapy in her left eye was changed to dorzolamide three times daily only.

■ PMH

Hypertension, well controlled on lisinopril for 6 years
Kidney stones (occurred while taking acetazolamide)
Depression; controlled with exercise and counseling only; has never taken medications for depression
Myopia; corrected with glasses
Astigmatism; corrected with glasses
Pseudophakia; cataract surgery 3 years ago

■ FH

Parents are both deceased; father had POAG requiring surgery and was blind in right eye; mother died of breast cancer; has one brother who is alive with myopia

■ SH

Nonsmoker; drinks one to two glasses of wine per week

■ ROS

Decreased energy with two falls in the last month at home. All other systems negative.

■ Meds

Latanoprost 0.005% one drop nightly OD
Combigan 0.2%/0.5% one drop twice daily OD
Dorzolamide 2% one drop three times daily OS
Lisinopril 20 mg PO once daily

■ All

Penicillin—rash

■ Physical Examination

VS

BP 112/72, P 82, R 18, T 36.4°C

Eyes

Visual acuity: ODcc: 20/25; OScc: 20/60 (cc = with glasses)
Intraocular pressure: OD: 23; OS: 24 (normal range: 10–21 mm Hg)
Central corneal thickness (CCT): OD: 515: OS: 510 (normal 540 μm)

Gonioscopy: Iridocorneal angle is open with ciliary body band visible OU (open angle)

Pupils: Equal round and reactive OU; no relative afferent pupillary defect (rAPD)

Extraocular movements: Full OU

Slit Lamp Exam

Lids: Normal

Conjunctiva: 1+ injection OU

Cornea: Clear OU

Anterior chamber: Deep and quiet OU

Iris: Round and reactive OU

Lens: Posterior chamber intraocular lens OU

Vitreous: Normal

Optic Nerve

OD: Superior and inferior rim thinning with focal notch superiorly; cup-to-disk (C/D) ratio 0.85

OS: Superior rim loss, inferior rim thinning; disk hemorrhage inferotemporal disk; C/D ratio 0.95 (normal C/D 0.25)

CN II–XII grossly intact

Humphrey Visual Fields

OD: Good reliability, inferior arcuate depression; stable

OS: Good reliability, denser superior altitudinal defect splitting fixation, decreased foveal threshold

■ Assessment

1. Advanced POAG

   OD: Stable visual field, IOP slightly higher today.

   OS: Dense visual field loss now affecting central vision. IOP improved from baseline; however, it remains elevated and patient continues to progress.

2. *Pseudophakia*: Excellent result of cataract surgery

3. Myopia/astigmatism

4. Decline in energy

5. Recent falls

6. Depression well controlled on lifestyle modifications

7. Hypertension well controlled on lisinopril

■ Plan

1. *Right eye*: Continue latanoprost nightly and Combigan 0.2%/0.5% twice daily.

2. *Left eye*: Discontinue dorzolamide. Add latanoprost nightly and Combigan 0.2%/0.5% twice daily.

3. Follow-up in 1 month for IOP check of both eyes. If pressure remains elevated OU, schedule for glaucoma laser surgery.

4. *Decline in energy and falls*: Refer to PCP for systemic evaluation including depression and falls. May need to consider adverse effects of β-blocker if workup is negative.

5. Hypertension well controlled. Continue current medication regimen.

QUESTIONS

Collect Information

1.a. What subjective an objective evidence indicates that this patient has primary open-angle glaucoma (POAG)? See Figs. 109-1 to 109-3.

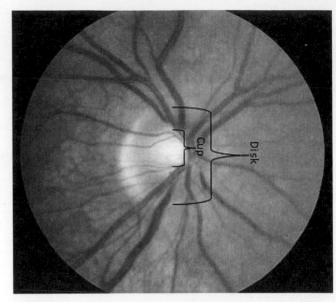

FIGURE 109-1. Normal optic nerve with cup-to-disk ratio (C/D) = 0.3.

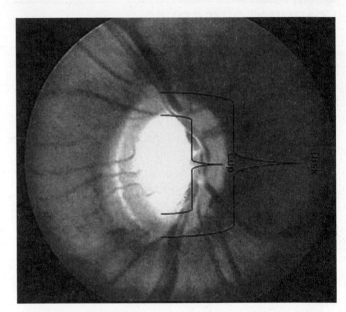

FIGURE 109-2. Abnormal, glaucomatous optic nerve with increased cup-to-disk ratio (C/D) = 0.8.

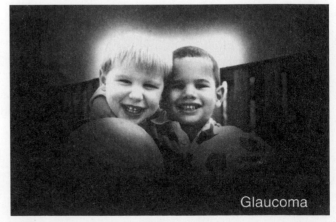

FIGURE 109-3. Simulated vision of patient with glaucoma. (Source: National Eye Institute, National Institutes of Health.)

1.b. What additional information is needed to fully assess this patient?

Assess the Information

2.a. What are this patient's risk factors for POAG?

2.b. Assess the severity of POAG based on the subjective and objective information available.

2.c. Create a list of the patient's drug therapy problems and prioritize them. Include assessment of medication appropriateness, effectiveness, safety, and patient adherence.

Develop a Care Plan

3.a. What are the goals of pharmacotherapy in this case?

3.b. What pharmacologic classes and individual agents are available to treat glaucoma?

3.c. How can glaucoma medications be combined to improve patient adherence?

3.d. If this patient were diagnosed today, what would be the optimal first-line pharmacologic therapy?

3.e. What surgical treatments might be useful for this patient?

3.f. During what phase of this patient's disease case are surgical treatments indicated?

3.g. Create an individualized, patient-centered, team-based care plan for this patient's glaucoma. Include specific drugs, dosage forms, doses, schedules, and durations of therapy.

3.h. Which medications should be avoided in this patient?

Implement the Care Plan

4.a. What information should the patient receive about the disease of glaucoma, proper medication administration technique, and possible adverse effects of treatment?

4.b. Describe how care should be coordinated with other healthcare providers.

Follow-Up: Monitor and Evaluate

5. Explain how to monitor and evaluate the care plan for medication appropriateness, effectiveness, safety, and patient adherence by using clinical and laboratory data, patient feedback, and other information.

■ SELF-STUDY ASSIGNMENTS

1. Perform a literature search on the reason why antimetabolites such as mitomycin C and 5-fluorouracil (5-FU) are used in glaucoma surgery. What is the mechanism of action of these antimetabolites in trabeculectomy pressure-lowering surgery?

2. Discuss the mechanism of action of latanoprostene bunod (Vyzulta) and netarsudil (Rhopressa). How does their efficacy compare to timolol?

CLINICAL PEARL

Glaucoma is a silent and generally slowly progressive optic neuropathy. Optimizing pharmacotherapy of glaucoma must consider systemic medical conditions, social situations, and environmental factors that may limit adherence. Patients should be monitored regularly for disease progression because many continue to progress on treatment despite "normal pressures."

REFERENCES

1. Heijl A, Leske MC, Bengtsson B, et al. Reduction of intraocular pressure and glaucoma progression: results from the Early Manifest Glaucoma Trial. Arch Ophthalmol. 2002;120:1268–1279.

2. Gordon MO, Beiser JA, Brandt JA, et al. The Ocular Hypertension Treatment Study: baseline factors that predict the onset of primary open-angle glaucoma. Arch Ophthalmol. 2002;120:714–720.

3. Drance S, Anderson DR, Schulzer M. Collaborative Normal-Tension Glaucoma Study. Risk factors for progression of visual field abnormalities in normal-tension glaucoma. Am J Ophthalmol. 2001;131:699–708.

4. Tielsch JM, Katz J, Sommer A, Quigley HA, Javitt JC. Family history and risk of primary open angle glaucoma. The Baltimore Eye Survey. Arch Ophthalmol. 1994;112(1):69–73.

5. Newman-Casey PA, Blachley T, Lee PP, et al. Patterns of glaucoma medication adherence over four years of follow-up. Ophthalmology. 2015;122:2010–2021.

6. Weinreb RN, Sforzolini BS, Vittitow J, Liebmann J. Latanoprostene bunod 0.024% versus timolol maleate 0.5% in subjects with open-angle glaucoma or ocular hypertension: the APOLLO study. Ophthalmology. 2016;123(5):965–973.

7. Serle JB, Katz LJ, McLaurin E, et al; Rocket-1 and Rocket-2 Study Groups. Two phase 3 clinical trials comparing the safety and efficacy of netarsudil to timolol in patients with elevated intraocular pressure: Rho Kinase Elevated IOP Treatment Trial 1 and 2 (ROCKET 1 and ROCKET-2). Am J Ophthalmol. 2018;186:116–127.

8. Higginbotham EJ. Considerations in glaucoma therapy: fixed combination versus their component medications. Clin Ophthalmol. 2010;4:1–9.

9. Gross RL. Current medical management of glaucoma. In: Yanoff M, Duker J, et al, eds. Ophthalmology. 3rd ed. Oxford, UK: Mosby–Elsevier; 2009:1220–1225.

10. Katz LJ, Steinmann WC, Kabir A, et al. Selective laser trabeculoplasty versus medical therapy as initial treatment of glaucoma: a prospective randomized trial. J Glaucoma. 2012;21:460–468.

110

ALLERGIC RHINITIS

Congested Beyond Relief . . . . Level I

Jon P. Wietholter, PharmD, BCPS, FCCP

LEARNING OBJECTIVES

After completing this case study, the reader should be able to:

- Discuss common signs and symptoms associated with allergic rhinitis.

- Choose appropriate measures to limit or avoid exposure to specific allergens.

- Select an appropriate pharmacotherapeutic regimen for managing allergic rhinitis.

- Construct a plan for patients with allergic rhinitis on appropriate medication use, including instillation technique for an intranasal medication.

PATIENT PRESENTATION

■ Chief Complaint

"I can't breathe!"

■ HPI

A 27-year-old man presents to an outpatient internal medicine clinic with complaints of severe congestion, intermittent bilateral rhinorrhea, and persistent sneezing. He states that symptoms are at their worst when he is outdoors, particularly after it rains. Because he spends time outdoors daily for work, the symptoms have been bothering him consistently over the past 1–2 months. Additionally, he is having trouble sleeping due to nasal congestion. He has struggled with these symptoms since he was a child, but they have significantly worsened over the past 2 years after he moved to West Virginia from California. He hasn't noticed a fever or a sore throat, but the symptoms are becoming troublesome. He is seeking advice on how to cope with and manage these symptoms.

■ PMH

Moderate asthma (diagnosed when he was 16)

■ FH

Father, age 54, with a history of asthma and allergic rhinitis. Mother, age 48, with a history of migraines.

■ SH

Works in construction; (–) tobacco, (–) illicit drugs, (+) social alcohol use (primarily on weekends with friends); has two cats and two dogs.

■ Meds

Diphenhydramine 25 mg PO Q 8 H PRN for allergy symptoms
Budesonide 80 mcg/formoterol 4.5 mcg MDI two puffs Q 6 H PRN for asthma reliever therapy; uses infrequently
Budesonide 80 mcg/formoterol 4.5 mcg MDI two puffs Q 12 H for asthma maintenance therapy

■ All

Penicillin (hives); cephalexin (trouble breathing)

■ ROS

Denies headaches; no shortness of breath, wheezing, chest pain, or abdominal discomfort

■ Physical Examination

Gen

Appears tired and sounds congested. Although sneezing and rhinorrhea are complaints, they are not actively ongoing during this evaluation.

VS

BP 112/74 mm Hg, P 68 bpm, RR 18, T 36.9°C; Wt 155 lb (70.5 kg), Ht 5′8″ (173 cm)

Skin

Turgor normal, no rashes or lesions

HEENT

NC/AT; PERRLA; EOMI; (–) periorbital edema or discoloration; TMs are intact; (+) swollen nasal mucous membranes and nasal turbinates with a pale, bluish hue and discharge down the posterior pharynx; (–) tenderness over frontal and maxillary sinuses; (–) oropharyngeal lesions; throat is nonerythematous

Neck/Lymph Nodes

No lymphadenopathy or thyromegaly

Chest

CTA bilaterally; no noticeable wheezing or coughing

CV

RRR without murmur or rub

Abd

Soft, nontender, (+) BS

MS/Ext

No erythema, pain, or edema; pulses 2+

Neuro

A&O × 3; CN: visual fields and hearing intact; 5/5 strength throughout

■ Labs

Na 140 mEq/L	Hgb 15.4 g/dL
K 3.9 mEq/L	Hct 45.3%
Cl 108 mEq/L	Plt 391 × 10³/mm³
CO_2 28 mEq/L	WBC 9.6 × 10³/mm³
BUN 10 mg/dL	
SCr 0.7 mg/dL	
Glu 88 mg/dL	

■ Other

Peak expiratory flow (PEF): Patient states home readings are always >80% of personal best.

■ Assessment

This is a 27-year-old man complaining of signs and symptoms consistent with moderate–severe persistent allergic rhinitis.

QUESTIONS

Collect Information

1.a. What subjective and objective information indicates the presence of allergic rhinitis?

1.b. What additional information is needed to fully assess this patient's allergic rhinitis?

Assess the Information

2.a. Assess the severity of allergic rhinitis based on the subjective and objective information available.

2.b. Create a list of the patient's drug therapy problems and prioritize them. Include assessment of medication appropriateness, effectiveness, safety, and patient adherence.

Develop a Care Plan

3.a. What are the goals of pharmacotherapy for allergic rhinitis in this case?

3.b. What nondrug therapies might be useful for this patient's allergic rhinitis?

3.c. What feasible pharmacotherapeutic options are available for treating this patient's allergic rhinitis?

3.d. Create an individualized, patient-centered, team-based care plan to optimize medication therapy for this patient's allergic rhinitis and other drug therapy problems. Include specific drugs, dosage forms, doses, schedules, and durations of therapy.

Implement the Care Plan

4.a. What information should be provided to the patient to enhance adherence, ensure successful therapy, and minimize adverse effects?

4.b. Describe how care should be coordinated with other healthcare providers.

Follow-Up: Monitor and Evaluate

5. Explain how to monitor and evaluate the care plan for medication appropriateness, effectiveness, safety, and patient adherence by using clinical and laboratory data, patient feedback, and other information.

■ CLINICAL COURSE: ALTERNATIVE THERAPY

The patient reports that he has read about butterbur extract being helpful for allergy symptoms. He asks whether it would be okay to use it in addition to his prescription medications. See Section 19 of this Casebook for questions regarding the use of butterbur extract for allergy symptoms.

■ SELF-STUDY ASSIGNMENTS

1. Review the emerging evidence base for both subcutaneous and sublingual allergen immunotherapy (SCIT and SLIT) including

patient populations most likely to benefit from them and potential adverse effects with each treatment modality.

2. Describe a situation where monotherapy with an antihistamine or decongestant would be appropriate or preferred for managing allergic rhinitis. Support your recommendations with efficacy and safety data.

CLINICAL PEARL

Intranasal corticosteroids and intranasal antihistamines are excellent monotherapy options for many patients with allergic rhinitis. When used in combination, they are even more effective than monotherapy and are quicker acting with an onset of about 5 minutes.

REFERENCES

1. Seidman MD, Gurgel RK, Lin SY, et al. Clinical practice guideline: allergic rhinitis. Otolaryngol Head Neck Surg. 2015;152(IS):S1–S43.

2. Bousquet J, Anto JM, Bachert C, et al. Allergic rhinitis. Nat Rev Dis Primers. 2020 Dec 3;6(1):95.

3. Dykewicz MS, Wallace DV, Amrol DJ, et al. Rhinitis 2020: a practice parameter update. J Allergy Clin Immunol. 2020 Oct;146(4):721–767.

4. Dykewicz MS, Wallace DV, Baroody F, et al. Treatment of seasonal allergic rhinitis: an evidence-based focused 2017 guideline update. Ann Allergy Asthma Immunol. 2017;119(6):489–511.

5. Wheatley LM, Togias A. Clinical practice. Allergic rhinitis. N Engl J Med. 2015;372:456–463.

6. Brozek JL, Bousquet J, Agache I, et al. Allergic rhinitis and its impact on asthma (ARIA) guidelines: 2016 revision. J Allergy Clin Immunol. 2017;140:950–958.

7. Sur DKC, Plesa ML. Treatment of allergic rhinitis. Am Fam Physician 2015;92(11):985–992.

8. Bousquet J, Schunemann HJ, Hellings PW, et al. MACVIA clinical decision algorithm in adolescents and adults with allergic rhinitis. J Allergy Clin Immunol. 2016;138(2):367–374.

111

ACNE VULGARIS

The Graduate...............................Level II

Rebecca M. Law, BS Pharm, PharmD

Wayne P. Gulliver, MD, FRCPC

LEARNING OBJECTIVES

After completing this case study, the reader should be able to:

- Understand risk factors and aggravating factors in the pathogenesis of acne vulgaris.

- Understand the treatment strategies for acne, including appropriate situations for using nonprescription and prescription medications and use of topical and systemic therapies.

- Educate patients with acne on systemic therapies.

- Monitor the safety and efficacy of selected systemic therapies.

PATIENT PRESENTATION

■ Chief Complaint

"I can't stand this acne!"

■ HPI

This is an 18-year-old woman with a history of facial acne since age 15. One month ago, she completed a 3-month course of minocycline in combination with Differin (adapalene). Her acne has flared up again, and she presents again to her family physician for treatment.

■ PMH

She has irregular menses as a result of polycystic ovary syndrome diagnosed 3 years ago, which has not required medical treatment. However, it has resulted in an acne condition that was initially quite mild; she responded well to nonprescription topical products. In the past 2 years, the number of facial lesions has increased despite OTC and, later, prescription drug treatments. Initially, her physician prescribed Benzamycin Gel (benzoyl peroxide 5%/erythromycin 3%), which was beneficial, but this had to be discontinued because of excessive drying. Differin XP (adapalene 0.3% gel) was used next, and it controlled her condition for about 6 months; then the acne worsened and oral antibiotics were added. Most recently, she has received two 3-month courses of minocycline over the past year. She has also noted some scarring and cysts in the past few months.

■ FH

Her parents are alive and well; she has two older brothers (ages 21 and 25). Her father had acne with residual scarring.

■ SH

The patient is under some stress because she is graduating from high school in a few weeks. She wants to do well in school so she will qualify for the best colleges. Both of her brothers graduated with honors. She has been sexually active for the past 2 months, and her boyfriend uses condoms.

■ Meds

None currently

■ All

NKDA

■ ROS

In addition to the complaints noted above, the patient has irregular menstrual periods and mild hirsutism

■ Physical Examination

Gen

Alert, moderately anxious teenager in NAD

VS

BP 110/70 mm Hg, RR 15, T 37°C; Wt 45 kg, Ht 5'2"

Skin

Ten to fifteen comedones on forehead, nose, and chin; four to five papules and pustules on the nose and malar area. A few healing cysts on the chin. Superficial scars on malar area. Increased facial hair.

HEENT

PERRLA, EOMI, fundi benign, TMs intact

Chest

CTA bilaterally

Cor

RRR without MRG, S_1 and S_2 normal

Abd

(+) BS, soft, nontender, no masses

MS/Ext

No joint aches or pains; peripheral pulses present

Neuro

CN II–XII intact

■ Labs

Na 140 mEq/L	Hgb 13.0 g/dL	AST 21 IU/L	T. chol 170 mg/dL
K 3.7 mEq/L	Hct 38%	ALT 39 IU/L	LDL-C 90 mg/dL
Cl 100 mEq/L	Plt 300 × 10³/mm³	LDH 105 IU/L	Trig 90 mg/dL
CO_2 25 mEq/L	WBC 7.0 × 10³/mm³	Alk phos 89 IU/L	HDL 45 mg/dL
BUN 12 mg/dL		T. bili 1.0 mg/dL	FSH 30 mIU/mL
SCr 1.0 mg/dL		Alb 3.9 g/dL	LH 150 mIU/mL
Glu 100 mg/dL			DHEAS
			221 mcg/dL
			(6 μmol/L)
			Testosterone (free)
			2.3 ng/mL
			Prolactin
			15 ng/mL

QUESTIONS

Collect Information

1.a. What subjective and objective information indicates the presence of acne vulgaris?

1.b. What additional information is needed to fully assess this patient's acne?

Assess the Information

2.a. Assess the severity of acne vulgaris based on the subjective and objective information available.

2.b. Create a list of the patient's drug therapy problems and prioritize them. Include assessment of medication appropriateness, effectiveness, safety, and patient adherence.

2.c. How does polycystic ovary syndrome contribute to this patient's acne and other physical findings?

Develop a Care Plan

3.a. What are the goals of pharmacotherapy in this case?

3.b. What nondrug therapies might be useful for this patient?

3.c. What feasible pharmacotherapeutic alternatives are available for treating acne vulgaris?

3.d. Create an individualized, patient-centered, team-based care plan to optimize medication therapy for this patient's acne and other drug therapy problems. Include specific drugs, dosage forms, doses, schedules, and durations of therapy.

Implement the Care Plan

4.a. What information should be provided to the patient to enhance compliance, ensure successful therapy, and minimize adverse effects?

4.b. Describe how care should be coordinated with other healthcare providers.

Follow-Up: Monitor and Evaluate

5. Explain how to monitor and evaluate the care plan for medication appropriateness, effectiveness, safety, and patient adherence by using clinical and laboratory data, patient feedback, and other information.

■ CLINICAL COURSE

Two months later, the patient's acne is improving, but she has developed bloating, weight gain, and increased appetite, likely related to the therapy prescribed. She also reveals that her maternal grandmother and aunt both died of melanoma, and a friend told her that she should not be using her new therapy.

■ FOLLOW-UP QUESTION

1. Based on this new information, what is the most appropriate course of action?

■ SELF-STUDY ASSIGNMENTS

1. Review the dysmorphic syndrome associated with acne.

2. Review the nonpharmacologic management of acne, including stress reduction and dietary changes.

CLINICAL PEARL

In females with acne, scarring + cysts + two courses of oral antibiotics means hormonal therapy and "consider isotretinoin."

REFERENCES

1. Dreno B, Pecastaings S, Corvec S, et al. *Cutibacterium acnes (Propionibacterium acnes)* and acne vulgaris: a brief look at the latest updates. J Eur Acad Dermatol Venereol. 2018;32(Suppl 2):5–14.

2. Eichenfield LF, Krakowski AC, Piggott C, et al. Evidence-based recommendations for the diagnosis and treatment of pediatric acne. Pediatrics 2013;131:S163–S186. Available at: *https://pediatrics.aappublications.org/content/pediatrics/131/Supplement_3/S163.full.pdf*. Accessed February 22, 2019.

3. Nast A, Dreno B, Bettoli V, et al. European evidence-based (S3) guidelines for the treatment of acne—update 2016—short version. J Eur Acad Dermatol Venereol. 2016;30(8):1261–1268.

4. Asai Y, Baibergenova A, Dutil M, et al. Management of acne: Canadian clinical practice guideline. CMAJ 2016;188(2):118–126.

5. Thiboutot D, Dreno B, Abanmi A, et al. Practical management of acne for clinicians: an international consensus from the Global Alliance to Improve Outcomes in Acne. J Am Acad Dermatol. 2018;78:S1–S23.

6. Polycystic Ovary Syndrome. Office of Women's Health, US Department of Health & Human Services. October 22, 2018. Available at: *https://www.womenshealth.gov/a-z-topics/polycystic-ovary-syndrome*. Accessed March 7, 2019.

7. Gollnick H, Cunliffe W, Berson D, et al. Management of acne: a report from a Global Alliance to Improve Outcomes in Acne. J Am Acad Dermatol. 2003;49(1 Suppl):S1–S37.

8. Law RM. The pharmacist's role in the treatment of acne. America's Pharmacist. 2003;125:35–42.

9. Zaenglein AL, Pathy AL, Schlosser BJ, et al. Guidelines of care for the management of acne vulgaris. J Am Acad Dermatol. 2016;74(5):945–973.

10. Santhosh P, George M. Clascoterone: a new topical anti-androgen for acne management. Int J Dermatol. 2021;60(12):1561–1565.

11. Tan J. Dapsone 5% gel: a new option in topical therapy for acne. Skin Therapy Lett. 2012;17(8):1–3.

12. Chung JP, Yiu AK, Chung TK, et al. A randomized crossover study of medroxyprogesterone acetate and Diane-35 in adolescent girls with polycystic ovarian syndrome. J Pediatr Adolesc Gynecol. 2014;27:166–171.

13. Karagas MR, Stukel TA, Dykes J, et al. A pooled analysis of 10 case-control studies of melanoma and oral contraceptive use. Br J Cancer. 2002;86:1085–1092.

112

PSORIASIS

The Harried School Teacher..................... Level II

Rebecca M. Law, BS Pharm, PharmD

Wayne P. Gulliver, MD, FRCPC

LEARNING OBJECTIVES

After completing this case study, students should be able to:

- Describe the pathophysiology and clinical presentation of plaque psoriasis.

- Discuss the appropriate use of topical, photochemical, and systemic treatment modalities including biologic agents for psoriasis, based on disease severity.

- Compare the efficacy and adverse effects of systemic therapies for psoriasis, including first-line standard therapies (methotrexate, acitretin, cyclosporine), second-line therapies (azathioprine, hydroxyurea, sulfasalazine), and the biologic agents (TNF-alpha inhibitors, ustekinumab, IL-17 inhibitors, and IL-23 inhibitors).

- Select appropriate therapeutic regimens for patients with plaque psoriasis based on disease severity and patient-specific considerations such as organ dysfunction.

- Educate patients with psoriasis about proper use of pharmacotherapy, potential adverse effects, and necessary precautions.

PATIENT PRESENTATION

■ Chief Complaint

"Nothing is helping my psoriasis."

■ HPI

A 50-year-old man with a 27-year history of psoriasis presented to the outpatient dermatology clinic 2 days ago with another flare-up of his psoriasis. He was admitted to the inpatient dermatology service for a severe flare of plaque psoriasis involving his arms, legs, elbows, knees, palms, abdomen, back, and scalp (Fig. 112-1).

The patient was diagnosed with plaque psoriasis at age 23. He initially responded to topical therapy with medium-potency topical corticosteroids, later to calcipotriol. He subsequently required photo-chemotherapy using psoralens with UVA phototherapy (PUVA) to control the condition. PUVA eventually became ineffective, and about 10 years ago he was started on oral methotrexate 5 mg once weekly. Dosage escalations kept the condition under fairly good control for about 5 years. Flare-ups during that period were initially managed with SCAT (short-contact anthralin therapy), but they eventually became more frequent and lesions were more widespread despite increasing the methotrexate dose. A liver biopsy performed about 5 years ago showed no evidence of fibrosis, hepatitis, or cirrhosis.

After requiring two SCAT treatments in a 4-month period, along with methotrexate 25 mg once weekly orally (given as two doses of 12.5 mg 12 hours apart), a change in therapy was considered

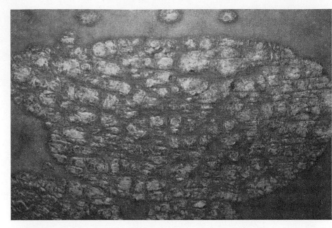

FIGURE 112-1. Plaque psoriasis. This papulosquamous skin disease is characterized by small and large erythematous papules and plaques with overlying adherent silvery scale. (Adapted with permission from Yancey KB, Lawley, TJ. Approach to the patient with a skin disorder. In: Jameson J, Fauci AS, Kasper DL, et al, eds. *Harrison's Principles of Internal Medicine.* 20th ed. 2018. New York, NY: McGraw-Hill Education; 2018. *https://accesspharmacy.com.* Accessed April 12, 2019.)

necessary at that time. Because he was receiving the maximum recommended methotrexate dose and had already reached a lifetime cumulative methotrexate dose of 2.2 grams, he was changed to a cyclic regimen of cyclosporine microemulsion (Neoral) 75 mg orally twice daily for 3 months, followed by acitretin (Soriatane) 25 mg orally once daily with dinner for 3 months, and repeat. He found the acitretin drying, so after 6 months he was changed to the current regimen of only cyclosporine microemulsion 75 mg orally twice daily. This appeared to work. Flare-ups had become infrequent and were again successfully managed by SCAT for over 1 year. However, in the past 6 months, he has already required two SCAT treatments for flare-ups, and this is his third and most severe flare-up.

■ PMH

One episode of major depressive illness triggered by the death of his first wife, which occurred 16 years ago (age 34). He was treated by his family physician who prescribed fluoxetine for 6 months. He has had no recurrences. He has no other chronic medical conditions and no other acute or recent illnesses.

■ FH

Parents alive and well. Father has HTN and type 2 diabetes. Has two older sisters and a younger brother. Younger brother was diagnosed with psoriasis about 5 years ago. No history of other immune disorders or malignancy.

■ SH

Patient is an elementary school teacher. He is currently a nonsmoker but used to be a heavy smoker in his younger years (20s and 30s); social use of alcohol (glass of wine with dinner). He is married and has two children ages 10 and 12 with his second wife. There has been an increased workload for the past year because of teacher layoffs at his school.

■ Meds

Neoral 75 mg PO twice daily
Acetaminophen for occasional headaches

■ **All**

NKDA

■ **ROS**

Skin feels very itchy despite using a nonmedicated moisturizer TID. No joint aches or pains. No complaints of shortness of breath. Occasional nausea associated with a cyclosporine dose. Has been feeling stressed because of tensions at work but does not feel depressed.

■ **Physical Examination**

Gen

Alert, mildly anxious 50-year-old man in NAD

VS

BP 129/83 mm Hg, P 88 bpm, T 37°C; Wt 75 kg, Ht 5'9"

Skin

Confluent plaque psoriasis with extensive lesions on abdomen, arms, legs, back, and scalp. Thick crusted lesions on elbows, knees, palms, and soles. Lesions are red to violet in color, with sharply demarcated borders except where confluent, and are loosely covered with silvery-white scales. There are no pustules or vesicles. There are excoriations on trunk and extremities consistent with scratching.

HEENT

PERRLA, EOMI, fundi benign, TMs intact; extensive scaly lesions on scalp as noted

Neck/Lymph Nodes

No lymphadenopathy; thyroid nonpalpable

Chest

CTA bilaterally

CV

RRR without MRG; S_1 and S_2 normal

Abd

(+) BS, soft, nontender, no masses; extensive scaly lesions and excoriations on skin as noted above

MS/Ext

No joint swelling, warmth, or tenderness; skin lesions as noted above; no nail involvement; peripheral pulses 2+ throughout

Neuro

A&O × 3; CN II–XII intact; DTRs 2+ toes downgoing

■ **Labs**

Na 139 mEq/L	Hgb 13.5 g/dL	AST 22 IU/L
K 4.0 mEq/L	Hct 35.0%	ALT 38 IU/L
Cl 102 mEq/L	Plt 255 × 10^3/mm³	LDH 107 IU/L
CO_2 25 mEq/L	WBC 6.0 × 10^3/mm³	Alk phos 98 IU/L
BUN 14 mg/dL		T. bili 1.0 mg/dL
SCr 1.0 mg/dL		Alb 3.7 g/dL
Glu 98 mg/dL		Uric acid 4 mg/dL
		T. chol 180 mg/dL

QUESTIONS

Collect Information

1.a. What subjective and objective information indicates the presence of plaque psoriasis?

1.b. What comorbidities does this patient have that are associated with psoriasis?

1.c. What additional information is needed to fully assess this patient?

1.d. What risk factors for developing psoriasis or experiencing a disease flare-up are present in this patient?

Assess the Information

2.a. Assess the severity of psoriasis based on the subjective and objective information available.

2.b. Create a list of the patient's drug therapy problems and prioritize them. Include assessment of medication appropriateness, effectiveness, safety, and patient adherence.

Develop a Care Plan

3.a. What are the goals of pharmacotherapy for this patient's plaque psoriasis and other drug therapy problems?

3.b. What nondrug therapies might be useful for managing this patient's psoriasis and related drug therapy problems?

3.c. What feasible pharmacotherapeutic alternatives are available for managing this patient's psoriasis and related drug therapy problems?

3.d. Create an individualized, patient-centered, team-based care plan to optimize medication therapy for this patient's plaque psoriasis and related drug therapy problems. Include specific drugs, dosage forms, doses, schedules, and durations of therapy.

Implement the Care Plan

4.a. What information should be provided to the patient to enhance compliance, ensure successful therapy, and minimize adverse effects?

4.b. Describe how care should be coordinated with other healthcare providers.

Follow-Up: Monitor and Evaluate

5. Explain how to monitor and evaluate the care plan for medication appropriateness, effectiveness, safety, and patient adherence by using clinical and laboratory data, patient feedback, and other information.

■ SELF-STUDY ASSIGNMENTS

1. Perform a literature search to identify potential future therapies for psoriasis: topical therapies such as NSAIDs, protein kinase C inhibitors, methotrexate gel, an implantable 5-fluorouracil formulation; systemic therapies such as glucosamine, monoclonal antibodies, and cytokines.

2. Perform a literature search to review the current guidelines, opinions, and evidence regarding liver biopsies and long-term methotrexate use for patients with psoriasis.

CLINICAL PEARL

Provide patient-specific therapies and always consider any psychosocial effects, debilities, and comorbidities related to the patient's psoriasis.

REFERENCES

1. Kim WB, Jerome D, Yeung J. Diagnosis and management of psoriasis. Can Fam Physician. 2017;63(4):278–285.
2. Papp KA, Gulliver W, Lynde CW, Poulin Y (Steering Committee). Canadian Guidelines for the Management of Plaque Psoriasis. 1st ed. June 2009. Available at: *https://dermatology.ca/dermatologists/guidelines/psoriasis*. Also see: Canadian Psoriasis Guidelines Addendum Committee. Addendum to the Canadian Guidelines for the Management of Plaque Psoriasis, May 2016. J Cutan Med Surg. 2016;20(5):375–431. Available at: *https://www.ncbi.nlm.nih.gov/pmc/articles/PMC5014087/*. Accessed April 30, 2022.
3. Elmets CA, Korman NJ, Prater EF, et al. Joint American Academy of Dermatology–National Psoriasis Foundation guidelines of care for the management and treatment of psoriasis with topical therapy and alternative medicine modalities for psoriasis severity measures. J Am Acad Dermatol. 2021;84:430–470.
4. Menter A, Cordoro KM, Davis DMR, et al. Joint American Academy of Dermatology–National Psoriasis Foundation guidelines of care for the management and treatment of psoriasis in pediatric patients. J Am Acad Dermatol. 2020;82:161–201.
5. Menter A, Gelfand JM, Connor C, et al. Joint American Academy of Dermatology–National Psoriasis Foundation guidelines of care for the management of psoriasis with systemic nonbiologic therapies. J Am Acad Dermatol. 2020;82:1445–1486.
6. Elmets CA, Lim HW, Stoff B, et al. Joint American Academy of Dermatology–National Psoriasis Foundation guidelines of care for the management of psoriasis with phototherapy. J Am Acad Dermatol. 2019;81:775–804.
7. Rosmarin DM, Lebwohl M, Elewski BE, et al. Cyclosporine and psoriasis: 2008 National Psoriasis Foundation Consensus Conference. J Am Acad Dermatol. 2010;62:838–853.
8. Kalb RE, Strober B, Weinstein G, Lebwohl M. Methotrexate and psoriasis: 2009 National Psoriasis Foundation Consensus Conference. J Am Acad Dermatol. 2009;60:824–837.
9. European S3-Guidelines on the systemic treatment of psoriasis vulgaris. Updated 2015. EDF in cooperation with EADV and IPC. J Eur Acad Dermatol Venereol. 2015;29(12):e1–22.
10. Smith CH, Jabbar-Lopez ZK, Yiu ZZ, et al. British Association of Dermatologists guidelines for biologic therapy for psoriasis 2017. Br J Dermatol. 2017;177(3):628–636.
11. Menter A, Strober BE, Kaplan DH, et al. Joint AAD-NPF guidelines of care for the management and treatment of psoriasis with biologics. J Am Acad Dermatol. 2019;80(4):1029–1072.
12. Elmets CA, Leonardi CL, Davis DMR, et al. Joint AAD-NPF guidelines of care for the management and treatment of psoriasis with awareness and attention to comorbidities. J Am Acad Dermatol. 2019;80(4):1073–1113.
13. Armstrong AW, Siegel MP, Bagel J, et al. From the Medical Board of the National Psoriasis Foundation: treatment targets for plaque psoriasis. J Am Acad Dermatol. 2017;76(2):290–298.

113

ATOPIC DERMATITIS

The Itch That Erupts When Scratched . . . . Level I

Rebecca M. Law, BS Pharm, PharmD

Howard I. Maibach, MD

LEARNING OBJECTIVES

After completing this case study, students should be able to:

- Understand risk factors and aggravating factors in the pathophysiology of atopic dermatitis.
- Understand treatment strategies for atopic dermatitis, including nonpharmacologic management.
- Educate patients and their caregivers about management of atopic dermatitis.
- Monitor the safety and efficacy of selected pharmacologic therapies.

PATIENT PRESENTATION

■ Chief Complaint

As stated by the patient's mother, "My child constantly wants to scratch her skin, and she can't sleep well during the night."

■ HPI

A 3½-year-old girl started attending daycare about 1 month ago. She did not want to go and still exhibits a lot of clinging behavior when her mother tries to leave; she still cries when her mother eventually does manage to leave. Her mother says that the child's atopic dermatitis has flared up again. She has had atopic dermatitis since she was about 6 months old. It had been well controlled by topical corticosteroids and liberal use of moisturizers. Her recent flare-up began about 2–3 weeks ago. She has not been sleeping well and is constantly trying to scratch her skin at night. Her mother has been using 100% cotton sheets for her bed since she was an infant. She has sewn mittens on 100% cotton pajamas to prevent scratching because she had previously caused excoriations from scratching, which then became infected. During the day, the patient constantly wants to scratch but has been told to just "pat" the itchy area. The caregivers at the daycare center keep an eye on her scratching behavior as well but are not always able to prevent her from scratching herself. They also inform her mother that the child likes to eat food shared by other children.

■ PMH

The patient was breast-fed from birth for a total of 8 weeks, when her mother decided to return to work. She was then cared for at home by a babysitter and fed cow's milk, with oatmeal cereal being introduced as the first solid food. She was fed lemon meringue pie (made with egg white) once, and developed generalized hives, which led to the recognition of an egg allergy. This was confirmed by prick testing. The parents recently became aware that the babysitter left her alone a lot (sitting on the floor/carpet to play by herself). That was the major reason for sending her to a daycare center.

■ SH

The patient is the only child of a professional couple. Her father is an engineer, and her mother is a litigation lawyer who often works long hours. The couple has a stressful lifestyle, and it appears that the stress is reflected in her care. For example, she sometimes would be driven to one or another babysitter's homes at the last minute, when something urgent arose that the couple had to take care of. There is little family time. Unfortunately, their relatives do not live in the same city, and there is little social support for the child on a day-to-day basis. The parents were hoping that the daycare center would be helpful, but so far that has proven to be another issue for her. She does not want to participate in activities there and has frequent temper tantrums. She does not play well with other children. She had been toilet-trained but has now lost her toilet training and is using diapers again. The mother started smoking again due to the recent stress; her child keeps her up at night, and the mother is having difficulty dealing with her child's multiple issues at home and at the daycare center.

■ FH

There is a strong family history of atopy. The father has a severe allergy to shellfish, and the mother has a history of hay fever. The father's sister has multiple food allergies. The maternal grandmother had asthma. The paternal first cousin had infantile eczema. The maternal first cousin has a severe peanut allergy (generalized hives).

■ Meds

Hydrocortisone 1% cream applied to affected areas two to four times a day; although twice daily is her usual maintenance dose, she currently needs it three to four times a day.

Vaseline ad lib

Diphenhydramine 0.5 teaspoonful PO at bedtime as needed (when skin is excessively itchy, to allow her to sleep)

■ All

NKDA. Multiple food allergies: egg (hives, developed allergy as an infant), strawberries, raspberries, and tomatoes.

■ ROS

Not obtained

■ Physical Examination

Gen

Unhappy, cranky, thin, clinging girl who keeps sucking her thumb

VS

BP 98/50, HR 96, RR 18, T 37°C; Wt 12.2 kg (10th percentile), Ht 98 cm (38.6″; 50th percentile), head circumference 49.5 cm (19.5″; 50th percentile)

Skin

Generally dry over entire body. Eczematous skin lesions on her cheeks and in flexure areas (behind ears, wrist joints, elbows, knees). Numerous pruritic papules in flexure areas with mild excoriations seen from scratching. Some spots of bleeding seen, but there is no crusting and the skin does not appear infected. Some cracking skin lesions seen behind the ears and knees. No lichenification. There are no lesions on the extensor parts of her body, the top of her nose, or in the diaper area.

The remainder of the physical exam was normal.

■ Labs

Na 135 mEq/L	Hgb 12.0 g/dL	WBC differential	AST 20 IU/L
K 4.0 mEq/L	Hct 35%	Neutros 50%	ALT 7 IU/L
Cl 102 mEq/L	Plt 230 × 10³/mm³	Bands 3%	IgE 300 IU/mL
CO₂ 26 mEq/L	WBC 5.0 × 10³/mm³	Eosinophils 18%	D-dimer 90 ng/mL
BUN 8 mg/dL		Lymphs 27%	INR 1.1
SCr 0.2 mg/dL		Basophils 1%	aPTT 30 seconds
		Monos 1%	

Allergen-specific serum IgE tests: Elevated for egg, strawberries, raspberries

Note: Reference ranges at age 3.5—BUN 8–20 mg/dL, SCr 0.2–0.8 mg/dL, AST 20–60 IU/L, ALT 0–37 IU/L, and IgE 0–25 IU/mL; WBC differential—neutros 20–65%, eos 0–15%, basos 0–2%, lymphs 20–60%, and monos 0–10%.

Swab of skin lesion where there is bleeding: No growth

■ Assessment

This is a 3½-year-old child with an exacerbation of atopic dermatitis, likely stress induced.

QUESTIONS

Collect Information

1.a. What subjective and objective information indicates the presence of atopic dermatitis?

1.b. What additional information is needed to fully assess this patient's atopic dermatitis?

Assess the Information

2.a. Assess the severity of atopic dermatitis based on the subjective and objective information available.

2.b. What risk factors or aggravating factors may have contributed to the patient's atopic dermatitis flare?

2.c. Create a list of the patient's drug therapy problems and prioritize them. Include assessment of medication appropriateness, effectiveness, safety, and patient adherence.

Develop a Care Plan

3.a. What are the goals of pharmacotherapy for atopic dermatitis and related concerns (behavior issues, caregiver stress) in this case?

3.b. What nondrug therapies might be useful to manage this patient's pruritus, atopic dermatitis, behavioral issues, and her caregivers' stress?

3.c. What feasible pharmacotherapeutic alternatives are available to manage this patient's pruritus, atopic dermatitis, behavioral issues, and caregiver stress?

3.d. Create an individualized, patient-centered, team-based care plan to optimize medication therapy for this patient's atopic dermatitis and other drug therapy problems. Include specific drugs, dosage forms, doses, schedules, and durations of therapy.

Implement the Care Plan

4.a. How would you inform the patient's caregiver about the atopic dermatitis treatment regimen to enhance adherence, ensure successful therapy, and minimize adverse effects?

4.b. Describe how care should be coordinated with other healthcare providers.

Follow-Up: Monitor and Evaluate

5. Explain how to monitor and evaluate the care plan for medication appropriateness, effectiveness, safety, and patient adherence by using clinical and laboratory data, patient feedback, and other information.

■ SELF-STUDY ASSIGNMENTS

1. Review the use of phototherapy for atopic dermatitis.

2. Discuss how the clinical presentation and treatment strategies for an 8-month-old infant with atopic dermatitis might differ from those of a 3½-year-old child.

CLINICAL PEARL

In atopic dermatitis, minimizing preventable risk factors such as stress, eliminating triggers, providing appropriate skin care, and controlling the itch are as important as pharmacologic treatment.

ACKNOWLEDGMENT

This case is based on the patient case co-authored for previous editions with Po Gin Kwa, MD, FRCPC.

REFERENCES

1. Wollenberg A, Barbarot S, Bieber T, et al. Consensus-based European guidelines for treatment of atopic eczema (atopic dermatitis) in adults and children: part I & part II. J Eur Acad Dermatol Venereol. 2018;32(5): 657–682, 850–878.

2. Wong ITY, Tsuyuki RT, Cresswell-Melville A, et al. Guidelines for the management of atopic dermatitis (eczema) for pharmacists. Can Pharm J. (Ott) 2017;150(5):285–297.

3. Kim BS. Atopic Dermatitis. Medscape eMedicine updated October 30, 2018. Available at: http://emedicine.medscape.com/article/1049085-overview. Accessed November 19, 2018.

4. Eichenfield LE, Tom WL, Chamlin SI, et al. Guidelines of care for the management of atopic dermatitis. Section 1. Diagnosis and assessment of atopic dermatitis. J Am Acad Dermatol. 2014;70:338–351.

5. Sidbury R, Tom WL, Bergman JN, et al. Guidelines of care for the management of atopic dermatitis. Section 4. Prevention of disease flares and use of adjunctive therapies and approaches. J Am Acad Dermatol. 2014;71(6):1218–1233.

6. DaVeiga SP. Epidemiology of atopic dermatitis: a review. Allergy Asthma Proc. 2012;23:227–234.

7. Koblenzer CS. Itching and the atopic skin. J Allergy Clin Immunol. 1999;104(3 Pt 2):S109–S113.

8. Eichenfield LF, Tom WL, Berger TG, et al. Guidelines of care for the management of atopic dermatitis. Section 2. Management and treatment of atopic dermatitis with topical therapies. J Am Acad Dermatol. 2014;71(1):116–132.

9. Eichenfield LF, Boguniewicz M, Simpson EL, et al. Translating atopic dermatitis management guidelines into practice for primary care providers. Pediatrics 2015;136(3):554–565.

10. Sidbury R, Davis DM, Cohen DE, et al. Guidelines of care for the management of atopic dermatitis. Section 3. Management and treatment with phototherapy and systemic agents. J Am Acad Dermatol. 2014;71:327–349.

11. Gooderham M, Lynde CW, Papp K, et al. Review of systemic treatment options for adult atopic dermatitis. J Cutan Med Surg. 2017;21(1):31–39.

12. Le M, Berman-Rosa M, Ghazawi FM, et al. Systematic review on the efficacy and safety of oral Janus kinase inhibitors for the treatment of atopic dermatitis. Front Med. 2021 Sep 1;8:682547. doi: 10.3389/fmed.2021.682547.

13. Patel R, DuPont HL. New approaches for bacteriotherapy: prebiotics, new-generation probiotics, and synbiotics. Clin Infect Dis. 2015;60(Suppl 2):S108–S121.

114

DERMATOLOGIC DRUG REACTION

A Case of TEN..................................Level III

Rebecca M. Law, BS Pharm, PharmD

Howard I. Maibach, MD

LEARNING OBJECTIVES

After completing this case study, the reader should be able to:

- Describe the approach to identifying or ruling out a suspected drug-induced skin reaction.

- Recognize the signs and symptoms of drug-induced Stevens–Johnson syndrome (SJS) and toxic epidermal necrolysis (TEN).

- Name the drugs most commonly implicated in causing SJS and TEN.

- Determine an appropriate course of action for a patient with a suspected drug-induced skin reaction.

- Discuss the treatment approach for a patient with TEN, including nonpharmacologic and pharmacologic therapies.

- Participate in a collaborative interprofessional team approach when managing a patient with TEN.

- Educate patients with suspected drug-induced SJS or TEN about the nature of the reaction and necessary precautions, including which medications to avoid in the future.

- Identify patients with potentially serious skin reactions who should be referred for further medical evaluation and treatment.

PATIENT PRESENTATION

■ Chief Complaint

"My child has a blistering rash all over her body and is really sick!"

■ HPI

A 14-year-old girl presents to the ED with a high fever, vomiting, diarrhea, and a 3-day history of a skin rash. The rash is maculopapular with blisters and has spread to involve 75% of her body surface area. She had a UTI about 1.5 weeks ago and was prescribed a 7-day course of TMP/SMX. She adhered to the regimen; her urinary tract symptoms of dysuria and frequency and her abdominal discomfort resolved within 2–3 days. This was her first UTI. She continued to take the TMP/SMX as directed. Seven days after starting therapy, she noticed red spots on her arms and legs that began to spread over the whole body. The rash began to blister. She became febrile, and last night she began vomiting and had two bouts of diarrhea. This morning her mother brought her to the ED where she was assessed by physical exam and quickly transferred to the ICU. She was then immediately intubated to protect her airway patency. The rash was continuing to spread with additional blisters observed.

■ PMH

Unremarkable

■ FH

Parents A&W, no siblings

■ SH

The patient is a student who just began taking jazz classes about 2 months ago. She is not sexually active, does not smoke, and does not use alcohol. There have been no recent changes in diet or in her living environment.

■ Meds

Just completed a 7-day course of TMP/SMX. No additional drugs taken including OTCs, vitamins, herbals, or drugs of abuse. Not on oral contraceptives.

■ Meds in Hospital

For intubation: Ketamine 40 mg IV × 1, midazolam 1 mg IV × 1, propofol 120 mg IV × 1
For BP support: Dopamine IV infusion at 12 mcg/kg/min

■ All

NKDA

■ ROS

Skin is tender to the touch, with rash and blisters. Continues to have loose BM. Vomited × 1 in ED. Otherwise negative except for complaints noted above.

■ Physical Examination (in ICU)

Gen

Fairly anxious 14-year-old girl looking acutely ill

VS

BP 90/50 mm Hg, HR 90, RR 25, T 40.1°C

Skin

Extensive maculopapular rash over 75% of BSA. Blisters involve over 30% of BSA and are still spreading—additional blisters have appeared since her initial arrival to the ED. Some blisters have become confluent, and there is detachment of the epidermis. Small blisters on discrete dark red purpuric macules symmetrically over face, hands, feet, limbs, and trunk with widespread erythema. Blisters and intensely red oozing erosions over lips (especially vermilion border), oral mucosa, and vaginal area. Some ruptured blisters on skin and some with necrotic centers. Positive Nikolsky's sign. Skin is tender to the touch.

HEENT

PERRLA, EOMI, fundi benign, TMs intact. Corneal abrasions but no blisters. Conjunctivitis with some debris collecting under eyelids.

External nares clear. Blisters in oral cavity and ulceration on lower lip. Pharynx erythematous and blistering.

Chest

Upper airway congestion; debris and ulceration in mouth, throat, and epiglottis

Cor

RRR without murmurs, rubs, or gallops; S_1 and S_2 normal

Abd

(+) BS, soft, nontender, no masses

Genitourinary

Blistering in vaginal area. Foley catheter inserted—urine output approximately 40–50 mL/hr.

MS/Ext

Maculopapular rash and some blisters on arms and legs. Bilateral arthralgias and myalgias. Peripheral pulses present.

Neuro

Oriented × 3. No signs of confusion.

■ Labs

Na 140 mEq/L	Glucose	WBC 11 × 10³/mm³	Hgb 12 g/dL
K 4.0 mEq/L	95 mg/dL	PMNs 65%	Hct 31%
Cl 101 mEq/L	BUN 9 mg/dL	Bands 5%	Plt 239 × 10³/mm³
CO₂ 32 mEq/L	SCr 0.7 mg/dL	Eos 8%	INR 1.24
PO₄ 2.2 mg/dL	AST 15 IU/L	Monos 1%	aPTT
T. protein 6.5 g/dL	ALT 22 IU/L	Basos 1%	32.4 seconds
Albumin 3.1 g/dL	LDH 120 IU/L	Lymphs 20%	ESR 35 mm/hr
			RF negative

Urinalysis: No protein, ketones, blood, WBC, or bacteria

■ Chest X-Ray

WNL

■ Clinical Course

Day 2 of Admission

Urine output still 40–50 mL/hr; 1050 mL/previous 24 hr.

Day 3 of Admission

Histopathology of biopsy specimen from lesion on lip: Epidermal degeneration with intraepidermal vesiculation and subepidermal bullae. Mild perivascular lymphocytic infiltrate.
Direct immunofluorescence of biopsy specimen from lip lesion: Negative.
Swab from blisters on arm: Coagulase-negative *Staphylococcus*, *Pseudomonas aeruginosa*.
Blood cultures: (+) Coagulase-negative *Staphylococcus*, sensitive to vancomycin.
Urine culture (midstream urine): No growth.

■ Assessment

This is a 14-year-old girl with TEN, likely drug induced, who has developed secondary *Staphylococcus epidermidis* bacteremia.

QUESTIONS

Collect Information

1.a. What subjective and objective information indicates the presence of TEN?

1.b. What additional information is needed to fully assess this patient's skin disorder?

Assess the Information

2.a. What subjective and objective information correlates with TEN disease severity and a worse prognosis?

2.b. Create a list of the patient's drug therapy problems and prioritize them. Include assessment of medication appropriateness, effectiveness, safety, and patient adherence.

Develop a Care Plan

3.a. What are the goals of pharmacotherapy in this case?

3.b. What nondrug therapies might be useful for managing TEN in this patient?

3.c. What feasible pharmacotherapeutic alternatives are available for treating TEN?

3.d. Create an individualized, patient-centered, team-based care plan to optimize medication therapy for this patient. Include specific drugs, dosage forms, doses, schedules, and durations of therapy.

Implement the Care Plan

4.a. What information should be provided to the patient to enhance adherence, ensure successful therapy, and minimize adverse effects?

4.b. Describe how care should be coordinated with other healthcare providers.

Follow-Up: Monitor and Evaluate

5. Explain how to monitor and evaluate the care plan for medication appropriateness, effectiveness, safety, and patient adherence by using clinical and laboratory data, patient feedback, and other information.

■ SELF-STUDY ASSIGNMENTS

1. Differentiate among the various types, terminology, and manifestations of cutaneous drug reactions, including irritant drug reactions, fixed drug reactions, maculopapular skin reactions, photoallergic and phototoxic reactions, bullous reactions, morbilliform and urticarial reactions, pigmentation, lichenoid eruptions, SJS, TEN, drug hypersensitivity syndrome, and vasculitis.

2. If this patient had SJS, how would the clinical presentation, disease course, and treatment differ from those of TEN?

3. Obtain information on the anticonvulsants and NSAIDs that have been most commonly implicated in causing SJS/TEN.

4. Review the pharmacogenomics of drug hypersensitivity, in particular with regard to SCARs such as TEN. Association with specific genetic markers (eg, HLA-B*15:01 and HLA-B*15:02 alleles) are discussed in the corresponding textbook chapter.

CLINICAL PEARL

Aggressive and vigilant nondrug supportive therapies are vital to the effective management of TEN.

REFERENCES

1. Schwartz RA, McDonough PH, Lee BW. CME: toxic epidermal necrolysis. Part I. Introduction, history, classification, clinical features, systemic manifestations, etiology, and immunopathogenesis. Part II. Prognosis, sequelae, diagnosis, differential diagnosis, prevention, and treatment. J Am Acad Dermatol. 2013;69:173.e1–e11 (part 1), 187.e1–e16 (part 2).

2. Cohen V. Toxic epidermal necrolysis. eMedicine, updated December 1, 2017. Available at: *http://emedicine.medscape.com/article/229698-overview*. Accessed September 13, 2018.

3. Roujeau J-C, Bricard G, Nicolas J-F. Drug-induced epidermal necrolysis: important new piece to end the puzzle. J Allergy Clin Immunol. 2011;128:1277–1278.

4. Gerull R, Nelle M, Schaible T. Toxic epidermal necrolysis and Stevens-Johnson syndrome: a review. Crit Care Med. 2011;39(6):1521–1532.

5. Mockenhaupt M, Viboud C, Dunant A, et al. Stevens–Johnson syndrome and toxic epidermal necrolysis: assessment of medication risks with emphasis on recently marketed drugs. The EuroSCAR–Study. J Invest Dermatol. 2008;128:35–44.

6. Schnyder B, Pichler WJ. Allergy to sulfonamides. J Allergy Clin Immunol. 2013;131(1):256–257.e1–e5. doi: 10.1016/j.jaci.2012.10.003.

7. Schynder B. Approach to the patient with drug allergy. Med Clin N Am. 2010;94(4):665–679.

8. Creamer D, Walsh SA, Dziewulski P, Exton LS. Guidelines for the management of Stevens-Johnson syndrome/toxic epidermal necrosis in adults. Br J Dermatol. 2016;174(6):1194–1227.

9. Wang C-W, Yang L-Y, Chen CB, et al. Randomized, controlled trial of TNF-alpha antagonist in CTL-mediated severe cutaneous adverse reactions. J Clin Invest. 2018;128(3):985–996.

10. Lee HY, Walsh, SA, Creamer D. Long-term complications of Stevens-Johnson syndrome/toxic epidermal necrolysis (SJS/TEN): the spectrum of chronic problems in patients who survive an episode of SJS/TEN necessitates multidisciplinary follow-up. Br J Dermatol. 2017;177(4):924–935.

115

IRON DEFICIENCY ANEMIA

Iron It Out . . . . Level I

Elizabeth M. Bald, PharmD, BCACP

Matthew A. Cantrell, PharmD, BCPS

LEARNING OBJECTIVES

After completing this case study, the reader should be able to:

- Identify the signs, symptoms, and laboratory manifestations of IDA.

- Select appropriate iron therapies for the treatment of IDA.

- Understand the monitoring parameters for both short- and long-term treatment of IDA.

- Inform patients of the potential adverse effects of iron therapy.

- Educate patients about the importance of adherence to their iron therapy regimen.

PATIENT PRESENTATION

■ Chief Complaint

"I feel tired all the time."

■ HPI

A 42-year-old man presents to his primary care provider with the above complaint. With further questioning, he reveals that he first noticed these symptoms approximately 3 weeks ago. He initially believed they were related to longer work hours at his new job; however, the symptoms have worsened in the past 2 weeks, and he has also been experiencing epigastric pain and nausea. He denies any signs of bleeding but does acknowledge that his appetite has been decreased due to the nausea. He finished a course of azithromycin for community-acquired pneumonia approximately 1 month ago.

■ PMH

Type 2 DM × 3 years

■ FH

Mother alive age 61 with HTN, type 2 DM, and depression; father died of colon cancer at age 62.

■ SH

Never smoker; drinks a glass of wine with dinner two nights per week; married with two children.

■ ROS

No fever or chills; (–) burning pain in stomach after meals; (–) heartburn; (–) melena; (+) reduced appetite; has one BM daily; no significant weight changes over past 5 years; (+) dry mouth; (+) fatigue, tires easily; (–) paralysis, fainting, numbness, paresthesia, or tremor; (–) headache; has myopic vision; (–) tinnitus or vertigo; has hay fever in spring; (–) wheezing; denies chest pain, edema; (–) dyspnea and orthopnea; denies nocturia, hematuria, dysuria, or history of stones

■ Meds

Dulaglutide 1.5 mg subQ once weekly
Empagliflozin 25 mg PO once daily
Metformin XR 1000 mg PO twice daily

■ All

Codeine (upset stomach)
Penicillin (rash)

■ Physical Examination

Gen

The patient is in no acute distress and appears his stated age.

VS

BP 124/78 mm Hg, P 82 bpm, RR 18, T 36.2°C, pulse oximetry 96% in room air; Wt 66.8 kg, Ht 5′5″

HEENT

PERRL; EOMI; conjunctivae are pale; mucous membranes pale and dry; normal funduscopic examination; deviated nasal septum; no sinus tenderness; oropharynx clear

Neck/Lymph Nodes

Neck supple without masses; trachea midline; no thyromegaly, no JVD

CV

RRR

Abd

Moderate epigastric pain on palpation; (+) BS

Genit/Rect

Rectal examination (–)

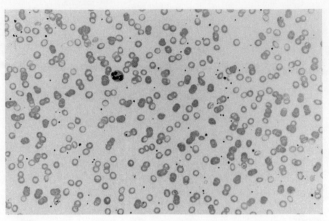

FIGURE 115-1. Blood smear with hypochromic, microcytic red blood cells (Wright–Giemsa × 330). (Photo courtesy of Lydia C. Contis, MD.)

MS/Ext

Spoon-shaped nails (koilonychia) on the second and fourth fingers

Neuro

A&O × 3; DTR 2+; normal gait

■ Other Information

H. pylori Urea Breath Test: positive
Peripheral blood smear: hypochromic, microcytic red blood cells (Fig. 115-1)

■ Labs

See Table 115-1.

■ Assessment

1. Moderate IDA possibly secondary to poor absorption with *H. pylori* infection

QUESTIONS

Collect Information

1.a. What subjective and objective information indicates the presence of iron deficiency anemia (IDA)?

1.b. What additional information is needed to fully assess this patient's IDA?

Assess the Information

2.a. Assess the severity of IDA based on the subjective and objective information available.

2.b. Create a list of the patient's drug therapy problems and prioritize them. Include assessment of medication appropriateness, effectiveness, safety, and patient adherence.

Develop a Care Plan

3.a. What are the goals of pharmacotherapy for this patient's anemia?

3.b. What nondrug therapy may be effective for managing this anemia?

3.c. What oral and parenteral pharmacotherapeutic alternatives could be used to treat this patient's anemia?

3.d. Create an individualized, patient-centered, team-based care plan to optimize medication therapy for this patient's drug therapy problems. Include specific drugs, dosage forms, doses, schedules, and durations of therapy.

Implement the Care Plan

4.a. What information should be provided to the patient to enhance adherence, ensure successful therapy, and minimize adverse effects?

4.b. Describe how care should be coordinated with other healthcare providers.

Follow-Up: Monitor and Evaluate

5. Explain how to monitor and evaluate the care plan for medication appropriateness, effectiveness, safety, and patient adherence by using clinical and laboratory data, patient feedback, and other information.

■ SELF-STUDY ASSIGNMENTS

1. Make a list of oral medications that should not be taken close to the time of oral iron administration; note the medications for which ferrous salts may interfere with their absorption.

2. Perform a literature search to determine the evidence supporting use of various sustained-release iron preparations, and determine the incremental cost of such products.

3. Calculate the correct total dose of parenteral iron dextran (ie, total dose iron dextran) for this patient, and write a comprehensive order for its administration.

CLINICAL PEARL

Indications for parenteral iron therapy include failure or intolerance to oral iron therapy or when a quicker recovery is necessary.

TABLE 115-1	Laboratory Values		
Na 136 mEq/L	Hgb 11.4 g/dL	WBC 10.53× 10³/mm³	Ca 9.2 mg/dL
K 4.0 mEq/L	Hct 39.7%	Lymphs 21.7%	Iron 19 mcg/dL
Cl 106 mEq/L	RBC 5.63 × 10⁶/mm³	Monos 5.7%	TIBC 440 mcg/dL
CO₂ 22 mEq/L	MCV 70.5 μm³	Eos 20.2%	Transferrin sat 4%
BUN 14 mg/dL	MCH 20.2 pg	Basos 1.2%	Ferritin 2 ng/mL
SCr 0.79 mg/dL	MCHC 28.7 g/dL		B₁₂ 680 pg/mL
Glucose 137 mg/dL	RDW 19.4%		Folic acid 8.2 ng/mL
A1C 8.7%	MPV 0.8 fL		

REFERENCES

1. Ko CW, Siddique SM, Patel A, et al. AGA clinical practice guidelines on the gastrointestinal evaluation of iron deficiency anemia. Gastroenterology. 2020;159(3):1085–1094.

2. Camaschella C. Iron-deficiency anemia. N Engl J Med. 2015;372: 1832–1843.

3. Chey WD, Leontiadis GI, Howden CW, Moss SF. ACG clinical guideline: treatment of *Helicobacter pylori* infection. Am J Gastroenterol. 2017;112(2):212–239 [published correction appears in Am J Gastroenterol. 2018;113(7):1102].

4. WHO. Haemoglobin concentrations for the diagnosis of anaemia and assessment of severity. Vitamin and Mineral Nutrition Information System. Geneva, World Health Organization, 2011 (WHO/NMH/NHD/MNM/11.1). Available at: *http://www.who.int/vmnis/indicators/haemoglobin.pdf*. Accessed November 24, 2021.

5. American Diabetes Association. 9. Pharmacologic approaches to glycemic treatment: standards of medical care in diabetes–2021. Diabetes Care. 2021;44(Suppl 1):S111–S124.

6. Grundy SM, Stone NJ, Bailey AL, et al. 2018 AHA/ACC/AACVPR/AAPA/ABC/ACPM/ADA/AGS/APhA/ASPC/NLA/PCNA guideline on the management of blood cholesterol: a report of the American College of Cardiology/American Heart Association Task Force on Clinical Practice Guidelines Circulation 2019;139(25):e1082–e1143 [published correction appears in Circulation 2019;139(25):e1182–e1186].

7. Stoffel NU, Cercamondi CI, Brittenham G, et al. Iron absorption from oral iron supplements given on consecutive versus alternate days and as single morning doses versus twice-daily split dosing in iron-depleted women: two open-label, randomised controlled trials. Lancet Haematol. 2017;4(11):e524–e533.

8. Auerbach M, Adamson JW. How we diagnose and treat iron deficiency anemia. Am J Hematol. 2016;91(1):31–38.

9. Monoferric (ferric derisomaltose) Prescribing Information; Pharmacosmos Therapeutics Inc., Morristown, NJ; 2020.

116

VITAMIN B$_{12}$ DEFICIENCY

Seriously Lacking Motivation.................... Level II

Jon P. Wietholter, PharmD, BCPS, FCCP

*Notice to the reader: the case author provided suggested answers to the questions related to this case in **Appendix D** to give students an example of how case answers should be constructed.*

LEARNING OBJECTIVES

After completing this case study, the reader should be able to:

- Determine signs, symptoms, and laboratory abnormalities associated with vitamin B$_{12}$ deficiency.

- Discuss appropriate vitamin B$_{12}$ pharmacotherapy recommendations.

- Select an appropriate regimen for treatment of vitamin B$_{12}$ deficiency.

- Choose appropriate monitoring parameters for initial and subsequent evaluations of patients with vitamin B$_{12}$ deficiency.

PATIENT PRESENTATION

■ Chief Complaint

"I feel like I'm constantly tired and fatigued. Also, my tongue is sore and swollen and feels like I burned it on a piece of hot pizza, making it hard for me to eat or drink anything."

■ HPI

A 55-year-old woman presents to your outpatient clinic with her husband. She reports that she has been somewhat fatigued and lethargic for 10+ years, but her symptoms have worsened over the last 4–5 months to the point that she constantly feels tired. Additionally, she states that over the past 2–3 weeks, her tongue has become very painful and swollen and that she struggles to eat. She tries to avoid eating anything that could worsen her pain, and she feels "fuller" more quickly than usual when eating. On questioning, she mentions a slight tingling and numbness in her feet that seems to worsen when finishing any physical activity. The patient has lost about 10 lb over the past 3 months and states that she feels like she is running a constant low-grade fever.

■ PMH

Type 2 diabetes mellitus
GERD

■ FH

Father alive (78 yo) with CAD, HTN, and type 2 DM
Mother alive (77 yo) with HTN and COPD

■ SH

Lives with her husband; (–) tobacco, alcohol, or illicit drugs

■ Meds

Metformin 1000 mg PO Q 12 H
Omeprazole 20 mg PO daily

■ All

Penicillin (hives)
Levofloxacin (anaphylaxis)

■ ROS

Complains of tongue pain and slight tingling sensation in her toes; (–) polyuria or polydipsia; denies any visual changes, constipation, or urinary retention

■ Physical Examination

Gen

Woman in no acute distress with normal affect and speech; appears fatigued

VS

BP 123/77 mm Hg, P 106 bpm, RR 16, T 37.8°C; O$_2$ sat 96% on room air; Wt 82 kg, Ht 5'9"

Skin

Pale, turgor normal, no rashes or lesions

HEENT

PERRLA; EOMI; (+) red, smooth, swollen, sore tongue with loss of papillae; TMs normal

Neck

Supple; no masses, lymphadenopathy, or thyromegaly

Chest

Normal bilateral breath sounds; (–) wheezing on auscultation

CV

Regular rhythm; no murmurs or gallops; (+) mild tachycardia

Abd

Soft, nontender; mild splenomegaly; no masses; normal bowel sounds

Ext

No erythema, pain, or edema; normal pulses; (+) paresthesias; (–) joint redness or swelling; (–) limb weakness; reflexes intact

Neuro

A&O × 3; CN: visual fields and hearing intact; coordination intact; decreased pinprick in both lower extremities; decreased vibratory sensation in both lower extremities; decreased temperature sensation in both lower extremities; (–) ataxia or lightheadedness

■ Labs (All Fasting)

Na 136 mEq/L	Hgb 8.4 g/dL	AST 30 IU/L	Iron 124 mcg/dL
K 3.5 mEq/L	Hct 25.3%	ALT 24 IU/L	Ferritin
Cl 108 mEq/L	RBC $2.09 \times 10^6/mm^3$	Alk phos 79 IU/L	100 ng/mL
CO_2 24 mEq/L	Plt $91 \times 10^3/mm^3$	T. bili 0.8 mg/dL	Transferrin
BUN 11 mg/dL	WBC $5.5 \times 10^3/mm^3$	D. bili 0.4 mg/dL	229 mg/dL
SCr 0.7 mg/dL	MCV 121 μm³		LDH 140 IU/L
Glu 134 mg/dL	MCH 40 pg		B_{12} 101 pg/mL
A1C 6.8%	MCHC 33.2 g/dL		Folate 12.3 ng/mL
TSH 3.4 mIU/L			

■ Peripheral Blood Smear Morphology

Macro-ovalocytosis, hypersegmented granulocytes, large platelets, macrocytic red blood cells with megaloblastic changes (Fig. 116-1).

■ Assessment

1. Macrocytic anemia consistent with vitamin B_{12} deficiency of unknown origin

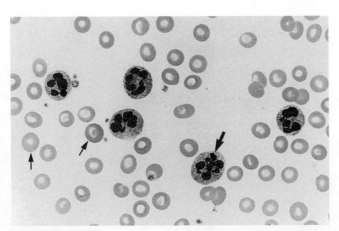

FIGURE 116-1. Blood smear with enlarged hypersegmented neutrophils, one with eight nuclear lobes (*large arrow*) and macrocytes (*small arrows*) (Wright–Giemsa × 1650). (Photo courtesy of Lydia C. Contis, MD.)

2. Atrophic glossitis and peripheral sensory neuropathy possibly associated with vitamin B_{12} deficiency
3. Type 2 diabetes mellitus (controlled)
4. GERD (uncertain control)

QUESTIONS

Collect Information

1.a. What subjective and objective information indicates the presence of vitamin B_{12} deficiency?

1.b. What additional information is needed to fully assess this patient's vitamin B_{12} deficiency?

Assess the Information

2.a. Assess the severity of vitamin B_{12} deficiency based on the subjective and objective information available.

2.b. Create a list of the patient's drug therapy problems and prioritize them. Include assessment of medication appropriateness, effectiveness, safety, and patient adherence.

Develop a Care Plan

3.a. What are the goals of pharmacotherapy for vitamin B_{12} deficiency in this case?

3.b. What nondrug therapies might be useful for this patient's vitamin B_{12} deficiency?

3.c. What feasible pharmacotherapeutic options are available for treating vitamin B_{12} deficiency?

3.d. Create an individualized, patient-centered, team-based care plan to optimize medication therapy for the vitamin B_{12} deficiency and other drug therapy problems. Include specific drugs, dosage forms, doses, schedules, and durations of therapy.

Implement the Care Plan

4.a. What information should be provided to the patient to enhance adherence, ensure successful therapy, and minimize adverse effects?

4.b. Describe how care should be coordinated with other healthcare providers.

Follow-Up: Monitor and Evaluate

5. Explain how to monitor and evaluate the care plan for medication appropriateness, effectiveness, safety, and patient adherence by using clinical and laboratory data, patient feedback, and other information.

■ SELF-STUDY ASSIGNMENTS

1. A serum vitamin B_{12} level is not the most reliable laboratory test for evaluating vitamin B_{12} deficiency. Review the diagnostic tests that are more commonly used and provide a rationale for their use.

2. The anemia resulting from vitamin B_{12} deficiency can be corrected by simply giving patients folic acid. Discuss why it's important to differentiate between these two common causes of macrocytic anemia (folic acid deficiency and vitamin B_{12} deficiency) instead of simply treating all patients with folic acid monotherapy.

CLINICAL PEARL

Multiple medications have been linked to vitamin B_{12} deficiency, including acid-suppressive agents via their impairment of cobalamin release from dietary protein sources. However, vitamin B_{12} repletion can still be achieved in these patients with oral cyanocobalamin since this formulation is not protein bound.

REFERENCES

1. Green R. Vitamin B_{12} deficiency from the perspective of a practicing hematologist. Blood. 2017;129(19):2603–2611.
2. Langan RC, Goodbred AJ. Vitamin B_{12} deficiency: recognition and management. Am Fam Physician. 2017 Sep 15;96(6):384–389.
3. Briani C, Dalla Torre C, Citton V, et al. Cobalamin deficiency: clinical picture and radiological findings. Nutrients. 2013;5:4521–4539.
4. Miller JW. Proton pump inhibitors, H_2-receptor antagonists, metformin, and vitamin B-12 deficiency: clinical implications. Adv Nutr. 2018 Jul 1;9(4):511S–518S.
5. Chan CQ, Low LL, Lee KH. Oral vitamin B_{12} replacement for the treatment of pernicious anemia. Front Med. (Lausanne) 2016;3(38):1–6.
6. Oberley MJ, Yang DT. Laboratory testing for cobalamin deficiency in megaloblastic anemia. Am J Hematol. 2013;88:522–526.
7. Wang H, Li L, Qin LL, Song Y, Vidal-Alaball J, Liu TH. Oral vitamin B_{12} versus intramuscular vitamin B_{12} for vitamin B_{12} deficiency. Cochrane Database Syst Rev. 2018 Mar 15;3(3):CD004655.
8. Liu Q, Li S, Quan H, Li J. Vitamin B_{12} status in metformin treated patients: systematic review. PLoS One 2014;9(6):e100379. doi: 10.1371/journal.pone.0100379.

117

FOLIC ACID DEFICIENCY

More Wine, Anyone?............................Level I

Jonathan M. Kline, PharmD, BCPS, CDE

Amber Nicole Chiplinski, PharmD, BCPS

LEARNING OBJECTIVES

After completing this case study, the reader should be able to:

- Recognize the signs, symptoms, and laboratory abnormalities associated with folic acid deficiency.

- Identify the confounding factors that may contribute to the development of folic acid deficiency (eg, medications, concurrent disease states, and dietary habits).

- Recommend an appropriate treatment regimen to correct anemia resulting from folic acid deficiency.

- Educate patients with folic acid deficiency regarding pharmacologic and nonpharmacologic interventions used to correct folic acid deficiency.

- Describe appropriate monitoring parameters for initial and subsequent monitoring of folic acid deficiency.

PATIENT PRESENTATION

■ Chief Complaint

"My stomach hurts and I have been throwing up today."

■ HPI

A 43-year-old woman presents with a 1-day history of vomiting and mild abdominal pain along with some chest discomfort late in the day. The pain radiates down to the lower abdominal quadrants bilaterally. They deny any fevers, chills, or similar pains in the past. They also complain of loose stools and chronic fatigue for the past 2–3 months.

■ PMH

Celiac disease
Hypothyroidism
Osteopenia

■ FH

Mother positive for lupus; sister with Crohn disease; negative for DM, CAD, CVA, CA

■ SH

Married; (+) alcohol—three to four glasses of wine per day, increased recently from one to two glasses after her mother-in-law moved in

■ Meds

Levothyroxine 100 mcg PO daily
Ortho Tri-Cyclen Lo 1 tab PO daily

■ All

Doxycycline—rash

■ ROS

(+) Generalized weakness; (–) dizziness; (–) weight gain or loss; (–) fever; (–) vision or hearing changes; (–) cough, chest pain, palpitations; (–) shortness of breath; (+) nausea/vomiting, abdominal pain, loose stools; (–) rectal bleeding; (–) nocturia or dysuria; (+) bilateral lower extremity weakness; (–) edema, rashes, or petechiae; (–) symptoms of depression or anxiety; (–) history of bleeding problems or VTE

■ Physical Examination

Gen

Appears generally ill

VS

BP 135/90 mm Hg, P 82 bpm, RR 40, T 35.5°C; Ht 64", Wt 52 kg

Skin

No petechiae, rashes, ecchymoses, or active lesions; decreased skin turgor

HEENT

PERRLA; tongue is large and erythematous; dry mucous membranes

Neck/Lymph Nodes

Normal ROM; no JVD, adenopathy, thyromegaly, or bruits

Lung/Thorax

Lungs CTA bilaterally

CV

RRR; no murmurs, gallops, or rubs

Abd

Soft, nondistended, with midepigastric and right flank and right lower quadrant tenderness; (+) bowel sounds

MS/Ext

Lower extremities warm with 2+ bipedal pulses; no clubbing, cyanosis, or edema

Neuro

CN II–XII grossly intact; decreased muscle strength 3/5 bilaterally in upper and lower extremities; DTRs 2+ throughout

■ Labs

Na 138 mEq/L	Hgb 12.6 g/dL	AST 128 IU/L	Folate 2.8 ng/mL
K 4.2 mEq/L	Hct 37.2%	ALT 52 IU/L	B_{12} 242 pg/mL
Cl 102 mEq/L	RBC $3.78 \times 10^6/mm^3$	Alk phos 142 IU/L	
CO_2 21 mEq/L	Plt $217 \times 10^3/mm^3$	GGT 288 IU/L	
BUN 7 mg/dL	WBC $6.3 \times 10^3/mm^3$	T. bili 2.1 mg/dL	
SCr 0.52 mg/dL	MCV 120.4 μm^3	Alb 3.4 g/dL	
Glu 89 mg/dL	MCH 40.5 pg	TSH 2.06 mIU/L	
Amylase 404 IU/L	MCHC 33.6 g/dL	T_4, free 1.2 ng/dL	
Lipase 679 IU/L	RDW 12.1%		

■ Assessment

Acute pancreatitis secondary to alcohol use
Dehydration
Macrocytic anemia secondary to folate deficiency

QUESTIONS

Collect Information

1.a. What subjective and objective information indicates the presence of anemia secondary to folate deficiency?

1.b. What additional information is needed to fully assess this patient's anemia?

Assess the Information

2.a. Assess the severity of the anemia based on the subjective and objective information available.

2.b. Create a list of the patient's drug therapy problems and prioritize them. Include assessment of medication appropriateness, effectiveness, safety, and patient adherence.

2.c. Could the patient's folate deficiency have been caused by drug therapy or comorbidity?

2.d. Why is it important to differentiate folate deficiency from vitamin B_{12} deficiency, and how is this accomplished?

Develop a Care Plan

3.a. What are the goals of pharmacotherapy for this patient's anemia?

3.b. What nondrug therapies may be used to correct this patient's folic acid deficiency?

3.c. What feasible pharmacotherapeutic alternatives are available for treating this patient's anemia?

3.d. Create an individualized, patient-centered, team-based care plan to optimize medication therapy for this patient. Include specific drugs, dosage forms, doses, schedules, and durations of therapy.

Implement the Care Plan

4.a. What information should be provided to the patient to enhance adherence, ensure successful therapy, and minimize adverse effects?

4.b. Describe how care should be coordinated with other healthcare providers.

Follow-Up: Monitor and Evaluate

5. Explain how to monitor and evaluate the care plan for medication appropriateness, effectiveness, safety, and patient adherence by using clinical and laboratory data, patient feedback, and other information.

■ SELF-STUDY ASSIGNMENTS

1. What are the advantages and disadvantages of folinic acid (leucovorin calcium) over standard folic acid, and why is this the preferred folate supplement in patients receiving high-dose methotrexate?

2. List and compare the mechanism for how the following drugs can lead to folic acid deficiency: azathioprine, trimethoprim, and phenytoin.

3. What is the role of folic acid in the management of methanol ingestion?

CLINICAL PEARL

Unlike dietary folate, supplemented folic acid (pteroylglutamic acid) is absorbed even with abnormal function of GI mucosal cells. Likewise, persistent alcohol ingestion or the use of drugs affecting folic acid absorption, folate transport, or dihydrofolate reductase will not prevent a sufficient therapeutic response to oral supplementation.

REFERENCES

1. McCleery J, Abraham RP, Denton DA, et al. Vitamin and mineral supplementation for preventing dementia or delaying cognitive decline in people with mild cognitive impairment. Cochrane Database Syst Rev. 2018;11(11):CD01905. doi: 10.1002/14651858.CD011905.pub2.

2. Snow CF. Laboratory diagnosis of vitamin B_{12} and folate deficiency: a guide for the primary care physician. Arch Intern Med. 1999;159:1289–1298.

3. Nagao T, Hirokawa M. Diagnosis and treatment of macrocytic anemia in adults. J Gen Fam Med. 2017;18(5):200–204.

4. Medici V, Halstead CH. Folate, alcohol, and liver disease. Mol Nutr Food Res. 2013;57(4):596–606.

5. Devalia V, Hamilton MS, Molloy AM. Guidelines for the diagnosis and treatment of cobalamin and folate disorders. Br J Haematol. 2014;166(4):496–513.

6. Hesdorffer CS, Longo DL. Drug-induced megaloblastic anemia. N Engl J Med. 2015;373(17):1649–1658.

7. Shere M, Bapat P, Nickel C, Koren G, Bushan K, Koren G. Association between use of oral contraceptives and folate status: a systematic review and meta-analysis. J Obstet Gynaecol Can. 2015;37(5):430–438.

8. Ashok T, Puttam H, Tarnate VCA, et al. Role of vitamin B2 and folate in metabolic syndrome. Cureus 2021;13(10):e18521.

9. Theisen-Toupal J, Horowitz G, Breu A. Low yield of outpatient serum testing: eleven years of experience. JAMA Intern Med. 2014;174(10):1696–1697.

10. Caron P, Grunenwald S, Persani L, Borson-Chazot F, Leroy R, Duntas L. Factors influencing the levothyroxine dose in the hormone replacement therapy of primary hypothyroidism in adults. Rev Endocr Metab Disord. 2021. doi: 10.1007/s11154-021-09691-9.

118

SICKLE CELL ANEMIA

The Misunderstood Pain Crisis . . . . Level I

Jamal Brown, PharmD, BCGP

Tamara Richards, PharmD, BCPS

LEARNING OBJECTIVES

After completing this case study, the reader should be able to:

- Recognize the clinical characteristics associated with an acute sickle cell crisis.

- Discuss the presentation of acute chest syndrome and treatment options.

- Recommend optimal analgesic therapy based on patient-specific information.

- Identify optimal endpoints of pharmacotherapy in sickle cell anemia patients.

- Recommend treatment to reduce the frequency of sickle cell crises.

PATIENT PRESENTATION

■ Chief Complaint

"I'm in pain all over and no one believes me! I can't breathe ... and I don't like being considered an addict!"

■ HPI

A 21-year-old African American man with a history of sickle cell anemia presents to the local community hospital ED frustrated and in pain. On waking up 3 days prior to admission, he experienced a sudden onset of pain in his hands, legs, and lower back. He began taking oxycodone 15 mg orally every 2 hours at that time with limited pain relief. When reaching out to his physician for additional pain medication, he was denied due to a disbelief of the patient's recently reported pain. His primary physician said that he was taking much larger doses of opioids than the physician's other patients. The ED physician questioned his level of pain and the opioid doses that he reported taking at home. This morning he had a temperature of 102°F, progressive shortness of breath, and priapism, which caused him to seek treatment at the ED. The patient acknowledged having sick contacts at his workplace.

■ PMH

Sickle cell anemia (hemoglobin SS disease) diagnosed before the age of 1 with approximately seven to eight crises per year requiring hospitalization

Acute chest syndrome 2 years ago that required intubation

Transfusion exchange with PRBC during the intubation admission

Several episodes of priapism, usually associated with sickle cell pain crisis

■ FH

Mother and father are alive and well, both with sickle cell trait. Patient has one sister with sickle cell trait.

■ SH

College student who is struggling to pass courses due to frequent missing of school for hospitalizations; depressed because sickle cell is affecting his life including limitation in sports and social activities. Struggling financially to keep up with hospital bills due to lapses in insurance.

■ Meds

Folic acid 1 mg PO daily
Hydroxyurea 500 mg PO daily
Oxycodone 15 mg PO Q 2 H PRN pain

■ All

Sulfa (reported rash when very young)
Codeine (nausea and dysphoria)

■ ROS

Denies nausea, vomiting, or diarrhea. Cannot remember his last bowel movement but believes he has not had one in the last 3 days. Has had fever with some chills and sweats; no cough, nasal discharge, rashes, or skin lesions. Reports stuttering priapism with recurring episodes each lasting approximately 1 hour, with no intervention.

■ Physical Examination

Gen

Thin, well-developed, diaphoretic African American man in acute distress

VS

BP 115/72 mm Hg, P 110 bpm, RR 20, T 101.3°F (38.5°C); Wt 72 kg; Ht 5′8″; 72 kg; O_2 sat 84% on room air improving to 97% on 4 L O_2

HEENT

PERRL; EOMI; oral mucosa soft and moist; scleral icterus and funduscopic examination; no sinus tenderness

Skin

Normal turgor; no rashes or lesions

Neck

Supple; nontender, no lymphadenopathy or thyromegaly

CV

RRR; II/VI SEM; no rubs or gallops

Lungs

Crackles in both bases on auscultation; dullness to percussion

Abd

Voluntary guarding, mild distention, hypoactive bowel sounds, no palpable spleen; no hepatomegaly or masses

Genitourinary

Priapism evident

Ext

No edema; notable tenderness in right shoulder and elbow

Neuro

A&O × 3; normal strength, reflexes intact

■ Labs

Na 143 mEq/L	Hgb 7.7 g/dL	AST 40 IU/L	Ca 8.8 mg/dL
K 4.2 mEq/L	Hct 20.8%	ALT 28 IU/L	Mg 1.9 mEq/L
Cl 112 mEq/L	Plt 480 × 10³/mm³	Alk phos 77 IU/L	Phos 3.9 mg/dL
CO₂ 28 mEq/L	MCV 88 μm³	LDH 1215 IU/L	(+) Anti-E red
BUN 50 mg/dL	Retic 18.2%	T. bili 5.0 mg/dL	cell antibody
SCr 1.4 mg/dL	WBC 18.2 × 10³/mm³	D. bili 0.8 mg/dL	
Glu 92 mg/dL	Segs 74%	Alb 3.4 g/dL	
	Bands 7.5%		
	Eos 1.5%		
	Lymphs 14%		
	Monos 3%		

■ Other

Arterial blood gas: pH 7.49, $PaCO_2$ 38 mm Hg, PaO_2 72 mm Hg, bicarb 30 mEq/L, O_2 sat 96% on oxygen

Sputum culture: Mixed flora

Hgb electrophoresis: Hgb A_2 3%; Hgb F 8%; Hgb S 89%

Peripheral blood smear: Sickle forms and target cells present (Fig. 118-1).

■ Chest X-Ray

This is a portable chest X-ray remarkable for diffuse interstitial infiltrates in both lung fields consistent with acute chest syndrome (Fig. 118-2). Cardiomegaly is also notable.

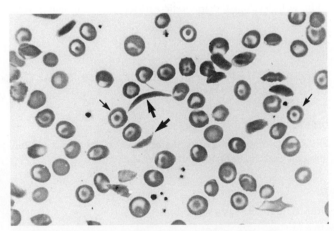

FIGURE 118-1. Peripheral blood with sickle cells (*large arrows*) and target cells (*small arrows*) (Wright–Giemsa ×1650). (Photo courtesy of Lydia C. Contis, MD.)

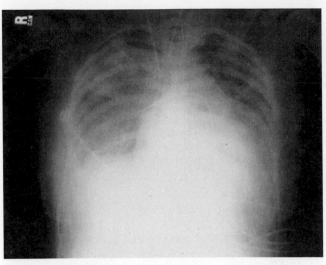

FIGURE 118-2. Lung radiograph of patient with acute chest syndrome secondary to sickle cell anemia. (Photo courtesy of Kenneth I. Ataga, MD.)

■ ECG

Normal sinus rhythm

■ Echocardiogram

Normal LV function

■ Assessment

A 21-year-old African American man in sickle cell crisis with probable acute chest syndrome, priapism, and constipation. Patient complains of severe pain but there are questions about the actual level of pain and the intensity of his home opioid regimen.

QUESTIONS

Collect Information

1.a. What subjective and objective information is consistent with an acute sickle cell crisis in this patient?

1.b. What information supports a diagnosis of acute chest syndrome in this patient?

1.c. What additional information is needed to fully assess this patient's acute sickle cell crisis?

Assess the Information

2.a. Assess the severity of this patient's acute sickle cell crisis based on the subjective and objective information available.

2.b. Create a list of the patient's drug therapy problems and prioritize them. Include assessment of medication appropriateness, effectiveness, safety, and patient adherence.

2.c. If healthcare providers incorrectly assume that a patient in sickle cell crisis who requests opioid analgesics is exhibiting drug-seeking behavior, how can that affect the provider's assessment and treatment of the patient's pain?

Develop a Care Plan

3.a. What are the goals of pharmacotherapy in this case?

3.b. What nondrug therapies might be useful for this patient?

3.c. What feasible pharmacotherapeutic alternatives are available for treating the patient's pain?

3.d. What feasible pharmacotherapeutic alternatives are available for treating opioid-induced constipation?

3.e. Create an individualized, patient-centered, team-based care plan to resolve this patient's medical problems. Include specific drugs, dosage forms, doses, schedules, and durations of therapy.

Implement the Care Plan

4.a. What information should be provided to the patient to enhance adherence, ensure successful therapy, and minimize adverse effects?

4.b. Describe how care should be coordinated with other healthcare providers.

Follow-Up: Monitor and Evaluate

5.a. Explain how to monitor and evaluate the care plan for medication appropriateness, effectiveness, safety, and patient adherence by using clinical and laboratory data, patient feedback, and other information.

■ CLINICAL COURSE

The plans you recommended have been initiated, and on the fourth day of hospitalization, the patient's pain is markedly improved, oxygen saturation improved to 98% on room air, he is afebrile, and his priapism has resolved. He has had two bowel movements but still feels his bowel habits have not yet returned to normal. He is only using two to three demands on his PCA per day and is asking to switch back to oral medication.

5.b. Considering this information, what changes (if any) in the pharmacotherapeutic plan are warranted while the patient is hospitalized?

5.c. What evidence suggests that the patient is adherent to hydroxyurea therapy, and how should this therapy continue to be monitored?

5.d. Develop a plan for follow-up that includes appropriate time frames to assess progress toward achievement of the goals of therapy.

■ SELF-STUDY ASSIGNMENTS

1. Determine the likelihood of a patient's offspring having sickle cell trait and/or disease if the patient has:

   a. Normal hemoglobin

   b. Sickle cell trait

   c. Sickle cell disease

2. Describe the complications associated with frequent crises in each organ system.

3. Discuss the differences between sickle cell anemia and β-thalassemia in terms of etiologies, laboratory abnormalities, and disease complications.

4. Discuss bias in sickle cell patients based on the article entitled, "Do Words Matter? Stigmatizing Language and the Transmission of Bias in the Medical Record."[3] How can you avoid bias in treating these patients and educating providers on this issue?

CLINICAL PEARL

Vaccination with pneumococcal conjugate 13-valent (PCV13) vaccine is necessary in addition to the 23-valent pneumococcal polysaccharide vaccine (PPSV23) for all adult sickle cell anemia patients with functional or anatomic asplenia if they have not received it previously. The PCV13 should be given at least 1 year after the last PPSV23 dose. For patients who have not received any pneumococcal vaccine, they should receive the PCV13 first, then the PPSV23 at least 8 weeks after receiving the PCV13, and a second dose 5 years after the first dose.

ACKNOWLEDGMENT

This case is based on the patient case written for the 10th edition by Sheh-Li-Chen, PharmD, BCOP.

REFERENCES

1. Vichinsky EP, Neumayr LD, Earles AN, et al. Causes and outcomes of the acute chest syndrome in sickle cell disease. National Acute Chest Syndrome Study Group. N Engl J Med 2000;342:1855–1865.

2. Goddu A, O'Conor KJ, Lanzkron S, et al. Do words matter? Stigmatizing language and the transmission of bias in the medical record. J Gen Intern Med. 2018;33(5):685–691.

3. Yawn BP, Buchanan GR, Afenyi-Annan AN, et al. Management of sickle cell disease: summary of the 2014 evidence-based report by expert panel members. JAMA. 2014;312(10):1033–1048.

4. Demerol (meperidine hydrochloride) [Package insert]. Parsippany, NJ, Validus Pharmaceuticals, LLC, August 2017. Available at: https://www.accessdata.fda.gov/drugsatfda_docs/label/2017/005010s055lbl.pdf. Accessed November 27, 2018.

5. Baddam S, Aban I, Hilliard L, Howard T, Askenazi D, Lebensburger JD. Acute kidney injury during a pediatric sickle cell vaso-occlusive pain crisis. Pediatr. Nephrol. 2017;32(8):1451–1456.

6. Niihara Y, Miller ST, Kanter J, et al. A phase 3 trial of L-glutamine in sickle cell disease. N Engl J Med. 2018;379(3):226–235.

7. Vichinsky E, Hoppe CC, Ataga KI, et al. A phase III randomized trial of voxelotor in sickle cell disease. N Engl J Med. 2019;381(6):509–519.

8. Ataga K, Kutlar A, Kanter J, et al. Crizanlizumab for the prevention of pain crises in sickle cell disease. N Engl J Med. 2017;376:429–439.

9. Argoff CE, Brennan MJ, Camilleri M, et al. Consensus recommendations on initiating prescription therapies for opioid-induced constipation. Pain Med. 2015;16(12):2324–2337.

10. Metlay JP, Waterer GW, Long AC, et al. Diagnosis and treatment of adults with community-acquired pneumonia. Am J Respir Crit Care Med. 2019;299(7):e45–e67.

119

USING LABORATORY TESTS IN INFECTIOUS DISEASES

Chief of Staph . . . . Level III

Anthony J. Guarascio, PharmD, BCPS

Branden D. Nemecek, PharmD, BCPS

LEARNING OBJECTIVES

After completing this case study, the reader should be able to:

- Discuss the possible etiology of bacterial disease following a viral illness such as influenza.

- Discuss the use of rapid diagnostic testing methods that help differentiate bacterial species as well as determine organism-specific antibiotic resistance profiles.

- Evaluate culture and sensitivity results, and determine the clinical significance of the minimum inhibitory concentration.

- Design an evidence-based care plan to treat a bloodstream infection based on laboratory information.

- Recommend a plan for monitoring efficacy and adverse reactions of an antimicrobial therapy regimen.

PATIENT PRESENTATION

■ Chief Complaint

Patient's wife states that, "Lately he (patient) has not been acting like himself. He has been very dizzy, tired, and has not been eating or drinking well."

■ HPI

A 68-year-old man came to the ED via ambulance. The patient's history is obtained from their wife. She describes a change in his mental status with lethargy and shortness of breath, along with a significant decrease in activity and nutritional intake. Over the past 24 hours, he became very nauseated and developed a fever (39°C). The symptoms started 3 days ago and have progressively worsened. He was seen by his primary care physician 6 days ago (last week) and determined to have a positive influenza-A nasal swab. He was prescribed oseltamivir and recently completed his 5-day treatment course.

■ PMH

Chronic kidney disease (Stage 3a)
Diabetes mellitus
Resistant hypertension
Influenza pneumonia

■ FH

Both parents are deceased (mother age 88 of PE; father age 71 of stroke). He is married without any children.

■ SH

Retired steel mill worker and union chief, distant history of tobacco and alcohol use with no current use.

■ Meds

Amlodipine 10 mg PO daily
Empagliflozin 25 mg PO daily
Glyburide 5 mg PO daily
Lisinopril 40 mg PO Q HS
Metformin 1000 mg PO BID
Spironolactone 25 mg PO daily

■ All

Penicillin: hives when he was a child
Morphine: itching

■ ROS

Patient's primary complaint is of nausea and dizziness, but due to current status, unable to review further.

■ Physical Examination

Gen

The patient is clearly fatigued and appearing in respiratory distress.

VS

BP 108/58, P 108, RR 36, T 39°C; Wt 64.2 kg, Ht 68″

Skin

Warm and diaphoretic

HEENT

PERRLA; EOM intact; dry mucous membranes, teeth clean and intact, pharynx negative

Neck/Lymph Nodes

No nodules, negative lymphadenopathy

Chest

Respiratory distress with marked effort and use of accessory muscles; generalized bilateral wheezing

CV

Tachycardic; normal S_1 and S_2; no heaves, thrills, or bruits

Abd

Soft, nondistended; nontender, no splenomegaly

Genit/Rect

Deferred

MS/Ext

Deferred

Neuro

Decreased responses; delayed recognition; responds to painful stimuli

■ Labs

From PCP Visit 6 Days Ago

Na 140 mEq/L	Hgb 11.2 g/dL	INR 1.1
K 4.5 mEq/L	Hct 32.1%	Influenza A/B PCR:
Cl 100 mEq/L	RBC $3.68 \times 10^6/mm^3$	positive A
CO_2 22 mEq/L	Plt $360 \times 10^3/mm^3$	
BUN 22 mg/dL	WBC $14.8 \times 10^3/mm^3$	
SCr 1.6 mg/dL	MCV 84.6 fL	
Glu 168 mg/dL		

Today's Values

Na 144 mEq/L	Hgb 10.6 g/dL	WBC 16.3 ×	INR 1.2
K 4.6 mEq/L	Hct 29.8%	$10^3/mm^3$	Influenza A/B PCR:
Cl 102 mEq/L	RBC $3.34 \times 10^6/mm^3$	Segs 70%	negative
CO_2 18 mEq/L	Plt $280 \times 10^3/mm^3$	Bands 22%	D-dimer
BUN 28 mg/dL	MCV 86.1 fL	Lymphs 6%	0.2 mcg/mL
SCr 1.3 mg/dL		Monos 2%	Nares MRSA swab:
Glu 58 mg/dL			positive
			O_2 saturation 92%

■ Urinalysis

Color, yellow; specific gravity, 1.170; pH 5; +2 protein; glucose positive, negative nitrites; negative LE; 15–20 RBC; few bacteria; 0–3/HPF WBC

■ Chest X-Ray

Patchy infiltrates with left lower lobe consolidation

■ Electrocardiogram

Normal sinus rhythm, heart rate 108 bpm, no axis deviation, no peaked T waves or T-wave inversion. No prior ECG for comparison.

■ Assessment

1. Respiratory distress with differential diagnosis pneumonia versus pulmonary embolus

2. Lab abnormalities (hypoglycemia)

■ Plan

1. Collect two sets of blood cultures and a sputum specimen. Collect urine sample for urinalysis and culture.

2. Start empiric vancomycin and cefepime per pharmacy to dose protocol.

3. Begin fluid resuscitation for hypotension and hypoglycemia.

QUESTIONS

Collect Information

1.a. What subjective and objective information indicates either the presence or absence of infection?

1.b. What additional information is needed to fully assess this patient's infection?

Assess the Information

2.a. Assess the severity of infection based on the subjective and objective information available.

2.b. Create a list of the patient's drug therapy problems and prioritize them. Include assessment of medication appropriateness, effectiveness, safety, and patient adherence.

Develop a Care Plan

3.a. What are the goals of pharmacotherapy for infection in this case?

3.b. What nondrug therapies might be useful for this patient's infection?

3.c. What feasible pharmacotherapeutic options are available for empirically treating infection in this patient?

■ CLINICAL COURSE

In the ED, the patient responds well to IV fluids with normalization of potassium and improvement in blood pressure and blood glucose. Shortly after the patient arrived on the medical floor, the microbiology lab calls the physician and reports that the patient's Gram stain from both blood cultures reveal Gram-positive cocci in clusters. GeneXpert MRSA/SA blood culture assay has returned as presumptive positive for MRSA. Sputum culture also reveals preliminary results of Gram-positive cocci in clusters. Final culture and susceptibility results are pending. The following day, blood and sputum culture and susceptibility results become available. Table 119-1 depicts the final culture susceptibility report that is identical for both sputum and blood isolates.

Develop a Care Plan (continued)

3.d. Based on this new information (microbiology lab report), create an individualized, patient-centered care plan to optimize medication therapy for the infection and this patient's other drug therapy problems. Include specific drugs, dosage forms, doses, schedules, and durations of therapy.

TABLE 119-1	*S. aureus* Susceptibility Report
Antibiotic	**MIC/Interpretation**
Clindamycin	≤0.25/susceptible[a]
Erythromycin	≥8/resistant
Gentamicin	≤0.5/susceptible
Levofloxacin	0.25/susceptible
Oxacillin	≥4/resistant
Penicillin	≥0.5/resistant
Rifampin	≤0.5/susceptible
Trimethoprim/sulfamethoxazole	≤10/susceptible
Vancomycin	1/susceptible
Tetracycline	≤1/susceptible

[a]Positive for inducible clindamycin resistance.

Implement the Care Plan

4.a. What information should be provided to the patient to enhance adherence, ensure successful therapy, and minimize adverse effects?

4.b. Describe how care should be coordinated with other healthcare providers.

Follow-Up: Monitor and Evaluate

5. Explain how to monitor and evaluate the care plan for medication appropriateness, effectiveness, safety, and patient adherence by using clinical and laboratory data, patient feedback, and other information.

■ FOLLOW-UP QUESTIONS

1. Develop a plan for follow-up that includes appropriate time frames to assess progress toward achievement of the goals of therapy. This should include a discussion about the timing of serum vancomycin concentrations to determine the appropriateness of drug dosing, appropriate frequency of serum vancomycin concentration assessments, and goal trough serum concentration in this patient.

2. How can laboratory data be used to assess chronic kidney disease for this patient?

3. When should the patient's blood cultures have been drawn in relation to antibiotic administration?

4. What is the clinical advantage of using a rapid identification test, such as a polymerase chain reaction (PCR) test, to help determine the staphylococcal species?

5. What effect does the organism's MIC have on the current treatment plan?

■ SELF-STUDY ASSIGNMENTS

1. Identify the organisms that most frequently represent contaminants in blood cultures.

2. Define the role of rapid diagnostic testing in the treatment of bloodstream infections.

3. Explain how a clinician interprets MRSA nasal swab surveillance results.

4. Describe how the management of this patient would change if kidney injury progressed to necessitate hemodialysis.

CLINICAL PEARL

Optimizing vancomycin for systemic MRSA infections requires targeting an individualized, patient-specific dose and interval that achieves a 24-hour AUC value of 400–600. This target maximizes both efficacy and safety, while assuming a vancomycin MIC of 1mg/L to achieve this AUC/MIC ratio.

REFERENCES

1. Sobel JD, Kaye D. Chapter 72 Urinary tract infections. In: Bennett JE, Dolin R, Blaser MJ, eds. Mandell, Douglas, and Bennett's Principles and Practice of Infectious Diseases. 9th ed. Philadelphia, PA, Saunders Elsevier; 2014:886–913.

2. Metersky ML, Masterson RG, Lode H, File TM Jr, Babinchak T. Epidemiology, microbiology, and treatment considerations for bacterial pneumonia complicating influenza. Int J Infect Dis. 2012;16(5):e321–e331.

3. Polenakovik HM, Pleiman CM. Ceftaroline for methicillin-resistant Staphylococcus aureus bacteraemia: case series and review of the literature. Int J Antimicrob Agents. 2013;42(5):450–455.

4. Liu C, Bayer A, Cosgrove SE, et al. Clinical practice guidelines by the Infectious Diseases Society of America for the treatment of methicillin-resistant Staphylococcus aureus infections in adults and children. Clin Infect Dis. 2011;52:1–38.

5. Rybak MJ, Le J, Lodise TP, et al. Therapeutic monitoring of vancomycin for serious methicillin-resistant Staphylococcus aureus infections: a revised consensus guideline and review by the American Society of Health-System Pharmacists, the Infectious Diseases Society of America, the Pediatric Infectious Diseases Society, and the Society of Infectious Diseases Pharmacists. Am J Health Syst Pharm. 2020;77(11):835–864.

6. Gilbert JS, Weiner DE, Bomback AS, Perazella MA, Tonelli M, eds. National Kidney Foundation's Primer on Kidney Diseases. 7th ed. Philadelphia, PA, Saunders Elsevier; 2018:326–336, 448–457.

7. Prybylski JP. Vancomycin trough concentration as a predictor of clinical outcomes in patients with Staphylococcus aureus bacteremia: a meta-analysis of observational studies. Pharmacotherapy. 2015;35(10):889–898.

8. Goff DA, Jankowski C, Tenover FC. Using rapid diagnostic tests to optimize antimicrobial selection in antimicrobial stewardship programs. Pharmacotherapy. 2012;32(8):677–687.

9. CLSI. Performance Standards for Antimicrobial Susceptibility Testing. 31st ed. CLSI Supplement M100. Clinical and Laboratory Standards Institute; 2021.

120

BACTERIAL MENINGITIS

This Is Spinal Tap. . . . . Level II

S. Travis King, PharmD, BCPS

Elizabeth A. Cady, PharmD, BCPS

LEARNING OBJECTIVES

After completing this case study, the reader should be able to:

- List risk factors and common presenting signs and symptoms of bacterial meningitis in infants and children.

- Differentiate common bacterial pathogens associated with meningitis in children of different ages.

- Recommend appropriate empiric and definitive antimicrobial and adjunctive therapy for bacterial meningitis.

- Identify appropriate monitoring parameters for antimicrobial therapy of bacterial meningitis.

PATIENT PRESENTATION

■ Chief Complaint

From mom: "Why is my baby so sleepy? And what is this purple rash?"

■ HPI

The patient is a 2-year-old, 13.6-kg male toddler who presented to the emergency department with his mother. Mom reports that she noticed him sleeping longer than normal since yesterday evening after returning from daycare, as well as this morning. She also reports that he had a poorer than normal appetite at dinner and breakfast. She also notes the rapid appearance of a purplish rash on his extremities, trunk, and back. At 08:00, she checked his temperature, which was of 39.1°C. At that point, the mother called her sister who is a nurse, who told her to go straight to the emergency room. When aroused prior to transport, he was irritable and crying frequently. During transport, he was in and out of sleep and did not respond well to normal stimuli. There was one episode of slight vomiting during transit.

■ PMH

The patient was born via an uncomplicated vaginal delivery at 39 weeks. Mother reports one episode of otitis media at 13 months of age, treated with amoxicillin.

■ FH

Mother is in good health; father has hypercholesterolemia; maternal grandparents both with metabolic syndrome; paternal grandfather in good health; maternal grandmother alive, history of breast cancer.

■ SH

Lives with mother and father. Father is a rock musician, and mother is a teacher. Patient began attending daycare 3 months ago. Father is a smoker. No pets in the home.

■ Meds

None; immunizations up to date per the US CDC Advisory Committee for Immunization Practices (ACIP)

■ All

NKDA

■ Review of Systems

Refer to HPI

■ Physical Examination

Gen

Lethargic toddler with generalized rash in mild–moderate distress

VS

SBP 75, HR 152, RR 48, T 39.4°C; Wt 13.6 kg, SatO$_2$ (RA): 98%

HEENT

PERRLA, tympanic membranes erythematous bilaterally

Chest

Lungs clear bilaterally

CV

Sinus tachycardia, regular rhythm, no murmurs, rubs, gallops

Abd

Soft, distended, (+) BS, (+) purpuric rash

Extremities

Capillary refill 4 seconds, extremities mottled and cool to the touch; (+) mildly blanching, purpuric rash is present; petechial lesions noted.

Neuro

Listless; arousable to strong stimuli only, (–) Brudzinski's, (–) Kernig's, (+) Babinski

■ Labs

Na 135 mEq/L	Hgb 13.2 g/dL	Ca 9.2 mg/dL	Arterial blood gases
K 3.9 mEq/L	Hct 39.6%	Mg 1.4 mEq/L	pH 7.32
Cl 110 mEq/L	Plt 160 × 10³/mm³	PO$_4$ 4.2 mg/dL	PaO$_2$ 80 mm Hg
CO$_2$ 14 mEq/L	WBC 25 × 10³/mm³	T. prot 6.6 g/dL	PaCO$_2$ 40 mm Hg
SCr 0.9 mg/dL	Neutros 70%	Alb 4.1 g/dL	HCO$_3$ 15 mEq/L
BUN 19 mg/dL	Bands 16%	Bili 0.7 mg/dL	Base excess
Glucose	Lymphs 10%	AST 86 IU/L	5.3 mEq/L
130 mg/dL	Monos 2%	ALT 20 IU/L	Procalcitonin:
	Eos 1%	ALP 285 IU/L	20.2 ng/mL
	Basos 1%		

■ CSF Serology/Urine Antigen Testing

Haemophilus influenzae type B (–); *Streptococcus pneumoniae* (–); group B *Streptococcus* (–)

■ CSF Analysis

Color/appearance: straw/cloudy, glucose 38 mg/dL, protein 315 mg/dL, WBC 420/mm³ (2% lymphs, 2% monos, 96% neutros), RBC 500/mm³

CSF Gram stain: Gram-negative diplococci

■ Cultures

Blood, urine, and CSF cultures: pending

■ Chest X-Ray

No acute cardiopulmonary process noted

■ Assessment

1. Acute bacterial meningitis, suspected meningococcal
2. Hypotension/metabolic acidosis

QUESTIONS

Collect Information

1.a. What subjective and objective information indicates the presence of meningitis?

1.b. What additional information is needed to fully assess this patient's meningitis?

Assess the Information

2.a. Assess the severity of meningitis based on the subjective and objective information available.

2.b. Create a list of the patient's drug therapy problems and prioritize them. Include assessment of medication appropriateness, effectiveness, safety, and patient adherence.

Develop a Care Plan

3.a. What are the goals of pharmacotherapy for meningitis in this case?

3.b. What nondrug therapies might be useful for managing this patient's meningitis?

3.c. What feasible pharmacotherapeutic options are available for treating this case of meningitis?

3.d. Create an individualized, patient-centered, team-based care plan to optimize medication therapy for meningitis and this patient's other drug therapy problems. Include specific drugs, dosage forms, doses, schedules, and durations of therapy.

3.e. What alternatives would be appropriate if the initial therapy fails or cannot be used?

Implement the Care Plan

4.a. What information should be provided to the patient to enhance compliance, ensure successful therapy, and minimize adverse effects?

4.b. Describe how care should be coordinated with other healthcare providers.

Follow-Up: Monitor and Evaluate

5. Explain how to monitor and evaluate the care plan for medication appropriateness, effectiveness, safety, and patient adherence by using clinical laboratory data, patient feedback, and other information.

■ CLINICAL COURSE

The patient received fluids, supportive care, and empiric antibiotics according to the hospital sepsis protocol. The patient was begun on vancomycin and ceftriaxone empirically. He also received dexamethasone (0.15 mg/kg every 6 hours starting with the first dose of antibiotics). Blood cultures returned positive for *Neisseria meningitidis*. CSF cultures return positive for *N. meningitidis*. Urine cultures remain negative.

Susceptibility testing of *N. meningitidis* from CSF culture demonstrates the following profile:

Penicillin MIC: 0.1 mcg/mL
Ceftriaxone MIC: 0.06 mcg/mL
Rifampin MIC: 0.25 mcg/mL
Ciprofloxacin MIC: 0.03 mcg/mL
Repeat procalcitonin on day 3 of admission is 6.3 ng/mL.
Repeat CBC at that time revealed: Hgb 13.5 g/dL, Hct 40.5%, platelets $225 \times 10^3/mm^3$, and WBC $12 \times 10^3/mm^3$ (66% Neutros, 32% Lymphs, 1% Basos, 1% Eos).

■ FOLLOW-UP QUESTION

1. Given the culture report, what changes, if any, should be made to the patient's antimicrobial or adjunctive regimen?

■ SELF-STUDY ASSIGNMENTS

1. Discuss the impact of vaccination on reducing the rates of meningitis and other invasive diseases in pediatric patients. What impact may be anticipated after FDA approval of the *N. meningitidis*, serotype B vaccine?

2. Describe the pharmacokinetic properties that influence the ability of antimicrobials to penetrate the blood–brain barrier.

3. Discuss the role of procalcitonin in the evaluation of bacterial versus aseptic meningitis.

4. Discuss the management alternatives when treating meningitis caused by drug-resistant meningococcal and pneumococcal pathogens.

CLINICAL PEARL

The *N. meningitis*, serotype B vaccine may be administered in addition to the quadrivalent vaccine to patients between the ages of 16 and 23 years. If patients age ≥10 years are deemed to be at risk for meningococcal disease (asplenia, complement deficiency, microbiology lab personnel), they should receive the serotype B vaccine.

REFERENCES

1. Tunkel AR, Hartman BJ, Kaplan SL, et al. Practice guidelines for the management of bacterial meningitis. Clin Infect Dis. 2004;39:1267–1284.
2. Chavez-Bueno S, McCracken GH. Bacterial meningitis in children. Pediatr Clin North Am. 2005;52:795–810.
3. Brouwer MC, Tunkel AR, van de Beek D. Epidemiology, diagnosis, and antimicrobial treatment of acute bacterial meningitis. Clin Microbiol Rev. 2010;23(3):467–492.
4. Bonadio W. Pediatric lumbar puncture and cerebrospinal fluid analysis. J Emerg Med. 2014;46(1):141–150.
5. Alkholi UM, Abd Al-Monem N, Abd El-Azim AA, Sultan MH. Serum procalcitonin in viral and bacterial meningitis. J Glob Infect Dis. 2011;3(1):14–18.
6. Centers for Disease Control and Prevention. Prevention and Control of Meningococcal Disease Recommendations of the Advisory Committee on Immunization Practices (ACIP). MMWR 2013;62(No. RR02):1–22.
7. Cohn A, MacNeil J. The changing epidemiology of meningococcal disease. Infect Dis Clin North Am. 2015;29(4):667–677.
8. Harcourt BH, Anderson RD, Wu HM, et al. Population-based surveillance of *Neisseria meningitidis* antimicrobial resistance in the United States. Open Forum Infect Dis. 2015 Aug 13;2(3):ofv117.
9. Brouwer MC, McIntyre P, Prasad K, van de Beek D. Corticosteroids for acute bacterial meningitis. Cochrane Database Syst Rev. 2015;(9):CD004405.
10. Wall EC, Ajdukiewicz KM, Heyderman RS, Garner P. Osmotic therapies added to antibiotics for acute bacterial meningitis. Cochrane Database Syst Rev. 2013;(3):CD008806.

121

COMMUNITY-ACQUIRED PNEUMONIA

The Coughing Conundrum . . . . Level II

Cole D. Luty, PharmD, BCPS

Trent G. Towne, PharmD, BCPS, BCIDP

LEARNING OBJECTIVES

After completing this case study, the reader should be able to:

• Recognize the common signs, symptoms, physical examination, laboratory, and radiographic findings in a patient with community-acquired pneumonia (CAP).

• Describe the most common causative pathogens of CAP, including their frequency of occurrence and susceptibility to frequently used antimicrobials.

- Discuss the risk stratification strategies that can be employed to determine whether a patient with CAP should be treated as an inpatient or outpatient.

- Provide recommendations for initial empiric antibiotic therapy for an inpatient or outpatient with CAP based on clinical presentation, severity of infection, age, allergies, and comorbidities.

- Define the goals of antimicrobial therapy for a patient with CAP, as well as the monitoring parameters that should be used to assess the response to therapy, conversion from IV to PO therapy (where warranted), and the occurrence of adverse medication reactions.

PATIENT PRESENTATION

■ Chief Complaint

"I have been short of breath and have been coughing up rust-colored phlegm for the past 3 days."

■ HPI

A 55-year-old man with a 3-day history of worsening shortness of breath, subjective fevers, chills, right-sided chest pain, and a productive cough presents to the ED. The patient states that his initial symptom of shortness of breath began approximately 1 week ago after delivering mail on an extremely cold winter day. He has been taking ibuprofen and an over-the-counter cough and cold preparation but feels that his symptoms are getting "much worse."

■ PMH

Hypertension × 15 years
Dyslipidemia × 15 years
Type 2 diabetes mellitus × 10 years

■ FH

Adopted; unknown birth parents

■ SH

Lives with wife and four children
Employed as a mail carrier for the US Postal Service
Denies alcohol, tobacco, or intravenous drug use

■ Medications

Prescription

Lisinopril 10 mg PO once daily
Hydrochlorothiazide 25 mg PO once daily
Atorvastatin 20 mg PO once daily
Metformin 1000 mg PO twice daily

Over-the-Counter

Ibuprofen 200 mg PO Q 6 H as needed for pain and fever
Guaifenesin/dextromethorphan (100 mg/10 mg/5 mL) two teaspoonfuls every 4 hours as needed for cough

■ All

NKDA

■ ROS

Patient is a good historian. He has been experiencing shortness of breath, a productive cough with rust-colored sputum, subjective fevers, chills, and pleuritic chest pain that is "on the right side of my chest." He denies any nausea, vomiting, constipation, or problems urinating.

■ Physical Examination

Gen

Patient is a well-developed, well-nourished man in moderate respiratory distress appearing somewhat anxious and uncomfortable.

■ VS

BP 155/85 mm Hg, P 127 bpm, RR 30, T 39.5°C; Wt 110 kg, Ht 5′11″

Skin

Warm to the touch; poor skin turgor

HEENT

PERRLA; EOMI; dry mucous membranes

Neck/Lymph Nodes

No JVD; full range of motion; no neck stiffness; no masses or thyromegaly; no cervical lymphadenopathy

Lungs/Thorax

Tachypnic, labored breathing; coarse rhonchi throughout right lung fields; decreased breath sounds in right middle and right lower lung fields

CV

Audible S_1 and S_2; tachycardic with regular rate and rhythm; no MRG

Abd

NTND; (+) bowel sounds

Genit/Rect

Deferred

Extremities

No CCE; 5/5 grip strength; 2+ pulses bilaterally

Neuro

A&O × 3; CN II–XII intact

■ Labs on Admission

Na 140 mEq/L	Hgb 12.1 g/dL	WBC 23.1 × 10³/mm³
K 4.3 mEq/L	Hct 35%	Neutrophils 67%
Cl 102 mEq/L	RBC 3.8 × 10⁶/mm³	Bands 15%
CO_2 22 mEq/L	Plt 220 × 10³/mm³	Lymphs 12%
BUN 42 mg/dL	MCV 91 μm³	Monos 6%
SCr 1.4 mg/dL	MCHC 35 g/dL	Procalcitonin 1.9 ng/mL
Glu 295 mg/dL		Lactic acid 2.3 mmol/L

■ ABG

pH 7.38; $PaCO_2$ 29; PaO_2 70 with 87% O_2 saturation on room air

■ Chest X-Ray

Right middle and right lower lobe consolidative airspace disease, likely pneumonia. Left lung is clear. Heart size is normal.

■ Chest CT Scan Without Contrast

No axillary, mediastinal, or hilar lymphadenopathy. The heart size is normal. There is consolidation of the right lower lobe and lateral segment of the middle lobe, with air bronchograms. No significant pleural effusions. The left lung is clear.

■ **Sputum Gram Stain**

>25 WBCs/hpf, <10 epithelial cells/hpf, many gram (+) cocci in pairs

■ **Sputum Culture**

Pending

■ **Blood Cultures × Two Sets**

Pending

■ **Other Lab Tests**

Streptococcus pneumoniae urine antigen—Pending
Legionella pneumophila urine antigen—Pending

■ **Assessment**

Probable multilobar CAP involving the RML and RLL

QUESTIONS

Collect Information

1.a. What subjective and objective information indicates the presence of CAP?

1.b. What additional information is needed to fully assess this patient's CAP?

Assess the Information

2.a. Assess the severity of this patient's CAP based on subjective and objective information available [use this information to decide on the site of care (inpatient or outpatient)].

2.b. Create a list of the patient's drug therapy problems and prioritize them. Include assessment of medication appropriateness, effectiveness, safety, and patient adherence.

Develop a Care Plan

3.a. What are the goals of pharmacotherapy for CAP in this case?

3.b. What nondrug therapies might be useful for this patient's CAP?

3.c. What feasible pharmacotherapeutic options are available for treating CAP?

3.d. Create an individualized, patient-centered, team-based care plan to optimize medication therapy for CAP and this patient's other drug therapy problems, including specific drugs, dosage forms, doses, schedules, and durations of therapy.

Implement the Care Plan

4.a. What information should be provided to the patient to enhance adherence, ensure successful therapy, and minimize adverse effects?

4.b. Describe how care should be coordinated with other healthcare providers.

Follow-Up: Monitor and Evaluate

5. Explain how to monitor and evaluate the care plan for medication appropriateness, effectiveness, safety, and patient adherence by using clinical and laboratory data, patient feedback, and other information.

■ **CLINICAL COURSE**

While in the ED, the patient was placed on 4 L of O_2 by nasal cannula, and his oxygen saturation improved to 98%. The patient was initiated on ceftriaxone 1 g IV daily and azithromycin 500 mg IV daily and admitted to the hospital. Over the next 48 hours, the patient's clinical status improved with decreasing fever, tachypnea, tachycardia, and shortness of breath. On hospital day 2, the *S. pneumoniae* urine antigen was positive, and the sputum culture demonstrated the growth of *S. pneumoniae*, resistant to erythromycin (MIC ≥1 mcg/mL), but susceptible to penicillin (MIC ≤2 mcg/mL), ceftriaxone (MIC ≤1 mcg/mL), levofloxacin (MIC ≤0.5 mcg/mL), and vancomycin (MIC ≤1 mcg/mL).

■ **FOLLOW-UP QUESTIONS**

1. Given this new information (at hospital day 2), what changes in the antimicrobial therapy would you recommend?

2. What oral antibiotic would be suitable to complete the course of therapy for CAP in this patient? When is it appropriate to convert a patient from IV to oral therapy for the treatment of CAP?

3. By hospital day 4, the patient's clinical symptoms of pneumonia had almost completely resolved, and the patient was discharged home on oral antibiotics to complete a 7-day course of treatment. What information should be provided to the patient about his oral outpatient antibiotic therapy to enhance adherence, ensure successful therapy, and minimize adverse medication reactions?

■ **SELF-STUDY ASSIGNMENTS**

1. Describe the role of molecular diagnostic testing and microbiology in the diagnosis and treatment of patients with CAP?

2. Describe the role of procalcitonin testing in the decision to initiate and de-escalation of antibiotics in patients with CAP.

3. Describe the role of short-course (5-day) antibiotic therapy in the management of CAP.

CLINICAL PEARL

Influenza and pneumococcal vaccines for appropriate patient types are important components for preventing CAP as well as for reducing the morbidity and mortality associated with CAP. The influenza vaccine is recommended for all persons 6 months of age or older and who do not have a contraindication. The pneumococcal vaccine recommendations vary based on patient-specific factors. Administration of the pneumococcal vaccine is recommendation for the following groups: Ages 65 years or older; Ages 19 through 64 years with chronic heart, lung, or liver conditions, diabetes, alcoholism, or cigarette smoking; Ages 19 years or older with immunocompromising conditions, cerebrospinal fluid leak, or cochlear implants.

REFERENCES

1. Metlay JP, Waterer GW, Long AC, et al. Diagnosis and treatment of adults with community-acquired pneumonia. An official clinical practice guideline of the American Thoracic Society and Infectious Diseases Society of America. Am J Respir Crit Care Med. 2019;200(7):e45–e67.

2. Mandell LA, Wunderink R. Pneumonia. In: Jameson J, Fauci AS, Kasper DL, et al, eds. Harrison's Principles of Internal Medicine, 20th ed. McGraw Hill; 2018. Available at: *https://accesspharmacy.mhmedical.com/content.aspx?bookid=2129&sectionid=184041853*. Accessed January 18, 2022.

3. Aliberti S, Dela Cruz CS, Amati F, et al. Community-acquired pneumonia. Lancet 2021;398:906–919.

4. Fine MJ, Auble TE, Yealy DM, et al. A prediction rule to identify low-risk patients with community-acquired pneumonia. N Engl J Med. 1997;336:243–250.

5. Lim WS, van der Eerden MM, Laing R, et al. Defining community-acquired pneumonia severity on presentation to hospital: an international derivation and validation study. Thorax. 2003;58:377–382.

6. Aujesky D, Auble TE, Yealy DM. Prospective comparison of three validated prediction rules for prognosis in community-acquired pneumonia. Am J Med. 2005;118:384–392.

7. Centers for Disease Control and Prevention. 2018. Active Bacterial Core Surveillance Report, Emerging Infections Program Network, *Streptococcus pneumoniae*, 2018. Available at: *http://www.cdc.gov/abcs/reports-findings/survreports/spneu18.pdf*. Accessed January 18, 2022.

122

HOSPITAL-ACQUIRED PNEUMONIA

The HAPpening............................... Level II

Kendra M. Damer, PharmD

LEARNING OBJECTIVES

After completing this case study, the reader should be able to:

- Recognize the signs and symptoms of hospital-acquired pneumonia (HAP).

- Identify the most common causative organisms associated with HAP, and recognize the impact of bacterial resistance on the etiology and treatment of HAP.

- Design an appropriate empiric antimicrobial therapy regimen for a patient with suspected HAP.

- Formulate a list of alternative antimicrobial therapy options for treating HAP based on the most common causative organisms.

- Recommend a directed/targeted antimicrobial therapy regimen for a patient with HAP based on patient-specific data and final microbiology culture and susceptibility results.

PATIENT PRESENTATION

■ Chief Complaint

"I can't catch my breath, and this cough is getting worse."

■ HPI

A 60-year-old man with a past medical history significant for MI was admitted to the hospital 5 days ago to undergo a scheduled surgical procedure following a recent diagnosis of colorectal adenocarcinoma with metastatic lesions to the liver. The patient was taken to the OR on hospital day 2 and underwent an exploratory laparotomy, diverting ileostomy, and Hickman catheter placement in preparation for chemotherapy. Postoperatively, the patient was transferred to the progressive ICU for recovery without complication. The patient had no new complaints until hospital day 5 when he complained of significant shortness of breath and a worsening cough with sputum production. He was noted to be in respiratory distress with an RR of 43 breaths/min, HR 147 bpm, BP 162/103 mm Hg, and O$_2$ saturation of 87%. He was transferred to the medical ICU and underwent endotracheal intubation due to worsening respiratory status. Imaging studies along with blood and sputum cultures were obtained after transfer.

■ PMH

CAD, S/P MI 3 years ago for which he did not undergo any surgical intervention
Colorectal carcinoma metastatic to liver (newly diagnosed)

■ SH

Lives with his wife; smokes one ppd × 40 years; denies alcohol or illicit drug use

■ Meds

Patient states that he did not take any medications at home. Hospital medications include (ICU medication list):

  Aspirin 81 mg PO daily
  Enoxaparin 40 mg subcutaneously every 24 hours
  Esomeprazole 40 mg PO daily
  Fentanyl 25 mcg/hr IV continuous infusion
  Lorazepam 2 mg/hr IV continuous infusion
  Metoprolol 25 mg PO every 12 hours
  Nicotine patch 21 mg per day applied daily

■ All

NKDA

■ ROS

Patient is experiencing significant shortness of breath and a cough with sputum production. He denies nausea, vomiting, or difficulty urinating. He complains of mild abdominal pain near his ostomy and incision sites.

■ Physical Examination

Gen

WDWN man, initially anxious, ill-appearing, and in moderate respiratory distress; now, S/P endotracheal intubation and in NAD

VS

BP 162/103 mm Hg, P 147 bpm, RR 43 breaths/min, T 38.5°C; Wt 70 kg, Ht 5'6"

Skin

Warm; no rash; no skin breakdown

HEENT

PERRLA; moist mucous membranes

Neck/Lymph Nodes

Supple; no lymphadenopathy

Lungs/Thorax

Scattered rhonchi with expiratory wheezing; diffuse bilateral crackles; decreased breath sounds in bilateral bases; right IJ Hickman catheter intact without erythema

CV

Tachycardic with regular rhythm; no MRG

Abd

Soft; mildly distended; hypoactive BS; large liver palpated in RUQ; ileostomy in RLQ is pink and functioning; surgical incision is C/D/I

Genit/Rect

Deferred

MS/Ext

1+ pitting edema; 2+ pulses bilaterally; good peripheral perfusion

Neuro

Prior to intubation, A&O × 3; CN II–XII intact; patient is now intubated and sedated.

■ Labs

Lab Parameter	Admission	Hospital Day 5
Na (mEq/L)	130	141
K (mEq/L)	4.1	5.1
Cl (mEq/L)	92	110
CO_2 (mEq/L)	24	19
BUN (mg/dL)	22	34
SCr (mg/dL)	1	1.1
Glu (mg/dL)	113	148
Ca (mg/dL)	9.4	9.2
WBC (cells/mm³)	9.5×10^3	17×10^3
Neutros (%)	89	88
Bands (%)	0	5
Lymphs (%)	5	4
Monos (%)	6	3
Eos (%)	0	0
Hgb (g/dL)	11.9	12.4
Hct (%)	35	37
Plts (cells/mm³)	448×10^3	584×10^3

■ ABG

Preintubation: pH 7.39; $PaCO_2$ 30; PaO_2 51 make HCO_3 25 mEq/L with 87% O_2 saturation on room air

Postintubation: pH 7.44; $PaCO_2$ 29; PaO_2 89 make HCO_3 23 mEq/L with 100% O_2 saturation on 40% inspired oxygen

■ Chest X-Ray

New bilateral opacities in the left upper lobe and right middle lobe; likely infectious process. Some increased alveolar infiltrates in the perihilar location and involving the lower lobes.

■ Chest CT Scan with IV Contrast

No evidence of pulmonary embolism. The heart size is normal. There are small mediastinal and axillary lymph nodes; none are pathologically enlarged. There are small bilateral pleural effusions with adjacent atelectasis. There are pleural-based airspace opacities within the left upper lobe and right middle lobe; this is most consistent with an acute infectious process.

■ Sputum Gram Stain

Greater than 25 WBC/hpf, <10 epithelial cells/hpf, 1+ (few) Gram-positive cocci, 3+ (many) Gram-negative rods

■ Sputum Culture

Pending

■ Blood Cultures × Two Sets

Pending

■ Assessment

Presumed bilobar HAP involving the LUL and RML

QUESTIONS

Collect Information

1.a. What subjective and objective information indicates the presence of HAP?

1.b. What additional information is needed to fully assess this patient's pneumonia?

Assess the Information

2.a. Assess the severity of HAP based on the subjective and objective information available.

2.b. Create a list of the patient's drug therapy problems and prioritize them. Include an assessment of medication appropriateness, effectiveness, safety, and patient adherence.

Develop a Care Plan

3.a. What are the goals of pharmacotherapy for HAP in this case?

3.b. What nondrug therapies might be useful for this patient's HAP?

3.c. What feasible pharmacotherapeutic options are available for treating HAP?

3.d. Create an individualized, patient-centered, team-based care plan to optimize medication therapy for this patient's HAP and other drug therapy problems. Include specific drugs, dosage forms, doses, schedules, and durations of therapy.

3.e. What alternatives would be appropriate if the initial care plan fails or cannot be used?

Implement the Care Plan

4.a. What information should be provided to the patient to enhance adherence, ensure successful therapy, and minimize adverse effects?

4.b. Describe how care should be coordinated with other healthcare professionals.

Follow-Up: Monitor and Evaluate

5. Explain how to monitor and evaluate the care plan for medication appropriateness, effectiveness, safety, and patient adherence by using clinical and laboratory data, patient feedback, and other information.

■ CLINICAL COURSE

Following endotracheal intubation and mechanical ventilation, the patient experienced improved oxygen saturation and a normalization of his respiratory and heart rates. He was started on appropriate empiric antimicrobial therapy while awaiting the results of sputum and blood cultures. The blood and sputum cultures revealed *Klebsiella pneumoniae*. The organism's susceptibility profile is provided below. Over the next 72 hours, the patient's clinical status improved with decreased sputum production, oxygen requirement, temperature, and WBC count. Improvement in chest X-ray findings was also noted, resulting in extubation on hospital day 8. The patient was transferred to the progressive ICU for his continued recovery.

Susceptibility Report for *Klebsiella pneumoniae*

Antimicrobial Agent	MIC (mg/L)	Interpretation
Ampicillin	≥32	Resistant
Ampicillin/sulbactam	≥32	Resistant
Piperacillin/tazobactam	≤4	Susceptible
Cefazolin	32	Resistant
Ceftriaxone	≤1	Susceptible
Cefepime	≤1	Susceptible
Meropenem	≤0.25	Susceptible
Gentamicin	≤1	Susceptible
Tobramycin	≤1	Susceptible
Ciprofloxacin	≤0.25	Susceptible
Levofloxacin	≤0.12	Susceptible
Trimethoprim/sulfamethoxazole	≥320	Resistant

■ FOLLOW-UP CASE QUESTION

1. Based on this new culture and susceptibility information, provide a recommendation for de-escalation of antimicrobial therapy from empiric to directed/targeted therapy. Include specific drugs, dosage forms, doses, schedules, and durations of therapy.

■ SELF-STUDY ASSIGNMENTS

1. Review national, regional, and local patterns of bacterial susceptibility for the most common causative organisms associated with HAP to determine appropriate empiric antimicrobial therapy choices for your geographic location.

2. Evaluate the literature to determine the most appropriate duration of therapy for HAP according to the causative microorganism.

3. Review the published literature to determine the role and utility of biomarkers (eg, procalcitonin [PCT]) and severity scoring (eg, acute physiologic assessment and chronic health evaluation II [APACHE II] and clinical pulmonary infection score [CPIS]) for the diagnosis and treatment of HAP.

4. Assess the patient's data and history to determine if he is eligible for any CDC-recommended immunizations against vaccine-preventable diseases.

5. Given the patient's past history of MI, evaluate the literature to determine the most appropriate recommendations for the medical management of CAD both as an inpatient and upon hospital discharge.

CLINICAL PEARL

Delays in initiation of appropriate empiric antimicrobial therapy have been associated with significant increases in hospital lengths of stay, healthcare costs, and mortality among patients with HAP.

REFERENCES

1. Kalil AC, Metersky ML, Klompas M, et al. Management of adults with hospital-acquired and ventilator-associated pneumonia: 2016 clinical practice guidelines by the Infectious Diseases Society of America and the American Thoracic Society. Clin Infect Dis. 2016;63(5):e61–e111.

2. Cilloniz C, Martin-Loeches I, Garcia-Vidal C, et al. Microbial etiology of pneumonia: epidemiology, diagnosis and resistance patterns. Int J Mol Sci. 2016;17:1–18.

3. Zaragoza R, Vidal-Cortés P, Aguilar G, et al. Update of the treatment of nosocomial pneumonia in the ICU. Crit Care. 2020;24(1):383–396.

4. Modi AR and Kovacs CS. Hospital-acquired and ventilator-associated pneumonia: diagnosis, management, and prevention. Cleve Clin J Med. 2020;87(10):633–639.

5. Maruyama T, Fujisawa T, Ishida T, et al. A therapeutic strategy for all pneumonia patients: a 3-year prospective multicenter cohort study using risk factors for multidrug-resistant pathogens to select initial empiric therapy. Clin Infect Dis. 2018;68(7):1080–1088.

6. Jean SS, Chang YC, Lin WC, et al. Epidemiology, treatment, and prevention of nosocomial bacterial pneumonia. J Clin Med. 2020;9(1):275–296.

7. Martin-Loeches I, Deja M, Koulenti D, et al. Potentially resistant microorganisms in intubated patients with hospital-acquired pneumonia: the interaction of ecology, shock and risk factors. Intensive Care Med. 2013;39:672–681.

8. Rybak MJ, Le J, Lodise TP, et al. Therapeutic monitoring of vancomycin for serious methicillin-resistant *Staphylococcus aureus* infections: a revised consensus guideline and review by the American Society of Health-System Pharmacists, the Infectious Diseases Society of America, the Pediatric Infectious Diseases Society, and the Society of the Infectious Diseases Pharmacists. Am J Health-Syst Pharm. 2020;77(11):835–863.

9. Purrello SM, Garau J, Giamarellos E, et al. Methicillin-resistant *Staphylococcus aureus* infections: a review of the currently available treatment options. J Glob Antimicrob Resist. 2016;7:178–186.

10. Xu E, Pérez-Torres D, Fragkou PC, et al. Nosocomial pneumonia in the era of multi-drug resistance: updates in diagnosis and management. Microorganisms. 2021;9(3):534–573.

123

ACUTE BRONCHITIS

The Collegiate Cough. . . . . Level II

Jessica H. Brady, PharmD, BCPS

Rebecca Clawson, MAT, PA-C

LEARNING OBJECTIVES

After completing this case study, the reader should be able to:

- Identify signs and symptoms of acute bronchitis

- Discuss why obtaining sputum cultures and Gram stains is not relevant in evaluation and treatment of patients with uncomplicated acute bronchitis.

- Discuss why antibiotic treatment is not indicated for uncomplicated acute bronchitis.

- Select nonpharmacologic and pharmacologic treatment alternatives for supportive care, incorporating data regarding efficacy.

PATIENT PRESENTATION

■ Chief Complaint

"I can't seem to stop coughing! It's keeping me and my roommate awake at night, not to mention totally disrupting my classes. My history professor even asked me to leave the class when I couldn't stop coughing! And now my throat is also sore. Everyone thinks I have COVID, though I assure them I've tested negative. I even tried my roommate's asthma inhaler hoping that my cough would stop, but it didn't. I just want an antibiotic to make this all go away!"

HPI

A 21-year-old college student presents to her university's Student Health Center, for a follow-up appointment for complaints of a cough with yellow sputum and a sore throat for the past 10 days. She has visited twice during this time due to her ongoing symptoms. At the first visit, she was tested for COVID-19, with a negative rapid antigen test. With continued symptoms, a PCR test for COVID-19 was also negative at her last visit. On questioning, the patient denies that she has had any fever, chills, or myalgias. She admits to using her roommate's albuterol asthma inhaler with short-lived relief. While her throat is still sore, she is most concerned with her disruptive cough.

PMH

Irregular menstrual cycle, ranging from 25 to 40 days in length
Current with age-appropriate vaccinations, except for influenza and HPV
Completed COVID-19 vaccine series 1 month prior to the start of the school term

FH

Father, 51, has been diagnosed with hypertension and hyperlipidemia and has a distant history of alcohol abuse. Mother, 50, is menopausal. The patient also has two younger brothers, ages 16 and 18, with no health issues.

SH

The patient lives in a university dorm with a suitemate. She denies alcohol use, due to her father's history of alcohol abuse, and tobacco use. She also denies any illicit drug use. She is currently a junior kinesiology major and hopes to attend physician assistant school on completion of her degree. She is also on the university dance line. The patient states that she is sexually active with her boyfriend of 8 months. They use condoms as a method of birth control, although inconsistently.

Meds

Acetaminophen 500 mg PO PRN headache or menstrual cramps

All

Penicillin—"all-over body rash"

ROS

General: denies fever, chills, and myalgia
Cardiovascular: denies chest pain and shortness of breath
Gastrointestinal: denies nausea, vomiting, and diarrhea

Physical Examination

Gen

Well-developed, thin woman in NAD

VS

BP 104/68 mm Hg, P 64 bpm, RR 14, T 97.9°F; Wt 126 lbs, Ht 5′6″

HEENT

PERRLA, conjunctivae clear, TMs intact. No epistaxis or nasal discharge. No sinus swelling or tenderness, and mucous membranes are moist. There are no oropharyngeal lesions.

Neck/Lymph Nodes

Supple without adenopathy or thyromegaly

Chest

(−) Rhonchi, rales, increased fremitus, wheezing, or egophony; negative bronchophony

CV

RRR without MRG

Abd

Soft, nontender, (+) and normoactive BS

Genit/Rect

Deferred

MS/Ext

Pulses 2+ throughout

Neuro

A&O × 3; 2+ reflexes throughout, 5/5 strength; CN II–XII intact

Labs

Na 140 mEq/L	Hgb 14 g/dL	WBC 6 × 10³/mm³
K 4.5 mEq/L	Hct 38%	Segs 55%
Cl 102 mEq/L	RBC 5.0 × 10⁶/mm³	Bands 3%
HCO₃ 24 mEq/L	Plt 250 × 10³/mm³	Lymphs 33%
BUN 14 mg/dL		Monos 6%
SCr 0.7 mg/dL		Eos 2%
FPG 88 mg/dL		Basos 1%

Assessment

1. Uncomplicated acute bronchitis.

2. Sexual/reproductive health issues should be further explored and addressed, particularly reliable birth control methods.

3. Need for updated immunizations.

QUESTIONS

Collect Information

1.a. What subjective and objective information indicates the presence of acute bronchitis?

1.b. What additional information is needed to fully assess this patient's acute bronchitis?

Assess the Information

2.a. Assess the severity of acute bronchitis based on the subjective and objective information available.

2.b. Create a list of the patient's drug therapy problems and prioritize them. Include assessment of medication appropriateness, effectiveness, safety, and patient adherence.

2.c. What psychosocial considerations are applicable to this patient?

Develop a Care Plan

3.a. What are the goals of pharmacotherapy for acute bronchitis in this case?

3.b. What nondrug therapies might be useful for this patient's acute bronchitis?

3.c. What feasible pharmacotherapeutic options are available for treating uncomplicated acute bronchitis?

3.d. Create an individualized, patient-centered, team-based care plan to optimize medication therapy for this patient's acute bronchitis and other drug therapy problems. Include specific drugs, dosage forms, doses, schedules, and durations of therapy.

Implement the Care Plan

4.a. What information should be provided to the patient to enhance adherence, ensure successful therapy, and minimize adverse effects?

4.b. Describe how care should be coordinated with other healthcare providers.

Follow-Up: Monitor and Evaluate

5. Explain how to monitor and evaluate the care plan for medication appropriateness, effectiveness, safety, and patient adherence by using clinical and laboratory data, patient feedback, and other information.

■ SELF-STUDY ASSIGNMENTS

1. Outline a treatment plan for a patient with chronic bronchitis presenting with an acute exacerbation, and contrast how this treatment would differ from treatment for a patient with a new diagnosis of uncomplicated acute bronchitis.

2. Prepare a patient education pamphlet on acute bronchitis. Be sure to address why antibiotics are not usually first-line therapy for uncomplicated acute bronchitis.

3. Discuss the differences in presentation and treatment of uncomplicated acute bronchitis for a child versus an adult versus an elderly patient.

CLINICAL PEARL

Even though over 90% of uncomplicated acute bronchitis cases are caused by viruses, many patients who present with symptoms of acute bronchitis expect to receive an antibiotic. Therefore, time should be spent with the patient explaining the decision not to prescribe an antibiotic and why excessive use of unnecessary antibiotics could harm the community at large.

REFERENCES

1. Woodhead M, Blasi F, Ewig S, et al. Joint Taskforce of the European Respiratory Society and European Society for Clinical Microbiology and Infectious Diseases. Guidelines for the management of adult lower respiratory tract infections-full version. Clin Microbiol Infect. 2011;17(Suppl 6):E1–E59.

2. Kinkade S, Long NA. Acute bronchitis. Am Fam Physician 2016;94(7):560–565.

3. Harris AM, Hicks LA, Qaseem A. Appropriate antibiotic use for acute respiratory tract infection in adults: advice for high-value care from the American College of Physicians and the Centers for Disease Control and Prevention. Ann Intern Med. 2016;164:425–434.

4. Tackett KL, Atkins A. Evidence-based acute bronchitis therapy. J Pharm Pract. 2012;25(6):586–590.

5. Smith SM, Fahey T, Smucny J, Becker LA. Antibiotics for acute bronchitis. Cochrane Database Syst Rev. 2017;(6):CD000245.

6. Becker LA, Hom J, Villasis-Keever M, van der Wouden JC. Beta2-agonists for acute bronchitis. Cochrane Database Syst Rev. 2011;(7):CD001726.

7. Smith SM, Schroeder K, Fahey T. Over-the-counter (OTC) medications for acute cough in children and adults in community settings. Cochrane Database Syst Rev. 2014;(11):CD001831.

8. Meites E, Szilagyi PG, Chesson HW, Unger ER, Romero JR, Markowitz LE. Human papillomavirus vaccination for adults: updated recommendations of the Advisory Committee on Immunization Practices. MMWR. 2019;68(32);698–702.

9. Saslow D, Andrews KS, Manassaram-Baptiste D, Smith RA, Fontham ETH. Human papillomavirus vaccination 2020 guideline update; American Cancer Society Guideline Adaptation. CA Cancer J Clin. 2020;70:274–280.

124

OTITIS MEDIA

Up to My Ears With Ear Infections . . . . Level II

Lauren Camaione, PharmD, BCPPS

Rochelle Rubin, PharmD, BCPS, CDCES

LEARNING OBJECTIVES

After completing this case study, the reader should be able to:

• Identify the signs and symptoms of acute otitis media (AOM).

• Discuss risk factors associated with an increased incidence of AOM.

• Identify the pathogens that most commonly cause AOM.

• Recommend an effective and economical treatment regimen, including specific agent(s), route of administration, and dose(s) of antibiotics and analgesic medications.

• State the role of delaying antibiotic therapy for AOM.

• Educate parents about recommended drug therapy using appropriate nontechnical terminology.

PATIENT PRESENTATION

■ Chief Complaint

Per patient's mom: "I've had it up to my ears with his ear infections!"

■ HPI

The patient is a 16-month-old boy who is brought to his pediatrician by his distraught mother on a Monday morning in early March. Mom describes a 2-day history of tugging at his right ear and crying, decreased appetite, decreased playfulness, and difficulty sleeping. Mom states that his temperature last night was elevated by electronic axial thermometer (39.5°C), so she gave him 5 mL of ibuprofen every 12 hours × 2 doses. Mom requests all recommendations be written as prescriptions (even ibuprofen) for day care administration. She also notes that it is tax season, and she needs the patient to be able to return to day care immediately so she can return to work as an accountant.

PMH

Former full-term, NSVD, 4-kg healthy infant at birth, breast-fed for 6 months. His immunizations are up-to-date, including four doses of 13-valent pneumococcal conjugate vaccination (Prevnar-13). His first episode of AOM at age 4 months treated with amoxicillin without adverse reactions. He had recurrent AOM × 3 over the past year; most recent episode 2 weeks ago treated with high-dose amoxicillin for 10 days without adverse reactions. The patient was seen approximately 1 month ago for persistent nonproductive cough of 5-day duration. A diagnosis of acute bronchiolitis was made, and symptoms improved with ibuprofen, fluids, and rest.

FH

Both parents in good health. Two siblings, 3 and 6 years old, in good health.

SH

The patient lives at home with his parents and two sisters. Both parents are employed and work out of the house. He and his 3-year-old sister attend day care. His elder sister attends elementary school. There is a pet dog in the home. The patient uses a pacifier regularly throughout the day. There is no smoking in the house.

Meds

Ibuprofen suspension 100 mg/5 mL, 100 mg (5 mL) PO Q 12 H × 2 doses in the past 24 hours

All

NKDA

ROS

Head: Otorrhea noted; ears tender to the touch
Respiratory: (per mom) denies wheezing. Lingering, mild cough still present, no sputum production

Physical Examination

Gen

WDWN 16-month-old male, now crying

VS

BP 104/60, HR 130 bpm, RR 26, T 39.1°C; Wt 10 kg, Ht 30″

Skin

Warm and dry; no rashes

HEENT

Both TMs erythematous (with R > L); right TM with moderate bulging and limited mobility; copious cerumen and purulent fluid behind TM; otorrhea noted; left TM landmarks appear normal including the pars flaccida, the malleus, and the light reflex below the umbo. However, the right TM landmarks are difficult to visualize, and fluid is obstructing visualization of the umbo. Throat is erythematous; nares patent.

Neck/Lymph Nodes

Supple; no lymphadenopathy

Chest

Mild crackles at bases bilaterally, improved since bronchiolitis visit 1 month ago

CV

RRR, no murmurs

Abd

Soft, nontender

Genit/Rect

Tanner stage I; rectal exam not performed

S/Ext

No CCE; moves all extremities well; warm, pink, no rashes; normal range of motion

Neuro

Responsive to stimulation, DTR 2+ no clonus, CN intact

Labs

None obtained

Assessment

Right ear AOM

QUESTIONS

Collect Information

1.a. What subjective and objective information indicates the presence of AOM?

1.b. What additional information is needed to fully assess this patient's AOM?

Assess the Information

2.a. Assess the severity of AOM based on the subjective and objective information available.

2.b. Create a list of the patient's drug therapy problems and prioritize them. Include assessment of medication appropriateness, effectiveness, safety, and patient adherence.

Develop a Care Plan

3.a. What are the goals of pharmacotherapy for AOM in this case?

3.b. What nondrug therapies might be useful for this patient's AOM?

3.c. What feasible pharmacotherapeutic options are available for treating AOM?

3.d. Create an individualized, patient-centered, team-based care plan to optimize medication therapy for the AOM and other drug therapy problems. Include the specific drugs, dosage forms, doses, schedules, and durations of therapy.

Implement the Care Plan

4.a. What information should be provided to the patient to enhance adherence, ensure successful therapy, and minimize adverse effects?

4.b. Describe how care should be coordinated with other healthcare providers.

Follow Up: Monitor and Evaluate

5. Explain how to monitor and evaluate the care plan for medication appropriateness, effectiveness, safety, and patient adherence by using clinical and laboratory data, patient feedback, and other information.

■ SELF-STUDY ASSIGNMENTS

1. Describe a scenario in which it would be appropriate to use azithromycin to treat AOM.

CLINICAL PEARL

Cefdinir administration should be separated from administration of iron supplements, iron-containing vitamins, or antacids containing magnesium or aluminum by 2 hours to prevent decreased absorption of cefdinir. Additionally, the concurrent use of cefdinir with iron-containing infant formulas can result in reddish color stool, but does not appear to decrease absorption of cefdinir.

REFERENCES

1. Lieberthal AS, Carroll AE, Chonmaitree T, et al. Clinical practice guideline: diagnosis and management of acute otitis media. Pediatrics. 2013;131:e964–e999.

2. American Academy of Otolaryngology—Head and Neck Surgery Foundation, American Academy of Pediatrics, American Academy of Family Physicians. Clinical Practice Guideline: Otitis Media with Effusion (Update). 2016;154(IS):S1-S41.

3. Neto JFL, Hemb L, Silva DB. Systematic literature review of modifiable risk factors for recurrent otitis media in childhood. J Pediatr. 2006;82:87–96.

4. Kaur R, Morris M, Pichichero M. Epidemiology of acute otitis media in the post pneumococcal conjugate vaccine era. Pediatrics. 2017;140(3):1–11.

5. Venekamp RP, Sanders S, Glasziou PP, et al. Antibiotics for acute otitis media in children. Cochrane Database Syst Rev. 2013;(1):CD000219.

6. Spiro DM, Tay KY, Arnold DH, Dziura JD, Baker MD, Shapiro ED. Wait-and-see prescription for the treatment of acute otitis media. JAMA. 2006;196:1235–1241.

7. Centers for Disease Control and Prevention. Active Bacterial Core Surveillance Report, Emerging Infections Program Network, *Streptococcus pneumoniae*, 2019. Atlanta, GA: Centers for Disease Control and Prevention; 2019. Available at: *https://www.cdc.gov/abcs/downloads/SPN_Surveillance_Report_2019.pdf*. Accessed January 14, 2022.

8. Bertin L, Pons G, d'Athis P, et al. A randomized, double-blind, multicentre controlled trial of ibuprofen versus acetaminophen and placebo for symptoms of acute otitis media in children. Fundam Clin Pharmacol. 1996;10:387–392.

125

RHINOSINUSITIS

Sick Sinus. . . . . Level II

Michael B. Kays, PharmD, FCCP, BCIDP

LEARNING OBJECTIVES

After completing this case study, the reader should be able to:

- Compare and contrast the signs and symptoms of acute viral and bacterial rhinosinusitis in a given patient, noting the cardinal symptoms of acute bacterial rhinosinusitis.

- Differentiate viral from bacterial etiology in rhinosinusitis based on a patient's symptoms.

- Identify the most common pathogens causing acute bacterial rhinosinusitis.

- Identify adult patients with a diagnosis of acute bacterial rhinosinusitis who may be candidates for observation without use of antibiotics.

- Formulate a treatment plan for a patient with acute bacterial rhinosinusitis based on duration of symptoms, severity of symptoms, and history of previous antibiotic use.

- Revise the treatment plan for a patient who fails the initially prescribed therapy.

PATIENT PRESENTATION

■ Chief Complaint

"I feel awful and congested, and my head hurts. I was starting to feel better, but now I think my sinus infection is back."

■ HPI

A 54-year-old man presents to his primary care physician with fever, purulent nasal discharge from the left naris, facial pain (L > R), nasal congestion, headache, and fatigue. He states that his symptoms of runny nose, congestion, fever, and malaise began 8 days ago, and the symptoms initially improved over the first 4–5 days. However, the symptoms have become progressively worse over the past few days. He also complains of intense facial pressure when he bends forward to tie his shoes or to pick up something. He has noticed a decreased sense of smell and states that foods do not taste the same as before. He has experienced occasional episodes of nausea, dizziness, tremors, and palpitations for the past week, and states that he has had difficulty sleeping the past few nights. He has been taking ibuprofen as needed and loratadine 5 mg/pseudoephedrine sulfate 120 mg every 12 hours but has received little relief from his symptoms. He states that he was treated for a sinus infection about 4 weeks ago. When questioned further, he states that he presented to an urgent care clinic complaining of a runny nose, congestion, sneezing, cough, and a mild sore throat of 2–3 days duration. He was leaving the following day for a business trip and asked the physician for an antibiotic prescription. He told the physician that azithromycin has always worked for him, so he was prescribed azithromycin 500 mg PO daily for 3 days. His symptoms slowly improved over 7–10 days, and he was symptom-free for a several days before his current symptoms began 8 days ago. He states that he only gets sick occasionally and has not had an infection in the past year prior to these episodes.

■ PMH

Sinus infection 4 weeks ago
Hypertension (well controlled with medication)
Hypercholesterolemia (well controlled with medication)

■ FH

Father died of MI at 64 years of age
Mother with hypertension and diabetes mellitus

■ SH

Smokes cigars on occasion (1–2 per week). Denies cigarette smoking and illicit drug use. Drinks socially (3–4 beers and 1 bottle of red wine per week)

He is divorced with two children (27-year-old son, 24-year-old daughter)

■ Meds

Lisinopril 20 mg PO daily

Hydrochlorothiazide 25 mg PO daily

Atorvastatin 40 mg PO daily

Ibuprofen 200–400 mg PO as needed

Claritin-D 12 hours (loratadine 5 mg/pseudoephedrine sulfate 120 mg) PO Q 12 H

■ All

None

■ ROS

Patient with an 8-day history of runny nose, congestion, fever, and malaise now with fever, purulent nasal drainage, congestion, facial pain, headache, fatigue, hyposmia, occasional nausea, dizziness, and palpitations. The symptoms improved initially but have progressively worsened over the past few days. In addition, the patient complains of insomnia, which may be contributing to the fatigue. He denies vomiting, diarrhea, chills, diaphoresis, dyspnea, productive cough, or allergies.

■ Physical Examination

Gen

Tired-looking, overweight man in mild distress; appears uncomfortable

VS

BP 158/102, P 98 bpm, RR 16, T 39.3°C; Wt 118 kg, Ht 73″

Skin

Warm to touch; good skin turgor; no other abnormalities

HEENT

NC/AT; PERRLA; EOMI; funduscopic exam normal; injected conjunctivae; anicteric sclerae. Thick, purulent, yellow-green nasal discharge; mucosal hypertrophy (L > R) without evidence of nasal polyps. Facial pain over left maxillary and frontal sinuses. No oral lesions; no periorbital swelling. Tympanic membranes intact, nonerythematous, nonbulging. Throat erythematous.

Neck/Lymph Nodes

Supple, no JVD, mild lymphadenopathy

Lungs/Thorax

CTA; no crackles or wheezing

CV

Tachycardic; normal S_1 and S_2, no MRG

Abd

Soft, nontender; bowel sounds present; no masses

Genit/Rect

Deferred

MS/Ext

No CCE

Neuro

A&O × 3; CN II–XII intact

■ Labs

None obtained

■ Assessment

1. Recurrent rhinosinusitis—patient is able to afford medications and states that he took all of his previous antibiotic prescription as directed

2. Dizziness, tremors, palpitations

3. Hypertension

4. Hypercholesterolemia

QUESTIONS

Collect Information

1.a. What subjective and objective information indicates the presence of rhinosinusitis?

1.b. What additional information is needed to fully assess this patient's rhinosinusitis?

Assess the Information

2.a. Assess the severity of rhinosinusitis based on the subjective and objective information available.

2.b. Create a list of the patient's drug therapy problems and prioritize them. Include assessment of medication appropriateness, effectiveness, safety, and patient adherence.

Develop a Care Plan

3.a. What are the goals of pharmacotherapy for acute rhinosinusitis in this case?

3.b. What nondrug therapies might be useful for this patient's acute rhinosinusitis?

3.c. What feasible pharmacotherapeutic options are available for treating acute bacterial rhinosinusitis?

3.d. Create an individualized, patient-centered, team-based care plan to optimize medication therapy for this patient's acute bacterial rhinosinusitis and other drug therapy problems. Include specific drugs, dosage forms, doses, schedules, and durations of therapy.

3.e. What alternatives would be appropriate if the initial care plan fails or cannot be used?

Implement the Care Plan

4.a. What information should be provided to the patient to enhance adherence, ensure successful therapy, and minimize adverse effects?

4.b. Describe how care should be coordinated with other healthcare providers.

Follow-Up: Monitor and Evaluate

5. Explain how to monitor and evaluate the care plan for medication appropriateness, effectiveness, safety, and patient adherence by using clinical and laboratory data, patient feedback, and other information.

■ SELF-STUDY ASSIGNMENTS

1. Determine if a change in mucus color from clear to yellow or green is an indication of a bacterial infection or if it is the natural course of a viral infection.

2. If the patient had a reported penicillin allergy, review appropriate questions for assessing the severity of the patient's allergy and the likelihood of an allergic reaction if he received a cephalosporin.

3. Review the pharmacokinetic and pharmacodynamic properties of antibacterial agents commonly used in the treatment of acute bacterial rhinosinusitis.

4. Review the prevalence and most common mechanisms of bacterial resistance in pathogens frequently encountered in acute bacterial rhinosinusitis.

CLINICAL PEARL

In patients with a clinical diagnosis of acute bacterial rhinosinusitis, the spontaneous resolution rate is 50–60%. Antibiotics, if prescribed, should be administered for the shortest effective duration.

REFERENCES

1. Chow AW, Benninger MS, Brook I, et al. IDSA clinical practice guideline for acute bacterial rhinosinusitis in children and adults. Clin Infect Dis. 2012;54:e72–e112.

2. Rosenfeld RM, Piccirillo JF, Chandrasekhar SS, et al. Clinical practice guideline (update): adult sinusitis. Otolaryngol Head Neck Surg. 2015;152 (2 Suppl):S1–S39.

3. Rosenfeld RM. Acute sinusitis in adults. New Engl J Med. 2016;375:962–970.

4. Benninger MS, Payne SC, Ferguson BJ, Hadley JA, Ahmad N. Endoscopically directed middle meatal cultures versus maxillary sinus taps in acute bacterial maxillary rhinosinusitis: a meta-analysis. Otolaryngol Head Neck Surg. 2006;134:3–9.

5. Fleming-Dutra KE, Hersh AL, Shapiro DJ, et al. Prevalence of inappropriate antibiotic prescriptions among US ambulatory care visits, 2010–2011. JAMA. 2016;315:1864–1873.

6. Benninger MS, Holy CE, Trask DK. Acute rhinosinusitis: prescription patterns in a real-world setting. Otolaryngol Head Neck Surg. 2016;154:957–962.

7. Benninger M, Brook I, Farrell DJ. Disease severity in acute bacterial rhinosinusitis is greater in patients infected with *Streptococcus pneumoniae* than in those infected with *Haemophilus influenzae*. Otolaryngol Head Neck Surg. 2006;135:523–528.

8. Matho A, Mulqueen M, Tanina M, et al. High-dose versus standard-dose amoxicillin/clavulanate for clinically-diagnosed acute bacterial sinusitis: a randomized clinical trial. PLoS One. 2018;13(5):e0196734.

9. FDA Drug Safety Communication: FDA advises restricting fluoroquinolone antibiotic use for certain uncomplicated infections; warns about disabling side effects that can occur together. Available at: *https://www.fda.gov/Drugs/DrugSafety/ucm500143.htm*. Accessed January 9, 2022.

10. Sader HS, Mendes RE, Le J, Denys G, Flamm RK, Jones RN. Antimicrobial susceptibility of *Streptococcus pneumoniae* from North America, Europe, Latin America, and the Asia-Pacific region: results from 20 years of the SENTRY Antimicrobial Surveillance Program (1997–2016). Open Forum Infect Dis. 2019;6:S14–S22.

126

ACUTE PHARYNGITIS

A Hard Pill to Swallow......................... Level II

Anthony J. Guarascio, PharmD, BCPS

Autumn Stewart-Lynch, PharmD, BCACP, CTTS

LEARNING OBJECTIVES

After completing this case study, the reader should be able to:

- List the subjective and objective information that a healthcare professional must gather from a patient with pharyngitis.

- Assess the need for antibiotic therapy in a patient with pharyngitis based on signs and symptoms and the results from microbiological and immunologic diagnostic studies.

- Prepare an evidence-based care plan for a patient with acute pharyngitis that is individualized to the patient's current presentation, past medical history, and concurrent medications.

- Identify the key educational and counseling points needed by the patient and/or caregivers to safely and effectively implement the therapeutic plan and to prevent disease transmission.

- List the parameters monitored by the healthcare professional to ensure clinical resolution and the prevention of suppurative and nonsuppurative complications of acute pharyngitis.

PATIENT PRESENTATION

■ Chief Complaint

"It hurts to swallow."

■ HPI

A 16-year-old girl presents to her community pharmacy complaining of sore throat and requests help finding an over-the-counter product to alleviate her symptoms. Her mother reports a fever of 102°F (38.9°C) on and off for the past 24 hours, and observes that she has been more tired over the past 2 days. She has been drinking only liquids since this time. She endorses a bumpy rash on her face and neck that has spread to her chest and arms. She denies cough, shortness of breath, or difficulty breathing. The patient complains of nausea and headaches but denies vomiting. Mother notes no recent illness in the family.

■ PMH

The patient has had prior cases of otitis media as a young child. Six months ago, she was diagnosed with primary dysmenorrhea. Otherwise, she is healthy. Immunization records indicate receipt of the following immunizations:

HepB: four doses (last dose age 12 months)
DTaP: five doses (last dose age 4 years)
Tdap: one dose given at age 11
Hib: four doses (last dose age 12 months)
PCV: four doses (last dose age 12 months)
IPV: four doses (last dose age 4 years)

MMR: two doses (last dose age 12 months)
Varicella: two doses (last dose age 12 months)
MenACWY-D: one dose given at age 11
Influenza IIV/LAIV: last received at age 15
COVID-19 VACCINE, mRNA: two doses (last dose age 16 years)

■ FH

Noncontributory

■ SH

She lives with her parents and 12-year-old twin sisters. She started high school 2 years ago and is on the varsity lacrosse team. She denies the use of tobacco, alcohol, marijuana, or other substances.

■ Meds

Ethinyl estradiol 20 mcg/levonorgestrel 0.1 mg (21 days active-7 days placebo): one tablet by mouth daily
Naproxen 500 mg by mouth twice daily for 5 days (begin 2 days before menses)

■ All

Penicillin: reaction unknown

■ ROS

Negative except for complaints noted in the HPI

■ Physical Examination

Gen

WDWN 16-year-old girl, clearly fatigued

VS

BP 104/70, P 92, RR 22, T 38.8°C, Wt 50 kg, Ht 63″

Skin

Warm, faint scarlatiniform rash on face, neck, and arms that blanches with pressure

HEENT

Tonsils erythematous with associated white exudates; uvula edematous; soft palate with notable petechiae (see Figure 126-1). Otherwise unremarkable.

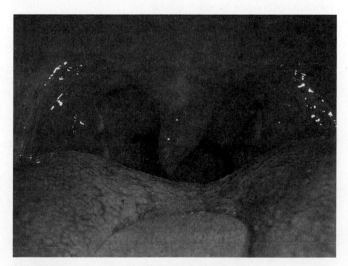

FIGURE 126-1. Image of patient's oral cavity and tonsils.

Neck/Lymph Nodes

Multiple enlarged anterior cervical lymph nodes

Genit/Rect

Deferred; LMP 3 weeks ago; not sexually active

■ Labs

Point of Care Rapid Streptococcal Antigen Detection Test (RADT): negative

■ Assessment

A 16-year-old girl presents with suspected group A *Streptococcus* (GAS) pharyngitis.

QUESTIONS

Collect Information

1.a. What subjective and objective information indicates the presence of GAS pharyngitis versus viral pharyngitis?

1.b. What additional information is needed to fully assess this patient's acute pharyngitis?

1.c. What additional information is needed to adequately assess this patient's penicillin allergy?

Assess the Information

2.a. Assess the severity of acute pharyngitis based on the subjective and objective information available.

2.b. Create a list of the patient's drug therapy problems and prioritize them. Include assessment of medication appropriateness, effectiveness, safety, and patient adherence.

Develop a Care Plan

3.a. What are the goals of pharmacotherapy for GAS Pharyngitis in this case if the throat culture returns positive for GAS?

3.b. What nondrug therapies might be useful for this patient's acute pharyngitis?

3.c. What feasible pharmacotherapeutic options are available for treating GAS acute pharyngitis?

3.d. Create an individualized, patient-centered, team-based care plan to optimize medication therapy for acute pharyngitis and this patient's other drug therapy problems. Include specific drugs, dosage forms, doses, schedules, and durations of therapy.

Implement the Care Plan

4.a. What information should be provided to the patient and caregivers to enhance adherence, ensure successful therapy, minimize adverse effects, and prevent disease transmission to others?

4.b. Describe how care should be coordinated with other healthcare providers.

Follow-Up: Monitor and Evaluate

5. Explain how to monitor and evaluate the care plan for medication appropriateness, effectiveness, safety, and patient adherence by using clinical and laboratory data, patient feedback, and other information.

■ ADDITIONAL CASE QUESTIONS

1. What is the clinical significance of potential drug interactions between the patient's drug therapy for GAS pharyngitis and current medications?

2. The patient's mother is concerned about transmission to household contacts and requests antibiotic prescriptions for her siblings. Explain whether or not this would be necessary.

■ SELF-STUDY ASSIGNMENTS

1. Create a table that lists the preferred and alternative therapeutic options for GAS pharyngitis and includes the following comparative data: Drug name, dose, frequency, duration, available dosage forms, adverse effects, and cost.

2. Prepare a one-page paper that describes the incidence, risk factors, signs/symptoms, onset, and possible complications of scarlet fever, rheumatic fever, and poststreptococcal glomerulonephritis.

CLINICAL PEARL

While early initiation of antibiotic therapy can reduce the duration of GAS symptoms, withholding antibiotics until laboratory confirmation of GAS bacterial disease in the majority of clinical circumstances can reduce the potential for inappropriate antibiotic therapy while still preventing the spread of GAS to others and prevent development of complications. Negative RADT in the presence of clinical signs and symptoms strongly suggestive of GAS requires confirmatory throat culture.

REFERENCES

1. Gerber MA, Baltimore RS, Eaton CB, et al. Prevention of rheumatic fever and diagnosis and treatment of acute streptococcal pharyngitis. Circulation. 2009;119:1541–1551.

2. Shulman ST, Bisno AL, Clegg HW, et al. Practice guidelines for the diagnosis and management of group A streptococcal pharyngitis: 2012 update by the Infectious Diseases Society of America. Clin Infect Dis. 2012;55:1279–1282.

3. Wessels MR. Streptococcal pharyngitis. N Engl J Med. 2011;364:648–655.

4. Bilir SP, Kruger S, Faller M, et al. US cost-effectiveness and budget impact of point-of-care NAAT for Streptococcus. Am J Manag Care. 2021;27(5):e157–e163.

5. Fine AM, Nizet V, Mandl KD. Large-scale validation of the Centor and McIsaac scores to predict group A streptococcal pharyngitis. Arch Intern Med. 2012;172(11):847–852.

6. National Committee for Quality Assurance. Quality ID #66: Appropriate Testing for Children with Pharyngitis Available at: *https://qpp.cms.gov/docs/QPP_quality_measure_specifications/CQM-Measures/2020_Measure_066_MIPSCQM_v4.1.pdf*. Accessed January 27, 2022.

7. Centers for Disease Control and Prevention. Strep Throat: All You Need to Know. Available at: *https://www.cdc.gov/groupastrep/diseases-public/strep-throat.html*. Accessed March 18, 2022.

8. Centers for Disease Control and Prevention. Pharyngitis (strep throat): information for Clinicians. Available at: *https://www.cdc.gov/groupastrep/diseases-hcp/strep-throat.html*. Accessed January 27, 2022.

9. ACOG Committee on Practice Bulletins-Gynecology. ACOG Practice Bulletin No. 73: use of hormonal contraception in women with coexisting medical conditions. Obstet Gynecol. 2006 Jun;107:1453.

10. Curtis KM, Tepper NK, Jatlaoui TC, et al. U.S. medical eligibility criteria for contraceptive use, 2016. MMWR Recomm Rep. 2016;65(No. RR-3):1–104.

127

INFLUENZA

Run Over by the Flu. . . . . Level II

Christo L. Cimino, PharmD, BCPS, BCIDP

Douglas Slain, PharmD, BCPS, FCCP, FASHP

LEARNING OBJECTIVES

After completing this case study, the reader should be able to:

- Recognize the clinical presentation of influenza.

- Discuss influenza-related complications.

- Develop a patient-specific treatment plan for influenza.

- Identify appropriate target populations for vaccination against influenza.

- Compare and contrast available options for preventing influenza.

- Discuss strategies to control influenza outbreaks.

PATIENT PRESENTATION

■ Chief Complaint

"I feel like a truck ran over me. Every muscle and bone hurts, and I am burning up."

■ HPI

A 67-year-old male presents in mid-December to an urgent care clinic with complaints of 1-day history of fever, up to 39°C (102.2°F), muscle and bone aches, feeling tired, and headache. He has not had anything to eat in the past 12 hours due to loss of appetite and has not taken his glyburide this morning. He has been in his usual state of health previously and reports that some of his coworkers have been sick with the "flu." He decided to come to the clinic in hopes that an antibiotic can allow him to recover sooner since his son is getting married next weekend. He missed his regular appointment 1 month ago because he was "too busy."

■ PMH

Type 2 DM for 14 years
Hyperlipidemia
Hypertension

■ FH

Father and sister with type 2 DM

■ SH

Lives at home with his wife; works full time; quit smoking 10 years ago, but smokes occasionally when really stressed or in a social setting; drinks alcohol in a social setting.

■ Meds

Aspirin 81 mg PO daily
Hydrochlorothiazide 25 mg PO daily
Glyburide 5 mg PO every morning

Metformin 1 g PO twice daily
Lantus 35 units SC at bedtime
Atorvastatin 10 mg PO daily
Centrum Silver one tablet PO daily

■ All

NKDA

■ Review of Systems

Complains of severe fatigue, body aches, alternating between being too cold and sweating, sore throat, nonproductive cough, and a headache. He denies nasal congestion, nausea, vomiting, or diarrhea.

■ Physical Examination

Gen

WDWN overweight man in NAD

VS

BP 150/90 (patient reports similar readings at home), P 95 bpm, RR 18, T 38.5°C; Wt 95.5 kg, Ht 5′10″

Skin

Warm and moist secondary to diaphoresis, no lesions

HEENT

PERRLA; EOMI; TMs intact; wears dentures; mild pharyngeal erythema with no exudates

Neck/Lymph Nodes

Neck is supple and without adenopathy; no JVD

Lungs/Thorax

CTA; no crackles or wheezing

CV

RRR; normal S_1, S_2; no murmurs

Abd

Soft, obese; NT/ND; normal BS

Genit/Rect

Not performed

MS/Ext

Muscle strength and tone 4–5/5; no CCE

Neuro

A&O × 3; CN II–XII intact; decreased sensation to light touch of the lower extremities (both feet)

■ Labs

BMP	CBC	Fasting Lipid Profile	Other
Na 138 mEq/L	WBC 10 × 10³/mm³	T. chol 177 mg/dL	A1C 7.1%
K 3.8 mEq/L	Neutros 50%	LDL 110 mg/dL	
Cl 98 mEq/L	Bands 4%	HDL 35 mg/dL	
CO₂ 24 mEq/L	Eos 0%	Trig 160 mg/dL	
BUN 26 mg/dL	Lymphs 39%		
SCr 1.3 mg/dL	Hgb 13.2 g/dL		
Glu 135 mg/dL	Hct 41%		
	Plt 275 × 10³/mm³		

■ Diagnostic Tests

QuickVue rapid influenza test—positive
Abbott BinaxNOW rapid COVID-19 test—negative

■ Assessment

A 67-year-old man with diabetes, hypertension, and hyperlipidemia presents with influenza.

QUESTIONS

Collect Information

1.a. What subjective and objective information indicates the presence of influenza?

1.b. What additional information is needed to fully assess this patient's influenza?

Assess the Information

2.a. Assess the severity of influenza infection based on the subjective and objective information available.

2.b. Create a list of the patient's drug therapy problems and prioritize them. Include assessment of medication appropriateness, effectiveness, safety, and patient adherence.

Develop a Care Plan

3.a. What are the goals of pharmacotherapy in this case?

3.b. What nondrug therapies might be useful for this patient's influenza?

3.c. What feasible pharmacotherapeutic options are available for treating influenza infection? Include the drug name, dose, dosage form, route, frequency, and treatment duration. Are these options affected by the type of influenza that this patient is experiencing and the time since onset of illness?

3.d. Create an individualized, patient-centered, team-based care plan to optimize medication therapy for influenza and this patient's drug therapy problems. Include specific drugs, dosage forms, doses, schedules, and durations of therapy.

Implement the Care Plan

4.a. What information should be provided to the patient to enhance adherence, ensure successful therapy, and minimize adverse effects?

4.b. Describe how care should be coordinated with other healthcare providers.

Follow-Up: Monitor and Evaluate

5. Explain how to monitor and evaluate the care plan for medication appropriateness, effectiveness, safety, and patient adherence by using clinical and laboratory data, patient feedback, and other information.

■ CLINICAL COURSE

In October of the following year, the patient presents for his routine physical exam. He has been doing very well. His diabetes, hypertension, and hyperlipidemia are well controlled.

■ FOLLOW-UP QUESTIONS

1. What indications does this patient have for administration of the seasonal influenza vaccine?

2. If the vaccine is desirable, what is the optimal time frame for this patient to receive vaccination(s)?

3. What are all available options for vaccination against seasonal influenza?

4. Provide your individualized recommendations for protecting this patient against influenza virus infections.

5. Should all patients with confirmed influenza receive treatment with antiviral medications?

■ CLINICAL COURSE: ALTERNATIVE THERAPY

As the patient is leaving, he thanks you and promises to follow your recommendations. He states that he is worried about making anyone else sick, because of his son's upcoming wedding. "My cousins keep telling me they use elderberry syrup to keep from getting sick during flu season. Could that help keep my wife from getting this flu?" See Section 19 in this Casebook for information regarding the use of elderberry for influenza treatment and prevention.

■ SELF-STUDY ASSIGNMENTS

1. Prepare an educational pamphlet on influenza prevention and treatment directed at both patients and general practice physicians. Include recommendations for controlling influenza outbreaks.

2. Investigate the role of pharmacists as immunization providers.

3. Investigate the threat of human infection with avian influenza viruses. Are currently available influenza prevention strategies effective against avian flu?

CLINICAL PEARL

Development of antibodies takes approximately 2 weeks after influenza vaccination in adults, during which time they remain at high risk for influenza infection. If the immunization occurs during an influenza outbreak, chemoprophylaxis with antiviral agents can be administered for 2 weeks immediately after vaccination to minimize the risk of infection. The live attenuated influenza vaccine (LAIV) can cause a false-positive result for up to 7 days on a rapid influenza diagnostic test since these tests cannot differentiate between live attenuated and wild-type influenza viruses.

REFERENCES

1. Uyeki TM, Bernstein HH, Bradley JS, et al. Clinical practice guidelines by the Infectious Diseases Society of America: 2018 update on diagnosis, treatment, chemoprophylaxis, and institutional outbreak management of seasonal influenza. Clin Infect Dis. 2019;68(6):895–902.

2. United States Centers for Disease Control and Prevention. Guidance for clinicians on the use of rapid influenza diagnostic tests. Available at: http://www.cdc.gov/flu/professionals/diagnosis/clinician_guidance_ridt. htm. Accessed January 30, 2022.

3. United States Centers for Disease Control and Prevention. FDA-cleared RT-PCR assays and other molecular assays for influenza viruses. Available at: http://www.cdc.gov/flu/pdf/professionals/diagnosis/table1-molecular-assays.pdf. Accessed January 30, 2022.

4. Center for Disease Control and Prevention. Influenza antiviral medications: summary for clinicians. Available at: https://www.cdc.gov/flu/professionals/antivirals/summary-clinicians.htm. Accessed January 30, 2022.

5. Louie JK, Yang S, Acosta M, et al. Treatment with neuraminidase inhibitors for critically ill patients with influenza A (H1N1) pdm09. Clin Infect Dis. 2012;55(9):1198–1204.

6. Slain D. Intravenous zanamivir: a viable option for critically ill patients with influenza. Ann Pharmacother. 2021;55(6):760–771.

7. Grohskopf LA, Alyanak E, Ferdinands JM, et al. Prevention and control of seasonal influenza with vaccines: recommendations of the Advisory Committee on Immunization Practices, United States, 2021–22 Influenza Season. MMWR Recomm Rep. 2021;70(No. RR-5):1–28.

8. Whelton PK, Carey RM, Aronow WS, et al. 2017 ACC/AHA/AAPA/ABC/ACPM/AGS/APhA/ASH/ASPC/NMA/PCNA guideline for the prevention, detection, evaluation, and management of high blood pressure in adults: a report of the American College of Cardiology/American Heart Association Task Force on Clinical Practice Guidelines. Circulation. 2018 Oct 23;138(17):e484–e594.

9. Grundy SM, Stone NJ, Bailey AL, et al. 2018 AHA/ACC/AACVPR/AAPA/ABC/ACPM/ADA/AGS/APhA/ASPC/NLA/PCNA guideline on the management of blood cholesterol: a report of the American College of Cardiology/American Heart Association Task Force on Clinical Practice Guidelines. Circulation. 2019;139(25):e1082–e1143.

10. Black S, Nicolay U, Del Giudice G, Rappuoli R. Influence of statins on influenza vaccine response in elderly individuals. J Infect Dis. 2015;213(8):1224–1228.

128

CORONAVIRUS VACCINATION AND TREATMENT

The Cough Before the Storm. Level II

Siddharth F. Swamy, PharmD, BCPS, BCIDP

LEARNING OBJECTIVES

After completing this case study, the reader should be able to:

- Recognize the signs and symptoms of COVID-19 in individual patients.

- Evaluate the severity of COVID-19 based on subjective and objective information.

- Construct a treatment regimen for COVID-19 based on patient location and severity of disease.

- Formulate a monitoring plan for a hospitalized patient with COVID-19.

- Discuss the benefits of SARS-CoV-2 vaccination after recovery from COVID-19.

PATIENT PRESENTATION

■ Chief Complaint

"I'm having a really hard time breathing properly. It feels as if I can't catch my breath at all."

HPI

A 71-year-old man with multiple comorbidities was admitted with an 8-day history of fever, cough, headache, myalgia, diarrhea, and loss of taste and smell. He states these symptoms began about 5 days after Thanksgiving when he and his wife hosted a family gathering for their children and grandchildren. Some family members (including his wife) have since fallen ill and have recently tested positive for COVID-19. His shortness of breath worsened significantly over the last 2 days and this prompted him to seek hospital care. Of note, he is not vaccinated against COVID-19. He states that he was concerned about the rapidity with which the vaccines were developed and felt that "natural immunity should be enough." In the Emergency Department, his oxygen saturation on room air was in the range of 89–92% and he was initiated on supplemental oxygen via face mask at a rate of 6 liters per minute.

PMH

Obesity
Coronary artery disease
Hypertension
Type 2 diabetes mellitus

FH

Noncontributory

SH

Lives with wife
Currently retired (formerly employed as a high school track and field coach)
Endorses occasional alcohol use (1–2 drinks per week)
Denies tobacco or intravenous drug use
Former cigarette smoker; quit 5 years ago

Medications

Pravastatin 20 mg orally once daily at bedtime
Metoprolol 25 mg orally twice daily
Losartan 50 mg orally once daily
Metformin 1000 mg orally twice daily

Allergies

NKDA

ROS

Significant for fever, cough, shortness of breath (on exertion and at rest), fatigue, myalgia, loss of taste and smell, and diarrhea. Denies dizziness, chest pain or pressure, hemoptysis, lower extremity edema, or palpitations.

Physical Examination

Gen

Patient is an obese man in moderate respiratory distress who appears to be anxious and uncomfortable.

VS

BP 150/90, P 130 bpm, RR 28, T 38.3°C; Wt 109 kg, Ht 5′8″, SpO₂ of 89–92% on room air

Skin

Skin is warm and dry; capillary refill takes less than 2 seconds; no lesions

HEENT

Head normocephalic and atraumatic; PERRLA; EOMI; mucous membranes moist; moderate pharyngeal erythema

Neck/Lymph Nodes

Neck is supple; no cervical lymphadenopathy; no JVD

Lungs/Thorax

Tachypneic, labored breathing; on auscultation decreased breath sounds and rhonchi present; increased tactile fremitus on palpation

CV

Normal S_1 and S_2; tachycardic; regular rhythm

Abd

Soft; nondistended; normal bowel sounds

Genit/Rect

Deferred

MS/Ext

No lower extremity pain or edema; 5/5 grip strength; 2+ pulses bilaterally

Neuro

AAO × 3; CN II-XII intact

Labs

Na 142 mEq/L	Hgb 13 mg/dL	Monos 7%
K 4.4 mEq/L	Hct 39%	CRP 108 mg/L
Cl 105 mEq/L	RBC 4.2 × 10⁶/mm³	Ferritin 2,920 ng/mL
CO₂ 23 mmol/L	Plt 210 × 10³/mm³	D-Dimer 1.88 mcg/mL
BUN 38 mg/dL	MCV 90.4 μm³	Lactic acid 2.4 mmol/L
Scr 1.2 mg/dL	MCHC 35 g/dL	
Glu 203 mg/dL	WBC 5.6 × 10³/mm³	
T. bili 0.4 mg/dL	Neutrophils 76%	
AST 34 U/L	Bands 8%	
ALT 60 U/L	Lymphs 12%	

ABG

pH 7.38; PaCO₂ 27.2; PaO₂ 73.3 with 83% O₂ saturation on room air

Chest X-Ray

Scattered patchy bilateral peripheral lung disease and moderate-sized left upper lobe consolidation likely representative of bilateral pneumonia. No pneumothorax or pleural effusion identified.

Blood Cultures × Two Sets

Pending

Molecular Diagnostics

Influenza A by PCR—Not detected
Influenza B by PCR—Not detected
RSV by PCR—Not detected
SARS-CoV-2 by PCR—detected

Assessment

This is a 71-year-old male with multiple comorbidities who is admitted to the hospital with COVID-19. He is currently at day 8 of symptoms and has been initiated on oxygen supplementation via face mask at a rate of 6 L/min. He will be upgraded to a medical floor shortly.

QUESTIONS

Collect Information

1.a. What subjective and objective information indicates the presence of COVID-19?

1.b. What additional information is needed to fully assess this patient's COVID-19?

Assess the Information

2.a. Assess the severity of COVID-19 based on the subjective and objective information available.

2.b. Create a list of the patient's drug therapy problems and prioritize them. Include assessment of medication appropriateness, effectiveness, safety, and patient adherence.

2.c. What economic, psychosocial, cultural, racial, and ethical considerations are applicable to this patient?

Develop a Care Plan

3.a. What are the goals of pharmacotherapy for COVID-19 in this case?

3.b. What nondrug therapies might be useful for this patient's COVID-19?

3.c. What feasible pharmacotherapeutic options are available for treating COVID-19?

3.d. Create an individualized, patient-centered, team-based care plan to optimize medication therapy for COVID-19 and this patient's other drug therapy problems. Include specific drugs, dosage forms, doses, schedules, and durations of therapy.

Implement the Care Plan

4.a. What information should be provided to the patient to enhance adherence, ensure successful therapy, and minimize adverse effects?

4.b. Describe how care should be coordinated with other healthcare providers.

Follow up: Monitor and Evaluate

5. Explain how to monitor and evaluate the care plan for medication appropriateness, effectiveness, safety, and patient adherence by using clinical and laboratory data, patient feedback, and other information.

■ CLINICAL COURSE

The patient is transferred from the Emergency Department to a general medical floor in the hospital and is started on remdesivir and dexamethasone. Over the course of the next 48 hours, the patient's clinical status deteriorates due to progressive hypoxia and he is initiated on noninvasive ventilation with BiPAP. There is a concern that he may require intubation and he is transferred to a higher level of care (Intermediate Care Unit). A CT scan of the chest is performed and pulmonary embolism seems unlikely. There are no new localizing signs of new infection. Laboratory values have not changed significantly since hospital admission. The medical team feels that clinical deterioration is due to progression of COVID-19.

■ FOLLOW UP QUESTIONS

1. Given this new information (point at which he is put on BiPAP), how would you modify the treatment for COVID-19 in this patient?

2. What adverse reactions should be monitored for if the patient were to receive tocilizumab or baricitinib?

■ SELF-STUDY ASSIGNMENTS

1. Compare and contrast rapid antigen testing with nucleic acid amplification tests for SARS-CoV-2.

2. Describe the role of anti-SARS-CoV-2 monoclonal antibodies in the treatment and prevention of COVID-19.

3. Describe how motivational interviewing can be used to speak with unvaccinated patients about COVID-19 vaccines.

4. What are some of the reasons racial and ethnic minority groups are disproportionately affected by COVID-19?

CLINICAL PEARL

Data from November 2021 in the CDC's COVID Data Tracker suggest that unvaccinated individuals were four times more likely to test positive for COVID-19 and 15 times more likely to die from COVID-19 than fully vaccinated individuals. Even more impressively, unvaccinated individuals were 13 times more likely to test positive for COVID-19 and 68 times more likely to die from COVID-19 than fully vaccinated individuals who had also received booster doses. These findings again underscore the importance of completing the primary series of a SARS-CoV-2 vaccine and receiving a booster dose (when appropriate).

REFERENCES

1. COVID-19 Treatment Guidelines Panel. Coronavirus Disease 2019 (COVID-19) Treatment Guidelines. National Institutes of Health. Available at: *https://covid19treatmentguidelines.nih.gov/*. Accessed February 5, 2022.

2. Bhimraj A, Morgan RL, Shumaker AH, et al. Infectious Diseases Society of America Guidelines on the Treatment and Management of Patients with COVID-19. Infectious Diseases Society of America 2021; Version 5.6.0. Available at: *https://www.idsociety.org/practice-guideline/covid-19-guideline-treatment-and-management/*. Accessed February 5, 2022.

3. Centers for Disease Control and Prevention. People with Certain Medical Conditions. Available at: *https://www.cdc.gov/coronavirus/2019-ncov/need-extra-precautions/people-with-medical-conditions.html*. Accessed February 5, 2022.

4. Gupta A, Gonzalez-Rojas Y, Juarez E, et al. Early treatment for Covid-19 with SARS-CoV-2 neutralizing antibody sotrovimab. N Engl J Med. 2021;385(21):1941–1950.

5. Gottlieb RL, Vaca CE, Paredes R, et al. Early remdesivir to prevent progression to severe COVID-19 in outpatients. N Engl J Med. 2022;386(4):305–315.

6. Beigel JH, Tomashek KM, Dodd LE, et al. Remdesivir for the treatment of Covid-19—final report. N Engl J Med. 2020;383:1813–1826.

7. The RECOVERY Collaborative Group. Dexamethasone in hospitalized patients with Covid-19. N Engl J Med. 2021;384:693–704.

8. The REMAP-CAP Investigators. Interleukin-6 receptor antagonists in critically ill patients with Covid-19. N Engl J Med. 2021;384:1491–1502.

9. Marconi VC, Ramanan AV, de Bono S, et al. Efficacy and safety of baricitinib for the treatment of hospitalised adults with COVID-19 (COV-BARRIER): a randomised, double-blind, parallel-group, placebo-controlled phase 3 trial. Lancet Respir Med. 2021;9:1407–1418.

10. Centers for Disease Control and Prevention. Interim Clinical Considerations for Use of COVID-19 Vaccines Currently Authorized in the United States. Available at: *https://www.cdc.gov/vaccines/covid-19/clinical-considerations/covid-19-vaccines-us.html*. Accessed February 5, 2022.

129

SKIN AND SOFT TISSUE INFECTION

A Pain in the Butt . . . . Level I

Jarrett R. Amsden, PharmD, BCPS

LEARNING OBJECTIVES

After completing this case study, the reader should be able to:

- Evaluate the signs and symptoms of skin and soft tissue infections (SSTIs).

- Recommend appropriate empiric nonpharmacologic and pharmacologic treatment options for patients presenting with SSTIs.

- Differentiate between the definition and clinical manifestations of mild, moderate, and severe SSTI.

- Compare and contrast the clinical characteristics and presentation of a purulent vs nonpurulent SSTI.

- Design an antimicrobial treatment regimen for purulent and nonpurulent SSTIs that are mild, moderate, or severe.

- Develop monitoring parameters for nondrug and pharmacologic treatment of SSTIs.

PATIENT PRESENTATION

■ Chief Complaint

"I have a boil on my butt, and I cannot sit down for class."

■ HPI

A 19-year-old college student presents to the emergency department (ED) with a recurrent "boil" on his right buttock. The patient was seen in the ED 8 days ago where he had a similar area of fluctuance surgically drained. At that time, he was only given wound care instructions and was sent home, able to return to normal activities if the area remains covered. Today, he returns to the ED with a recurrent boil in the same right buttock area and states that "he cannot sit down for class." In addition, he reports mild fevers without chills, but he has not taken his temperature at home. Two sets of blood cultures were drawn and a second I&D of the area was performed and sent for culture and susceptibility, both of which are pending. The patient did have his nares and groin area swabbed for MRSA detection, and the results are pending. The ED provider does not think the patient needs to be admitted and can be safely treated as an outpatient.

■ PMH

I&D of the same buttock area 8 days ago

■ Surgical History

Appendectomy 4 years ago
Repair of left ACL tear 2 years ago

■ Social History

Denies any alcohol or illicit drug use

■ Meds

Clindamycin 300 mg PO QID × 7 days (prescribed at student health center visit 15 days ago for a similar SSTI; patient did not complete full course due to nausea)

■ All

Penicillin (hives as a child)

■ Immunizations

Up to date per student health center records

■ ROS

Negative except for complaints noted in HPI

■ Physical Examination

Gen

WDWN man in no acute distress, noticeable pain walking and sitting

VS

BP 129/74, P 81 bpm, RR 16, T 37.5°C; Wt 77.5 kg, Ht 6′0″

HEENT

PERRLA; EOMI, oropharynx clear

Neck/Lymph Nodes

Supple, no lymphadenopathy

Lungs/Thorax

CTA, no rales or wheezing

CV

RRR, no MRG

Abd

Soft, NT/ND; (+) BS

Genit/Rect

Deferred

Skin

Lateral right gluteal area: red, erythematous, warm, and tender to touch; localized fluid collection that appears fluctuant, consistent with a carbuncle and with minimal surrounding erythema

MS/Ext

Upper extremities: WNL
Lower extremities: Could not be adequately assessed due to patient's inability to sit; 3+ pulses bilaterally

Neuro

A&O × 3

■ **Labs**

Na 138 mEq/L
K 3.7 mEq/L
Cl 98 mEq/L
CO_2 23 mEq/L
BUN 23 mg/dL
SCr 0.8 mg/dL
Glu 95 mg/dL
Ca 9.4 mg/dL

Hgb 15.5 g/dL
Hct 44%
Plt 279 × 10³/mm³

WBC 11.3 × 10³/mm³
Neutros 89%
Lymphs 10%
Monos 1%

■ **Urine Drug Screen**

(–) Alcohol, (–) marijuana, (–) cocaine, and other substances

■ **Microbiology**

Blood cultures × two sets: *pending*
    Culture of abscess fluid from right buttock: *pending*
    MRSA nares swab: *pending*
    MRSA groin swab: *pending*

■ **Imaging Studies**

Negative for deep tissue involvement; localized area of inflammation and fluid measuring 2 cm × 4 cm; consistent with an abscess

■ **Assessment**

Recurrent right lateral gluteal SSTI with focal area of fluctuance/fluid that failed initial I&D

QUESTIONS

Collect Information

1.a. What subjective and objective information indicates the presence of a SSTI?

1.b. What additional information is needed to fully assess this patient's SSTI?

Assess the Information

2.a. Assess the severity (mild, moderate, or severe) of this patient's SSTI based on the subjective and objective information available.

2.b. Create a list of the patient's drug therapy problems and prioritize them. Include assessment of medication appropriateness, effectiveness, safety, and patient adherence.

2.c. What economic or psychosocial considerations are applicable to this patient?

Develop a Care Plan

3.a. What are the goals of pharmacotherapy for recurrent purulent SSTI in this case?

3.b. What nondrug therapies might be useful for this patient's recurrent purulent SSTI?

3.c. What feasible pharmacotherapeutic options are available for treating this patient's recurrent purulent SSTI?

3.d. Create an individualized, patient-centered, team-based care plan to optimize medication therapy for the SSTI and this patient's other drug therapy problems. Include specific drugs, dosage forms, doses, schedules, and durations of therapy.

3.e. What therapeutic alternatives, in order of preference, would be appropriate if the initial care plan fails or cannot be used and justify your selections.

Implement the Care Plan

4.a. What information should be provided to the patient to enhance adherence, ensure successful therapy, and minimize adverse effects?

4.b. Describe how care should be coordinated with other healthcare providers.

Follow-Up: Monitor and Evaluate

5. Explain how to monitor and evaluate the care plan for medication appropriateness, effectiveness, safety, and patient adherence by using clinical and laboratory data, patient feedback, and other information.

■ SELF-STUDY ASSIGNMENTS

1. Compare the therapeutic alternatives for treatment of mild, moderate, and severe SSTIs with purulence versus SSTIs without purulence.

2. Prepare a table that differentiates the presentation, signs, and symptoms of the patient in this case with those of a patient presenting with erysipelas, diabetic foot infection, and necrotizing fasciitis and also the organisms involved in each respective infection.

CLINICAL PEARL

Necrotizing fasciitis is a severe, progressing form of an SSTI that affects the subcutaneous tissues and moves along the superficial fascia. The infection may encompass all tissues from the skin to the muscle. The most commonly implicated organisms are *Streptococcus pyogenes* or *Clostridium perfringens*; however, in patients with exposures to fresh water *Aeromonas hydrophila* should be suspected, and for those with exposures to salt water, *Vibrio vulnificus* should be considered. The empiric treatment is doxycycline plus ciprofloxacin or doxycycline plus ceftazidime for *A. hydrophila* and *V. vulnificus*, respectively.[1]

REFERENCES

1. Stevens DL, Bisno AL, Chambers HF, et al. Practice guidelines for the diagnosis and management of skin and soft tissue infections: 2014 update by the Infectious Diseases Society of America. Clin Infect Dis. 2014;59(2):e10–e52.

2. Talan DA, Mower WR, Krishnadasan A, et al. Trimethoprim–sulfamethoxazole versus placebo for uncomplicated skin abscess. New Engl J Med. 2016;374(9):823–832.

3. Daum RS, Miller LG, Immergluck L, et al. A placebo-controlled trial of antibiotics for smaller skin abscesses. New Engl J Med. 2017;376(26):2545–2555.

4. Sharara SL, Maragakis LL, Cosgrove SE. Decolonization of *Staphylococcus aureus*. Infect Dis Clin North Am. 2021;35(1):107–133.

5. Fish DN. Skin and soft-tissue infections. In: DiPiro JT, Yee GC, Posey LM, Haines ST, Nolin TD, Ellingrod V, eds. Pharmacotherapy: A Pathophysiologic Approach. 11th ed. McGraw-Hill Education; 2020.

6. Liu C, Bayer A, Cosgrove SE, et al. Clinical practice guidelines by the Infectious Diseases Society of America for the treatment of methicillin-resistant *Staphylococcus aureus* infections in adults and children. Clin Infect Dis. 2011;52(3).

7. Raff AB, Kroshinsky D. Cellulitis: a review. JAMA. 2016;316(3):325–337.

8. McNeil JC, Fritz SA. Prevention strategies for recurrent community-associated *Staphylococcus aureus* skin and soft tissue infections. Curr Infect Dis Rep. 2019;21(4): Article 12.

9. Bidell MR, Lodise TP. Use of oral tetracyclines in the treatment of adult outpatients with skin and skin structure infections: Focus on doxycycline, minocycline, and omadacycline. Pharmacotherapy. 2021;(May):1–17.

10. Lake JG, Miller LG, Fritz SA. Antibiotic duration, but not abscess size, impacts clinical cure of limited skin and soft tissue infection after incision and drainage. Clin Infect Dis. 2020;71(3):661–663.

130

DIABETIC FOOT INFECTION

Let's Nail That Infection . . . . Level II

Renee-Claude Mercier, PharmD, BCPS-AQ ID, PhC, FCCP

Paulina Deming, PharmD, PhC

---

*Notice to the Reader: The case author provided suggested answers to the questions related to this case in **Appendix D** to give students an example of how case answers should be constructed.*

LEARNING OBJECTIVES

After completing this case study, the reader should be able to:

- Recognize the signs and symptoms of diabetic foot infections and identify the risk factors and the most likely pathogens associated with these infections.

- Recommend appropriate antimicrobial regimens for diabetic foot infections, including options for patients with drug allergies or renal insufficiency.

- Recommend appropriate home IV therapy and proper counseling to patients.

- Outline monitoring parameters for achievement of the desired pharmacotherapeutic outcomes and prevention of adverse medication reactions.

- Counsel diabetic patients about adequate blood glucose control as part of an overall plan for good foot health.

PATIENT PRESENTATION

■ Chief Complaint

"I had an ingrown toe nail that became infected several weeks ago, and now the whole foot is swollen."

■ HPI

A 67-year-old man presents to the ED complaining of a sore and swollen foot. Three weeks ago, he noticed that his right great toe became swollen and red due to an ingrown toenail. The patient tried to fix the nail with scissors and tweezers, but the swelling got worse, and thick, foul-smelling drainage became noticeable approximately 2 weeks ago. The patient was visiting family in Mexico at the time and now has just returned home to New Mexico. The primary care physician is Dr Martinez at First Choice Clinic, a Federally Qualified Health Center, in Albuquerque.

■ PMH

Type 2 DM × 18 years
Hospitalized 2 months ago for HHS
Left second toe amputation 1 year ago secondary to diabetic foot infection
Hyperlipidemia
Hypertension
Chronic renal insufficiency

■ FH

Father is deceased (56-year-old) secondary to MI, type 2 DM, HTN
Mother is deceased secondary to breast cancer (41-year-old)
One daughter, alive and well, 42-year-old

■ SH

The patient lives with his wife in Albuquerque, New Mexico. He denies tobacco and illicit drug use; however, he admits to a long history of drinking four to five beers per day. He admits to nonadherence with his medications and glucometer.

■ Meds

Lantus SoloStar 40 units once daily
Humalog KwikPen 12 units with each meal
Metformin 1000 mg PO twice daily
Aspirin 81 mg PO once daily
Lisinopril 20 mg PO once daily
Atorvastatin 40 mg PO daily

■ All

No known drug allergies

■ ROS

Negative except as noted in the HPI

■ Physical Examination

Gen

Patient is a thin man who appears very concerned about losing his foot.

VS

BP 126/79, P 92 bpm, RR 20, T 38.4°C; Wt 60 kg, Ht 5′10″

Skin

Warm, coarse, and very dry

HEENT

PERRLA; EOMI; funduscopic exam is normal with absence of hemorrhages or exudates. TMs are clouded bilaterally but with no erythema or bulging. Oropharynx shows poor dentition but is otherwise unremarkable.

Neck/Lymph Nodes

Neck is supple; normal thyroid; no JVD; no lymphadenopathy

Chest

CTA

CV

RRR, normal S_1 and S_2

Abd

Distended, (+) BS, no guarding, no hepatosplenomegaly or masses felt

Ext

2+ edema with markedly diminished sensation of the right foot. Significant swelling and induration extend from first metatarsal to midfoot (4 cm × 5 cm) consistent with cellulitis. Purulent foul-smelling drainage expressed from great toe wound. Wound probe 1.5 cm deep. Pedal pulses present but diminished. Normal range of motion. Poor nail care with some fungus and overgrown toenails.

Neuro

A&O × 3; CN II–XII intact. Motor system intact (overall muscle strength 4–5/5). Sensory system exam showed a decreased sensation to light touch of the lower extremities (both feet); intact upper body sensation.

■ Labs

Na 136 mEq/L	Hgb 14.1 g/dL
K 3.6 mEq/L	Hct 42.3%
Cl 98 mEq/L	Plt 390 × 10³/mm³
CO$_2$ 24 mEq/L	WBC 17.3 × 10³/mm³
BUN 30 mg/dL	PMNs 78%
SCr 2.4 mg/dL	Lymphs 17%
Glu 323 mg/dL	Monos 5%
A1C 11.8%	
ESR 73 mm/h	

■ X-Ray

Right foot: There is soft tissue swelling from first metatarsal to midfoot consistent with cellulitis. No fluid collection noted. No evidence of adjacent periosteal reactions or erosions to suggest radiographic evidence of osteomyelitis. No definite subcutaneous air is evident. Presence of vascular calcifications.

■ Assessment

Diabetic foot infection with significant cellulitis in a patient with poorly controlled diabetes mellitus.

■ Clinical Course

On the day of admission, the patient went to surgery for I&D. Blood and tissue specimens were sent for culture and sensitivity testing.

QUESTIONS

Collect Information

1.a. What subjective and objective information indicates the presence of a diabetic foot infection?

1.b. What additional information is needed to fully assess this patient's diabetic foot infection?

Assess the Information

2.a. Assess the severity of the diabetic foot infection based on the subjective and objective information available.

2.b. Create a list of the patient's drug therapy problems and prioritize them. Include assessment of medication appropriateness, effectiveness, safety, and patient adherence.

2.c. What economic and psychosocial considerations are applicable to this patient?

Develop a Care Plan

3.a. What are the goals of pharmacotherapy for diabetic foot infection in this case?

3.b. What nondrug therapies might be useful for this patient's diabetic foot infection?

3.c. What feasible pharmacotherapeutic options are available for the treatment of diabetic foot infection?

3.d. Create an individualized, patient-centered, team-based care plan to optimize medication therapy for diabetic foot infection and this patient's other drug therapy problems. Include specific drugs, dosage forms, doses, schedules, and durations of therapy.

3.e. What alternatives would be appropriate if the initial care plan for the infection fails or cannot be used?

Implement the Care Plan

4.a. What information should be provided to the patient to enhance adherence, ensure successful therapy, and minimize adverse effects?

4.b. Describe how care should be coordinated with other healthcare providers.

Follow-Up: Monitor and Evaluate

5. Explain how to monitor and evaluate the care plan for medication appropriateness, effectiveness, safety, and patient adherence by using clinical and laboratory data, patient feedback, and other information.

■ CLINICAL COURSE

The patient received the empiric therapy you recommended until the tissue cultures were reported positive for *Bacteroides fragilis* and *Staphylococcus aureus* (with susceptibility to vancomycin, linezolid, quinupristin/dalfopristin, and daptomycin and resistance to oxacillin, tetracycline, erythromycin, clindamycin, and sulfamethoxazole/trimethoprim). Susceptibilities are not available for *B. fragilis*. The blood cultures were all found to have no growth. The patient remained hospitalized for an additional 10 days and received a more *directed* antimicrobial regimen and multiple surgical debridements of the wound. The cellulitis slowly improved over this time, and multiple x-rays did not suggest osteomyelitis. He was then discharged to complete the antimicrobial regimen on an outpatient basis. Over the next 2 weeks, he received wound care at home and showed significant but slow progress in healing of the wound.

■ FOLLOW-UP CASE QUESTIONS

1. What therapeutic options are available for treating this patient after results of cultures are known to contain MRSA and *B. fragilis*?

2. Design an optimal drug treatment plan for treating the mixed infection while he remains hospitalized.

3. Design an optimal pharmacotherapeutic plan for completion of treatment after he is discharged from the hospital.

■ SELF-STUDY ASSIGNMENTS

1. Review in more detail different therapeutic options available for home IV therapy, including the antimicrobial agents suitable for use, types of IV lines available, and contraindications to home IV therapy.

2. Outline the patient counseling you would provide for successful home IV therapy.

3. Describe how you would educate this diabetic patient about proper foot care to prevent further skin or tissue breakdown.

CLINICAL PEARL

Treatment of diabetic foot infections with antimicrobial agents alone is often inadequate; local wound care (incision, drainage, debridement, and amputation), good glycemic control, and immobilization of the limb are often required.

REFERENCES

1. Lipsky BA, Berendt AR, Cornia PB, et al. 2012 Infectious Diseases Society of America clinical practice guideline for the diagnosis and treatment of diabetic foot infections. Clin Infect Dis. 2012;54:132–173.

2. Levin ME. Management of the diabetic foot: preventing amputation. South Med J. 2002;95:10–20.

3. Echániz-Aviles G, Velazquez-Meza ME, Vazquez-Larios Mdel R, Soto-Noguerón A, Hernández-Dueñas AM. Diabetic foot infection caused by community-associated methicillin-resistant *Staphylococcus aureus* (USA300). J Diabetes. 2015 Nov;7(6):891–892.

4. Lipsky BA, Cannon CM, Ramani A, et al. Ceftaroline fosamil for treatment of diabetic foot infections: the CAPTURE study experience. Diabetes Metab Res Rev. 2015;31(4):395–401.

5. Lipsky BA, Tabak YP, Johannes RS, Vo L, Hyde L, Weigelt JA. Skin and soft tissue infections in hospitalised patients with diabetes: culture isolates and risk factors associated with mortality, length of stay and cost. Diabetologia. 2010;53:914–923.

6. Liu C, Bayer A, Cosgrove SE, et al. Clinical practice guidelines by the Infectious Diseases Society of America for the treatment of methicillin-resistant *Staphylococcus aureus* infections in adults and children. Clin Infect Dis. 2011;52:1–38.

7. Martí-Carvajal AJ, Gluud C, Nicola S, et al. Growth factors for treating diabetic foot ulcers. Cochrane Database Syst Rev. 2015 Oct 28; 10:1–144.

8. Guillamet CV, Kollef MH. How to stratify patients at risk for resistant bugs in skin and soft tissue infections? Curr Opin Infect Dis. 2016;29(2):116–123.

9. Weigelt J, Itani K, Stevens D, Lau W, Dryden M, Knirsch C. Linezolid versus vancomycin in the treatment of complicated skin and soft tissue infections. Antimicrob Agents Chemother. 2005;46:2260–2266.

10. Nicolau DP, Stein GE. Therapeutic options for diabetic foot infections: a review with an emphasis on tissue penetration characteristics. J Am Podiatr Med Assoc. 2010;100:52–63.

131

INFECTIVE ENDOCARDITIS

A Symptom of the Larger Disease . . . . Level II

Emily N. Drwiega, PharmD, BCIDP

Manjunath (Amit) P. Pai, PharmD, FCP

Keith A. Rodvold, PharmD, FCCP, FIDSA

LEARNING OBJECTIVES

After completing this case study, the reader should be able to:

- Identify major and minor diagnostic criteria for infective endocarditis.

- Select an appropriate empiric antibiotic regimen for presumed infective endocarditis.

- Design a pharmacotherapy regimen for endocarditis that accounts for patient-specific factors such as medication allergies, comorbidities, and social history.

- Recognize the psychosocial and ethical issues related to the treatment of infective endocarditis among intravenous drug users.

- Establish monitoring parameters for a selected drug therapy in the treatment of a patient with infective endocarditis.

PATIENT PRESENTATION

■ Chief Complaint

"Let me go home! I was just tired, nothing is wrong with me! Why am I here?"

■ HPI

A 27-year-old woman presents to the emergency department in police custody after being found unconscious outside the local gas station. She was only minimally responsive upon arrival of EMS but became combative in the field following a dose of naloxone. Upon arrival to the emergency department, she remains altered but is able to relay symptoms of cough, chest pain, and shaking chills.

■ PMH

Generalized anxiety disorder (diagnosed 5 years ago)
Chronic back pain (diagnosed 6 years ago, due to workplace-related injury)
Genital herpes (diagnosed 2 years ago)

■ FH

Mother: Depression, committed suicide 12 years ago

■ SH

Tobacco use, 1/2 ppd; "social" alcohol use; intravenous heroin "sometimes" including speedballing (mixed heroin with crack cocaine)

Meds

Amitriptyline 100 mg PO QHS
Ibuprofen 200 mg, two tablets PO Q 6 H PRN back pain
Sertraline 100 mg PO daily
Valacyclovir 500 mg PO daily

All

Amoxicillin (unknown reaction as a child)

ROS

Constitutional: Chills. Uncertain about fevers. No weight loss or appetite change.
HEENT: No visual disturbances, nose bleeds, recent cold symptoms, or voice changes.
Respiratory: Cough. No shortness of breath. No hemoptysis or wheezing.
Cardiovascular: Diffuse chest pain. No palpitations, orthopnea, or leg swelling.
GI: No diarrhea, stomach pain, nausea, vomiting, or blood in stools.
GU: No dysuria, hematuria, or frequent urination.
MS: No joint pain or swelling. No extremity weakness. (+) back pain.
Integumentary: No rash or jaundice.
Neuro: Questionable syncope, mild confusion. No dizziness or seizures.
Psych: Anxious. No depression, hallucinations, or insomnia.
Endo: No menstrual irregularities or intolerance to heat or cold.
Heme: No swollen glands or easy bruising.

Physical Examination

Gen

Patient is a woman in some distress; clothing is dirty and poorly maintained

VS

BP 85/60, HR 120 bpm, RR 24, T 39.5°C; Wt 55 kg, Ht 5'2"

Skin

Skin is clean, dry, and intact. No evidence of rash or petechiae. Track marks noted on the anterior arm bilaterally.

HEENT

PERRLA, EOMI, anicteric sclerae, no Roth spots, poor dentition

Neck/Lymph Nodes

No lymphadenopathy, JVD, or thyromegaly

Lungs

Trachea midline. Lungs clear to auscultation bilaterally; no wheezing, rales, or rhonchi.

CV

No tenderness with palpation of chest wall. RRR, normal S_1 and S_2, III/VI holosystolic murmur located over left sternal border.

Abd

Bowel sounds present in all four quadrants. Abdomen soft, non-tender, nondistended.

MS/Ext

Reflexes 2/4 in upper and lower extremities bilaterally; 5/5 muscle strength in all four extremities. No edema.

Neuro

Nonfocal; alert and oriented × 2; negative asterixis. CN II–XII intact.

Labs

Na 136 mEq/L	Hgb 9.8 g/dL	WBC 17.6×10^3/mm³
K 4.1 mEq/L	Hct 19.4%	Neutros 78%
Cl 102 mEq/L	Plt 200×10^3/mm³	Bands 8%
CO_2 25 mEq/L	RDW 14.2%	Lymphs 12%
BUN 15 mg/dL	MCV 81.1 mm³	Monos 2%
SCr 0.8 mg/dL	MCH 26.3 pg/cell	Alb 2.1 g/dL
Glu 98 mg/dL	MCHC 34 g/dL	INR 1.0
ESR 140 mm/hr	CRP 12 mg/L	Lactate 2.0 mmol/L

Urine Drug Screen

Positive for opiates, benzodiazepines, and cannabinoids.

Urine Pregnancy Screen

Negative

COVID-19 Nasal Swab PCR Testing

Negative

ECG

Sinus tachycardia. Nonspecific T-wave changes.

Chest X-Ray

Normal heart size. Small lower lobe infiltrates. Correlate clinically.

CT Chest

Multiple small nodular lesions consistent with septic pulmonary emboli

Blood Cultures

Two bottles from right hand, collected and pending (drawn @ 0100)
Two bottles from left antecubital, collected and pending (drawn @ 1400)

Assessment

A 27-year-old woman with recent intravenous drug use presenting s/p naloxone in the field with sepsis and probable infective endocarditis.

QUESTIONS

Collect Information

1.a. What subjective and objective information indicate the presence of infective endocarditis?

1.b. What additional information is needed to fully assess this patient's infective endocarditis?

■ CLINICAL COURSE (PART 1)

The patient is initiated on vancomycin, aztreonam, and tobramycin. Review of the electronic medical record reveals that she has received ceftriaxone in the past without a documented reaction. The

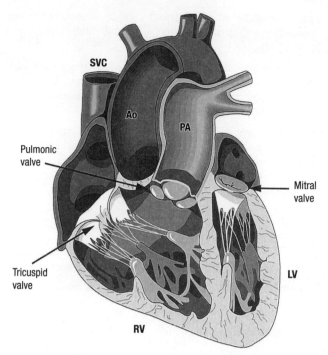

FIGURE 131-1. Diagram illustrating the location of the tricuspid, pulmonic, and mitral valves. Ao, aorta; LV, left ventricle; PA, pulmonary artery; RV, right ventricle; SVC, superior vena cava.

transthoracic echocardiogram demonstrates a 5-mm vegetation on the tricuspid valve with no evidence of valvular dysfunction or perivalvular abscess. Magnetic resonance imaging of the spine shows only chronic changes and no evidence of vertebral osteomyelitis. Four out of four blood culture sets result positive with Gram stain demonstrating Gram-positive cocci in clusters. The rapid diagnostic panel identifies the organism as *Staphylococcus aureus* and does not detect any resistance genes (MecA, VanA, VanB). The hepatitis C antibody test is negative and the fourth-generation HIV immunoassay is negative.

Assess the Information

2.a. Assess the location and severity of infective endocarditis based on the subjective and objective information available.

2.b. Create a list of the patient's drug therapy problems and prioritize them. Include assessment of medication appropriateness, effectiveness, safety, and patient adherence.

Develop a Care Plan

3.a. What are the goals of pharmacotherapy for infective endocarditis?

3.b. What nondrug therapies might be useful for this patient's infective endocarditis?

3.c. What feasible pharmacotherapeutic options are available for treating *Staphylococcus aureus* native valve infective endocarditis?

3.d. Create an individualized, patient-centered, team-based care plan to optimize medication therapy for this patient's drug therapy problems. Include specific drugs, dosage forms, schedules, and durations of therapy.

■ CLINICAL COURSE (PART 2)

On hospital day 3, the patient's vital signs have stabilized and she is transferred out of the intensive care unit to a floor bed. She refuses

to engage in any discussions regarding her substance use disorder and is adamant that she will leave against medical advice if she is not discharged soon. Additionally, she is refusing to take a penicillin due to concern regarding her allergy, which occurred during childhood. Cardiothoracic surgery has evaluated the patient and deemed her not to be a good surgical candidate at this time point due to a lack of functional impairment in the valve and high risk for reinfection of any implanted prosthesis.

3.e. If after educating the patient on penicillin allergies, she remains concerned, what non-beta-lactam IV treatment options are available?

Implement the Care Plan

4.a. What information should be provided to the patient to enhance adherence, ensure successful therapy, and minimize adverse effects?

4.b. Describe how care should be coordinated with other healthcare providers.

■ CLINICAL COURSE (PART 3)

The patient has not been accepted by any skilled nursing facilities due to her low acuity, substance use disorder, and lack of medical insurance. She has agreed to remain in the hospital for the remainder of her antibiotic therapy.

Follow-Up: Monitor and Evaluate

5. Explain how to monitor and evaluate the care plan for medication appropriateness, effectiveness, safety, and patient adherence by using clinical and laboratory data, patient feedback, and other information.

■ ADDITIONAL CASE QUESTIONS

1. Is it ethical to discharge this patient with an indwelling central venous catheter for outpatient parenteral antimicrobial therapy (OPAT)?

2. What ethical considerations are there regarding surgical management of this patient's infective endocarditis?

■ SELF-STUDY ASSIGNMENTS

1. Evaluate the clinical literature to identify studies assessing intravenous-to-oral antibiotic switch therapy for intravenous drug users with right-sided and left-sided infective endocarditis due to methicillin-susceptible *S. aureus*.

2. Review the clinical literature assessing cefazolin as compared to antistaphylococcal penicillins for the treatment of MSSA bacteremia and endocarditis.

3. Interpret existing data on daptomycin as an alternative treatment for infective endocarditis due to methicillin-susceptible *S. aureus* in patients with suspected or confirmed type I allergy to β-lactams.

4. Assess the clinical literature evaluating treatment options of right-sided endocarditis in IVDU due to MRSA.

CLINICAL PEARL

There is an option to use 2 weeks of an antistaphylococcal β-lactam or daptomycin for treatment of intravenous drug users with uncomplicated, right-sided infective endocarditis due to methicillin-susceptible *S. aureus*. Although not commonly employed in clinical practice, this regimen may help reduce the treatment burden in this challenging patient population.

REFERENCES

1. Baddour LM, Wilson WR, Bayer AS, et al. Infective endocarditis in adults: diagnosis, antimicrobial therapy, and management of complications. A scientific statement for healthcare professionals from The American Heart Association. Circulation. 2015;132:1435–1486.

2. Habib G, Lancellotti P, Antunes MJ, et al. 2015 ESC guidelines for the management of infective endocarditis: the Task Force for the Management of Infective Endocarditis of the European Society of Cardiology (ESC). Endorsed by: European Association for Cardio-Thoracic Surgery (EACTS), the European Association of Nuclear Medicine (EANM). Eur Heart J. 2015;36(44):3075–3128.

3. Fleischauer AT, Ruhl L, Rhea S, Barnes E. Hospitalizations for endocarditis and associated health care costs among persons with diagnosed drug dependence. MMWR Morb Mortal Wkly Rep. 2017;66(22):569–673.

4. Lefevre B, Hoen B, Goehringer F, et al. Antistaphylococcal penicillins vs. cefazolin in the treatment of methicillin-susceptible *Staphylococcus aureus* infective endocarditis: a quasi-experimental monocentre study. Eur J Clin Microbiol Infect Dis. 2021;40(12):2605–2616.

5. Eljaaly K, Alshehri S, Erstad BL. Systematic review and meta-analysis of the safety of antistaphylococcal penicillins compared to cefazolin. Antimicrob Agents Chemother. 2018;62(4):e01816–17.

6. Spellberg B, Chambers HF, Musher DM, et al. Evaluation of a paradigm shift from intravenous antibiotics to oral step-down therapy for the treatment of infective endocarditis—A narrative review. JAMA Intern Med. 2020;180(5):769–777.

7. Gudiol C, Cuervo G, Shaw E, Pujol M, Carratala J. Pharmacotherapeutic options for treating *Staphylococcus aureus* bacteremia. Expert Opin Pharmacother. 2017;18(18):1947–1963.

8. Sakoulas G, Geriak M, Nizet V. Is a reported penicillin allergy sufficient grounds to forgo the multidimensional antimicrobial benefits of β-lactam antibiotics? Clin Infect Dis. 2019;68(1):157–164.

9. McDanel JS, Perencevich EN, Diekema DJ, et al. Comparative effectiveness of beta-lactams versus vancomycin for treatment of methicillin-susceptible *Staphylococcus aureus* bloodstream infections among 122 hospitals. Clin Infect Dis. 2015;61(3):361–367.

10. Crass RL, Powell KL, Huang AM. Daptomycin for the treatment of *Staphylococcus aureus* infections complicated by pulmonary septic emboli. Diag Microbiol Infect Dis. 2019;93(2):131–135.

132

TUBERCULOSIS

Close Encounters............................ Level II

Vanthida Huang, PharmD, FCCP

LEARNING OBJECTIVES

After completing this case study, the reader should be able to:

- Recognize the common signs and symptoms, physical examination, laboratory, and radiographic findings in a patient with active pulmonary tuberculosis.

- Design a therapeutic regimen for treatment of a patient with newly diagnosed active pulmonary tuberculosis based on clinical presentation, patient-specific history and physical characteristics, subjective and objective findings, comorbidities, and desired clinical response.

- Define the goals of therapy for a patient with active pulmonary tuberculosis, as well as the monitoring parameters that should be used to assess the response to therapy and to prevent/minimize the occurrence of adverse reactions.

- Provide patient education on the proper administration of drug therapy for active pulmonary tuberculosis including directions for use, administration of therapy in relation to meals, the importance of adherence, and potential adverse reactions of the medications.

- Recognize potential drug interactions that may occur with anti-tuberculosis medication.

PATIENT PRESENTATION

■ Chief Complaint

"I have been coughing up blood for the past 3 days."

■ HPI

A 35-year-old man who presents to the ED with a 3–4-week history of a productive cough, originally yellow sputum which is now accompanied by the presence of blood streaks in the sputum for the past 3 days. He also complains of fevers, chills, night sweats, dyspnea that worsens on exertion, fatigue, and an unintentional 20-lb weight loss over the past several weeks.

■ PMH

None

■ FH

None

■ SH

The patient immigrated to the United States from South America 3 years ago but has not recently traveled. Patient has a 10-pack-year history of smoking but quit several weeks ago. Patient drinks alcohol socially on weekends. He is a laborer and is currently working for cash on home construction. Patient shares an apartment with his coworkers who recently moved to the United States from South America and experiences similar respiratory symptoms.

■ Meds

Acetaminophen 650 mg PO q6h PRN for fever
Guaifenesin/dextromethorphan (400 mg/20 mg) 20 mL PO q4h PRN for cough, which have not provided any relief

■ All

Penicillin: rash

■ ROS

Negative except for the complaints noted above

■ Physical Examination

Gen

Somewhat thin-appearing, fatigued man in mild respiratory distress

VS

BP 131/70, P 100 bpm, RR 24, T 38.8°C, 93% O$_2$ saturation on room air; Wt 65 kg, Ht 5'9"

Skin

No lesions

HEENT

PERRLA, EOMI, no scleral icterus

Neck/Lymph Nodes

Supple

Lungs/Thorax

Rhonchi and dullness to percussion in RUL, tachypneic, labored breathing

CV

Slightly tachycardic, no MRG

Abd

Soft NTND; (+) bowel movement

MS/Ext

No CCE, pulses 2+ throughout; full ROM

Neuro

A&O × 3; CN II–XII intact

■ Labs

Na 143 mEq/L	Hgb 11.6 g/dL	WBC 12.3 × 10³/mm³	Bili 0.6 mg/dL
K 3.7 mEq/L	Hct 34.8%	Neutros 74%	Alk phos
Cl 106 mEq/L	RBC 3.8 × 10⁶/mm³	Bands 8%	120 IU/L
CO₂ 22 mEq/L	Plt 269 × 10³/mm³	Lymphs 10%	ALT 45 IU/L
BUN 21 mg/dL	MCV 92 μm³	Monos 8%	AST 34 IU/L
SCr 0.9 mg/dL	MCHC 33 g/dL		
Glu 101 mg/dL			

Tuberculin skin test (TST) result: Pending
Interferon gamma release assay (IGRA): Pending
Sputum AFB smear: Numerous AFB (Fig. 132-1)
XPert® MTB/RIF real-time PCR: Pending
Sputum acid-fast bacillus (AFB) culture: Pending
HIV antibody test (fourth-generation HIV antibody/antigen ELISA + supplemental antibody differentiation immunoassay): Pending

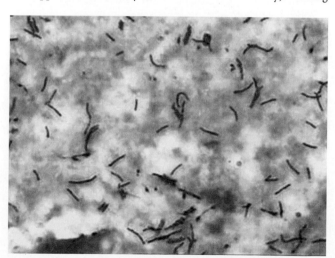

FIGURE 132-1. AFB smear. AFB (*shown as thin rods*) are tubercle bacilli.

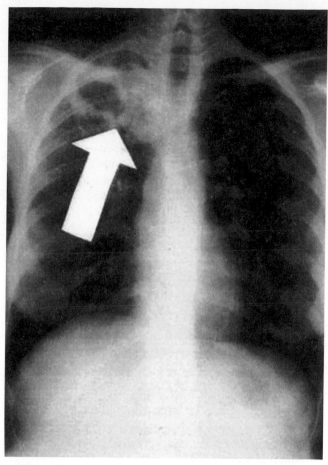

FIGURE 132-2. Chest radiograph. *Arrow* points to cavitation in patient's upper right lobe.

■ Radiology

CXR: RUL cavitary lesion with surrounding consolidation/air space disease (Fig. 132-2)

Chest CT: Focal airspace disease with tree-in-bud pattern in the RUL, including a cavitary lesion measuring 3.5 cm × 3.5 cm. Right hilar lymphadenopathy with scattered mediastinal lymphadenopathy. There is no pleural effusion or pneumothorax. Findings are consistent with active tuberculosis infection.

■ Assessment

Active pulmonary tuberculosis

QUESTIONS

Collect Information

1.a. What subjective and objective information indicates the presence of active pulmonary tuberculosis in this patient?

1.b. What additional information is needed to fully assess this patient's tuberculosis?

Assess the Information

2.a. Assess the severity of this patient's active pulmonary tuberculosis based on the subjective and objective information available.

2.b. Create a list of the patient's drug therapy problems and prioritize them. Include assessment of medication appropriateness, effectiveness, safety, and patient adherence.

2.c. What economic and social considerations are applicable to this patient?

Develop a Care Plan

3.a. What are the goals of pharmacotherapy for active pulmonary tuberculosis in this case?

3.b. What nondrug therapies might be useful for this patient's active pulmonary tuberculosis?

3.c. What feasible pharmacotherapeutic options are available for the treatment of active pulmonary tuberculosis?

3.d. Create an individualized, patient-centered, team-based care plan to optimize medication therapy for the pulmonary tuberculosis and this patient's other drug therapy problems. Include specific drugs, dosage forms, doses, schedules, and durations of therapy.

Implement the Care Plan

4.a. What information should be provided to the patient to enhance adherence and, ensure successful therapy, and minimize adverse effects?

4.b. Describe how care should be coordinated with other healthcare providers.

Follow-Up: Monitor and Evaluate

5. Explain how to monitor and evaluate the care plan for medication appropriateness, effectiveness, safety, and patient adherence using clinical and laboratory data, patient feedback, and other information.

■ CLINICAL COURSE

The patient was admitted to the hospital and placed into respiratory isolation in a negative-pressure room. Because the initial sputum sample demonstrated the presence of numerous AFB, the patient was started on the antituberculosis therapy you recommended while waiting for the results of culture and susceptibility tests. Later that day, the XPert® MTB/RIF real-time PCR result performed on the sputum smear sample revealed the presence of *Mycobacterium tuberculosis* complex, and rifampin resistance was not detected.

On hospital day 2, his TST was measured as 20 mm, the IGRA was positive, and his HIV test result was negative. The patient tolerated the antituberculosis regimen during the initial weeks of therapy, and subsequent sputum AFB smears became negative 2 weeks after initiation of therapy. The sputum AFB culture eventually grew *M. tuberculosis*, which was susceptible to isoniazid, rifampin, pyrazinamide, ethambutol, and streptomycin. During the third week of antituberculosis therapy, an increase in the patient's AST (140 IU/L) and ALT (120 IU/L) was noted, although the patient remained asymptomatic. The total bilirubin and alkaline phosphatase remained within normal limits. Follow-up mycobacterial sputum cultures obtained after 2 months of antituberculosis therapy were negative.

■ FOLLOW-UP CASE QUESTIONS

1. What factors place this patient at increased risk for acquiring TB?

2. How should other close contacts of the patient be evaluated and treated?

3. How should the results of the susceptibility report of this patient's *M. tuberculosis* isolate influence his drug therapy?

4. How should the increase in AST and ALT in this patient be managed? What changes should be made to the current antituberculosis regimen and/or monitoring plan?

5. How should AST and ALT elevations greater than five times the upper limit of normal be managed in a patient on antituberculosis therapy?

■ SELF-STUDY ASSIGNMENTS

1. Review the differences (eg, methodology, turnaround time, advantages, disadvantages, cost) between the TST and IGRAs in the diagnosis of active pulmonary and latent tuberculosis. Discuss the populations or scenarios where the IGRA may be preferred over the TST.

2. Review the safety and efficacy of rifapentine in managing active pulmonary tuberculosis and latent tuberculosis.

3. Perform a literature search to determine the national and regional rates of isoniazid resistance in clinical isolates of *M. tuberculosis*. How do these rates compare with those reported in other areas of the world where tuberculosis is endemic?

4. Review the management strategies of active drug-resistant pulmonary tuberculosis.

5. Review the management strategies of active pulmonary tuberculosis in an HIV-infected patient on antiretroviral therapy, with special attention to potential drug interactions between first-line antituberculosis agents and the non-nucleoside reverse transcriptase inhibitors or protease inhibitors.

6. Review the essential components of a public health program to prevent, control, and eliminate tuberculosis at a state and national levels.

CLINICAL PEARL

The treatment of tuberculosis in patients with HIV infection is often modified based on the many drug interactions that can occur among the rifamycins and antiretroviral agents.

ACKNOWLEDGMENT

This case is based on the patient case written for the 11th edition by Sharon M. Erdman, PharmD and Kendra M. Damer, PharmD.

REFERENCES

1. Sia IG, Wieland ML. Current concepts in the management of tuberculosis. Mayo Clin Proceed. 2011;86(4):348–361.

2. Lewinsohn DM, Leonard MK, LoBue PA, et al. Official American Thoracic Society/Infectious Diseases Society of America/Centers for Disease Control and Prevention clinical practice guidelines: diagnosis of tuberculosis in adults and children. Clin Infect Dis. 2017;64(2):111–115.

3. Nahid P, Dorman SE, Alipanah N, et al. Official American Thoracic Society/Centers for Disease Control and Prevention/Infectious Diseases Society of America clinical practice guidelines: treatment of drug-susceptible tuberculosis. Clin Infect Dis. 2016;63(7):e147–e195.

4. CDC. Guidelines for preventing the transmission of *Mycobacterium tuberculosis* in health-care settings, 2005. MMWR. 2005;54(No. RR-17).

5. Sterling TR, Njie G, Zenner D, et al. Guidelines for the treatment of latent tuberculosis infection: recommendations from the National Tuberculosis Controllers Association and CDC, 2020. MMWR Recomm Rep. 2020;69(1):1–11.

6. Nahid P, Mase SR, Migliori GB, et al. Treatment of drug-resistant tuberculosis. An official ATS/CDC/ERS/IDSA clinical practice guideline. Am J Respir Crit Care Med. 2020;201(4):500–501.

7. Singanayagam A, Sridhar S, Dhariwal J, et al. A comparison between two strategies for monitoring hepatic function during anti-tuberculosis therapy. Am J Respir Crit Care Med. 2012;185:653–659.

8. Saukkonen JJ, Cohn DL, Jasmer RM, et al. An official ATS statement: hepatoxicity of antituberculosis therapy. Am J Respir Crit Care Med. 2006;174:935–952.

9. Centers for Disease Control and Prevention. Managing Drug Interactions in the Treatment of HIV-Related Tuberculosis. Atlanta, GA: US Department of Health and Human Services, CDC 2013.

10. Cole B, Nilsen DM, Will L, Etkind SC, Burgos M, Chorba T. Essential Components of a Public Health Tuberculosis Prevention, Control, and Elimination Program: Recommendations of the Advisory Council for the Elimination of Tuberculosis and the National Tuberculosis Controllers Association. MMWR Recomm Rep. 2020;69(RR-7):1–27.

133

CLOSTRIDIOIDES DIFFICILE INFECTION

You Want to Transplant What?? .... Level II

Brandon Dionne, PharmD, BCPS-AQ ID, BCIDP, AAHIVP

Michael J. Gonyeau, BS, MEd, PharmD, FCCP, FNAP, BCPS

LEARNING OBJECTIVES

After completing this case study, the reader should be able to:

- Identify signs and symptoms of *Clostridioides difficile* infection (CDI).

- Discuss CDI complications and prevention strategies.

- Evaluate treatment options and develop an optimal patient-specific treatment plan for initial and recurrent CDI, including drug, dose, frequency, route of administration, and duration of therapy.

- Develop a pertinent monitoring plan for a CDI regimen from a therapeutic and toxic standpoint.

PATIENT PRESENTATION

■ Chief Complaint

"I have been having to go to the bathroom a lot more frequently, and my stomach hurts a lot."

■ HPI

A 68-year-old woman is transferred to your medical team from the MICU after being admitted for sepsis secondary to a urinary tract infection and hypotension requiring pressor support. Over the past 2 days, she has been complaining of frequent foul-smelling stools. One week prior to being transferred to your team, she was admitted to the hospital complaining of urinary frequency and urgency for 3 days, nausea, vomiting, and left-sided flank pain, as well as light-headedness and dizziness. In the ED, the patient was hypotensive (BP 92/63 mm Hg) and tachycardic (HR 112–124 bpm), with an elevated lactate level and leukocytosis. She was transferred to the MICU for pressor support and started on an empiric regimen of cefepime 2 g IV Q 12 H and vancomycin 1 g IV Q 12 H for suspected urosepsis. Urine (×2) and blood (×3) cultures were subsequently found to be growing *Escherichia coli* and enteric Gram-negative rods, respectively, and antibiotic coverage was narrowed to ceftriaxone 2 g IV daily on day 5 based on susceptibility. The patient's blood pressure was stabilized, no ileus was detected, and she was transferred to the internal medicine service on day 7 of hospitalization. She is now complaining of new-onset diarrhea and abdominal pain.

■ PMH

CDI 2 months ago, treated with vancomycin 125 mg PO every 6 hours for 10 days
Hyperlipidemia
HTN
s/p MI 2003

■ SH

Lives at home alone, lifetime smoker (half pack per day for 54 years), drinks alcohol socially

■ Medications

Metoprolol succinate 100 mg PO once daily
Lisinopril 10 mg PO once daily
Atorvastatin 10 mg PO once daily
Pantoprazole 40 mg PO once daily

■ All

NKDA

■ Physical Examination

Gen

Patient is overweight and complains of abdominal discomfort.

VS

BP 149/85, P 98 bpm, RR 20, T 38.8°C; Ht 5′8″, Wt 87.2 kg

Skin

Warm and moist secondary to diaphoresis, no lesions

HEENT

PERRLA; EOMI; TMs intact; clear oropharynx, moist oral mucosa

Neck/Lymph Nodes

Neck is supple and without adenopathy; no JVD

Lungs/Thorax

CTA

CV

RRR; normal S_1, S_2; no murmurs

Abd

Abdomen is soft and nondistended, diffusely tender to palpation. Slight rebound and guarding. Positive bowel sounds.

Genit/Rect

Not performed

MS/Ext

Muscle strength and tone 5/5 in upper and lower; no C/C/E

Neuro

A&O × 3; CN II–XII intact

■ Labs

Na 138 mEq/L	Hgb 16.1 g/dL	WBC 16.9 × 10³/mm³	T. chol 205 mg/dL
K 3.5 mEq/L	Hct 49.8%	Neutros 50%	LDL 137 mg/dL
Cl 102 mEq/L	Plt 375 × 10³/mm³	Bands 9%	HDL 29 mg/dL
CO_2 22 mEq/L	A1C 7.9%	Eos 0%	Trig 197 mg/dL
BUN 36 mg/dL		Lymphs 34%	
SCr 1.8 mg/dL		Monos 7%	
(baseline			
0.9 mg/dL)			
Glu 101 mg/dL			
Alb 1.9 mg/dL			

■ CXR

Clear

■ ECG

NSR, unchanged from previous

■ *Clostridioides difficile* GDH/toxin EIA test

GDH antigen and A/B toxin assay both positive

■ Assessment

A 68-year-old woman presents with frequent, foul-smelling stools for 2 days with recent history of receiving broad-spectrum antibiotics and currently receiving ceftriaxone for pyelonephritis and a bloodstream infection (day 9); *C. difficile* antigen/toxin positive.

QUESTIONS

Collect Information

1.a. What subjective and objective information indicates the presence of CDI?

1.b. What additional information is needed to fully assess this patient's CDI?

Assess the Information

2.a. Assess the severity of CDI based on the subjective and objective information available.

2.b. Create a list of the patient's drug therapy problems and prioritize them. Include assessment of medication appropriateness, effectiveness, safety, and patient adherence.

Develop a Care Plan

3.a. What are the goals of pharmacotherapy for CDI in this case?

3.b. What nondrug therapies might be useful for this patient's CDI?

3.c. What feasible pharmacotherapeutic options are available for treating CDI?

3.d. Create an individualized, patient-centered, team-based care plan to optimize medication therapy for the CDI and this

patient's other drug therapy problems. Include specific drugs, dosage forms, doses, schedules, and durations of therapy.

3.e. What alternatives would be appropriate if the initial care plan fails or cannot be used?

Implement the Care Plan

4.a. What information should be provided to the patient to enhance adherence, ensure successful therapy, and minimize adverse effects?

4.b. Describe how care should be coordinated with other healthcare providers.

Follow-Up: Monitor and Evaluate

5. Explain how to monitor and evaluate the care plan for medication appropriateness, effectiveness, safety, and patient adherence by using clinical and laboratory data, patient feedback, and other information.

■ ADDITIONAL CASE QUESTIONS

1. What should be done if the patient develops similar signs and symptoms 3 weeks after successful CDI treatment?

2. Your medical team wants to start the patient on loperamide 2 mg PO after each bowel movement to control diarrhea. Do you agree with this course of action? Why or why not?

■ SELF-STUDY ASSIGNMENTS

1. Evaluate the relationship between PPI use and CDI recurrence and develop a plan to assess patient need for PPI use on discharge.

2. Conduct a literature search and develop a policy regarding infection control procedures to reduce the risk of CDI.

3. Assess the potential use of probiotics as an adjunct in the treatment and prevention of recurrent CDI.

4. Conduct a literature search to assess the cost-effectiveness and/ or cost utility of fecal microbiota transplant in the treatment of recurrent CDI.

CLINICAL PEARL

While fidaxomicin has a higher drug cost than oral vancomycin, the higher rate of global cure may make it more cost-effective in patients at higher risk for recurrence due to decreased hospital readmissions. It is important to consider transitions of care (ie, ensuring that the patient will be able to afford the fidaxomicin) before initiating it.

REFERENCES

1. Bagdasarian N, Rao K, Malani PN. Diagnosis and treatment of *Clostridium difficile* in adults: a systematic review. JAMA. 2015;313:398–408.

2. McDonald LC, Gerding DN, Johnson S, et al. Clinical practice guidelines for *Clostridium difficile* infection in adults and children: 2017 update by the Infectious Diseases Society of America (IDSA) and Society for Healthcare Epidemiology of America (SHEA). Clin Infect Dis. 2018;66:987–994.

3. Flack JM, Calhoun D, Schiffrin EL. The New ACC/AHA hypertension guidelines for the prevention, detection, evaluation, and management of high blood pressure in adults. Am J Hypertens. 2018;31(2):133–135.

4. Johnson S, Lavergne V, Skinner AM, et al. Clinical practice guideline by the Infectious Diseases Society of America (IDSA) and Society for

Healthcare Epidemiology of America (SHEA): 2021 focused update guidelines on management of *Clostridioides difficile* infection in adults. Clin Infect Dis. 2021;73(5):e1029–e1044.

5. Kelly CR, Fischer M, Allegretti JR, et al. ACG Clinical guidelines: prevention, diagnosis, and treatment of *Clostridioides difficile* infections. Am J Gastroenterol. 2021;116(6):1124–1147.

6. Gallagher JC, Reilly JP, Navalkele B, et al. Clinical and economic benefits of fidaxomicin compared to vancomycin for *Clostridium difficile* infection. Antimicrob Agents Chemother. 2015;59:7007–7010.

7. Wilcox MH, Gerding DN, Poxton IR, et al. Bezlotoxumab for prevention of recurrent *Clostridium difficile* infection. N Engl J Med. 2017;376:305–317.

8. Grundy SM, Stone NJ, Bailey AL, et al. 2018 AHA/ACC/AACVPR/ AAPA/ABC/ACPM/ADA/AGS/APhA/ASPC/NLA/PCNA guideline on the management of blood cholesterol: a report of the American College of Cardiology/American Heart Association task force on clinical practice guidelines. Circulation. 2019;139:e1082–e1143

9. Azab M, Doo L, Doo DH, et al. Comparison of the hospital-acquired *Clostridium difficile* infection risk of using proton pump inhibitors versus histamine-2 receptor antagonists for prophylaxis and treatment of stress ulcers: a systematic review and meta-analysis. Gut Liver. 2017;11:781–788.

10. Song JH, Kim YS. Recurrent *Clostridium difficile* infection: Risk factors, treatment, and prevention. Gut Liver. 2019;13(1):16–24.

134

INTRA-ABDOMINAL INFECTION

Like Mother, Like Son . . . . Level II

Paulina Deming, PharmD, PhC

Renee-Claude Mercier, PharmD, BCPS, PhC

LEARNING OBJECTIVES

After completing this case study, the reader should be able to:

- Recognize the clinical manifestations of spontaneous bacterial peritonitis (SBP; also known as primary bacterial peritonitis).

- List the goals of antimicrobial therapy for SBP.

- Recommend appropriate therapy for SBP.

- Monitor therapy for SBP for safety and efficacy.

- Recommend secondary prophylaxis for SBP.

PATIENT PRESENTATION

■ Chief Complaint

"My belly hurts so bad I can barely move."

■ HPI

A 47-year-old man who was brought to the ED by his wife. She stated that he has been suffering from nausea, vomiting, and severe abdominal pain for the past 2–3 days. His intake of food and fluids has been minimal over the past several days.

■ PMH

Cirrhosis, diagnosed last year with onset of ascites
Cholecystectomy 15 years ago

■ FH

Mother had known alcohol dependence; died 10 years ago due to complications of cirrhosis. Father's history unknown.

■ SH

Retired construction worker; alcohol use disorder with 10–12 cans of beer per day × 25 years and occasional heavier use on weekends; denies use of tobacco or illicit drugs; inconsistent adherence to medications; per patient's wife, he avoids salt but confirms he eats fast food two to three times per week.

■ Meds

Furosemide 40 mg PO once daily
Acetaminophen 325 mg PO PRN for pain

■ All

NKDA

■ ROS

As noted in the HPI. Denies any hematemesis or melena.

■ Physical Examination

Gen

Thin man who appears older than his stated age, with a distended abdomen and in severe pain

VS

BP 154/82, P 102 bpm, RR 32, T 38.2°C; current Wt 92 kg, (IBW 68 kg), Ht 5'11"

Skin

Jaundiced, warm, coarse, and very dry. Spider angiomata present on chest, back, and arms.

HEENT

Yellow sclera; PERRLA; Oropharynges show poor dentition but are otherwise unremarkable.

Neck/Lymph Nodes

Supple; normal-size thyroid; no JVD or palpable lymph nodes

Chest

Lungs are CTA; shallow and frequent breathing

Heart

Tachycardia, normal S_1 and S_2 with no S_3 or S_4

Abd

Distended; pain on pressure or movements; pain is sharp and diffuses throughout abdomen; (+) guarding. (+) HSM. Decreased bowel sounds.

Genit/Rect

Prostate normal size; guaiac (−) stool

Ext

No clubbing or cyanosis; bilateral pitting pedal edema 1+

Neuro

Oriented to person and place; lethargic and apathetic, slumped posture, slowed movements

■ Labs

Na 142 mEq/L	Hgb 13.1 g/dL	AST 90 IU/L
K 3.9 mEq/L	Hct 40.6%	ALT 60 IU/L
Cl 96 mEq/L	Plt 65 × 10³/mm³	Alk phos 350 IU/L
CO_2 20 mEq/L	WBC 12.25 × 10³/mm³	T. bili 2.2 mg/dL
BUN 44 mg/dL	Neutros 73%	D. bili 1.8 mg/dL
SCr 1.2 mg/dL	Bands 9%	Albumin 2.8 g/dL
Glu 101 mg/dL	Lymphs 13%	INR 1.34
	Monos 5%	

■ Abdominal Ultrasound

Nodular liver consistent with cirrhosis; ascites; splenomegaly

■ Blood Cultures

Pending × 2

■ Paracentesis

Ascitic fluid: leukocytes 720/mm³, protein 2.8 g/dL, albumin 1.1 g/dL, pH 7.28, lactate 30 mg/dL. Gram stain: numerous PMNs, no organisms.

■ Assessment

SBP

QUESTIONS

Collect Information

1.a. What subjective and objective information indicates the presence of spontaneous bacterial peritonitis (SBP)?

1.b. What additional information is needed to fully assess this patient's SBP?

Assess the Information

2.a. Assess the severity of SBP based on the subjective and objective information available.

2.b. Create a list of the patient's drug therapy problems and prioritize them. Include assessment of medication appropriateness, effectiveness, safety, and patient adherence.

2.c. What economic, psychosocial, cultural, racial, and ethical considerations are applicable to this patient?

Develop a Care Plan

3.a. What are the goals of pharmacotherapy for SBP in this case?

3.b. What nondrug therapies might be useful for this patient's SBP or cirrhosis?

3.c. What feasible pharmacotherapeutic options are available for treating SBP?

3.d. Create an individualized, patient-centered, team-based care plan to optimize medication therapy for SBP and this patient's other drug therapy problems. Include specific drugs, dosage forms, doses, schedules, and durations of therapy.

3.e. What alternatives would be appropriate if the initial care plan for SBP fails or cannot be used?

Implement the Care Plan

4.a. What information should be provided to the patient to enhance adherence, ensure successful therapy, and minimize adverse effects?

4.b. Describe how care should be coordinated with other healthcare providers.

Follow-Up: Monitor and Evaluate

5. Explain how to monitor and evaluate the care plan for medication appropriateness, effectiveness, safety, and patient adherence by using clinical and laboratory data, patient feedback, and other information.

■ CLINICAL COURSE

The blood cultures were reported positive for *Klebsiella pneumoniae*; resistant to ampicillin and ampicillin/sulbactam; and sensitive to aztreonam, ceftriaxone, levofloxacin, gentamicin, and piperacillin/tazobactam. The ascitic fluid culture grew *K. pneumoniae* as well. The patient received cefotaxime 2 g IV Q 8 H for a total of 5 days. After 1 day of antimicrobial treatment, repeat blood cultures were negative. He rapidly improved, and on discharge, his mental status had returned to baseline.

■ SELF-STUDY ASSIGNMENTS

1. Develop a table that illustrates the primary differences (clinical manifestations, pathogens involved, diagnosis methods, and treatment) between primary and secondary bacterial peritonitis.

2. Describe the pathophysiologic changes that occur in cirrhosis that contribute to the development of ascites and SBP.

3. Develop a table that compares the pharmacotherapeutic options for patients to assist in reducing alcohol cravings and consumption.

4. Develop a plan for nonpharmacologic management of patients with cirrhosis.

CLINICAL PEARL

Bacteremia is present in up to 75% of patients with primary peritonitis caused by aerobic bacteria but is rarely found in those with peritonitis caused by anaerobes. Ascitic fluid cultures are often negative, and a diagnosis of SBP is frequently made based on ascitic fluid PMN counts and the patient's clinical presentation. Pharmacotherapy of SBP is thus often empiric, and should be re-assessed and broadened if patients do not show clinical response.

REFERENCES

1. Biggins SW, Angeli P, Garcia-Tsao G, et al. Diagnosis, evaluation, and management of ascites, spontaneous bacterial peritonitis and hepatorenal syndrome: 2021 practice guidance by the American Association for the Study of Liver Diseases. Hepatology. 2021;74:1014–1048.

2. Runyon BA, McHutchison JG, Antillon MR, Akriviadis EA, Montano AA. Short-course versus long-course antibiotic treatment of spontaneous bacterial peritonitis: a randomized controlled study of 100 patients. Gastroenterology. 1991;100:1737–1742.

3. Angeli P, Gines P, Wong F, et al. Diagnosis and management of acute kidney injury in patients with cirrhosis: revised consensus recommendations of the International Club of Ascites. Gut. 2015;64:531–537.

4. Fernandez J, Tandon P, Mensa J, Garcia-Tsao G. Antibiotic prophylaxis in cirrhosis: good and bad. Hepatology. 2016;63:2019–2031.

5. Crabb DW, IM GY, Szabo G, et al. Diagnosis and treatment of alcohol-associated liver disease: 2019 practice guidance from the American Association for the Study of Liver Diseases. Hepatology. 2020;71:306–333.

135

LOWER URINARY TRACT INFECTION

Where Is the Bathroom? . . . . Level I

Melissa E. Badowski, PharmD, MPH, FIDSA, FCCP, BCIDP, BCPS, AAHIVP

Sharon M. Erdman, PharmD, FIDP

Keith A. Rodvold, PharmD, FCCP, FIDSA

LEARNING OBJECTIVES

After completing this case study, the reader should be able to:

- Recognize common signs and symptoms of acute uncomplicated cystitis/urinary tract infections (UTIs) in females.

- Design a therapeutic regimen for the treatment of acute uncomplicated cystitis after consideration of symptoms, medical history, allergies, objective findings, drug–drug interactions, and desired clinical response.

- Describe parameters that should be monitored during the treatment of acute uncomplicated cystitis to ensure efficacy and minimize toxicity.

- Provide patient education on the proper administration of antibiotic therapy for acute uncomplicated cystitis, including directions for use, administration of therapy in relation to meals, importance of medication adherence (including the need to complete the entire prescribed course), proper storage, and potential adverse reactions of the medication.

PATIENT PRESENTATION

■ Chief Complaint

"It burns when I urinate. I am urinating all the time."

■ HPI

A 26-year-old woman presents to a family medicine clinic in Nashville with complaints of dysuria, urinary frequency and urgency, and suprapubic tenderness for the past 2 days.

■ PMH

Patient has been previously diagnosed with three UTIs over the past 8 months based on symptoms. Each episode was treated with oral trimethoprim (TMP)/sulfamethoxazole (SMX).

■ FH

Mother has DM; remainder of FH is noncontributory.

■ SH

Denies smoking but admits to occasional marijuana and social alcohol use. Patient has been sexually active with one partner for the past 9 months and typically uses spermicide-coated condoms for contraception.

■ Meds

None

■ All

No known allergies

■ ROS

Patient reports urethral pain and burning with urination, as well as mild suprapubic tenderness. She denies systemic symptoms such as fever, chills, vomiting, or back pain, and does not report any urethral or vaginal discharge. Upon further questioning, she notes that the UTIs started soon after she met her boyfriend, and she does not always completely empty her bladder after sexual intercourse.

■ Physical Examination

Gen

Cooperative woman in no acute distress

VS

BP 110/60 mmHg, P 68 bpm, RR 16, T 36.8°C; Wt 57 kg, Ht 5'5"

Skin

No skin lesions

HEENT

PERRLA; EOMI; TMs intact

Neck/Lymph Nodes

Supple without lymphadenopathy

Chest

CTA

CV

RRR, no MRG

Back

No CVA tenderness

Abd

Soft; (+) bowel sounds; no organomegaly or tenderness

Pelvic

No vaginal discharge or lesions; LMP 2 weeks ago; mild suprapubic tenderness

Ext

Pulses 2+ throughout; full ROM

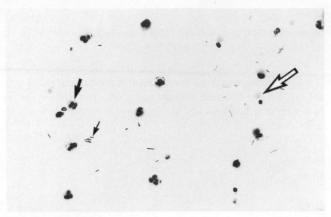

FIGURE 135-1. Urine sediment with neutrophils (*solid arrow*), bacteria (*small arrow*), and occasional red blood cells (*open arrow*) (Wright–Giemsa × 1650). (Photo courtesy of Lydia C. Contis, MD.)

Neuro

A&O × 3; CN II–XII intact; reflexes 2+; sensory and motor levels intact

■ Labs

Urinalysis

Yellow, cloudy; pH 5.0; WBC 50 cells/hpf; RBC 1–5 cells/hpf; protein (–); trace blood; glucose (–); leukocyte esterase (+); nitrite (+); many bacteria (Fig. 135-1)

Urine Culture

Not performed

■ Assessment

Acute uncomplicated cystitis

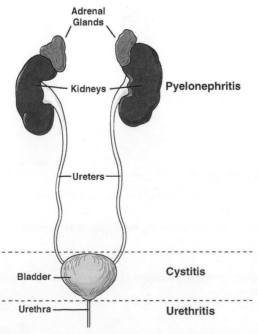

FIGURE 135-2. Anatomy and associated infections of the urinary tract.

QUESTIONS

Collect Information

1.a. What subjective and objective information indicates the presence of acute uncomplicated cystitis?

1.b. What additional information is needed to fully assess this patient's acute uncomplicated cystitis?

Assess the Information

2.a. Assess the severity of this episode of acute uncomplicated cystitis based on the subjective and objective information available.

2.b. Create a list of the patient's drug therapy problems and prioritize them. Include assessment of medication appropriateness, effectiveness, safety, and patient adherence.

Develop a Care Plan

3.a. What are the goals of pharmacotherapy for acute uncomplicated cystitis?

3.b. What nondrug therapies might be useful for this patient's acute uncomplicated cystitis?

3.c. What feasible pharmacotherapeutic options are available for empiric first- and second-line treatment of acute uncomplicated cystitis?

3.d. Create an individualized, patient-centered, team-based care plan to optimize medication therapy for this patient's acute uncomplicated cystitis and other drug therapy problems. Include specific drugs, dosage forms, doses, schedules, and durations of therapy.

3.e. What alternatives would be appropriate if the initial care plan for acute uncomplicated cystitis fails or cannot be used?

Implement the Care Plan

4.a. What information should be provided to the patient to enhance adherence, ensure successful therapy, and minimize adverse effects?

4.b. Describe how care should be coordinated with other healthcare providers.

Follow-Up: Monitor and Evaluate

5. Explain how to monitor and evaluate the care plan for medication appropriateness, effectiveness, safety, and patient adherence by using clinical and laboratory data, patient feedback, and other information.

■ ADDITIONAL CASE QUESTION

1. What long-term treatment strategies are available for this patient to prevent further episodes of acute uncomplicated cystitis?

■ SELF-STUDY ASSIGNMENTS

1. Review the safety and efficacy of single-dose, 3-, 5-, and 7-day antimicrobial therapy for the treatment of acute uncomplicated cystitis.

2. Perform a literature search to obtain current data on the national and regional rates of resistance of outpatient urinary tract isolates of *Escherichia coli* to TMP/SMX and fluoroquinolone antibiotics. How do these rates compare with those reported at your institution, your clinic, or your geographic area?

3. If this patient were pregnant, what antibiotics would be appropriate for treatment?

4. Differentiate between reinfection and relapse infection.

CLINICAL PEARL

UTIs occur rarely in young males, unless there is an underlying structural abnormality or instrumentation of the urinary tract.

REFERENCES

1. Gupta K, Hooton TM, Naber KG, et al. International clinical practice guidelines for the treatment of acute uncomplicated cystitis and pyelonephritis in women: a 2010 update by the Infectious Diseases Society of America and the European Society for Microbiology and Infectious Diseases. Clin Infect Dis. 2011;52:e103–e120.

2. Hooton TM. Clinical practice. Uncomplicated urinary tract infection. N Engl J Med. 2012;366:1028–1037.

3. Dielubanza EJ, Schaeffer AJ. Urinary tract infections in women. Med Clin North Am. 2011;95:27–41.

4. Walker E, Lyman A, Gupta K, Mahoney MV, Snyder GM, Hirsch EB. Clinical management of an increasing threat: outpatient urinary tract infections due to multidrug-resistant uropathogens. Clin Infect Dis. 2016;63:960–965.

5. Gupta K, Grigoryan L, Trautner B. Urinary tract infection. Ann Intern Med. 2017;167:ITC49–64.

6. Kaye KS, Gupta V, Mulgirigama A, et al. Antimicrobial resistance trends in urine Escherichia coli isolates from adult and adolescent females in the United States from 2011 to 2019: rising ESBL strains and impact on patient management. Clin Infect Dis. 2021;73:1992–1999.

7. Etienne M, Lefebvre E, Frebourg N, et al. Antibiotic treatment of acute uncomplicated cystitis based on rapid urine test and local epidemiology: lessons from a primary care series. BMC Infect Dis. 2014;14:137–144.

8. Stapleton AE, Dziura J, Hooton TM, et al. Recurrent urinary tract infection and urinary Escherichia coli in women ingesting cranberry juice daily: a randomized controlled trial. Mayo Clin Proc. 2012;87:143–150.

9. Cunha BA, Cunha CB, Lam B, et al. Nitrofurantoin safety and effectiveness in treating acute uncomplicated cystitis (AUC) in hospitalized adults with renal insufficiency: antibiotic stewardship implications. Eur J Clin Micrbiol Infect Dis. 2017;36:1213–1216.

10. Sanchez GV, Babiker A, Master RN, Luu T, Mathur A, Bordon J. Antibiotic resistance among urinary isolates from female outpatients in the United States in 2003 and 2012. Antimicrob Agents Chemother. 2016;60:2680–2683.

136

PYELONEPHRITIS

Resistant Rod............................... Level II

Elizabeth A. Coyle, PharmD, FCCM, BCPS

LEARNING OBJECTIVES

After completing this case study, the reader should be able to:

- Differentiate the signs, symptoms, and laboratory findings associated with pyelonephritis from those seen in lower urinary tract infections.

- Recommend appropriate empiric antimicrobial and symptomatic pharmacotherapy for a patient with suspected pyelonephritis.

- Make appropriate adjustments in pharmacotherapy based on patient response and culture results, recognizing the prevalence of *Escherichia coli* and the risk of resistance.

- Design a monitoring plan for a patient with pyelonephritis that allows objective assessment of the response to therapy.

PATIENT PRESENTATION

■ Chief Complaint

"I can't get warm and my back is killing me."

■ HPI

A 24-year-old female college student with type 1 diabetes, presents to the ED complaining that she has had pain in her right flank region over the last 24 hours, as well as pain in her abdomen. She complains of some nausea and reports that she woke up this morning with severe stomach and back pain, but has not vomited. The patient states she has not eaten for 24 hours, but has been able to drink water and non-diet soda, and has continued to keep her insulin pump on, but has not given any additional regular insulin. The patient reports she recently started treatment for a urinary tract infection about 2 days ago with trimethoprim/sulfamethoxazole. She states that she has been feeling feverish and has chills. She reports no substernal chest pain, shortness of breath, cough, or sputum production. She denies any diarrhea or rash.

■ PMH

Type 1 diabetes, diagnosed at age 11; has an insulin pump

■ FH

Mother and father are in their 40s and healthy; one sister with asthma, and an older brother with Crohn disease

■ SH

Nonsmoker, no IVDU, drinks alcohol socially. Single, but has a steady boyfriend and is sexually active. Currently is a first-year law student at the local university.

■ Meds

Ortho-Novum 7/7/7 one tablet PO daily
Insulin pump; regular insulin basal rate of 28 units per day
Regular insulin 2 units with breakfast, lunch, and supper
Trimethoprim/sulfamethoxazole one double-strength tablet twice daily for 3 days (she has completed 2 days of therapy)

■ All

No known drug allergies

■ ROS

She has a history of UTIs and has had two UTIs in the past year, the most recent 2 days ago.

■ Physical Examination

Gen

Conscious, alert, and oriented young woman in mild distress

VS

BP 120/72, P 68 bpm, RR 16, T 39.0°C, O$_2$ sat 98% room air; Wt 65 kg (IBW 61.1 kg), Ht 5'7"

Skin

No tenting; dry skin; no signs of redness or rash

HEENT

EOMI; funduscopic examination WNL; pharynx clear and dry

Neck

Supple, no JVD

Chest

CTA

CV

RRR

Abd

Soft with suprapubic tenderness to deep palpation; no rebound or guarding; active bowel sounds. There is no hepatosplenomegaly or masses.

Back

No paraspinal or spinal tenderness

Genit/Rect

Normal female genitalia; no abnormal vaginal discharge; normal sphincter tone; last menstrual period 1 week ago

Ext

No CCE; pulses 2+ bilaterally

Neuro

A&O × 3; CN II–XII intact; sensory and perception intact

■ Labs and UA on Admission

See Table 136-1.

■ Chest X-Ray

No infiltrates, no consolidation seen

■ CT Abdomen With Contrast

Findings: Liver, gallbladder, pancreas, spleen, and adrenals are unremarkable. No evidence of ascites or focal areas of fluid collection. The left kidney is unremarkable. A hypoattenuating lesion is seen involving the right kidney from mid- to lower pole.

Impression: Hypoattenuating lesion in right kidney consistent with pyelonephritis; correlate with clinical picture.

■ Abdominal Ultrasound

Findings: There is a hypoechoic region within the lateral cortex of the right kidney, which does not display through transmission.

Impression: Focal cortical thickening with decreased echogenicity involving the mid right renal cortex, similar to the recent CT scan, most likely representing focal pyelonephritis. No renal abscess identified. No hydronephrosis.

■ Urine Gram Stain

Many Gram-negative rods

TABLE 136-1	Laboratory Tests and Urinalyses on Days 1–3 of Hospitalization		
Parameter (Units)	**Day 1**	**Day 2**	**Day 3**
Serum chemistry			
Na (mEq/L)	141	139	141
K (mEq/L)	3.9	4.0	4.1
Cl (mEq/L)	99	101	102
CO_2 (mEq/L)	27	28	28
BUN (mg/dL)	25	18	12
SCr (mg/dL)	1.2	1.0	1.0
Glucose (mg/dL)	60	80	85
Hematology			
Hgb (g/dL)	13.9	13.8	13.6
Hct (%)	40.6	40.3	40.5
Plt (×10³/mm³)	275	276	276
WBC (×10³/mm³)	22.3	18.5	11.9
PMN/B/L/M (%)	80/13/7/0	85/10/5/0	86/6/7/1
Urinalysis			
Appearance	Hazy		
Color	Amber		
pH	5.0		
Specific gravity	1.017		
Blood	2+		
Ketones	Negative		
Leukocyte esterase	3+		
Nitrites	2+		
Urine protein, qualitative	Trace		
Urine glucose, qualitative	Trace		
WBC/hpf	625		
RBC/hpf	102		
Bacteria	Many		
WBC casts	2+		

B, bands; L, lymphocytes; M, monocytes; PMN, polymorphonuclear leukocytes.

■ Blood Culture

Many Gram-negative rods

■ Vaginal Swab

Negative

■ Assessment

1. Pyelonephritis
2. Bacteremia
3. Type 1 diabetes

QUESTIONS

Collect Information

1.a. What subjective and objective information indicates the presence of pyelonephritis?

1.b. What additional information is needed to fully assess this patient's pyelonephritis?

Assess the Information

2.a. Assess the severity of the pyelonephritis based on the subjective and objective information available.

2.b. Create a list of the patient's drug therapy problems and prioritize them. Include assessment of medication appropriateness, effectiveness safety, and patient adherence.

Develop a Care Plan

3.a. What are the goals of pharmacotherapy for pyelonephritis in this case?

3.b. What nondrug therapies might be useful for this patient's pyelonephritis?

3.c. What feasible pharmacotherapeutic options are available for treating pyelonephritis?

3.d. Create an individualized, patient-centered, team-based care plan to optimize medication therapy for pyelonephritis and this patient's other drug therapy problems. Include specific drugs, dosage forms, doses, schedules, and durations of therapy.

Implement the Care Plan

4.a. What information should be provided to the patient to enhance adherence, ensure successful therapy, and minimize adverse effects?

4.b. Describe how care should be coordinated with other healthcare providers.

Follow-Up: Monitor and Evaluate

5. Explain how to monitor and evaluate the care plan for medication appropriateness, effectiveness, safety, and patient adherence by using clinical and laboratory data, patient feedback, and other information.

■ CLINICAL COURSE

The patient was admitted to the hospital and started on the empiric antimicrobial regimen you recommended. She was given acetaminophen Q 6 H for pain. Her fevers subsided with the initiation of acetaminophen and antibiotics. On day 3 of hospitalization, she was much improved and was ready for discharge. Laboratory tests for days 2 and 3 are included in Table 136-1. Culture results from admission were finalized on day 3 (late in the day) and are shown in Table 136-2.

■ FOLLOW-UP CASE QUESTION

1. Given this new information, what recommendations, if any, do you have for changes in the initial drug regimen?

■ SELF-STUDY ASSIGNMENTS

1. Develop a protocol for switching patients from IV to oral therapy when treating pyelonephritis.

2. Perform a literature search to find clinical trials comparing drug therapy in pyelonephritis, and compare inclusion criteria, drug regimens, outcomes, and costs of therapy.

3. Develop a clinical pathway that could be used for managing suspected pyelonephritis.

CLINICAL PEARL

Pyelonephritis can be managed with many different drugs; choose drugs that are bactericidal and cleared in the active form by the kidney. Drugs suitable for once-daily therapy help to reduce treatment costs.

TABLE 136-2   Results of Urine and Blood Cultures Taken on Day 1 and Reported on Day 3

Urine Culture
Result: >100,000 cfu/mL *Escherichia coli*

Antibiotic	Kirby–Bauer Interpretation
Ampicillin/sulbactam	Resistant
Ampicillin	Resistant
Cefazolin	Resistant
Cefuroxime	Sensitive
Ceftriaxone	Sensitive
Levofloxacin	Sensitive
Piperacillin/tazobactam	Sensitive
Imipenem	Sensitive
Tobramycin	Sensitive
Fosfomycin	Sensitive
Nitrofurantoin	Sensitive
TMP/SMX	Resistant

Day 1 blood cultures × 2 sets
Result: Many *E. coli*

Antibiotic	Kirby–Bauer Interpretation
Ampicillin/sulbactam	Resistant
Ampicillin	Resistant
Cefazolin	Resistant
Cefuroxime	Sensitive
Ceftriaxone	Sensitive
Levofloxacin	Sensitive
Piperacillin/tazobactam	Sensitive
Imipenem	Sensitive
Tobramycin	Sensitive
TMP/SMX	Resistant

Vaginal swab
No growth × 3 days
Day 2 blood cultures
Results: No growth to date
Day 3 blood cultures
Results: No growth to date

REFERENCES

1. Sader HS, Castanheira M, Flamm RK, Jones RN. Antimicrobial activities of ceftazidime-avibactam and comparator agents against gram-negative organisms isolated from patients with urinary tract infections in U.S. medical centers, 2012 to 2014. Antimicrob Agents Chemother. 2016;60(7):4355–4360.

2. Keepers TR, Gomez M, Celeri C, Krause KM, Biek D, Critchley I. Fosfomycin and comparator activity against select Enterobacteriaceae, *Pseudomonas*, and *Enterococcus* urinary tract infection isolates from the United States in 2012. Infect Dis Ther. 2017;6(2):233–243.

3. Gupta K, Hooton TM, Naber KG, et al. International clinical practice guidelines for the treatment of acute uncomplicated cystitis and pyelonephritis in women: a 2010 update by the Infectious Diseases Society of America and the European Society for Microbiology and Infectious Diseases. Clin Infect Dis. 2011;52(5):e103–e120.

4. Colgan R, Williams M. Diagnosis and treatment of acute pyelonephritis in women. Am Fam Physician. 2011;84(5):519–526.

5. Eliakim-Raz N, Yahav D, Paul M, Leibovici L. Duration of antibiotic treatment for acute pyelonephritis and septic urinary tract infection—7 days versus longer treatment: systemic review and meta-analysis of randomized controlled trials. J Antimcrob Chemother. 2013;68:2183–2191.

6. Sandberg T, Skoog G, Hermansson AB, et al. Ciprofloxacin for 7 days versus 14 days in women with acute pyelonephritis: a randomized, open-label and double-blind, placebo-controlled, non-inferiority trial. Lancet. 2012;380(9840):484–490.

7. Abbo LM, Hooten TM. Antimicrobial stewardship and urinary tract infections. Antibiotics. 2014;3:174–192.

8. Wagenlehner F, Umeh O, Steenbergen J, Yuan G, Darouiche RO. Ceftolozane-tazobactam compared with levofloxacin in the treatment of complicated urinary-tract infections, including pyelonephritis: a randomized, double-blind, phase 3 trial (ASPECT-cUTI). Lancet 2015;385:1949–1956.

9. Wagenlehner FM, Sobel JD, Newell P, et al. Ceftazidime-avibactam versus doripenem for the treatment of complicated UTIs, including acute pyelonephritis: RECAPTURE, a Phase 3 Randomized Trial Program. Clin Infect Dis. 2016;63(6):754–762.

10. Dhillon S. Meropenem/vaborbactam: a review in complicated urinary tract infections. Drugs 2018;78:1259–1270.

137

PELVIC INFLAMMATORY DISEASE AND OTHER SEXUALLY TRANSMITTED INFECTIONS

Stealth Infections............................. Level II

Neha Sheth Pandit, PharmD, AAHIVP, BCPS

Jennifer Hoffmann, MS, CRNP-BC, MPH

LEARNING OBJECTIVES

After completing this case study, the reader should be able to:

- Identify relevant information from patient history, physical examination, and laboratory data suggestive of the diagnosis of a sexually transmitted infection (STI).

- List major complications of STIs and appropriate strategies for prevention and/or treatment.

- Discuss other health issues that may be present in patients referred for treatment of STIs, including immunization needs and risk reduction.

- Provide appropriate treatment plans for patients with STIs, including location of treatment, medication(s), dosage form, doses, route of administration, frequency, duration, and monitoring for efficacy and toxicities.

- Develop patient counseling strategies regarding drug treatment and possible adverse reactions.

PATIENT PRESENTATION

■ Chief Complaint

"I'm here for my yearly check-up."

■ HPI

A 23-year-old nulligravida female presents to a health clinic for annual pelvic exam. Her last menstrual period (LMP) started 10 days ago and lasted 4 days. She reports normal vaginal discharge with mild intermittent dyspareunia for approximately a month. She is heterosexual, sexually active with 2–3 concurrent partners, and admits to unprotected sex "at least once" in the past 2 weeks. She endorses vaginal, oral, and rectal intercourse. She does not know the sexual histories of her current or past sexual partners or their sexual partners. She reports 15 lifetime sexual partners.

■ PMH

She reports no history of sexually transmitted infections and has not undergone testing for HIV. She has been immunized against hepatitis B but not against human papillomavirus. She is unaware of hepatitis A or C as infectious diseases, asking "Do you get that from sex or restaurant food?"

No active medical problems.

■ FH

Noncontributory

■ SH

Denies IV or recreational drug use; smokes 5–10 cigarettes daily; has 2–4 drinks "on weekends." She is employed full-time.

■ Meds

She has a levonorgestrel intrauterine device (IUD) that was inserted 2 years ago without complications.

■ All

Ciprofloxacin ("makes me dizzy")

■ ROS

Occasional painful menses self-treated with brand name menstrual treatment (Pamprin or Midol—she does not recall exactly)

■ Physical Examination

Gen

Well-developed woman in no acute distress

VS

BP 110/76 mm Hg, Pulse 80 bpm, RR 16 breaths/min, T 37.1°C; Ht 158 cm, Wt 62 kg

Skin

Warm, dry, no rashes

HEENT

No erythema of pharynx or oral ulcers

Neck/Lymph Nodes

No lymphadenopathy; neck supple

Chest

Unlabored respiratory effort, clear to auscultation bilaterally

Breast

No mass or discharge

CV

Regular rate and rhythm; no murmurs

Abd

No tenderness or rebound; no HSM

Genit/Rect

Pubic hair Tanner stage V; no genital or perianal ulcers present; vulva with no ulcers, erythema, or excoriations. Vaginal area with large amount of thick yellow-white discharge. Cervix shows erythema and extensive yellow-white discharge; cervical friability; no masses on bimanual examination; cervical motion tenderness; adnexal tenderness and fullness on right. No genital growths visualized.

MS/Ext

No adenopathy, lesions, or rashes; no arthritis or tenosynovitis

Neuro

CN II–XII intact, DTRs 2+ and symmetric bilaterally

Psych

Awake, alert, and oriented. Appropriate mood and affect.

■ Labs

Na 138 mEq/L	Hgb 12.2 g/dL	WBC 12.75 × 10³/mm³
K 4.2 mEq/L	Hct 37%	Neutros 66%
Cl 102 mEq/L	Plt 250 × 10³/mm³	Bands 12%
BUN 22 mg/dL	SCr 0.9 mg/dL	Lymphs 10%
Glu 106 mg/dL		Monos 12%

■ Other Tests

Vaginal Saline Wet Preparation and KOH

Examination of vaginal discharge: Increased WBCs (too numerous to count), pH 5.0, no yeast or hyphae seen; "whiff" test positive with KOH preparation; many clue cells present.

Urine Dipstick

Leukocytes and nitrites neg; protein 100 mg/dL; otherwise unremarkable

Urine Pregnancy Test

Negative

Vaginal Specimen

Sent for NAAT for *Neisseria gonorrhoeae, Chlamydia trachomatis, Trichomonas vaginalis,* and *Mycoplasma genitalium*

Cervical Specimen

Sent for PAP and high-risk HPV test

Blood Specimen

Sent for RPR, HCV antibody reflex RNA, and 4th generation HIV test

■ Assessment

Pelvic Inflammatory Disease (infection of the upper genital tract and cervicitis)
Bacterial vaginosis

QUESTIONS

Collect Information

1.a. What subjective and objective information indicates the presence of sexually transmitted infections (STIs) and pelvic inflammatory disease (PID)?

1.b. What additional information is needed to fully assess this patient's STIs and PID?

Assess the Information

2.a. Assess the severity of PID based on the subjective and objective information available.

2.b. Create a list of drug therapy problems and prioritize them. Include assessment of medication appropriateness, effectiveness, safety, and patient adherence.

Develop a Care Plan

3.a. What are the goals of pharmacotherapy for PID in this case?

3.b. What nondrug therapies might be useful for this patient's PID?

3.c. What feasible pharmacotherapeutic options are available for treating PID?

3.d. Create an individualized, patient-centered, team-based care plan to optimize medication therapy for PID and other drug therapy problems. Include specific drugs, dosage forms, schedules, and durations of therapy.

Implement the Care Plan

4.a. What information should be provided to the patient to enhance adherence, ensure successful therapy, and minimize adverse effects?

4.b. Describe how care should be coordinated with other healthcare providers.

Follow-Up: Monitor and Evaluate

5. Explain how to monitor and evaluate the care plan for medication appropriateness, effectiveness, safety, and patient adherence by using clinical and laboratory data, patient feedback, and other information.

■ CLINICAL COURSE

Three days later, *N. gonorrhoeae, C. trachomatis,* and *M. genitalium* NAAT tests returned positive. *T. vaginalis* is negative.

■ FOLLOW-UP CASE QUESTION

1. What changes, if any, in anti-infective therapy are required (after the positive NAAT tests)? Include specific drugs, dosage forms, doses, schedules, and durations of therapy.

■ SELF-STUDY ASSIGNMENTS

1. Review the legal status of expedited partner therapy (EPT) in your area of practice. Discuss the ethical implications of this practice (see *https://www.cdc.gov/std/ept*).

2. Survey 10 local community pharmacists to assess their knowledge of EPT. Would they dispense the ordered medications?

3. Review nonprescription brand name products for management of dysmenorrhea and accompanying pain for ingredients, effectiveness, and cost. Develop recommendations for the most cost-effective therapy.

4. Review the current preexposure prophylaxis (PrEP) guidelines for HIV to see if this patient would be a good candidate for prophylaxis medication. If so, develop recommendations for PrEP with an appropriate monitoring plan.

CLINICAL PEARLS

1. Although partner notification and treatment may be enhanced through EPT strategies, misconceptions regarding legality and ethics of this practice limit implementation of this public health initiative.

2. Healthcare providers should view a diagnosis of STI as an immunization opportunity to enhance care of the individual while furthering public health initiatives for disease prevention.

REFERENCES

1. Workowski KA, Bachmann LH, Chan PA, et al. Sexually transmitted infections treatment guidelines, 2021. MMWR Recomm Rep. 2021;70(4):1–187.

2. Papp JR, Schachter J, Gaydos CA, Van Der Pol B. Recommendations for the laboratory-based detection of *Chlamydia trachomatis* and *Neisseria gonorrhoeae*—2014. MMWR Recomm Rep. 2014;63(RR-02):1–19.

3. Brunham RC, Gottlieb SL, Paavonen J. Pelvic inflammatory disease. N Engl J Med. 2015;372(21):2039–2048.

4. Soper DE and Wiesenfeld HC. The continued challenges in the diagnosis of acute pelvic inflammatory disease: focus on clinically mild disease. J Infect Dis 2021;224(S2):S75–S79.

5. Llata E, Bernstein KT, Kerani RP, et al. Management of pelvic inflammatory disease in selected U.S. sexually transmitted disease clinics: sexually transmitted disease surveillance network, January 2010–December 2011. Sex Transm Dis. 2015;42(8):429–433.

6. Centers for Disease Control and Prevention: Screening for HIV. Available at: *https://www.cdc.gov/hiv/clinicians/screening/index.html.* Accessed January 29, 2022.

7. Meites E, Kempe A, Markowitz LE. Use of a 2-dose schedule for human papillomavirus vaccination—updated recommendations of the Advisory Committee on Immunization Practices. MMWR Morb Mortal Wkly Rep. 2016;65(49):1405–1408.

8. Centers for Disease Control and Prevention. Expedited Partner Therapy. Available at: *https://www.cdc.gov/std/ept/default.htm.* Accessed January 30, 2022.

9. US Preventive Services Task Force Recommendation State. Behavioral counseling interventions to prevent sexually transmitted infections. JAMA 2020;324(7):674–681.

138

SYPHILIS

Here Today … Gone Tomorrow? . . . . Level I

Craig Martin, PharmD, BCPS, MBA

LEARNING OBJECTIVES

After completing this case study, the reader should be able to:

- Discuss the diagnosis of syphilis and differentiate among the temporal stages of the disease.

- Develop a treatment plan individualized for the patient's stage of syphilis.

- Recommend alternative treatment regimens when the primary therapeutic option is contraindicated.

- Describe appropriate monitoring, follow-up, and counseling of patients with a syphilitic infection to ensure treatment success.

PATIENT PRESENTATION

■ Chief Complaint

"This rash started 3–4 days ago on my back and stomach. My whole left side has been hurting, and I've also been feeling weaker than usual lately."

■ HPI

A 27-year-old man with a past medical history of HIV presents with left upper quadrant/left back/left side pain and a diffuse rash. He states the rash started 3–4 days ago and is mostly on his chest, abdomen, and arms. He also has several macules on his scalp. The rash is nonpainful and nonpruritic, except on his scalp, where he has developed a few scabs from scratching. No drainage from any lesions is noted. He also has been having some chest pain that is worse with breathing. He notes nausea, though no vomiting, and reports ongoing non-bloody diarrhea for months. He presents to the ED primarily because of pain in his upper left back radiating around his left side. His urine is very dark, brownish-red; however, he has no dysuria. The patient also states he has felt weaker than usual for the past few days.

■ PMH

HIV diagnosed 6 months ago, on antiretroviral therapy

■ FH

Both parents have hypertension, still living

■ SH

Cigarette smoking 1.5 ppd since early teens; social alcohol usage (average four drinks per week); occasional methamphetamine use—both smoked and injected (with clean needles); MSM (four partners in last 6 months) with inconsistent use of condoms

■ Meds

Bictegravir/tenofovir alafenamide/emtricitabine 50/25/200 mg (coformulated tablet) PO once daily
Acetaminophen–hydrocodone 325/5 mg PO Q 6 H PRN

■ All

NKDA

■ ROS

Constitutional: reports weakness and malaise; denies fever
Eyes: denies vision changes
Ears, nose, and throat: denies sore throat, rhinorrhea, or sinus pressure
Lymphatic: denies lymph node swelling
Respiratory: denies shortness of breath, dyspnea on exertion, or cough
Cardiovascular: reports some chest pain on inspiration
Gastrointestinal: reports intermittent nausea, no vomiting, and consistent diarrhea
Neurologic: denies neuropathy symptoms
Musculoskeletal: reports arthralgias and myalgias
Skin: rash on scalp, abdomen, arms, and legs present
Pain: reports persistent abdominal and left-sided pain

Physical Examination

Gen

Awake and alert, NAD. Appropriate. He is oriented to person, place, and year.

VS

T 98.4°F, BP 114/70, HR 92, RR 16, O$_2$ sat 98; Ht 61″, Wt 59 kg

Skin

Numerous palpable, blanchable macules, mostly ~5 mm with one area of confluence on the left lower abdomen. Macules are present on both arms, chest, and back—four to five scabs with surrounding erythema on the scalp.

HEENT

Moist mucous membranes, neck supple. No cervical, postauricular, or supraclavicular lymphadenopathy. No apparent oral lesions. Mild icterus.

Neck/Lymph Nodes

Supple; no lymphadenopathy, bruits, JVD, or thyromegaly

Chest

CTA bilaterally. No crackles or wheezes.

CV

RRR; S$_1$, S$_2$; no m/r/g

Abd

Soft, nondistended. Diffuse tenderness with minimal localization to the RUQ and more prominent on the epigastrium, LUQ, and back. (+) BS. No rebound or guarding.

Extremities

Warm, well perfused, no edema. 2+ DP and PT pulses

GU

Rash extending to the penis; no other lesions present. Moderate inguinal lymphadenopathy.

Rectal

Scar from recently healed ulcer noted

Musculoskeletal

No joint swelling or effusions

Neuro

CN II–XII grossly intact. No dysmetria. Strength 5/5 on all four extremities.

Labs

Na 138 mEq/L	Hgb 12.3 g/dL	AST 95 IU/L	HIV viral load
K 3.9 mEq/L	Hct 36.9%	ALT 66 IU/L	<20 copies/mL
Cl 96 mEq/L	WBC 9.3 × 10³/mm³	Alk phos	HCV RNA
CO$_2$ 28 mEq/L	CD4 460 cells/mm³	1271 IU/L	negative
BUN 7 mg/dL	Plt 391 × 10³/mm³	T. bili 5.0 mg/dL	RPR titer positive
SCr 0.7 mg/dL			at 1:256
Glu 100 mg/dL			FTA-ABS positive

CT Abdomen and Pelvis

Mild hepatosplenomegaly with minimal intrahepatic biliary ductal dilatation and prominence of the common duct. There are multiple tortuous perirectal vessels that may represent varices secondary to portal hypertension. Proctitis is present with innumerable reactive perirectal and pelvic lymph nodes.

Assessment

HIV-infected patient with newly diagnosed syphilis (appears to be in a secondary stage)

QUESTIONS

Collect Information

1.a. What subjective and objective information indicates the presence of syphilis?

1.b. What additional information is needed to fully assess this patient's syphilis?

Assess the Information

2.a. Assess the severity of syphilis based on the subjective and objective information available.

2.b. Create a list of the patient's drug therapy problems and prioritize them. Include an assessment of medication appropriateness, effectiveness, safety, and patient adherence.

Develop a Care Plan

3.a. What are the goals of pharmacotherapy for syphilis in this case?

3.b. What nondrug therapies might be useful for this patient's syphilis?

3.c. What feasible pharmacotherapeutic options are available for treating syphilis?

3.d. Create an individualized, patient-centered, team-based care plan to optimize medication therapy for syphilis and this patient's other drug therapy problems. Include specific drugs, dosage forms, doses, schedules, and duration of therapy.

Implement the Care Plan

4.a. What information should be provided to the patient to enhance adherence, ensure successful therapy, and minimize adverse effects?

4.b. Describe how care should be coordinated with other healthcare providers.

Follow-Up: Monitor and Evaluate

5. Explain how to monitor and evaluate the care plan for medication appropriateness, effectiveness, safety, and patient adherence by using clinical and laboratory data, patient feedback, and other information.

■ SELF-STUDY ASSIGNMENTS

1. Describe the differences in syphilis presentation as a reflection of disease progression.

2. Discuss the tests or procedures that should be used to diagnose and monitor the progression/regression of syphilis over time.

3. Identify potential confounding factors that may impact test results in HIV-infected patients with syphilis.

Patients undergoing penicillin therapy for syphilis frequently experience the Jarisch–Herxheimer reaction within the first 24 hours of treatment. This is an inflammatory response to the breakdown of spirochetes and the subsequent release of endotoxins. Usually manifesting as fever, chills, myalgias, arthralgias, and headache, it is generally self-limiting and may be treated with analgesics and antipyretics as needed.

REFERENCES

1. Centers for Disease Control and Prevention. Sexually Transmitted Disease Surveillance, 2013. Atlanta, GA: U.S. Department of Health and Human Services; December 2014. Available at: *http://www.cdc.gov/std/stats13/syphilis.htm*. Accessed January 15, 2022.
2. Centers for Disease Control and Prevention. Sexually transmitted diseases treatment guidelines, 2021. MMWR Morb Mortal Wkly Rep. 2021;70(4):1–187.
3. Radolf JD, Tramont EC, Salazar JC. Syphilis (*Treponema pallidum*). In: Mandell GL, Bennett JE, Dolin R, eds. Principles and Practice of Infectious Diseases. 8th ed. Philadelphia, PA: Churchill Livingstone; Volume 2, 2015:2684–2709.
4. Panel on Opportunistic Infections in HIV-infected Adults and Adolescents. Guidelines for the prevention and treatment of opportunistic infections in HIV-infected adults and adolescents: recommendations from CDC, the National Institutes of Health, and the HIV Medicine Association of the Infectious Diseases Society of America, November 2021. Available at: *https://clinicalinfo.hiv.gov/en/guidelines/adult-and-adolescent-opportunistic-infection/whats-new-guidelines*. Accessed January 15, 2022.
5. Bai ZG, Wang B, Yang K, et al. Azithromycin versus penicillin G benzathine for early syphilis. Cochrane Database Syst Rev. 2012;6:CD007270.
6. Warwick Z, Dean G, Fisher M. Should syphilis be treated differently in HIV-positive and HIV-negative individuals? Treatment outcomes at a university hospital, Brighton, UK. Int J STD AIDS. 2009;20(4):229–230.
7. See S, Scott EK, Levin MW. Penicillin-induced Jarisch-Herxheimer reaction. Ann Pharmacother. 2005;39(12):2128–2130.

139

GENITAL HERPES, GONOCOCCAL, AND CHLAMYDIAL INFECTIONS

Triple Threat . . . . Level II

Albert T. Bach, PharmD, APh

Karl M. Hess, PharmD, APh, CTH, CMWA, FCPhA, FAPhA

LEARNING OBJECTIVES

After completing this case study, the reader should be able to:

- Identify subjective and objective data consistent with genital herpes, gonorrhea, and chlamydia.

- Recommend appropriate therapies for treating genital herpes, gonorrhea, and chlamydia.

- Provide effective and comprehensive counseling for patients with genital herpes, gonorrhea, and chlamydia.

- List the treatment goals for a patient with genital herpes, gonorrhea, and chlamydia

PATIENT PRESENTATION

■ Chief Complaint

"I have painful sores in my genital area, and I have terrible headaches and muscle aches."

■ HPI

A 19-year-old nulligravida woman who presents to the county health STD clinic for evaluation of genital lesions that have been present for 3 days. She has also noticed a white non-odorous vaginal discharge that has lasted 14 days. She admits to anal and vaginal intercourse with two regular partners in the past 60 days. It has been 5 days since her last sexual encounter.

■ PMH

Recurrent UTIs; most recent 3 months ago
Vaginal candidiasis; most recent 6 months ago
Gonorrhea 5 years ago
Trichomonas vaginalis 2 years ago

■ FH

Mother with type 2 DM; father died at age 50 of an acute MI

■ SH

Lives with her boyfriend and works at a local grocery store. She admits to occasional use of alcohol and marijuana.

■ Meds

Ethinyl estradiol and norethindrone (Junel) 21 1/20 one tablet PO daily
Multivitamin with iron one tablet PO daily
Ibuprofen 200 mg PO Q 6 H PRN headache
Nitrofurantoin 100 mg PO once daily for recurrent UTI prophylaxis

■ All

Trimethoprim/sulfamethoxazole (hives and tongue swelling)

■ ROS

(–) Cough, night sweats, weight loss, dysuria, or urinary frequency; (+) anorectal pain; last menstrual period 6 weeks ago

■ Physical Examination

Gen

Thin, young woman in NAD

VS

BP 136/71 mm Hg, P 78 bpm, RR 17 breaths/min, T 37.8°C; Wt 51 kg, Ht 5'5"

Skin

Dry, no lesions, normal color and temperature

HEENT

PERRLA, EOMI without nystagmus

Neck

Supple; no adenopathy, JVD, or thyromegaly

Chest

Air entry equal; no crepitations or wheezing

CV

RRR, normal S_1 and S_2; no S_3 or S_4; no murmurs or rubs

Abd

Soft, mild tenderness to palpation in RLQ, (+) bowel sounds

Genit/Rect

Tender inguinal adenopathy. External exam clear for nits and lice, several extensive shallow small painful vesicular lesions over vulva and labia, swollen and red. Vagina red, rugated, moderate amounts of creamy white discharge. Cervix pink, covered with above discharge, nontender, about 3 cm. Corpus nontender, no palpable masses. Adnexa with no palpable masses or tenderness. Rectum with no external lesions; (+) diffuse inflammation and friability internally, no masses.

Ext

Peripheral pulses 2+ bilaterally, DTRs 2+, no joint swelling or tenderness

Neuro

Alert and oriented, CN II–XII intact

■ Labs

Na 135 mEq/L	Hgb 12.9 g/dL	WBC 6.3×10^3/mm³	RPR nonreactive
K 4.0 mEq/L	Hct 37.3%	PMNs 64%	Preg test: hCG
Cl 102 mEq/L	Plt 255 ×	Bands 2%	pending
CO_2 27 mEq/L	10^3/mm³	Eos 1%	HIV serology: ELISA
BUN 11 mg/dL		Lymphs 24%	pending
SCr 0.9 mg/dL		Monos 9%	
Glu 72 mg/dL			

■ Other

Vaginal discharge: Whiff test (–); pH <4.5; wet mount *Trichomonas* (–), clue cells (–), yeast (+)

■ Clinical Course

The following results were reported 2 days later:

Vulval swab DFA monoclonal stain: HSV-2 isolated

Vaginal and rectal swab gonorrhea NAAT (PCR): *Neisseria gonorrhoeae* (+)

Vaginal and rectal swab chlamydia NAAT (PCR): *Chlamydia trachomatis* (+)

■ Assessment

A 19-year-old woman who may be pregnant and has primary genital HSV-2 infection, vaginal candidiasis, and gonococcal and chlamydial infections of the vagina, cervix, and rectum. Adherent to all current medications.

QUESTIONS

Collect Information

1.a. What subjective and objective information indicates the presence of sexually transmitted infections (STIs)?

1.b. What additional information is needed to fully assess this patient's STIs?

Assess the Information

2.a. Assess the classification of genital herpes infection based on the subjective and objective information available.

2.b. Create a list of the patient's drug therapy problems and prioritize them. Include assessment of medication appropriateness, effectiveness, safety, and patient adherence.

Develop a Care Plan

3.a. What are the goals of pharmacotherapy for STIs in this case?

3.b. What nondrug therapies might be useful for this patient's STIs?

3.c. What feasible pharmacotherapeutic options are available for treatment of genital herpes, chlamydia, and gonorrhea?

3.d. Create an individualized, patient-centered, team-based care plan to optimize medication therapy for the STIs and other drug therapy problems. Include specific drugs, dosage forms, doses, schedules, and durations of therapy.

3.e. What alternatives would be appropriate if the initial care plan fails or cannot be used?

Implement the Care Plan

4.a. What information should be provided to the patient to enhance adherence, ensure successful therapy, and minimize adverse effects?

4.b. Describe how care should be coordinated with other healthcare providers.

Follow-Up: Monitor and Evaluate

5. Explain how to monitor and evaluate the care plan for medication appropriateness, effectiveness, safety, and patient adherence by using clinical and laboratory data, patient feedback, and other information.

■ FOLLOW-UP QUESTIONS

1. Six months later, Megan calls the STD clinic complaining of genital lesions that look and feel the same as the lesions she had 6 months earlier when seen and treated in the clinic. Should this episode of recurrent genital herpes be treated? If so, what therapies would be appropriate?

2. Is daily suppressive therapy indicated because she had a recurrent episode?

3. When is herpes treatment indicated for sexual partners?

4. When is chlamydia and gonorrhea treatment indicated for sexual partners?

■ SELF-STUDY ASSIGNMENTS

1. Research the potential role of vaccines in the future management of herpes.

2. Recommend alternative agents for treating acyclovir-resistant herpes.

3. Explain the relationship between herpes and HIV infections. Is there a role for herpes simplex virus–suppressive therapy in preventing HIV transmission?

4. Describe complications of herpes that may require hospitalization, and recommend an appropriate treatment regimen.

CLINICAL PEARL

Most genital herpes infections are transmitted by persons who have asymptomatic viral shedding and are unaware that they have the infection. Systemic antiviral drugs control the signs and symptoms of genital herpes infection, but they do not eradicate latent virus.

ACKNOWLEDGMENT

This case is an updated version of a case created by Jonathan C. Cho, PharmD, MBA, BCIDP, BCPS in the 11th edition of this book.

REFERENCES

1. Workowski KA, Bachmann LH, Chan PA, et al. Sexually transmitted infections treatment guidelines, 2021. MMWR Recomm Rep. 2021;70(No. RR-4):1–187.
2. Valtrex (Valacyclovir) caplets package insert. Research Triangle Park, NC. GlaxoSmithKline. June 2021.
3. Famvir (Famciclovir) tablets package insert. East Hanover, NJ. Novartis Pharmaceuticals Corporation. September 2016.
4. Update to CDC's sexually transmitted diseases treatment guidelines, 2010: oral cephalosporins no longer a recommended treatment for gonococcal infections. MMWR Morb Mortal Wkly Rep. 2012 Aug 10;61(31):590–594.

140

OSTEOMYELITIS AND SEPTIC ARTHRITIS

I Must Be Getting Old . . . . Level II

R. Brigg Turner, PharmD

Gregory B. Tallman, PharmD, MS, BCPS, BCIDP

LEARNING OBJECTIVES

After completing this case study, the reader should be able to:

- Describe the most common presenting signs and symptoms of osteomyelitis.

- Recommend an antimicrobial treatment plan with empiric and definitive therapy for osteomyelitis.

- Develop alternative treatment approaches for osteomyelitis when the preferred regimen cannot be used.

- Identify monitoring parameters to evaluate the efficacy and toxicity of antimicrobial therapy for osteomyelitis.

- Provide patient education on the proper administration of home infusion antibiotics for osteomyelitis.

PATIENT PRESENTATION

■ Chief Complaint

"My back is hurting more and I just don't feel well."

■ HPI

A 52-year-old man with a history of chronic back pain presents with a 1-week history of acute back pain and spasms localized in the thoracic region. There is radiation of pain to his upper right leg with movement. On a scale of 1–10, the patient rates that pain as an 8. The patient also reports intermittent malaise, body aches, and intermittent chills.

■ PMH

Patient reports chronic back pain starting approximately 10 years ago. He does not routinely seek medical care and does not report any other chronic conditions.

■ FH

Noncontributory

■ SH

He has smoked one pack of cigarettes per day for the past 20 years. He admits to IV heroin use for the past 3–4 years.

■ Meds

Acetaminophen and ibuprofen as needed for back pain; he has increased use of these medications over the past week

■ All

No known allergies

■ ROS

He denies nausea, vomiting, fevers, chest pain, shortness of breath, and bowel or bladder incontinence. He reports decreased oral intake over the past week due to pain, general malaise, and intermittent chills.

■ Physical Examination

Gen

He does not appear to be in any acute distress.

VS

BP 152/109, P 84 bpm, RR 18, T 37.9°C; 96% SpO$_2$ on room air, Ht 5'8", Wt 90 kg

Skin

Intact

HEENT

PERRL, conjunctivae clear. Poor dentition noted.

Neck/Lymph Nodes

No lymphadenopathy

Lungs/Thorax

Clear to auscultation bilaterally, no wheezing, rhonchi, or rales

CV

Regular rate and rhythm; no appreciable murmurs, gallops, or rubs

Abd

Soft, nontender, nondistended; bowel sounds present

Genit/Rect

Deferred

MS/Ext

Decreased dorsiflexion on the left foot, which he states is chronic. Bilateral lower extremity strength is 5/5. He has reproducible pain in the thoracic spine.

Neurologic

Cranial nerves II–XII are intact

Psychiatric

Oriented to person, place, and time. Mood and affect are appropriate.

■ Labs

Na 136 mEq/L	Hgb 13.7 g/dL
K 4.0 mEq/L	Hct 41.1%
Cl 102 mEq/L	Plt 341 × 10³/mm³
CO_2 25 mEq/L	WBC 22.7 × 10³/mm³
BUN 18 mg/dL	Neutros 71%
SCr 0.87 mg/dL	Bands 17%
Glu 120 mg/dL	Lymphs 3%
Ca 9.4 mg/dL	Monos 9%
ESR 73 mm/hr	
CRP 84.2 mg/L	

■ Abdominal and Pelvic CT Scan

CT scan of abdomen and pelvis are unremarkable. Thoracic spine shows degenerative disk disease from T1 to T5.

■ MRI

MRI shows T2–T3 osteomyelitis and paravertebral abscess.

■ Blood Cultures × Two Sets

Pending

■ Other

HCV Ab negative; HIV nonreactive

■ Assessment

1. Paravertebral abscess and osteomyelitis in the presence of chronic back pain
2. Substance use disorder—heroin
3. Chronic tobacco smoker

QUESTIONS

Collect Information

1.a. What subjective and objective information indicates the presence of osteomyelitis?

1.b. What additional information is needed to fully assess this patient's osteomyelitis?

Assess the Information

2.a. Assess the severity of osteomyelitis based on the subjective and objective information available.

2.b. Create a list of the patient's drug therapy problems and prioritize them. Include assessment of medication appropriateness, effectiveness, safety, and patient adherence.

2.c. What economic, psychosocial, cultural, and ethical considerations are applicable to this patient?

Develop a Care Plan

3.a. What are the goals of pharmacotherapy for osteomyelitis in this case?

3.b. What nondrug therapies might be useful for this patient's osteomyelitis?

3.c. What feasible pharmacotherapeutic options are available for treating osteomyelitis?

3.d. Create an individualized, patient-centered, team-based care plan to optimize medication therapy for the osteomyelitis and this patient's other drug therapy problems. Include specific drugs, dosage forms, doses, schedules, and durations of therapy.

■ CLINICAL COURSE

The patient was taken to interventional radiology, and a culture from CT-guided aspiration of his paravertebral abscess was obtained. The patient was treated initially with empiric vancomycin plus cefepime. After 2 days, paravertebral abscess culture and blood cultures (2 out of 4) revealed *Staphylococcus aureus* with susceptibilities reported in Table 140-1. Repeat blood cultures were collected and a transthoracic echocardiogram reported an ejection fraction of approximately 65%, trace aortic and mitral regurgitation, and no evidence of vegetation or perivalvular abscess. The patient has improvement of symptoms, he is clinically stable, repeat blood cultures were negative, and the physician determines that discharge is appropriate and orders placement of a peripherally-inserted central catheter (PICC) for outpatient intravenous drug administration.

3.e. Given this new clinical information (after microbiology report), update your care plan to include targeted intravenous antimicrobial therapy against the causative pathogen.

TABLE 140-1	**Blood Culture Susceptibilities of *Staphylococcus aureus*: Final Report**
Cefazolin	Susceptible
Clindamycin	Susceptible
Oxacillin	Susceptible
Trimethoprim/sulfamethoxazole	Susceptible
Vancomycin	Susceptible, MIC = 0.5 mg/L

Implement the Care Plan

4.a. What information should be provided to the patient to enhance adherence, ensure successful therapy, and minimize adverse effects?

4.b. Describe how care should be coordinated with other healthcare providers.

Follow-Up: Monitor and Evaluate

5. Explain how to monitor and evaluate the care plan for medication appropriateness, effectiveness, safety, and patient adherence by using clinical and laboratory data, patient feedback, and other information.

■ SELF-STUDY ASSIGNMENTS

1. Devise alternative IV and oral treatment regimens if the patient was unable to tolerate the initial targeted antibiotic(s) used.

2. Discuss the considerations that need to be made when sending this patient home with a PICC line.

CLINICAL PEARL

Staphylococcus aureus is the most common organism causing osteomyelitis, and concurrent bacteremia is common. *S. aureus* bacteremia is a serious condition requiring specialized care. Consultation with infectious diseases specialists results in better patient care and outcomes. All patients should have a thorough physical exam to identify metastatic foci and an echocardiogram to detect vegetation, intracardiac abscess, or valvular perforation to aid in the diagnosis of infective endocarditis.

REFERENCES

1. Li HK, Rombach I, Zambellas R, et al. Oral versus intravenous antibiotics for bone and joint infection. N Engl J Med. 2019;380(5):425–436.

2. Berbari EF, Kanj SS, Kowalski TJ, et al. 2015 Infectious Diseases Society of America (IDSA) clinical practice guidelines for the diagnosis and treatment of native vertebral osteomyelitis in adults. Clin Infect Dis. 2015;61(6):e26–e46.

3. McHenry MC, Easley KA, Locker GA. Vertebral osteomyelitis: long-term outcome for 253 patients from 7 Cleveland-area hospitals. Clin Infect Dis. 2002;34(10):1342–1350.

4. Lipsky BA, Berendt AR, Cornia PB, et al. 2012 Infectious Diseases Society of America clinical practice guideline for the diagnosis and treatment of diabetic foot infections. Clin Infect Dis. 2012;54(12):e132–e173.

5. Tice AD, Rehm SJ, Dalovisio JR, et al. Practice guidelines for outpatient parenteral antimicrobial therapy. IDSA guidelines. Clin Infect Dis. 2004;38(12):1651–1672.

6. Norris AH, Shrestha NK, Allison GM, et al. 2018 Infectious Diseases Society of America clinical practice guideline for the management of outpatient parenteral antimicrobial therapy. Clin Infect Dis. 2019;68(1):e1–e35.

7. Suzuki J, Johnson J, Montgomery M, Hayden M, Price C. Outpatient parenteral antimicrobial therapy among people who inject drugs: a review of the literature. Open Forum Infect Dis. 2018;5(9):ofy194.

8. Weissman S, Parker RD, Siddiqui W, Dykema S, Horvath J. Vertebral osteomyelitis: retrospective review of 11 years of experience. Scand J Infect Dis. 2014;46(3):193–199.

9. Bidell MR, Patel N, O'Donnell JN. Optimal treatment of MSSA bacteraemias: a meta-analysis of cefazolin versus antistaphylococcal penicillins. J Antimicrob Chemother. 2018;73(10):2643–2651.

10. Babouee Flury B, Elzi L, Kolbe M, et al. Is switching to an oral antibiotic regimen safe after 2 weeks of intravenous treatment for primary bacterial vertebral osteomyelitis? BMC Infect Dis. 2014;14:226.

141

SEPSIS

Time Is of the Essence . . . . .Level III

Trisha N. Branan, PharmD, BCCCP

Susan E. Smith, PharmD, BCCCP, BCPS

LEARNING OBJECTIVES

After completing this case study, the reader should be able to:

• Recognize the signs and symptoms of sepsis and septic shock.

• State patient variables used to diagnose sepsis and septic shock.

• Identify the initial treatment goals for patients after the diagnosis of sepsis.

• Formulate a comprehensive treatment plan for the initial management of patients with sepsis.

• Recommend appropriate supportive care therapies for patients with sepsis.

PATIENT PRESENTATION

■ Chief Complaint

The patient presents from her nursing home with altered mental status and lethargy that has progressively worsened over the past 24 hours.

■ HPI

An 80-year-old woman who resides in a nursing home with a past medical history that includes hypertension, advanced dementia, depression, and GERD presents to the hospital. She was discharged last week from another hospital after being treated for 5 days for a urinary tract infection. She did well through the first 2 days after discharge but has become increasingly lethargic and drowsy in the past 24 hours. She is barely responsive at the time of assessment. She has had no reports of fever, nausea, vomiting, or pain.

■ PMH

HTN
Advanced dementia
Depression
GERD

■ PSH

Noncontributory

■ FH

No HTN, DM, CAD, cancer, or vascular disease

■ SH

Lives in a nursing home due to dementia
No tobacco, alcohol, or illicit drug use

■ Medications

Clonidine 0.2 mg/24 H transdermal patch every week

Acetaminophen 500 mg PO Q 6 H as needed for pain/fever

Lorazepam 0.5 mg PO Q HS

Hydralazine 50 mg PO TID

Omeprazole 20 mg PO QAM

Rivastigmine 4.6 mg/24 H transdermal patch Q HS

Levofloxacin 500 mg PO Q 24 H for 3 days (received 5 days of inpatient IV therapy; completed total course 2 days ago)

■ Allergies

NKDA

■ Review of Systems

Unable to obtain due to patient's mental status

■ Physical Examination

Gen

Unresponsive, thin appearing woman in acute distress

VS

BP 86/42 mm Hg, P 118–142 bpm, RR 14–35 breaths/min, T 35.6°C; SpO$_2$: 94% on 8L NC, Ht 5'3", Wt 50.8 kg

Skin

Skin is warm, dry and pink, intact with no rashes or lesions

HEENT

Normocephalic, no scleral icterus, no sinus tenderness

Neck/Lymph Nodes

Supple, nontender, no carotid bruits, no JVD, no lymphadenopathy

Lungs

Decreased air entry in the bases, otherwise clear, tachypnea

CV

Tachycardia, regular rhythm, no murmur, gallop, or edema

Abdomen

Soft, NT/ND, normal bowel sounds, no masses

Musculoskeletal

Normal range of motion and strength, no tenderness or swelling

Neuro

Responsive to painful stimuli at this time, unable to assess further

■ Labs

Na 135 mEq/L	Mg 2.2 mg/dL	WBC 19.3	Arterial blood gases
K 4.4 mEq/L	Phos 3.1 mg/dL	× 10^3/mm^3	pH 7.15
Cl 105 mEq/L	Alb 2.3 g/dL	PMNs 72%	PaCO$_2$ 28 mm Hg
CO$_2$ 12 mEq/L	Alk Phos 55 IU/L	Bands 18%	PaO$_2$ 165 mm Hg
BUN 42 mg/dL	T. bili 0.4 mg/dL	Lymphs 5%	HCO$_3$ 9.8 mEq/L
SCr 2.3 mg/dL	AST 15 IU/L	Monos 5%	Lactate 6.3 mmol/L
Glu 195 mg/dL	ALT 10 IU/L	Hgb 12.2 g/dL	
Ca 7.2 mg/dL		Hct 38%	
		Plt 205 × 10^3/mm^3	

■ Urinalysis

Color yellow, appearance cloudy, WBC 120/hpf, RBC 5/hpf, leukocyte esterase (+), nitrite (+), epithelial cells 3–5/hpf, pH 5, bacteria 15/hpf

■ Other

ECG: sinus tachycardia (HR 122), QRS 98/QT-QT$_c$ 358/425

■ Clinical Course

After several hours in the ED, the patient's blood pressure failed to improve despite receiving 2 L of normal saline. Her mental status did not improve, and her urinary output has been approximately 50 mL over past 3 hours (via foley catheter). She was intubated and placed on mechanical ventilation secondary to respiratory failure and concern for airway protection due to her mental status. The intensivist is called to evaluate the patient. The intravenous medications she received in the ED included:

Normal saline 2 L (bolus)

Etomidate 20 mg

Succinylcholine 75 mg

Midazolam 2 mg

Norepinephrine 15 mcg/min continuous infusion begun

Ceftriaxone 2 g × 1 dose

■ Assessment

An 80-year-old woman is admitted to the ICU with concerns of septic shock, respiratory failure, and acute kidney injury secondary to a UTI.

QUESTIONS

Collect Information

1.a. What subjective and objective information indicates the presence of septic shock?

1.b. What additional information is needed to fully assess this patient's septic shock?

Assess the Information

2.a. Assess the severity of septic shock based on the subjective and objective information available.

2.b. Create a list of the patient's drug therapy problems and prioritize them. Include assessment of medication appropriateness, effectiveness, safety, and patient adherence.

2.c. What ethical considerations are applicable to this patient?

Develop a Care Plan

3.a. What are the goals of pharmacotherapy for septic shock in this case?

3.b. What nondrug therapies might be useful for this patient's septic shock?

3.c. What feasible pharmacotherapeutic options are available for treating septic shock?

3.d. Create an individualized, patient-centered, team-based care plan to optimize medication therapy for septic shock and this patient's other drug therapy problems. Include specific drugs, dosage forms, doses, schedules, and durations of therapy.

3.e. What alternatives would be appropriate if the initial care plan fails or cannot be used?

Implement the Care Plan

4.a. What information should be provided to the patient to enhance adherence, ensure successful therapy, and minimize adverse effects?

4.b. Describe how care should be coordinated with other healthcare providers.

Follow-Up: Monitor and Evaluate

5. Explain how to monitor and evaluate the care plan for medication appropriateness, effectiveness, safety, and patient adherence by using clinical and laboratory data, patient feedback, and other information.

■ SELF-STUDY ASSIGNMENTS

1. Review the medical literature supporting use of regular insulin infusions to achieve glycemic control in patients with sepsis focusing on target blood glucose values.

2. Review the medical literature on use of corticosteroids in sepsis focusing on dosing, administration, and diagnosis of sepsis-induced adrenal insufficiency.

CLINICAL PEARL

Antibiograms are an important tool in antimicrobial selection in sepsis syndromes. Patients can present with sepsis from a variety of settings such as the community, nursing home, or in-hospital settings. By knowing the typical resistance patterns of the most common pathogens within a given setting, the most likely beneficial empiric regimen can be selected to ensure coverage of the infecting pathogen.

REFERENCES

1. Singer M, Deutschman C, Seymour CW, et al. The third international consensus definitions for sepsis and septic shock (sepsis-3). JAMA. 2016:315(8):801–810.

2. Evans L, Rhodes A, Alhazzani W, et al. Surviving sepsis campaign: international guidelines for management of sepsis and septic shock 2021. Crit Care Med. 2021;49(11):e1063–e1143.

3. Rivers E, Nguyen B, Havstad S, et al. Early goal-directed therapy in the treatment of severe sepsis and septic shock. N Engl J Med. 2001;345:1368–1377.

4. Yealy D, Kellum J, Huang D, et al. The ProCESS Investigators. A randomized trial of protocol-based care for early septic shock. N Engl J Med. 2014;370:1683–1693.

5. Peake S, Delaney A, Bailey M, et al. Goal-directed resuscitation for patients with early septic shock. N Engl J Med. 2014;371:1496–1506.

6. Mouncey P, Osborn T, Power S, et al. Trial of early, goal-directed resuscitation for septic shock. N Engl J Med. 2015;372:1301–1311.

7. Sprung CL, Annane D, Keh D, et al. Hydrocortisone therapy for patients with septic shock. N Engl J Med. 2008;358:111–124.

8. Annane D, Renault A, Brun-Buisson, C, et al. Hydrocortisone plus fludrocortisone for adults with septic shock. N Engl J Med. 2018;378:809–881.

9. Finfer S, Chittock DR, Su SY, et al; NICE-SUGAR Study Investigators. Intensive versus conventional glucose control in critically ill patients. N Engl J Med. 2009;360:1346–1349.

10. Gupta K, Hooton T, Naber K, et al. International clinical practice guidelines for the treatment of acute uncomplicated cystitis and pyelonephritis in women: a 2010 update by the Infectious Diseases Society of America and the European Society for Microbiology and Infectious Diseases. Clin Infect Dis. 2011;52(5):e103–e120.

142

DERMATOPHYTOSIS

Toeing the Line.................................Level I

Ryan Flynn, PharmD

Natalie R. Tucker, PharmD, BCPS, BCIDP

LEARNING OBJECTIVES

After completing this case study, the reader should be able to:

- Recognize the signs and symptoms of a dermatophyte infection.

- Describe nonpharmacologic options for managing dermatophyte infection.

- Recommend an appropriate treatment plan for a dermatophyte infection.

- Explain the best way for the patient to use a selected antifungal product.

PATIENT PRESENTATION

■ Chief Complaint

"My feet itch."

■ HPI

A 41-year-old man presents to a family medicine clinic because of recent itching on his feet. He is an assistant manager at a local retail store who plays basketball at the YMCA for exercise three times a week. He sweats profusely during games and always showers before going home. He has not changed laundry detergent recently, but he admits that he does not always wash his athletic clothes between workouts. He says his feet have always smelled bad, but he first started to notice the burning and itching about 6 weeks ago. He started applying some deodorizing spray to his feet a week ago, but thus far it has only made a slight improvement in itching. Now his groin is starting to itch as well.

■ PMH

Appendectomy 20 years ago
GERD diagnosed 5 years ago
Type 2 diabetes mellitus diagnosed 1 year ago
Dyslipidemia diagnosed 1 year ago

■ SH

Recent sexual activity (within past month); denies tobacco use; drinks beer on weekends and after games or practice

■ Meds

Pantoprazole 40 mg daily
Simvastatin 20 mg daily
Metformin 500 mg twice daily
Men's multivitamin daily

■ All

Penicillin (rash as a baby)

ROS

Denies fever and chills. Fatigued only after basketball practice. Reports frequent trauma to feet while playing in games. Complains of itching between his toes and groin area.

PE

Gen

An obese, but healthy-looking man wearing sandals, shorts, and a T-shirt. Oriented × 3, normal mood and affect.

VS

BP 118/78 mm Hg, P 60 bpm, RR 18; Wt 105 kg, Ht 5′11″

Skin

Visible regions are soft and moist

HEENT

Normocephalic, PERLA, EOMI, external auditory canals and tympanic membranes clear, hearing grossly; no nasal discharge; oral cavity and pharynx normal, no inflammation, swelling, or lesions

Neck/Lymph Nodes

Neck supple, nontender without lymphadenopathy

Lungs

Clear to auscultation and percussion

CV

Rhythm is regular. Extremities are warm and well perfused.

Abd

Fat rolls can be seen around his belly.

Genit/Rect

Not directly examined, but patient reports pruritus and burning of skin around groin, not on penis or scrotum. Redness can be seen on the medial aspects of the upper thighs.

MS/Ext

Foul-smelling, dry, scaling feet with white flaking between toes. Toenails on both feet appear to have yellow-brown discoloration. The nails of some of the toes are thicker than the rest, particularly on the right foot.

Neuro

CN II–XII normal. Sensation to pain, touch, and proprioception normal.

Labs

None available, but patient states his cholesterol and blood sugars are "good."

Assessment

1. Athlete's foot (tinea pedis)
2. Jock itch (tinea cruris)
3. Possible onychomycosis
4. Unsanitary foot and body hygiene

QUESTIONS

Collect Information

1.a. What subjective and objective information indicates the presence of dermatophytosis?

1.b. What additional information is needed to fully assess this patient's dermatophytosis?

Assess the Information

2.a. Assess the severity of dermatophytosis based on the subjective and objective information available.

2.b. Create a list of the patient's drug therapy problems and prioritize them. Include assessment of medication appropriateness, effectiveness, safety, and patient adherence.

Develop a Care Plan

3.a. What are the goals of pharmacotherapy for dermatophytosis?

3.b. What nondrug therapies might be useful for this patient's dermatophytosis?

3.c. What feasible pharmacotherapeutic options are available for treating dermatophytosis?

3.d. Create an individualized, patient-centered, team-based care plan to optimize medication therapy for dermatophytosis and this patient's other drug therapy problems. Include specific drugs, dosage forms, doses, schedules, and durations of therapy.

Implement the Care Plan

4.a. What information should be provided to the patient to enhance adherence, ensure successful therapy, and minimize adverse effects?

4.b. Describe how care should be coordinated with other healthcare providers.

Follow-Up: Monitor and Evaluate

5. Explain how to monitor and evaluate the care plan for medication appropriateness, effectiveness, safety, and patient adherence by using clinical and laboratory data, patient feedback, and other information.

■ CLINICAL COURSE

The patient returns to your clinic 2 months later. He tells you that his itching has stopped, but his toenails are still thick and crusty. They are also darker yellow than before. He has an appointment with his physician next week.

■ FOLLOW-UP QUESTIONS

1. What is "pulse" therapy for onychomycosis, and what are its advantages and disadvantages?

2. What are the differences between appropriate treatment of onychomycosis and tinea pedis?

3. If itraconazole had been prescribed for this patient, what could be some possible reasons for lack of efficacy?

■ SELF-STUDY ASSIGNMENTS

1. Explain the situations where it is necessary to refer a patient to a physician for the treatment of tinea infections and when oral therapy is preferred over topical agents.

2. Compare the mechanisms of action for the azole and allylamine antifungals.

3. Review the rates and precipitating factors of oral terbinafine- and itraconazole-associated hepatotoxicity.

CLINICAL PEARL

Tinea capitis should be treated with a systemic antifungal as topical agents do not penetrate the hair shaft. Topical products are used during the first 2 weeks only to decrease transmissibility to others.

REFERENCES

1. Sahoo AK, Mahajan R. Management of tinea corporis, tinea cruris, and tinea pedis: a comprehensive review. Indian Dermatol Online J. 2016;7(2):77–86.

2. Westerberg DP, Voyack MJ. Onychomycosis: current trends in diagnosis and treatment. Am Fam Physician. 2013;88(11):762–770.

3. Ely JW, Rosenfeld S, Seabury SM. Diagnosis and management of tinea infections. Am Fam Physician. 2014;90(10):702–710.

4. Gupta AK, Foley KA, Versteeg SG. New antifungal agents and new formulations against dermatophytes. Mycopathologia. 2017;182:127–141.

5. Ameen M, Lear JT, Madan V, Mustapa M, Richardson M. British Association of Dermatologists' guidelines for the management of onychomycosis. Br J Dermatol. 2014;171(5):937–958.

6. Saunders J, Maki K, Koski R, Nybo SE. Tavaborole, efinaconazole, and luliconazole: three new antimycotic agents for the treatment of dermatophytic fungi. J Pharm Pract. 2017;30(6):621–630.

143

BACTERIAL VAGINOSIS

Competition Among Bacteria . . . . Level I

Charles D. Ponte, BSc, PharmD, BC-ADM, BCPS, CDCES, CPE, FADCES, FAPhA, FASHP, FCCP, FNAP

LEARNING OBJECTIVES

After completing this case study, the reader should be able to:

• Identify predisposing factors associated with bacterial vaginosis.

• List the common clinical and diagnostic findings associated with bacterial vaginosis.

• Develop a therapeutic plan for the management of bacterial vaginosis.

• Describe the role of the pharmacist and other healthcare providers in the overall management of infectious vaginitis.

PATIENT PRESENTATION

■ Chief Complaint

"I think I might have a yeast infection."

■ HPI

A 30-year-old female graduate student comes to the family practice center for an acute care visit. She states that 1 month ago she was seen at an urgent care center for severe facial pain and headache. She was diagnosed with an acute sinus infection and given a prescription for a 2-week course of doxycycline (100 mg PO BID). During treatment, she developed a vaginal yeast infection. She self-treated it with a nonprescription antifungal cream that alleviated her symptoms. She states that she completed her course of doxycycline despite some mild diarrhea that she attributed to the drug. Presently, she complains of some mild vaginal discomfort (worse with intercourse) and a "fishy" vaginal odor. Her last period was approximately 5 weeks ago. She admits to inconsistent use of a diaphragm and foam for contraception.

■ PMH

Venereal warts—2011
GERD

■ FH

Noncontributory

■ SH

She is a graduate student in the College of Business and Economics. Has multiple sexual partners (including women); male partners rarely use condoms. Has smoked one pack of cigarettes per day since age 16. Alcohol use consists of a glass of wine nightly and occasional beer. Smokes an occasional marijuana joint.

■ Meds

Prilosec 20 mg PO Q HS
Multivitamin one PO daily
Calcium supplement with vitamin D one PO daily

■ All

Cats (itchy eyes and sneezing); house dust (watery eyes, sneezing); penicillin (hive-like pruritic rash, some tightness in her chest); topical clindamycin (facial rash when used to treat acne 15 years ago)

■ ROS

Noncontributory except that she has noticed a small amount of thin, white mucus on her underclothing and her period is approximately 7 days late.

■ Physical Examination

Limited because of acute visit for specific gynecologic complaint

Gen

Patient is a healthy-appearing 30-year-old woman in NAD.

VS

BP 130/75 mm Hg, P 90 bpm, RR 16, T 37.4°C; Wt 51.5 kg, Ht 5′3″

Genit/Rect

External genitalia WNL; no discharge expressed from the urethra, vagina with a small amount of thin white mucus; positive "whiff" test; pH 5.0. Cervix—not completely visualized; appears clear with a small amount of mucoid discharge from the os. Uterus is slightly enlarged, nontender, retroflexed, no cervical motion tenderness. Adnexa without tenderness or masses.

■ **Labs**

Microscopic examination of vaginal secretions: 20–25 WBC/hpf; 10–15 clue cells/hpf; 0 lactobacilli/hpf; 15–20 squamous epithelial cells/hpf

Serum pregnancy test—negative

■ **Assessment**

Vaginal candidiasis—resolved

Bacterial vaginosis

QUESTIONS

Collect Information

1.a. What subjective and objective information indicates the presence of bacterial vaginosis (consider Table 143-1)?

1.b. What additional information is needed to fully assess this patient's bacterial vaginosis?

Assess the Information

2.a. Assess the severity of bacterial vaginosis based on the subjective and objective information available.

2.b. Create a list of the patient's drug therapy problems and prioritize them. Include assessment of medication appropriateness, effectiveness, safety, and patient adherence.

Develop a Care Plan

3.a. What are the goals of pharmacotherapy for bacterial vaginosis in this case?

3.b. What nondrug therapies might be useful for this patient's bacterial vaginosis?

3.c. What feasible pharmacotherapeutic options are available for treating this patient's bacterial vaginosis?

3.d. Create an individualized, patient-centered, team-based care plan to optimize medication therapy for this patient's drug therapy problems. Include specific drugs, dosage forms, doses, schedules, and durations of therapy.

3.e. What alternatives would be appropriate if the initial care plan fails or cannot be used?

Implement the Care Plan

4.a. What information should be provided to the patient to enhance adherence, ensure successful therapy, and minimize adverse effects?

4.b. Describe how care should be coordinated with other healthcare providers.

Follow-Up: Monitor and Evaluate

5. Explain how to monitor and evaluate the care plan for medication appropriateness, effectiveness, safety, and patient adherence by using clinical and laboratory data, patient feedback, and other information.

■ CLINICAL COURSE

After completion of the treatment that you recommended, the patient returns to the clinic in 10 days for follow-up. She voices no complaints except that she has been experiencing some vaginal itching, dysuria, and continued painful intercourse. Physical examination reveals a thick, whitish material adherent to the vaginal mucosa. The vulva appears erythematous with excoriations on the labia majora. Microscopic analysis of vaginal secretions revealed hyphae and budding yeast. No white cells are noted. Vaginal pH is normal. The patient is diagnosed with vaginal candidiasis.

■ FOLLOW-UP QUESTION

1. What is the most likely cause of this patient's vaginal candidiasis?

■ SELF-STUDY ASSIGNMENTS

1. Discuss management of a patient who fails a specific course of treatment for bacterial vaginosis.

2. Discuss the pros and cons of screening asymptomatic pregnant women for the presence of bacterial vaginosis.

3. Describe the best therapeutic approach for a woman diagnosed with bacterial vaginosis who is breastfeeding her infant.

4. Discuss the role of sexual transmission in the pathogenesis of bacterial vaginosis.

CLINICAL PEARL

Historically, patients prescribed metronidazole were counseled to avoid alcohol. The drug was thought to cause a disulfiram-like reaction leading to flushing, GI distress, sweating, thirst, and blurred vision. Since the drug does not inhibit alcohol dehydrogenase, such a reaction is unlikely and is unsubstantiated in the literature. Advise patients that judicious use of alcohol is probably safe during the administration of metronidazole.

TABLE 143-1	Characteristics of Different Types of Vaginitis			
Characteristic	**Candida**	**Bacterial**	**Trichomonas**	**Chemical**
Pruritus	++	+/−	+/−	++
Erythema	+	+/−	+/−	+
Abnormal discharge	+	+	+/−	−
Viscosity	Thick	Thin	Thick/thin	−
Color	White	Gray	White, yellow, green-gray	−
Odor	None	Foul, "fishy"	Malodorous	−
Description	Curd-like	Homogeneous	Frothy	−
pH	3.8–5.0	>4.5	5.0–7.5	−
Diagnostic tests	Potassium hydroxide preparation shows long, thread-like fibers of mycelia microscopically	(+) "Whiff test," "clue cells"	Pear-shaped protozoa, cervical "strawberry" spots	−

REFERENCES

1. Coudray MS, Madhivanan P. Bacterial vaginosis—a brief synopsis of the literature. Eur J Obstet Gynecol Reprod Biol. 2020;245:143–148.
2. Allsworth JE, Peipert JF. Severity of bacterial vaginosis and the risk of sexually transmitted infection. Am J Obstet Gynecol. 2011;113:e1–e6.
3. Muzny CA, Kardas P. A narrative review of current challenges in the diagnosis and management of bacterial vaginosis. Sex Transm Dis. 2020;47:441–446.
4. Wang Z, He Y, Zheng Y. Probiotics for the treatment of bacterial vaginosis: a meta-analysis. Int J Environ Res Public Health. 2019;16(20):3859.
5. Centers for Disease Control and Prevention. Diseases characterized by vulvovaginal itching, burning, irritation, odor, or discharge. Sexually transmitted diseases treatment guidelines, 2021. MMWR Morb Mortal Wkly Rep. 2021;70:1–187. Available at: *www.cdc.gov/mmwr/volumes/70/rr/pdfs/rr7004a1-H.pdf.* Accessed January 30, 2022.
6. Screening for bacterial vaginosis in pregnant persons to prevent preterm delivery—US Preventive Services Task Force Recommendation Statement. JAMA. 2020;323:1286–1292.

144

CANDIDA VAGINITIS

It's Back. . . . . Level I

Linda Ou, BScPharm, PharmD, MSc

Rebecca M. Law, BScPharm, PharmD

LEARNING OBJECTIVES

After completing this case study, the reader should be able to:

- Distinguish *Candida* vaginitis (vulvovaginal candidiasis, VVC) from other types of vaginitis.

- Recognize when patients with symptoms of vaginitis should be referred to a physician for further evaluation and treatment.

- Recommend an appropriate treatment regimen for a patient with VVC.

- Evaluate appropriate treatment alternatives for a patient with recurrent VVC, while considering issues relating to non-*albicans* VVC.

- Educate patients with vaginitis about proper use of pharmacotherapeutic treatments and nonpharmacologic management strategies.

PATIENT PRESENTATION

Chief Complaint

"I'm having the same problem I had 2 weeks ago, and my doctor is away until next Monday. Can you give me some more of these suppositories?"

HPI

A 32-year-old woman presents to your pharmacy with the above complaint. Upon further questioning, you find that she was diagnosed 3 weeks ago by her physician as having another vaginal *Candida* infection. She was prescribed nystatin suppositories 100,000 units intravaginally for 14 nights, which was the same as what she had been prescribed for her previous episode of vaginal candidiasis 2 months earlier. She stated that she finished the prescription 1 week ago and felt better at the time. However, 3 days ago, she began to notice mild vaginal itching again. She thought it was her new control-top pantyhose and stopped wearing them, but the itching got worse and became more severe with a burning sensation. There was also a white, dry, curd-like vaginal discharge that was nonodorous. This seemed to be identical to what she had experienced 3 weeks ago. Her physician is away until next week, and she wondered if the pharmacy can give her some more suppositories. Last month, she began using tights (with an adjustable waist) to help prevent varicose veins.

PMH

Diabetes type 1 since age 11. Her blood glucose is well controlled, and her physician is keeping a close eye due to her pregnancy.

Recurrent leg ulcers and foot infections for which she has been prescribed antibiotics on a frequent basis. Currently, there are no ulcers or infections, and she is not on antibiotics.

SH

Nonsmoker; drinks alcohol in moderate amounts (one to two drinks maximum) at social functions. She is married and is 7½ months pregnant.

Meds

Insulin glargine 15 units SC Q AM for past year

Insulin lispro 6 units SC 15 minutes prior to breakfast, 8 units 15 minutes prior to lunch, and 10 units 15 minutes prior to dinner, for past 4 months

Maternal multivitamin 1 tablet PO Q AM

All

NKDA

ROS

Not performed

Physical Examination

VS

BP 120/78 mm Hg; Wt 70 kg, Ht 5'5"

Note: No further assessments performed

Labs

Not available

QUESTIONS

Collect Information

1.a. What subjective and objective information indicates the presence of vulvovaginal candidiasis (VVC, *Candida* vaginitis)?

1.b. What additional information is needed to fully assess this patient's VVC?

Assess the Information

2.a. Assess the severity of VVC based on the subjective and objective information available.

TABLE 144-1 Characteristics of Different Types of Vaginitis

Characteristic	*Candida*	Bacterial	*Trichomonas*	Chemical
Pruritus	++	+/–	+/–	++
Erythema	+	+/–	+/–	+
Abnormal discharge	+	+	+/–	–
Viscosity	Thick	Thin	Thick/thin	–
Color	White	Gray	White, yellow, green–gray	–
Odor	None	Foul, "fishy"	Malodorous	–
Description	Curd-like	Homogeneous	Frothy	–
pH	3.8–5.0	>4.5	5–7.5	–
Diagnostic tests	Potassium hydroxide prep. shows long, thread-like fibers of mycelia microscopically	+ Whiff test, clue cells	Pear–shaped protozoa, cervical "strawberry" spots	–

For some discussion of above conditions and diagnostic considerations, see: Diseases characterized by vaginal discharge: vulvovaginal candidiasis. CDC 2015 sexually transmitted diseases treatment guidelines. Available at: *http://www.cdc.gov/std/tg2015/candidiasis.htm* and STI-associated syndromes guide: Vaginitis. Government of Canada. Available at: *www.canada.ca/en/public-health/services/infectious-diseases/sexual-health-sexually-transmitted-infections/canadian-guidelines/sti-associated-syndromes/vaginitis.html*. Accessed March 16, 2022.

2.b. Create a list of the patient's drug therapy problems and prioritize them. Include assessment of medication appropriateness, effectiveness, safety, and patient adherence.

Develop a Care Plan

3.a. What are the goals of pharmacotherapy for VVC in this case?

3.b. What nondrug therapies might be useful for this patient's VVC?

3.c. What feasible pharmacotherapeutic options are available for treating VVC?

3.d. Create an individualized, patient-centered, team-based care plan to optimize medication therapy for this patient's VVC and other drug therapy problems. Include specific drugs, dosage forms, doses, schedules, and durations of therapy.

Implement the Care Plan

4.a. What information should be provided to the patient to enhance adherence, ensure successful therapy, and minimize adverse effects?

4.b. Describe how care should be coordinated with other healthcare providers.

Follow-Up: Monitor and Evaluate

5. Explain how to monitor and evaluate the care plan for medication appropriateness, effectiveness, safety, and patient adherence by using clinical and laboratory data, patient feedback, and other information.

■ CLINICAL COURSE

The recommended treatment was successful. Two months later, the patient had another episode of VVC, which was again successfully treated. She delivered a healthy 7-lb baby boy born at term. A month after that, she had another episode of VVC, and she is now nursing.

■ FOLLOW-UP CASE QUESTION

1. What is the most appropriate course of action for managing this patient's recurrent VVC?

■ SELF-STUDY ASSIGNMENTS

1. Obtain information on tests used to diagnose different types of vaginitis.

2. Compare the retail cost of nonprescription vaginitis treatments in your area.

3. Outline your plans for communicating your treatment recommendations to the patient's physician.

CLINICAL PEARL

Patients with symptoms suggestive of bacterial vaginosis or sexually transmitted infection (eg, fever, abdominal or back pain, foul-smelling discharge) should be referred to a physician for further evaluation and treatment.

REFERENCES

1. Workowski KA, Bachmann LH, Chan PA, et al. Sexually transmitted infections treatment guidelines, 2021. MMWR Recomm Rep. 2021;70(No. RR-4):1–187.
2. STI-associated syndromes guide: vaginitis. Government of Canada. Available at: *www.canada.ca/en/public-health/services/infectious-diseases/sexual-health-sexually-transmitted-infections/canadian-guidelines/sti-associated-syndromes/vaginitis.html*. Accessed March 16, 2022.
3. Falagas ME, Betsi GI, Athanasiou S. Probiotics for prevention of recurrent vulvovaginal candidiasis: a review. J Antimicrob Chemother. 2006;58:266–272.
4. Young G, Jewell D. Topical treatment for vaginal candidiasis (thrush) in pregnancy. Cochrane Database Syst Rev. 2001;(4):CD000225.
5. Sobel JD, Chaim W, Nagappan V, Leaman D. Treatment of vaginitis caused by Candida glabrata: use of topical boric acid and flucytosine. Am J Obstet Gynecol. 2003;189:1297–1300.
6. Wooltorton E. Drug advisory: the interaction between warfarin and vaginal miconazole. CMAJ. 2001;165(7):938.
7. Sanchez JM, Moya G. Fluconazole teratogenicity. Prenat Diagn. 1998;18:862–863.
8. Berard A, Sheehy O, Zhao J-P et al. Associations between low- and high-dose oral fluconazole and pregnancy outcomes: 3 nested case-control studies. CMAJ 2019;191(7):E179–E187.
9. Jick SS. Pregnancy outcomes after maternal exposure to fluconazole. Pharmacotherapy. 1999;19:221–222.
10. Ray D, Goswami R, Banerjee U, et al. Prevalence of Candida glabrata and its response to boric acid vaginal suppositories in comparison with oral fluconazole in patients with diabetes and vulvovaginal candidiasis. Diabetes Care. 2007;30:312–317.

145

INVASIVE FUNGAL INFECTIONS

The Brewer's Yeast .... Level II

Douglas Slain, PharmD, BCPS, FCCP, FASHP

LEARNING OBJECTIVES

After completing this case study, the reader should be able to:

- Construct a prudent empiric antifungal regimen for a patient with candidemia.

- Determine situations in which to use echinocandins for invasive *Candida* infections.

- Discuss how identification of non-albicans *Candida* species can influence antifungal selection.

PATIENT PRESENTATION

■ Chief Complaint

"I am burning up and feel like I have the flu."

■ HPI

A 50-year-old man who has been experiencing fever, chills, and has not been feeling well over the past 4 days was admitted to our hospital yesterday. He was at home receiving home therapy with daptomycin 700 mg IV once daily (day 12 of a 14-day course) via PICC line for MRSA bacteremia, which he developed after having an appendectomy at an outside community hospital about a month ago. During that hospitalization, he also received a course of piper-acillin–tazobactam for appendicitis. His postoperative stay was complicated by a surgical site infection and MRSA bacteremia. He had the catheter removed at that time and was started on vancomycin until he developed a rash and possible neutropenia. He was then switched to (and eventually sent home on) daptomycin. Prior to being discharged from the outside hospital, the patient also received 7 days of fluconazole 200 mg PO daily for a urine sample from a Foley catheter that grew 100,000 colonies/mL of *Candida glabrata*. He never grew *Candida* from any other site.

A set of blood cultures was drawn on this admission to our hospital and is showing no growth at 24 hours. His surgical site does not look infected. His PICC line was removed, and blood and urine cultures were drawn. Piperacillin–tazobactam was added to the dap-tomycin empirically on admission.

■ PMH

GERD
Hyperlipidemia
HTN

■ PSH

S/P hernia repair 2 years ago
S/P appendectomy 1 month ago

■ FH

Father died of CHF; mother still alive with no major medical problems.

■ SH

He is the brewmaster at the local brewery. Married; has four adult children. Denies smoking or excessive ethanol use.

■ Home Meds

Omeprazole 40 mg PO once daily
Simvastatin 40 mg PO once daily
Metoprolol XL 50 mg PO once daily
Ibuprofen 600 mg PO TID PRN

■ All

Vancomycin—reaction: neutropenia and rash.

■ Physical Examination

Gen

Patient is a 50-year-old Caucasian man who is resting somewhat comfortably in bed.

VS

BP 128/85 mm Hg, P 70 bpm, RR 20, T 38.5°C, O_2 sat 97; Wt 125 kg, Ht: 5′11″

Skin

Mildly clammy, no Janeway lesions or Osler nodes

HEENT

PERRLA, EOMI, nares patent

Neck/Lymph Nodes

Neck supple; no lymphadenopathy

Lungs/Thorax

CTA

Heart

ECG: Regular rate and rhythm. No murmurs.

Abd

Bowel sounds present. Last BM yesterday.

GU

Grossly normal, UA pending

MS/Ext

No abnormalities

Neuro

Intact

■ Labs

Na 137 mEq/L	Hgb 12.9 g/dL	WBC 13.4 × 10³/mm³	AST 35 IU/L
K 4.3 mEq/L	Hct 40%	PMNs 70%	ALT 30 IU/L
Cl 99 mEq/L	Plt 332	Bands 8%	Alk phos 140 IU/L
CO₂ 27 mEq/L	× 10³/mm³	Lymphs 16%	T. bili 1.1 mg/dL
BUN 7 mg/dL		Monos 5%	CK 56 IU/L
SCr 0.8 mg/dL		Eos 1%	Lipase 92 IU/L
Glu 98 mg/dL			Amylase 112 IU/L
Mg 2.2 mg/dL			

Serum (1-3)-β-d-glucan: 85 pg/mL (positive)

■ Blood Cultures

No growth at 24 hours

■ Chest X-Ray

No infiltrates

■ Assessment

1. Possible bacterial infection (new source vs nonresponding MRSA bacteremia)

2. Possible fungal infection

■ Plan

1. Continue daptomycin 700 mg IV daily and piperacillin–tazobactam 3.375 mg IV Q 8 H.

2. Start fluconazole 800 mg IV loading dose, then 400 mg IV daily.

3. Order abdominal CT scan.

4. Draw additional blood cultures.

QUESTIONS

Collect Information

1.a. What subjective and objective information indicates the presence of invasive fungal infection?

1.b. What additional information is needed to fully assess this patient's fungal infection?

Assess the Information

2.a. Assess the severity of the possible fungal infection based on the subjective and objective information available.

2.b. Create a list of the patient's drug therapy problems and prioritize them. Include assessment of medication appropriateness, effectiveness, safety, and patient adherence.

Develop a Care Plan

3.a. What are the goals of pharmacotherapy for the fungal infection in this case?

3.b. What nondrug therapies might be useful for this patient's fungal infection?

3.c. What feasible pharmacotherapeutic options are available for treating the fungal infection?

3.d. Create an individualized, patient-centered, team-based care plan to optimize medication therapy for the fungal infection and this patient's other drug therapy problems. Include specific drugs, dosage forms, doses, schedules, and durations of therapy.

Implement the Care Plan

4.a. What information should be provided to the patient to enhance adherence, ensure successful therapy, and minimize adverse effects?

4.b. Describe how care should be coordinated with other healthcare providers.

Follow-Up: Monitor and Evaluate

5. What clinical and laboratory parameters should be used to evaluate the therapy for achievement of the desired therapeutic outcome and to detect or prevent adverse effects?

■ CLINICAL COURSE

The abdominal CT scan showed no signs of intra-abdominal infection. Despite two more days of continued daptomycin therapy, the patient continues to be febrile with leukocytosis, but WBC is slightly improved.

Culture and sensitivity data are now available:

- *Blood cultures* positive at 72 hours (drawn on admission):
  - ✓ PICC line catheter: Rare budding yeast and rare coagulase-negative staphylococci
  - ✓ Left peripheral: Rare budding yeast

The team continued fluconazole and discontinued daptomycin and piperacillin–tazobactam. They also ordered a funduscopic eye exam to check for *Candida* endophthalmitis. A transesophageal echocardiogram (TEE) was ordered and showed no signs of vegetation.

■ FOLLOW-UP QUESTIONS

1. Given the microbiology results at 72 hours, what changes (if any) would you recommend?

2. If the funduscopic eye exam were to suggest endophthalmitis, what therapies would be best for treating the eye infection?

■ SELF-STUDY ASSIGNMENTS

1. Explain how the T2-*Candida* rapid diagnostic test works.

2. Search the medical literature to determine whether any antifungal agents have displayed useful activity against *Candida* in biofilm.

CLINICAL PEARL

Despite the general enhanced in vitro *Candida* activity of voriconazole over fluconazole, therapy with voriconazole may be affected by azole-class resistance mechanisms.

REFERENCES

1. Pappas PG, Kauffman CA, Andes D, et al. Clinical practice guidelines for the management of candidiasis: 2016 update by the Infectious Diseases Society of America. Clin Infect Dis. 2016;62(4):e1–e50.

2. Tortorano AM, Prigitano A, Morroni G, Brescini L, Barchiesi F. Candidemia: evolution of drug resistance and novel therapeutic approaches. Infect Drug Resist. 2021 Dec 19;14:5543–5553.

3. Gubbins PO, Heldenbrand S. Clinically relevant drug interactions of current antifungal agents. Mycoses. 2010;53:95–113.

4. Lionakis MS, Edwards Jr JE. Pathogenesis, diagnosis, and treatment of fungal infections. In: Loscalzo J, Fauci A, Kasper D, Hauser S, Longo D, Jameson J, eds. Harrison's Principles of Internal Medicine. 21st ed. McGraw Hill; 2022. Available at: *https://accesspharmacy-mhmedical-com.soleproxy.hsc.wvu.edu/content.aspx?bookid=3095&sectionid=263965855*. Accessed April 18, 2022.

5. Aguilar-Zapata D, Petraitiene R, Petraitis V. Echinocandins: the expanding antifungal armamentarium. Clin Infect Dis. 2015;61(S6):S604–S611.

6. Mahoney MV, Childs-Kean LM, Khan P, Rivera CG, Stevens RW, Ryan KL. Recent updates in antimicrobial stewardship in outpatient parenteral antimicrobial therapy. Curr Infect Dis Rep. 2021;23(12):24.

7. Khan FA, Slain D, Khakoo RA. Candida endophthalmitis: focus on current and future antifungal treatment options. Pharmacotherapy. 2007 Dec;27(12):1711–1721.

146

INFECTION IN AN IMMUNOCOMPROMISED PATIENT

Making a Rash Decision......................... Level II

Morgan Belling, PharmD, BCOP

Aaron Cumpston, PharmD, BCOP

LEARNING OBJECTIVES

After completing this case study, the reader should be able to:

- Construct a prudent empiric antibiotic regimen for a febrile neutropenic patient.

- Determine appropriate situations to use vancomycin in empiric antimicrobial regimens for treatment of febrile neutropenic episodes.

- Describe situations in which antibiotic monotherapy versus combination therapy would be warranted for empiric treatment of febrile neutropenia.

PATIENT PRESENTATION

■ Chief Complaint

"I have a fever and chills."

■ HPI

A 60-year-old female with a history of IgG kappa multiple myeloma who is undergoing an autologous hematopoietic cell transplant. Her stem cells were collected by peripheral blood collection, which were mobilized with cyclophosphamide and filgrastim. During collection, she developed a vesicular rash involving her left lower abdominal quadrant, which was documented by PCR analysis to be herpes zoster. This was treated with valacyclovir. Her preparative regimen for transplant was high-dose melphalan, followed by stem cell rescue with her peripheral blood stem cells. Eight days after stem cell infusion, she spiked a fever of 38.6°C (101.5°F). She now also complains of chills and nausea.

■ PMH

IgG kappa multiple myeloma
GERD
HTN
Hyperlipidemia
CAD
Peripheral neuropathy
Type 2 DM
Chronic back pain

■ FH

Mother died of CAD at early age; father died at age 67 from lung cancer; has one sister and one brother, both living and well

■ SH

High school cafeteria manager of 22 years; now retired. She is married and lives with her husband. She has three children. Denies smoking or alcohol use.

■ Meds

Esomeprazole 40 mg PO once daily
Atorvastatin 80 mg PO once daily
Fentanyl patch 75 mcg Q 48 H
Gabapentin 800 mg PO TID
Lisinopril 5 mg PO once daily
Metoprolol 75 mg PO BID
Multivitamin PO once daily
Oxycodone IR 15 mg Q 6 H PRN pain
Pioglitazone 15 mg PO once daily
Promethazine 25 mg PO Q 6 H PRN nausea
Valacyclovir 500 mg PO once daily, after previously completing 1000 mg TID × 7 days for treatment course
Fluconazole 400 mg PO once daily
Levofloxacin 500 mg PO once daily
Senna-docusate capsule one PO daily
Filgrastim 480 mcg subcutaneously daily

■ All

Ceftazidime—"bad rash"

■ ROS

(+) Fever/chills, (+) nausea; denies vomiting, cough, diarrhea

■ Physical Examination

Gen

Patient is a 60-year-old female who appears alert and oriented.

VS

BP 115/83 mm Hg, P 115 bpm, RR 16, T 38.6°C; O$_2$ sat 98%; Wt 191 lb, Ht 5'1"

Skin

Warm and dry. No erythema or induration around port on left chest. Resolving herpes zoster rash on abdomen; lesions are crusted and healing.

HEENT

PERRLA, EOMI, (–) tonsillar erythema, (–) rhinorrhea, (–) mucositis

Neck/Lymph Nodes

Neck supple; no lymphadenopathy

Lungs/Thorax

Normal; no wheezes, crackles, or rhonchi

CV

Tachycardic but regular rhythm; no murmurs, rubs, or gallops

Abd

Soft, NT, (+) bowel sounds

Genit/Rect

Deferred

MS/Ext

No deformity, mild weakness, no peripheral edema

Neuro

A&O × 3; CN II–XII grossly intact

■ Labs

Na 135 mEq/L	WBC $0.2 \times 10^3/mm^3$	AST 16 IU/L
K 3.6 mEq/L	Hgb 8.9 g/dL	ALT 15 IU/L
Cl 95 mEq/L	Hct 25.3%	Alk phos 38 IU/L
CO_2 21 mEq/L	Plt $21 \times 10^3/mm^3$	LDH 187 IU/L
BUN 16 mg/dL	ANC $0.05 \times 10^3/mm^3$	T. bili 0.6 mg/dL
SCr 1.0 mg/dL	A1C 6.7%	Albumin 2.8 g/dL
Glu 149 mg/dL		
Ca 8.0 mg/dL		

■ UA

Pending

■ Blood Cultures

PICC line: Pending
Peripheral: Pending

■ Chest X-Ray

Presence of a 2.2-cm oval-shaped density projecting at the level of the retrocardiac aspect of the medial left lung base

■ CT Scan With IV Contrast

Normal, no evidence of pulmonary nodule that was a concern on chest X-ray

■ Assessment

1. Multiple myeloma s/p autologous stem cell transplant
2. Neutropenic fever
3. Concern for possible pneumonia, despite CT scan findings

■ Initial Plan

1. Begin empiric piperacillin–tazobactam 4.5 g IV Q 6 H (infused over 30 minutes).
2. Discontinue prophylactic levofloxacin.
3. Monitor for rash due to history of ceftazidime allergy.
4. Monitor renal function and hydrate with IV fluids due to IV contrast with CT scan.
5. Continue home medications.

QUESTIONS

Collect Information

1.a. What subjective and objective information indicates the presence of neutropenic fever and possible infection?

1.b. What additional information is needed to fully assess this patient's possible infection?

Assess the Information

2.a. Assess the severity of the possible infection based on the subjective and objective information available.

2.b. Create a list of the patient's drug therapy problems and prioritize them. Include assessment of medication appropriateness, effectiveness, safety, and patient adherence.

Develop a Care Plan

3.a. What are the goals of pharmacotherapy for neutropenic fever in this case?

3.b. What nondrug therapies might be useful for this patient's possible infection?

3.c. What feasible pharmacotherapeutic options are available for treating the febrile neutropenic episode?

3.d. Create an individualized, patient-centered, team-based care plan to optimize medication therapy for neutropenic fever and this patient's other drug therapy problems. Include specific drugs, dosage forms, doses, schedules, and durations of therapy.

Implement the Care Plan

4.a. What information should be provided to the patient to enhance adherence, ensure successful therapy, and minimize adverse effects?

4.b. Describe how care should be coordinated with other healthcare providers.

Follow-Up: Monitor and Evaluate

5. Explain how to monitor and evaluate the care plan for medication appropriateness, effectiveness, safety, and patient adherence by using clinical and laboratory data, patient feedback, and other information.

■ CLINICAL COURSE

On day 2 of admission, the patient is still febrile and the following results are reported:

SCr 2.1 mg/dL	Hgb 8.4 g/dL
	Hct 22.8%
	Platelets $9 \times 10^3/mm^3$
	WBC $0.2 \times 10^3/mm^3$
BP 120/75, P 100, RR 18, T 38.3°C, O_2 sat 98% RA	
Urine and blood cultures (PICC line and peripheral): No growth at 24 hours	

The team continued to monitor the patient as planned. The patient started developing a systemic erythematous rash. On day 3, piperacillin–tazobactam was changed to imipenem–cilastatin due to the presumed drug rash. Her rash continued to worsen while taking imipenem. On day 5, the WBC was $0.3 \times 10^3/mm^3$, and caspofungin was added for empiric coverage for persistent fevers. On day 6, her WBC was $0.6 \times 10^3/mm^3$ with an ANC of $0.520 \times 10^3/mm^3$. At this time, blood cultures from the PICC line became positive for Gram-positive cocci in pairs and chains. The team added vancomycin 1500 mg Q 24 H and stopped the imipenem–cilastatin because the rash was still worsening and the patient was no longer neutropenic. The PICC line was removed, and caspofungin was discontinued the next day. Final identification of the organism in the blood was reported on day 8 as *Enterococcus faecalis*, sensitive to ampicillin and vancomycin. The patient became afebrile after initiation of vancomycin. Her creatinine had normalized by this time, she was no longer neutropenic, and her rash was starting to resolve. She was discharged to complete a 2-week course of vancomycin. All subsequent blood and urine cultures were negative for microbial growth.

FOLLOW-UP QUESTIONS

1. What other antibiotic therapies could have been used for the treatment of this patient's bacteremia?

2. What is the possibility of cross-reactivity between ceftazidime and aztreonam?

3. When should vancomycin be considered as an initial empiric agent in febrile neutropenic patients?

SELF-STUDY ASSIGNMENTS

1. Review the criteria for classification of febrile neutropenic patients as either "low" or "high" risk. What types of neutropenic patients would be considered "low risk" and might benefit from oral antibiotic regimens?

2. Construct a treatment algorithm for neutropenic patients with bloodstream infections caused by vancomycin-resistant *Enterococcus faecium* (VRE). The algorithm should include decisions based on renal function and drug contraindications.

CLINICAL PEARL

Bacterial infections in neutropenic patients have evolved from the historical isolation of Gram-negative pathogens to the most common bacteria isolated currently being Gram-positive organisms. This is especially true when fluoroquinolone prophylaxis is used.

REFERENCES

1. Freifeld AG, Bow EJ, Sepkowitz KA, et al. Clinical practice guideline for the use of antimicrobial agents in neutropenic patients with cancer: 2010 update by the Infectious Diseases Society of America. Clin Infect Dis. 2011;52:e56–e93.

2. Taplitz RA, Kennedy EB, Bow EJ, et al. Outpatient management of fever and neutropenia in adults treated for malignancy: American Society of Clinical Oncology and Infectious Diseases Society of America clinical practice guideline update. J Clin Oncol. 2018;36(14):1443–1453.

3. Shenoy ES, Macy E4, Rowe T, Blumenthal KG. Evaluation and management of penicillin allergy: a review. JAMA 2019;321(2):188–199.

4. Mermel LA, Farr BM, Sherertz RJ, et al. Guidelines for the management of intravascular catheter-related infections. Clin Infect Dis. 2009;49:1–45.

5. National Comprehensive Cancer Network (NCCN) Clinical Practice Guidelines in Oncology (v1.2019). Prevention and treatment of cancer-related infections. Available at: *https://www.nccn.org/professionals/physician_gls/pdf/infections.pdf*. Accessed January 30, 2022.

6. Paul M, Dickstein Y, Schlesinger A, Grozinsky-Glasberg S, Soares-Weiser K, Leibovici L. Beta-lactam versus beta-lactam-aminoglycoside combination therapy in cancer patients with neutropenia. Cochrane Database Syst Rev. 2013;29;(6):CD003038.

7. Rutter WC, Cox JN, Martin CA, Burgess DR, Burgess DS. Nephrotoxicity during vancomycin therapy in combination with piperacillin-tazobactam or cefepime. Antimicrob Agents Chemother. 2017;61(2):e02089–16.

8. Gilbert DN, Chambers HF, Eliopoulos GM, Saag MS, Pavia AT, eds. The Sanford Guide to Antimicrobial Therapy 2018. 48th ed. Sperryville, VA: Antimicrobial Therapy; 2018.

9. Terico AT, Gallagher JC. Beta-lactam hypersensitivity and cross-reactivity. J Pharm Pract. 2014;27(6):530–544.

10. Luther MK, Rice LB, LaPlante KL. Ampicillin in combination with ceftaroline, cefepime, or ceftriaxone demonstrates equivalent activities in a high-inoculum *Enterococcus faecalis* infection model. Antimicrob Agents Chemother. 2016 April 22;60(5):3178–3182.

147

ANTIMICROBIAL PROPHYLAXIS FOR SURGERY

Failing to Plan Is Planning to Fail .... Level II

Ryan P. Mynatt, PharmD, BCPS

LEARNING OBJECTIVES

After completing this case study, the reader should be able to:

• Recommend appropriate antimicrobial prophylaxis for a given surgical procedure.

• Discuss the timing of antimicrobial prophylaxis for surgery, including doses prior to and after surgery.

• Describe the controversy regarding mechanical bowel preparation prior to colorectal surgery.

• Identify the pros and cons of using oral antimicrobial decontamination prior to colorectal surgery.

• Evaluate the need for perioperative antiplatelet therapy in a specific surgical patient.

PATIENT PRESENTATION

■ Chief Complaint

"I have colon cancer and I'm here for surgery."

■ HPI

A 72-year-old man was recently diagnosed with anemia and generalized weakness. The patient's workup for anemia included a colonoscopy, which showed a malignant neoplasm of the proximal ascending colon. The neoplasm was identified, and the biopsy revealed moderately differentiated adenocarcinoma. The patient denies any current abdominal pain or change in bowel habits but reports a 20-lb, unintentional weight loss over the past several months. He is eating but has less of an appetite than normal.

■ PMH

Significant for HTN, CAD, TIA, and chronic rhinitis. History of gastritis and anemia.

■ PSH

Tonsillectomy, left inguinal hernia repair, colonoscopy with biopsy

■ SH

Positive for smoking history of one-half of a pack daily; quit 20 years ago

■ Meds

Metoprolol succinate 50 mg PO daily
Hydrochlorothiazide 12.5 mg PO daily
Atorvastatin 40 mg PO daily

Sertraline 100 mg PO daily
Omeprazole 20 mg PO daily
Aspirin 81 mg PO daily
Triamcinolone nasal spray, two sprays in the morning
Ferrous sulfate 325 mg PO TID
Multivitamin one PO once daily

■ All

None

■ ROS

Cardiopulmonary: Denies chest pain, shortness of breath, or wheezing
Gastrointestinal: Denies history of hepatitis, ulcers, or jaundice
Genitourinary: He has no history of hematuria or renal calculi
Psychiatric: Positive for depression

■ Physical Examination

Gen

He has the appearance of a normally developed man who appears his stated age. He is alert, awake, and in no obvious distress.

VS

BP 132/86 mm Hg, P 68 bpm, RR 11, T 37.1°C; Wt 69 kg, Ht 172.7 cm

Skin

Warm and dry. Multiple seborrheic dermatomes over the abdomen and chest.

HEENT

Face reveals no asymmetry. Pupils are equal. Eyes have no icterus or exophthalmus, extraocular movements intact. He is wearing corrective lenses.

Neck/Lymph Nodes

No adenopathy or thyromegaly. There is no jugular venous distention.

Lungs/Thorax

Clear to auscultation

CV

Regular rate and rhythm without murmurs

Abd

The patient has a faint, left inguinal scar from prior left inguinal hernia repair. The abdomen is without palpable masses, splenomegaly, or hepatomegaly. No tenderness noted.

Genit/Rect

Not examined

MS/Ext

No scoliosis. He has mild lordotic and kyphotic components to the vertebral curvature. No paravertebral tenderness or spasm. Leg lengths and shoulder heights are grossly equal. Extremities: no gross deformities, rashes, or ecchymoses. 2+ pulses in all four extremities.

Neuro

No gross motor or sensory deficits or hyperreflexia. Good grip strength bilaterally.

■ Labs

Na 132 mEq/L	Hgb 11.9 g/dL	WBC 6.0×10^3/mm³
K 4.1 mEq/L	Hct 39.2%	PMNs 70%
Cl 97 mEq/L	RBC 4.06×10^6/mm³	Bands 0%
CO$_2$ 26 mEq/L	Plt 324×10^3/mm³	Eos 5%
BUN 14 mg/dL	MCV 84 mcm³	Lymphs 13%
SCr 0.9 mg/dL	MCHC 34.8 g/dL	Monos 12%
Glu 93 mg/dL		
Alb 3.9 g/dL		

■ Assessment

1. Adenocarcinoma of the proximal ascending colon
2. Right hemicolectomy planned

QUESTIONS

Collect Information

1.a. Do guidelines recommend antimicrobial prophylaxis for the surgical procedure planned for this patient?

1.b. What additional information is needed to fully assess this patient's need for surgical antimicrobial prophylaxis?

Assess the Information

2.a. Based on the planned surgical procedure, what is the risk for a surgical wound infection in this patient postoperatively?

2.b. Create a list of the patient's drug therapy problems and prioritize them, including potential postoperative problems.

2.c. Will a mechanical bowel preparation prior to surgery benefit this patient?

2.d. What are the potential advantages and disadvantages associated with giving oral antibiotics prior to a colorectal surgical procedure?

Develop a Care Plan

3.a. What are the goals of antimicrobial pharmacotherapy for preventing a surgical wound infection?

3.b. What nondrug therapies might be useful for this patient?

3.c. What feasible pharmacotherapeutic options are available for surgical prophylaxis for this patient's type of surgery?

3.d. Create an individualized, patient-centered, team-based care plan to optimize medication therapy for this patient's drug therapy problems. Include specific drugs, dosage forms, doses, schedules, and durations of therapy.

Implement the Care Plan

4.a. What information should be provided to this patient regarding the risk of surgical wound infections and the use of antibiotics to prevent this risk?

4.b. Describe how care should be coordinated with other healthcare providers.

Follow-Up: Monitor and Evaluate

5. Explain how to monitor and evaluate the care plan for medication appropriateness, effectiveness, safety, and patient adherence by using clinical and laboratory data, patient feedback, and other information.

■ SELF-STUDY ASSIGNMENTS

1. Construct a chart listing surgical procedures requiring preoperative antimicrobial prophylaxis and the recommended agent(s) to use.

2. Perform a literature search and assess the current information regarding use of oral antibiotics and mechanical bowel preparations prior to colorectal surgery.

3. Perform a literature search and assess the current information regarding using antiplatelets perioperatively (based on both patient characteristics and surgical procedure).

4. Perform a literature search and assess the current information regarding the need to consider the impact of antimicrobial resistant pathogens on perioperative antimicrobial therapy (based on presumed pathogen and surgical procedure).

CLINICAL PEARL

Patients who receive antibiotics for surgical prophylaxis within 3 hours after the surgical incision have a three times higher risk of surgical wound infection compared to patients who receive antibiotics within 2 hours before the incision.

ACKNOWLEDGMENT

This case is based on the patient case written for the 11th edition by Curtis L. Smith, PharmD, FCCP, BCPS.

REFERENCES

1. Nelson RL, Gladman E, Barbateskovic M. Antimicrobial prophylaxis for colorectal surgery. Cochrane Database Syst Rev. 2014 May 9;5:CD001181.
2. Hawn MT, Richman JS, Vick CC, et al. Timing of surgical antibiotic prophylaxis and the risk of surgical site infection. JAMA Surg. 2013;148(7):649–657.
3. Bratzler DW, Dellinger EP, Olsen KM, et al. Clinical practice guidelines for antimicrobial prophylaxis in surgery. Am J Health Syst Pharm. 2013;70:195–283.
4. Fleisher LA, Fleischmann KE, Auerbach AD, et al. 2014 ACC/AHA guideline on perioperative cardiovascular evaluation and management of patients undergoing noncardiac surgery: a report of the American College of Cardiology/American Heart Association Task Force on Practice Guidelines. Circulation. 2014;130(24):e278–e333.
5. Levine GN, Bates ER, Bittl JA, et al. 2016 ACC/AHA guideline focused update on duration of dual antiplatelet therapy in patients with coronary artery disease: a report of the American College of Cardiology/American Heart Association Task Force on Clinical Practice Guidelines: an update of the 2014 ACC/AHA guideline on perioperative cardiovascular evaluation and management of patients undergoing noncardiac surgery. Circulation. 2016;134(10):e123–e155.
6. Deveraux PJ, Mirkobrada M, Sessler DI, et al. Aspirin in patients undergoing noncardiac surgery. N Engl J Med. 2014;370:1484–1503.
7. Gould MK, Garcia DA, Wren SM, et al. American College of Chest Physicians. Prevention of VTE in nonorthopedic surgical patients: Antithrombotic Therapy and Prevention of Thrombosis, 9th ed. American College of Chest Physicians Evidence-Based Clinical Practice Guidelines. Chest 2012;141(2 Suppl):e227S–e277S.
8. Rollins KE, Javanmard-Emamghissi H, Lobo DN. Impact of mechanical bowel preparation in elective colorectal surgery: a meta-analysis. World J Gastroenterol. 2018;24(4):519–536.
9. Classen DC, Evans RS, Pestotnik SL, Horn SD, Menlove RL, Burke JP. The timing of prophylactic administration of antibiotics and the risk of surgical-wound infection. N Engl J Med. 1992;326:281–286.
10. Berríos-Torres SI, Umscheid CA, Bratzler DW, et al. Centers for Disease Control and Prevention guideline for the prevention of surgical site infection, 2017. JAMA Surg. 2017;152(8):784–791.

148

PEDIATRIC IMMUNIZATION

Back to School.................................. Level II

Jean-Venable "Kelly" R. Goode, PharmD, BCPS, FAPhA, FCCP

LEARNING OBJECTIVES

After completing this case study, the reader should be able to:

• Develop a plan for administering any needed vaccines when given a patient's age, immunization history, and medical history.

• Describe appropriate use of pediatric vaccines.

• Educate a child's parents on the risks associated with pediatric vaccines and ways to minimize adverse effects.

• Recognize inappropriate reasons for deferring immunization.

PATIENT PRESENTATION

■ Chief Complaint

"My daughter is here for the 'Back to School' program."

■ HPI

A 5-year-old girl who is generally healthy presents today (August 30, 2022) to the pharmacy with her mother for evaluation and to receive any needed immunizations. She will be entering kindergarten in the fall, and she needs to have an updated immunization record.

■ PMH

Received prenatal care, delivered at 42 weeks' gestation via uncomplicated vaginal delivery; birth weight 7 lb, 4 oz. Mother states that her child has had a couple of ear infections (currently on day 4 of treatment) and three or four "colds," no other illnesses.

■ FH

Mother is 4 months pregnant.

■ SH

Lives with mother, age 30, and father, age 32. No siblings. Mother works part-time. Father works as an electrician. Both parents are Baptist.

■ Meds

Amoxicillin suspension 540 mg PO Q 8 H
No recent OTC medication use

All

NKDA

ROS

Negative

Physical Examination

Gen

Alert, happy, appropriately developed 5-year-old child in NAD.

VS

BP 105/65 mm Hg, P 110 bpm, RR 28, T 36.7°C (axillary); Wt 18 kg (75th percentile), Ht 40 in (50th percentile).

HEENT

AF open, flat; PERRL; funduscopic exam not performed; ears slightly red; normal looking TMs, landmarks visualized, no effusion present; nose clear; throat normal

Lungs

Clear bilaterally

CV

RRR, no murmurs

Abd

Soft, nontender, no masses or organomegaly; normal bowel sounds

Genit/Rect

Normal external genitalia; rectal exam deferred, no fissures noted

Ext

Normal

Neuro

Alert; normal DTRs bilaterally

Labs

See Table 148-1 for immunization record card.
No other labs obtained

TABLE 148-1 Immunization Record Card

Immunization Record Card Name: Allison Showalter				
Vaccine	**Dose/Route/Site**	**Date**	**Health Professional**	**VIS**
Hepatitis B	0.5 mL IM thigh	3/15/2017	Colter, RN	Hep B
Pediarix (DTaP, Hep B, IPV)	0.5 mL IM thigh	5/20/2017	Edwards, RN	DTaP, Hep B, IPV
PCV-13	0.5 mL IM thigh	5/20/2017	Edwards, RN	PCV
Hib (HibTITER)	0.5 mL IM thigh	5/20/2017	Edwards, RN	Hib
Pediarix	0.5 mL IM thigh	7/29/2017	Edwards, RN	DTaP, Hep B, IPV
PCV-13	0.5 mL IM thigh	7/29/2017	Edwards, RN	PCV
Hib (HibTITER)	0.5 mL IM thigh	7/29/2017	Edwards, RN	Hib
Pediarix	0.5 mL IM thigh	9/30/2017	Jones, RN	DTaP, Hep B, IPV
PCV-13	0.5 mL IM thigh	9/30/2017	Jones, RN	PCV
Hib (HibTITER)	0.5 mL IM thigh	9/30/2017	Jones, RN	Hib
Hib (HibTITER)	0.5 mL IM thigh	4/1/2018	Edwards, RN	Hib
PCV-13	0.5 mL IM thigh	4/1/2018	Edwards, RN	PCV

Assessment

Normal-appearing child, in need of immunizations

QUESTIONS

Collect Information

1.a. What subjective and objective information indicates needs, precautions, or contraindications to immunization?

1.b. What additional information is needed to fully assess this patient?

Assess the Information

2.a. How do healthcare providers determine which vaccines an infant or child needs?

2.b. Assess the urgency of the immunization needs based on the subjective and objective information available.

2.c. Create a list of the patient's drug therapy and immunization-related problems. Include assessment of medication appropriateness, effectiveness, safety, patient adherence, and any contraindications or precautions for vaccination.

2.d. What economic, psychosocial, cultural, and ethical considerations are applicable to this patient?

Develop a Care Plan

3.a. What are the goals of pharmacotherapy in this case?

3.b. What feasible pharmacotherapeutic options are available for pediatric immunizations?

3.c. Create an individualized, patient-centered, team-based care plan to optimize immunizations for this patient. Include the vaccines that should be administered to this child today, including dose, route, and schedule.

Implement the Care Plan

4.a. What information should be provided to the patient and parents/caregivers to enhance adherence, ensure successful therapy, and minimize adverse effects?

4.b. Describe how care should be coordinated with other healthcare providers.

Follow-Up: Monitor and Evaluate

5. Explain how to monitor and evaluate the care plan for response to immunization and to detect or prevent adverse reactions and appropriate follow-up for additional immunizations and achievement of a fully immunized patient.

ADDITIONAL CASE QUESTIONS

1. The next year, the mother brings the child to a pediatric influenza immunization clinic stating that the child was diagnosed with diabetes about 3 months ago. The child's immunization record reveals influenza vaccine 0.5 mL × 1 dose last fall. What is your recommendation for influenza vaccination for this child?

2. What other immunizations are indicated for this child who now has a chronic condition, diabetes mellitus?

3. What is the proper immunization administration technique for children, including location and needle size?

■ SELF-STUDY ASSIGNMENTS

1. Search the Internet for the immunization laws and allowed exemptions in your state. What vaccines are required for child-care and school entry?

2. Review the most current immunization recommendations for persons aged 0–18 years, and provide a summary of how your recommendations for this case would be different if a 6-month-old patient in need of immunizations came to your clinic today.

3. Search the Internet for immunization-related websites about vaccine-associated adverse effects; compare these sites and evaluate them against reliable websites for vaccine information.

CLINICAL PEARL

Pediatric patients may receive multiple vaccinations at the same visit, vaccines should never be mixed in the same syringe (unless manufactured as a combination vaccine), but should be administered using separate syringes, needles, and sites. Vaccinations should be administered on time to protect children against vaccine-preventable diseases.

REFERENCES

1. Centers for Disease Control and Prevention. Advisory Committee on Immunization Practices (ACIP). Recommended immunization schedules for persons aged 0–18 years—United States, 202. Available at (updated annually): *http://www.cdc.gov/vaccines/schedules/hcp/child-adolescent.html*. Accessed January 9, 2022.

2. Ventola CL. Immunization in the United States: recommendations, barriers, and measures to improve compliance. Part 1: childhood vaccinations. Pharmacol Ther. 2016;41(7):426–436.

3. Liang JL, Tiwari T, Moro P, et al. Prevention of pertussis, tetanus, and diphtheria with vaccines in the United States: recommendations of the Advisory Committee on Immunization Practices (ACIP). MMWR Recomm Rep. 2018;67(2):1–44.

4. Marin M, Broder KR, Temte JL, et al. Use of combination measles, mumps, rubella, and varicella vaccine. Recommendations of the Advisory Committee on Immunization Practices (ACIP). MMWR Recomm Rep. 2010;59:(RR-3)1–12.

5. Centers for Disease Control and Prevention. Interim clinical considerations for use of COVID-19 vaccines currently approved or authorized in the United States. January 6, 2022. Accessed January 9, 2022.

6. Das RR, Panigrahi I, Naik SS. The effect of prophylactic antipyretic administration on post-vaccination adverse reactions and antibody response in children: a systematic review. PLoS One. 2014;9(9):e106629.

7. Kroger A, Bahta L, Hunter P. General Best Practice Guidelines for Immunization. Best Practices Guidance of the Advisory Committee on Immunization Practices (ACIP). Available at: *https://www.cdc.gov/vaccines/hcp/acip-recs/general-recs/index.html*. Accessed January 9, 2022.

8. Grohskopf LA, Alyanak E, Ferdinands JM, et al. Prevention and control of seasonal influenza with vaccines: recommendations of the Advisory Committee on Immunization Practices—United States, 2021–22 Influenza Season. MMWR Recomm Rep. 2021;70(5):1–28.

9. Centers for Disease Control and Prevention. Prevention of pneumococcal disease among infants and children—use of 13-valent pneumococcal conjugate vaccine and 23-valent pneumococcal polysaccharide vaccine. MMWR. 2010;59(RR-11):1–18.

149

ADULT IMMUNIZATION

Immunizations: Not Just Kid Stuff . . . . Level II

Jean-Venable "Kelly" R. Goode, PharmD, BCPS, FAPhA, FCCP

LEARNING OBJECTIVES

After completing this case study, the reader should be able to:

- Develop a plan for administering any needed vaccines when given a patient's age, immunization history, and medical history.

- Recognize appropriate precautions and contraindications for vaccination, including inappropriate reasons for deferring vaccination.

- Explain appropriate administration of vaccines, including timing and spacing of both inactive and live attenuated vaccines.

- Recognize the differences in vaccines for young adults currently in use in the United States.

PATIENT PRESENTATION

■ Chief Complaint

"I'm here to get my new prescription filled."

■ HPI

A 23-year-old woman presents to your pharmacy in January with a new prescription for prednisone 40 mg PO BID for 10 days. She has had a moderate asthma exacerbation. She just started her new job as an elementary school teacher. She is a new patient to your pharmacy. She inquires about your "One Less" signs which refer to a national HPV vaccination campaign.

■ PMH

Moderate persistent asthma
Chickenpox at age 5 per patient
Splenectomy secondary to car accident 3 months ago

■ FH

One sister who is healthy; mother is healthy; father has type 2 diabetes.

■ SH

Does not smoke; drinks alcohol socially; has healthcare coverage through her employer; religious affiliation is Baptist.

■ Meds

Albuterol MDI two inhalations PRN
Pulmicort DPI two inhalations once daily

■ All

NKDA

■ **Immunization Record**

No vaccines since kindergarten except:

- Meningococcal vaccine before she started her freshman year in college
- One dose of hepatitis B vaccine before she started her freshman year in college
- MMR vaccine before she started her freshman year in college
- Td 10 years ago at her adolescent well checkup

■ **ROS**

WDWN woman in NAD

■ **Physical Examination**

Deferred

VS

BP 120/72 mm Hg (left arm, large cuff, seated), P 76 bpm; Wt 54 kg, Ht 5′5″

■ **Assessment**

A 23-year-old woman recently treated for a moderate asthma exacerbation. She is in need of immunizations today.

QUESTIONS

Collect Information

1.a. What subjective and objective information indicates needs, precautions, or contraindications to immunization?

1.b. What additional information is needed to fully assess this patient?

Assess the Information

2.a. How do healthcare providers determine which vaccines an adult needs?

2.b. Assess the urgency of the immunization needs based on the subjective and objective information available.

2.c. Create a list of the patient's drug therapy and immunization-related problems. Include assessment of medication appropriateness, effectiveness, safety, patient adherence, and including any contraindications or precautions for vaccination.

2.d. What economic and psychosocial considerations are applicable to this patient?

Develop a Care Plan

3.a. What are the goals of pharmacotherapy in this case?

3.b. What feasible options are available for adult immunizations?

3.c. Create an individualized, patient-centered, team-based care plan to optimize medication therapy and immunizations for this patient. Include the vaccines that should be administered today, including dose, route, and schedule.

Implement the Care Plan

4.a. What information should be provided to the patient to enhance adherence, ensure successful therapy, and minimize adverse effects?

4.b. Describe how care should be coordinated with other healthcare providers.

Follow-Up: Monitor and Evaluate

5. Explain how to monitor and evaluate the care plan for response to immunization and to detect or prevent adverse reactions and appropriate follow-up for additional immunizations and achievement of a fully immunized patient.

■ **ADDITIONAL CASE QUESTIONS**

1. What screening questions should a patient be asked prior to administering any vaccinations?

2. What must be documented after a healthcare practitioner administers a vaccination?

3. What is the proper immunization administration technique for adults, including location and needle size?

■ **SELF-STUDY ASSIGNMENTS**

1. Review the most current immunization recommendations for adults and provide a summary of how your recommendations for this case would be different if this person were 65 years of age.

2. Develop a list of diseases and medications indicating that a patient may be a candidate for immunization.

3. Research the laws in your state to verify which vaccines pharmacists may administer. Also, explore how to implement an immunization service in your practice.

4. Review the guidelines for vaccination of pregnant women.

5. Search the Internet for immunization-related websites about vaccine-associated adverse reactions; compare these sites and evaluate them against reliable websites for vaccine information.

CLINICAL PEARL

Delays in vaccination put patients at risk of vaccine-preventable diseases. However, there is no need to restart an immunization series if the interval between doses is longer than that recommended in the routine schedule. Instead of starting over, merely count the doses administered (provided that they were given at an acceptable minimum interval) and complete the series.

REFERENCES

1. Centers for Disease Control and Prevention. Advisory Committee on Immunization Practices. Recommended adult immunization schedule for immunization schedules for adults aged 19 years and older—United States, 2021. Available at (updated annually): *https://www.cdc.gov/vaccines/schedules/hcp/adult.html*. Accessed February 13, 2022.

2. Kobayashi M, Farrar JL, Gierke R, et al. Use of 15-valent pneumococcal conjugate vaccine and 20-valent pneumococcal polysaccharide vaccine among U.S. adults: updated recommendations of the Advisory Committee on Immunization Practices (ACIP). MMWR. 2032;71(4):109–117.

3. Mbaeyi SA, Bozio CH, Duffy J, et al. Meningococcal vaccination: Recommendations of the Advisory Committee on Immunization Practices (ACIP), United States, 2020. MMWR. 2020;69(9):1–41.

4. Centers for Disease Control and Prevention. Interim clinical considerations for use of COVID-19 vaccines currently approved or authorized in the United States. February 11, 2022. Accessed February 13, 2022.

5. Recommendations from the National Vaccine Advisory Committee: Standards for Adult Immunization Practices. Public Health Reports 2014 March–April;129:115–123.

6. Meites E, Szilagyi PG, Chesson HW, et al. Human papillomavirus vaccination for adults: updated recommendations of the Advisory Committee on Immunization Practices. MMWR. 2019;68(32):698–702.

7. Havers FP, Moro P, Hunter P, et al. Use of tetanus toxoid, reduced diphtheria toxoid, and acellular pertussis vaccines: updated recommendations of the Advisory Committee on Immunization Practices (ACIP)—United Staes, 2019. MMWR. 2020;69(3):77–83.

8. Centers for Disease Control and Prevention. Prevention and control of *Haemophilus influenza* type B disease: recommendations of the Advisory Committee on Immunization Practices (ACIP). MMWR. 2014;63(RR01):1–14.

9. Grohskopf LA, Alyanak E, Ferdinands JM, et al. Prevention and control of seasonal influenza with vaccines: recommendations of the Advisory Committee on Immunization Practices—United States 2021–22 Influenza Season. MMWR. 2021;70(5):1–28.

150

HIV INFECTION

The Antiretroviral-Naïve Patient . . . . Level II

Rodrigo M. Burgos, PharmD, MPH

Sarah M. Michienzi, PharmD, BCPS, AAHIVP

LEARNING OBJECTIVES

After completing this case study, the reader should be able to:

- Describe when antiretroviral therapy should be initiated in patients living with HIV.

- List the treatment goals of antiretroviral therapy.

- Design an appropriate antiretroviral regimen for an antiretroviral-naïve person living with HIV based on patient-specific data.

- Provide patient education on recommended antiretroviral agents to ensure adherence and minimize adverse reactions.

PATIENT PRESENTATION

Chief Complaint

"I am here for regular care. It hurts to swallow."

HPI

A 34-year-old woman, diagnosed with HIV infection 2 years ago during a routine exam, presents to the HIV Specialty Clinic for follow-up. She was asymptomatic at the time of diagnosis. She is currently antiretroviral therapy (ART) naïve, and since her diagnosis she has been following up regularly every 6 months. However, up to this point, she has not been ready to commit to ART. Today she reports painful and difficult swallowing over the past 2–3 weeks.

PMH

HIV positive, diagnosed 2 years ago; risk factor heterosexual contact

FH

Noncontributory

SH

Never used drugs or smoked cigarettes; 1–2 alcoholic drinks on weekends; unemployed, lives with partner; sexually active with stable HIV (-) partner, aware of her HIV status, 100% condom use

Medications

Oral contraceptive one tablet PO daily

All

TMP/SMX (rash)

ROS

Difficulty and pain on swallowing

Physical Examination

Gen

Well-developed woman in NAD, alert and oriented × 3

VS

BP 110/64 mm Hg, P 80 bpm, RR 18, T 35.9°C; Wt 58 kg, Ht 5'5"

Skin

Anicteric, no skin lesions noted

HEENT

(+) Oral lesions and white plaques, sinuses nontender, PERRLA, ears and nose clear

Neck/Lymph Nodes

Supple, no thyromegaly, (+) bilateral cervical lymph nodes 0.7 cm in diameter

Chest

Lungs clear to auscultation

Breasts

Soft and nontender without masses, discharge, or other lesions noted

CV

S_1, S_2 without S_3, S_4, or murmur

Abd

(+) BS, soft, nontender, without HSM; (+) bilateral inguinal lymph nodes 0.5 cm in diameter

Genit/Rect

WNL, no grossly visible lesions

MS/Ext

No wasting, no CCE

Neuro

No focal deficits

Labs

See Table 150-1.

Assessment

A 34-year-old ART-naïve woman living with HIV shows steady decline in CD4 cell count and rising levels of HIV viremia since

TABLE 150-1 Laboratory Values for the Previous Visit and for Subsequent Visits

Parameter (Units)	2 Years Ago	This Visit	6 Weeks Later	12 Weeks Later
Weight (kg)	65	58	57	60
Hematology:				
Hgb (g/dL)	10.9	11.1	12.2	12.9
Hct (%)	32.9	33.6	36.5	37.3
Plt (×10³/mm³)	234	287	298	311
WBC (×10³/mm³)	7.1	5.7	6.9	7.1
Lymphs (%)	47.3	45.5	44.9	47.3
Monos (%)	6.4	6.6	6.1	6.4
Eos (%)	3.5	0.9	2.0	3.5
Basos (%)	0.3	0.2	0.4	0.3
Neutros (%)	42.5	46.8	46.6	42.5
ANC (×10³/mm³)	3.0	2.7	3.2	3.0
Chemistry:				
BUN (mg/dL)	5	10	9	7
SCr (mg/dL)	0.8	0.9	0.9	0.8
T. bili (mg/dL)	0.5	1.6	0.6	–
Alb (g/dL)	3.3	3.8	3.4	–
AST (IU/L)	17	19	18	–
ALT (IU/L)	12	13	14	–
Fasting glucose	115	93	92	
Fasting lipid profile:				
T. chol	–	115	155	–
Triglycerides	–	41	93	–
LDL	–	67	108	–
HDL	–	40	28	–
Surrogate markers:				
CD4 (%)	20	12	–	13
CD4 (cells/mm³)	377	180	–	200
HIV RNA (RT-PCR)[a] (copies/mL)	25,000	155,000	154	<20
Antiviral resistance test (genotypic resistance test)	L63P	–	–	–
Serologies:				
HBV surface Ab	Negative	–	–	–
HBV core Ab total	Negative	–	–	–
HBV surface Ag	Negative	–	–	–
HCV Ab	Negative	–	–	–
HAV Ab	Positive	–	–	–
Measles Ab	Positive			
Mumps Ab	Positive			
Rubella Ab	Positive			
Other tests:				
Human chorionic gonadotropin (hCG)	Negative	Negative		
G6PD	Not deficient			
HLA-B*5701	Negative			

[a]Reverse transcriptase polymerase chain reaction assay.

her initial diagnosis 2 years ago, presenting with painful swallowing and white plaques on posterior pharynx, and mouth consistent with esophageal and oropharyngeal candidiasis.

QUESTIONS

Collect Information

1.a. What subjective and objective information indicates the presence of HIV/AIDS?

1.b. What additional information is needed to fully assess this patient's HIV/AIDS?

Assess the Information

2.a. Assess the severity of HIV/AIDS based on the subjective and objective information available.

2.b. Create a list of the patient's HIV-related drug therapy problems and prioritize them. Include assessment of medication appropriateness, effectiveness, safety, and patient adherence.

2.c. What economic, psychosocial, and ethical considerations are applicable to this patient?

Develop a Care Plan

3.a. What are the goals of pharmacotherapy for the HIV-related drug therapy in this case?

3.b. What nondrug therapies might be useful for this patient's HIV?

3.c. What feasible pharmacotherapeutic options are available for treating HIV?

3.d. Create an individualized, patient-centered, team-based care plan to optimize medication therapy for the HIV-related drug therapy problems. Include specific drugs, dosage forms, schedules, and durations of therapy.

Implement the Care Plan

4.a. What information should be provided to the patient to enhance adherence, ensure successful therapy, and minimize adverse effects?

4.b. Describe how care should be coordinated with other healthcare providers.

Follow-Up: Monitor and Evaluate

5. Explain how to monitor and evaluate the care plan for medication appropriateness, effectiveness, safety, and patient adherence by using clinical and laboratory data, patient feedback, and other information.

■ CLINICAL COURSE

The patient and care team accepted your treatment recommendations. The patient returns to the clinic for follow-up 6 and 12 weeks after treatment initiation. She reports nausea from her medications that resolved after several days of therapy. See Table 150-2 for her treatment flow sheet.

■ FOLLOW-UP CASE QUESTIONS

1. Provide an assessment of the ART regimen efficacy at each follow-up visit.

2. Identify potential problems with her concomitant medications and discuss alternatives.

■ SELF-STUDY ASSIGNMENTS

1. Review the current literature regarding management of treatment-experienced patients living with HIV in the setting of virologic failure and optimizing ART in the setting of virologic suppression.

2. Review the current literature regarding development of resistance to ART and strategies for preventing and managing resistance.

3. Review the current literature regarding survival and life expectancy for persons living with HIV/AIDS.

TABLE 150-2 Laboratory Values

Parameter	6 Weeks Later	12 Weeks Later
HIV RNA (RT-PCR) (copies/mL)	154	<20
CD4-lymphocyte count (cells/mm³)	NA	200
CD4-lymphocyte percent (%)	NA	13
Symptoms of HIV infection	Asymptomatic	Asymptomatic
Adverse events reported	Mild nausea, no vomiting	None
Concomitant medications	Oral contraceptive 1 tablet PO daily Dapsone 100 mg PO daily	Oral contraceptive 1 tablet PO daily Dapsone 100 mg PO daily

CLINICAL PEARL

Current guidelines recommend that ART be initiated in all patients living with HIV, regardless of CD4 count, to prevent transmission and improve clinical outcomes. In addition to medication potency and efficacy, clinicians should always individualize therapeutic choices based on available data and unique patient factors, including comorbid conditions, transmitted viral resistance, adherence, potential adverse reactions, drug–drug or drug–food interactions, and consequences of virologic failure.

REFERENCES

1. Centers for Disease Control and Prevention. Revised surveillance case definitions for HIV infection—United States, 2014. MMWR. 2014;63(RR-03):1–10.
2. Centers for Disease Control and Prevention. Appendix: Stage-3-defining opportunistic illness in HIV infection. MMWR. 2014;563(RR-03):11.
3. Panel on Guidelines for the Prevention and Treatment of Opportunistic Infections in Adults and Adolescents with HIV. Guidelines for the prevention and treatment of opportunistic infections in HIV-infected adults and adolescents: recommendations from the Centers for Disease Control and Prevention, the National Institutes of Health, and the HIV Medicine Association of the Infectious Diseases Society of America. Available at: *https://clinicalinfo.hiv.gov/en/guidelines/adult-and-adolescent-opportunistic-infection*. Accessed April 5, 2022.
4. Panel on Antiretroviral Guidelines for Adults and Adolescents. Guidelines for the use of antiretroviral agents in adults and adolescents with HIV. Department of Health and Human Services. Available at: *https://clinicalinfo.hiv.gov/en/guidelines/adult-and-adolescent-arv*. Accessed April 5, 2022.
5. Anon. U=U taking off in 2017. Lancet HIV. 2017;4(11):e475.

151

BREAST CANCER

An Opportunity Lost............................ Level II

Jonathan W. Malara, PharmD, BCOP

Caroline Quinn, PharmD, BCOP

LEARNING OBJECTIVES

After completing this case study, the reader should be able to:

- Design a pharmacotherapeutic plan for treatment of locally advanced breast cancer.

- Develop an appropriate monitoring plan for patients receiving adjuvant hormonal therapy for treatment of breast cancer.

- Establish appropriate follow-up for patients after definitive treatment of breast cancer.

- Provide patient education on the proper dosing, administration, and adverse effects of letrozole and palbociclib.

- Compare and contrast the goals of treatment for locally advanced breast cancer versus metastatic breast cancer.

PATIENT PRESENTATION

■ Chief Complaint

"I have a lump in my breast."

■ HPI

A 61-year-old woman presents to the oncology clinic for evaluation of a new mass in her left breast. She first noticed a palpable breast mass on self-examination approximately 14 months ago but was unable to have it further investigated due to loss of health insurance. The patient describes the mass as intermittently painful. A mammogram was performed prior to her current visit, which was suspicious for malignancy.

■ PMH

Musculoskeletal injury 6 years ago. Fell from a chair while at work and suffered injuries to her cervical spine. The patient has required bone grafting from her right hip to her cervical spine. She has been prescribed multiple as-needed medications for pain control but uses them infrequently.

Depression (diagnosed 7 years ago)

■ FH

Sister diagnosed with breast cancer at age 60, now 5 years postsurgery. The patient was unable to recall any further details. No other significant cancer history is noted.

■ SH

Lives with and acts as primary caretaker for her mother, who has dementia. Denies alcohol use and is a nonsmoker. Has a 35-year-old daughter who also lives with her.

■ Endocrine History

Menarche age 13; menopause age 55; first child age 26; $G_1P_1A_0$. Last Pap smear at age 40. Took Premarin as HRT for 5 years after the onset of menopause.

■ Meds

Protonix 40 mg PO once daily
Zoloft 50 mg PO once daily
Neurontin 300 mg PO TID
Hydrocodone/acetaminophen 5 mg/300 mg, one to two tablets PO Q 6 H PRN pain

■ All

NKDA

■ ROS

Negative except for complaints noted above

■ Physical Examination

Gen

WDWN 61-year-old woman. Awake, alert, in NAD.

VS

BP 127/71 mm Hg, P 89 bpm, RR 16, T 36.7°C; Wt 137 lb, Ht 5'1"

HEENT

NC/AT; PERRLA; EOMI; ear, nose, and throat are clear

Neck/Lymph Nodes

Supple. No lymphadenopathy, thyromegaly, or masses. No supraclavicular or infraclavicular adenopathy.

Lungs

CTA and percussion

Breasts

Left: Notable for a 2.5-cm mass at the 6 o'clock position, approximately 3 cm from the nipple margin, not fixated to skin; no nipple retraction or discharge is visualized; the mass is not tender to palpation; 1.5-cm, nontender, palpable mass in the axilla noted.
Right: Without mass or lymphadenopathy.

CV

RRR; no murmurs, rubs, or gallops

Abd

Soft, NT/ND, normoactive bowel sounds. No appreciable hepatosplenomegaly.

Spine

Slight tenderness to percussion

Ext

No CCE

Neuro

No deficits noted

■ Labs

Na 142 mEq/L	Hgb 12.9 g/dL	WBC 8.7	AST 36 IU/L
K 3.7 mEq/L	Hct 37.6%	$\times 10^3/mm^3$	ALT 17 IU/L
Cl 102 mEq/L	RBC 4.13 × 10⁶/mm³	Neutros 55%	LDH 488 IU/L
CO₂ 26 mEq/L	Plt 410 × 10³/mm³	Lymphs 35%	T. bili 0.2 mg/dL
BUN 9 mg/dL	PT 11.9 seconds	Monos 8%	
SCr 0.7 mg/dL	INR 1.09	Eos 2%	
Glu 83 mg/dL	aPTT 30.1 seconds		

■ Chest X-Ray

Lungs are clear.

■ Other Diagnostic Tests

Diagnostic Bilateral Mammogram (Fig. 151-1)

1. American College of Radiology category V, highly suspicious for malignancy in the left breast. There is a high-density, irregular mass measuring 2.2 cm with indistinct margins seen in the left breast lower hemisphere at 6 o'clock located 3 cm from the nipple.

2. In the right breast, no dominant mass, distortion, or suspicious calcifications are identified.

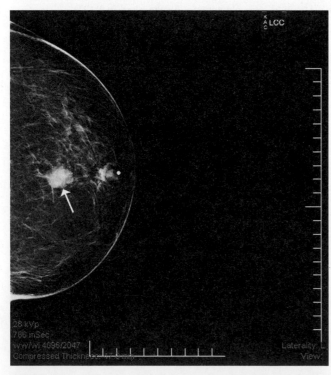

FIGURE 151-1. Mammogram of left breast. *Arrow* indicates area of abnormality highly suspicious for malignancy.

Unilateral Ultrasound Left Breast and Left Axilla with Biopsy

1. An ill-defined, hypoechoic mass is noted in the 5:00–6:00 region. This measures approximately 2.5 cm × 2.3 cm × 1.5 cm and is located 3 cm from the nipple. A core biopsy of this mass was performed.

2. Suspicious lymph nodes are noted in the axilla. The largest node measures 1.8 cm × 1.8 cm × 1.4 cm. FNA of this lymph node was performed. In the infraclavicular region, a few hypoechoic lymph nodes were also seen and were located in the lateral aspect. The largest node measured 0.8 cm × 0.8 cm × 0.8 cm. FNA of this infraclavicular lymph node was performed. No suspicious internal mammary or supraclavicular lymph nodes were seen.

Core needle Biopsy of Left Breast Mass

Left breast, 6 o'clock: infiltrating ductal carcinoma, modified Black's nuclear grade II (moderately differentiated), ER 95%, PR 95%, HER2 overexpression 2+, HER2 FISH negative (no amplification), and Ki-67 30% (moderate)

FNA of Left Axillary and Infraclavicular Lymph Nodes

1. Left axillary lymph node: metastatic adenocarcinoma consistent with breast primary

2. Left infraclavicular lymph node: metastatic adenocarcinoma consistent with breast primary

Bone Scan

1. No definite evidence of osseous metastases

2. Abnormality in cervical spine consistent with previous history of bone grafting

CT Abdomen

No lesions suggestive of metastases

CT Chest

No evidence of metastases

■ Assessment

A 61-year-old woman who has newly diagnosed breast cancer.

QUESTIONS

Collect Information

1. What subjective and objective information indicates the presence of breast cancer?

Assess the Information

2.a. Based on the information available, what is this patient's clinical stage of breast cancer?

2.b. In addition to the stage of disease, what other factors are important for determining the prognosis for breast cancer?

2.c. Create a list of the patient's drug therapy problems and prioritize them. Include assessment of medication appropriateness, effectiveness, safety, and patient adherence.

Develop a Care Plan

3.a. What is the primary goal for cancer treatment in this patient?

3.b. What nondrug therapies might be useful for treating this patient's breast cancer?

3.c. What feasible pharmacotherapeutic options are available for treating this patient's breast cancer prior to surgery?

3.d. Create an individualized, patient-centered, team-based care plan to treat this patient's breast cancer and optimize all medication therapy. Include specific drugs, dosage forms, doses, schedules, and durations of therapy.

Implement the Care Plan

4.a. What information should be provided to the patient to enhance adherence, ensure successful therapy, and minimize adverse effects?

4.b. Describe how care should be coordinated with other healthcare providers.

Follow-Up: Monitor and Evaluate

5. Explain how to monitor and evaluate the care plan for medication appropriateness, effectiveness, safety, and patient adherence by using clinical and laboratory data, patient feedback, and other information.

■ CLINICAL COURSE

The patient tolerated your treatment plan well. Twelve months after its completion, she returns to clinic complaining of lower back pain for the past 3–4 weeks. She has been taking hydrocodone/acetaminophen more regularly, "about two or three pills per day." This is a significant change since previously she reported not taking any. She is restaged with a bone scan, chest X-ray, abdominal CT, chest CT, and laboratory tests. Bone scan reveals metastases to the lumbar spine without spinal cord compression. Chest X-ray is negative. Abdominal CT shows a solitary liver metastasis. Chest CT is negative for metastases. LFTs are within normal limits. CA 27.29 is 100.7 U/mL. Biopsy of the liver lesion confirms recurrence of ER-positive, PR-positive, and HER2-negative breast cancer. The physician concludes that this patient's breast cancer is now metastatic to the bone and liver. The previous therapy is discontinued, and the patient is started on palbociclib and letrozole. The patient's updated information is as follows.

Labs

Na 140 mEq/L   Hgb 12.5 g/dL   WBC $6.7 \times 10^3/mm^3$ AST 40 IU/L
K 3.9 mEq/L   Hct 36.4%   Neutros 64%   ALT 24 IU/L
Cl 103 mEq/L   RBC $4.1 \times 10^6/mm^3$ Lymphs 30%   LDH 502 IU/L
CO_2 28 mEq/L   Plt $356 \times 10^3/mm^3$ Monos 3%   T. bili 0.5 mg/dL
BUN 11 mg/dL   Eos 3%
SCr 0.65 mg/dL
Glu 92 mg/dL

Meds

Cardizem CD 180 mg PO once daily
Protonix 40 mg PO once daily
Zoloft 50 mg PO once daily
Hydrocodone/acetaminophen 5 mg/300 mg, one to two tablets PO Q 6 H PRN pain

■ FOLLOW-UP QUESTIONS

1. What is this patient's current clinical stage of breast cancer, and what is the primary goal for cancer treatment for this patient now?

2. Based on the patient's current medication list, create a list of potential drug therapy problems as she begins a new therapy for cancer.

3. Since the patient has developed bone metastases, what other medication should be added to her treatment plan? At what dose and schedule?

4. What information should be provided to the patient regarding her new chemotherapy for breast cancer?

■ SELF-STUDY ASSIGNMENTS

1. Perform a literature search to obtain recent information regarding clinical trials utilizing trastuzumab and pertuzumab in patients with HER2 overexpressing breast cancer.

2. Perform a literature search to obtain recent information regarding clinical trials using aromatase inhibitors (anastrozole, letrozole, or exemestane) in patients with early-stage hormone receptor–positive breast cancer.

3. Develop a treatment plan for a patient presenting to the emergency center with febrile neutropenia after administration of chemotherapy.

4. Provide educational information regarding genetic testing for a patient with a family history of breast cancer.

CLINICAL PEARL

CDK 4/6 inhibitors cause neutropenia via temporary cell-cycle arrest of neutrophils and precursors. This allows for rapid recovery after interruption of treatment and results in lower rates of febrile neutropenia compared to cytotoxic chemotherapy, which causes direct damage to circulating neutrophils and bone marrow cells.

REFERENCES

1. Hortobagyi GN, Connolly JL, D'Orsi CJ, et al. Breast. In: Amin EB, Edge SB, Gress DM, et al, eds. AJCC Cancer Staging Manual. 8th ed. Chicago, IL: Springer; 2017:589–638.

2. Peto R, Davies D, Godwin J, et al. Comparisons between different polychemotherapy regimens for early breast cancer: meta-analyses of long-term outcome among 100,000 women in 123 randomised trials. Lancet. 2012;379(9814):432–444.

3. De Laurentiis M, Cancello G, D'Agostino D, et al. Taxane-based combinations as adjuvant chemotherapy of early breast cancer: a meta-analysis of randomized trials. J Clin Oncol. 2008;26:44–53.

4. Early Breast Cancer Trialists' Collaborative Group (EBCTCG). Aromatase inhibitors versus tamoxifen in early breast cancer: patient-level meta-analysis of the randomized trials. Lancet. 2015;386(10001):1341–1352.

5. Davies C, Pan H, Godwin J, et al. Long-term effects of continuing adjuvant tamoxifen to 10 years versus stopping at 5 years after diagnosis of oestrogen receptor-positive breast cancer: ATLAS, a randomised trial. Lancet. 2013;381:805–816.

6. Pan K, Bosserman LD, Chlebowski RT. Ovarian suppression in adjuvant endocrine therapy for premenopausal breast cancer. J Clin Oncol. 2019;37(11):858–861.

7. Khatcheressian JL, Hurley P, Bantug E, et al. Breast cancer follow-up and management after primary treatment: American Society of Clinical Oncology clinical practice guideline update. J Clin Oncol. 2013;31(7):961–965.

8. NCCN Clinical Practice Guidelines in Oncology (NCCN Guidelines®) for Breast Cancer V.8.2021 © National Comprehensive Cancer Network, Inc., 2019. Available at: https://www.nccn.org/professionals/physician_gls/pdf/breast.pdf. Accessed October 15, 2021.

9. Van Poznak C, Somerfield MR, Barlow WE, et al. Role of bone-modifying agents in metastatic breast cancer: an American Society of Clinical Oncology-Cancer Care Ontario Focused Guideline Update. J Clin Oncol. 2017;35(35):3978–3986.

10. Ibrance Package Insert. New York, NY: Pfizer Laboratories, Inc.; 2019.

152

NON–SMALL CELL LUNG CANCER

It Takes Your Breath Away .... Level II

Ronni Miller, PharmD, BCOP

Katelyn Gardner, PharmD

LEARNING OBJECTIVES

After completing this case study, the reader should be able to:

- Recognize the most common symptoms of non–small cell lung cancer (NSCLC).

- Design a treatment plan for patients with NSCLC.

- Design a pharmacotherapeutic plan for the treatment of hypercalcemia.

- Describe appropriate treatment strategies for brain metastases in NSCLC.

- Educate patients on the anticipated adverse effects of carboplatin, paclitaxel, docetaxel, and ramucirumab therapy.

PATIENT PRESENTATION

■ Chief Complaint

"I have been coughing up blood."

■ HPI

A 66-year-old woman presents to her PCP with complaints of a dry, nonproductive cough for 2.5 months, dyspnea on exertion, and hemoptysis for 1 week.

■ PMH

HTN
Anemia of unknown etiology × 1 year
Type 2 diabetes mellitus (T2DM)
PPD (–)

■ FH

Father died of colorectal cancer at age 68
Aunt died of breast cancer at age 70

■ SH

Married, lives with spouse; 30 pack-year cigarette smoking history (approximately 1 ppd × 30 years); occasional ETOH use; no known recent exposure to TB

■ Meds

Folic acid 1 mg PO daily
Ferrous sulfate 325 mg PO TID
Metformin 500 mg PO BID
Pantoprazole 40 mg PO daily

■ All

Penicillin (rash)
Sulfa (rash)

■ ROS

(+) For pulmonary symptoms as noted in HPI; no headaches, dizziness, or blurred vision

■ Physical Examination

Gen

Mildly overweight woman in slight distress. ECOG performance status of 1.

VS

BP 169/100 mmHg, P 90 bpm, RR 30, T 37.2°C; Wt 82 kg, Ht 5′6″

Skin

Patches of dry skin; no lesions

HEENT

PERRLA; EOMI; fundi benign; TMs intact

Neck/Lymph Nodes

No lymphadenopathy; neck supple

Lungs

Wheezing in RUL; remainder of lung fields clear

Heart

RRR; normal S_1, S_2

Abd

Soft, nontender; no splenomegaly or hepatomegaly

Genit/Rect

Normal female genitalia; guaiac (–) stool

Neuro

A&O × 3; sensory and motor intact, 5/5 upper, 4/5 lower; CN II–XII intact; (–) Babinski

■ Labs

Na 138 mEq/L	Hgb 10.7 g/dL	Ca 9.7 mg/dL
K 3.6 mEq/L	Hct 34.6%	Mg 2.0 mg/dL
Cl 101 mEq/L	Plt 255 × 10³/mm³	
CO₂ 23 mEq/L	WBC 9.9 × 10³/mm³	
BUN 11 mg/dL		
SCr 1.1 mg/dL		
Glu 182 mg/dL		

■ Chest X-Ray

PA and lateral views reveal a possible mass in right upper lobe (Fig. 152-1).

■ Assessment

A 66-year-old woman with new-onset hemoptysis is admitted for workup of a possible lung mass. She has anemia and a history of T2DM and HTN.

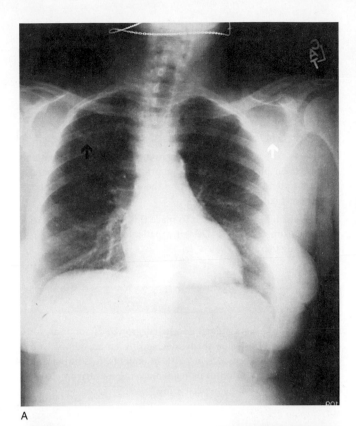

A

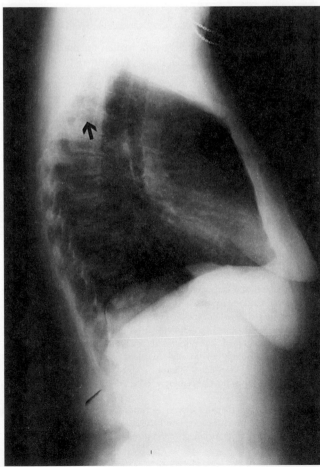

B

FIGURE 152-1. Chest X-ray with PA *(A)* and lateral *(B)* views showing a possible mass in the right upper lobe *(arrows)*.

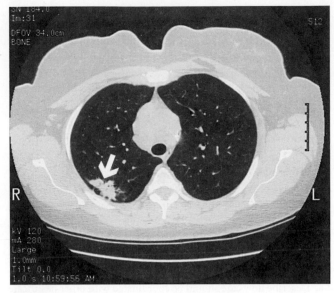

FIGURE 152-2. CT scan of the chest revealing a 2.5- × 2-cm right lung mass *(arrow)*.

CLINICAL COURSE (PART 1)

The patient was further evaluated for lung cancer on an outpatient basis. A bronchoscopy (with biopsy) was performed that identified adenocarcinoma. The chest CT scan revealed a 3- × 2-cm right lung mass (Fig. 152-2). A mediastinoscopy was performed to determine the resectability of the tumor. The mediastinoscopy and biopsy revealed unresectable stage IIIB (T_2N_3) NSCLC with metastases to the contralateral mediastinal nodes. A brain MRI was negative for disease. Tumor EGFR status was positive by IHC (nonsensitizing), and *EML4-ALK* and *ROS1* gene rearrangement were negative. Additional testing showed the tumor to have 5% PD-L1 expression and V600E mutation negative. PFTs included FEV_1 1.49 L and FVC 1.9 L. An echocardiogram showed mild LVH with an LVEF of 55%. Patient has an EGOG performance status of 1.

QUESTIONS

Collect Information

1.a. What subjective and objective information indicates the presence of non–small cell lung cancer (NSCLC) in this patient?

1.b. What additional information is needed to fully assess this patient's lung cancer?

Assess the Information

2.a. Assess the severity of the NSCLC based on the subjective and objective information available.

2.b. Create a list of the patient's drug therapy problems and prioritize them. Include assessment of medication appropriateness, effectiveness, safety, and patient adherence.

Develop a Care Plan

3.a. What is the goal for treating NSCLC in this patient? What is the likelihood of achieving this goal?

3.b. What nondrug therapies might be useful for treating NSCLC?

3.c. What feasible pharmacotherapeutic options are available for treating stage IIIB NSCLC?

3.d. Create an individualized, patient-centered, team-based care plan to optimize medication therapy for this patient's drug therapy problems. For NSCLC chemotherapy, include specific drugs, dosage forms, doses, schedules, and durations of therapy.

3.e. In addition to chemotherapy, what measures should be taken to ensure the tolerability of the NSCLC regimen and to prevent adverse effects?

Implement the Care Plan

4.a. What additional laboratory and clinical information are needed before administration of the chemotherapy?

4.b. Calculate the patient's BSA, creatinine clearance, and the amount of each drug to be administered based on the regimen chosen.

4.c. What information should be provided to the patient to enhance adherence, ensure successful therapy, and minimize adverse effects?

4.d. Describe how care should be coordinated with other healthcare providers.

4.e. Would the treatment plan for this patient change if she had presented initially with stage IIB NSCLC that was positive for a sensitizing EGFR mutation? If so, what would the treatment be?

Follow-Up: Monitor and Evaluate

5. Explain how to monitor and evaluate the care plan for medication appropriateness, effectiveness, safety, and patient adherence by using clinical and laboratory data, patient feedback, and other information.

■ CLINICAL COURSE (PART 2)

The patient's subsequent courses were complicated by the occurrence of DVT, weight loss, neutropenic fever, anemia, nausea/vomiting, and infections. At one point, she presented with a serum calcium level of 11.3 mg/dL and an albumin of 1.2 g/dL, with symptoms of weakness, confusion, nausea, and vomiting.

■ FOLLOW-UP QUESTIONS

1. Calculate the patient's corrected calcium level and provide an interpretation of that value.

2. What treatment modalities may be used to correct hypercalcemia?

■ CLINICAL COURSE (PART 3)

The patient completed concurrent chemotherapy with radiation followed by two cycles of carboplatin and paclitaxel. A repeat chest CT showed enlargement of the initial lesion, and a PET-CT demonstrated a 2- × 2-cm suspicious lesion in the liver. Her performance status remains an ECOG of 1.

■ FOLLOW-UP QUESTIONS

3. What treatment options are available for the patient at this time?

4. Design a specific chemotherapeutic regimen to treat this patient.

■ CLINICAL COURSE (PART 4)

Seven weeks after beginning the new chemotherapy regimen, the patient presents to the ED with complaints of headache and mental status changes as per the patient's husband and caregiver. An MRI of the head reveals multiple lesions, most likely brain metastases.

■ FOLLOW-UP QUESTIONS

5. Briefly discuss options (drug and nondrug) to treat brain metastases.

6. What is the role of anticonvulsant agents in the setting of brain metastases?

■ SELF-STUDY ASSIGNMENTS

1. Review clinically important drug interactions for cancer patients started on phenytoin. Include appropriate monitoring parameters. Extend your review beyond the medications this patient is currently receiving.

2. The oncologist has decided to place this patient on docetaxel + ramucirumab therapy. Design a patient education session for this drug therapy.

CLINICAL PEARL

Ramucirumab is a vascular endothelial growth factor receptor 2 (VEGFR2) inhibitor. Due to its mechanistic target, ramucirumab can increase blood pressure in ~20% of patients. It is important to monitor for hypertension in patients receiving ramucirumab, especially those with baseline hypertension.

ACKNOWLEDGMENT

This case is based on the patient case written for the 11th edition by Michelle L. Rockey, PharmD, BCOP, FHOPA and Julianna, V.F. Roddy, PharmD, BCOP.

REFERENCES

1. National Comprehensive Cancer Network Clinical Practice Guidelines in Oncology. Non-small cell lung cancer, version 7, 2021. Available at: *https://www.nccn.org/professionals/physician_gls/pdf/nscl.pdf*. Accessed October 29, 2021.

2. Wu YL, Tsuboi M, He J, et al. Osimertinib in resected EGFR-mutated non-small cell lung cancer. N Engl J Med. 2020;383:1711–1723.

3. Faivre-Finn C, Vicente D, Kurata T, et al. Four-year survival with durvalumab after chemoradiotherapy in stage III NSCLC- an update from the PACIFIC Trial. J Thorac Oncol. 2021;16(5):860–867.

4. Belani CP, Choy H, Bonomi P, et al. Combined chemotherapy regimens of paclitaxel and carboplatin for locally advanced non-small-cell lung cancer: a randomized phase II locally advanced multi-modality protocol. J Clin Oncol. 2005;23:5883–5891.

5. Fournel P, Robinet G, Thomas P, et al. Randomized phase III trial of sequential chemoradiotherapy compared with concurrent chemoradiotherapy in locally advanced non-small-cell lung cancer: Groupe Lyon-Saint-Etienne d'Oncologie Thoracique-Groupe Francis de Pneumo-Cancerologie NPC 95-01 study. J Clin Oncol. 2005;23:5910–5917.

6. National Comprehensive Cancer Network Clinical Practice Guidelines in Oncology. Antiemesis, version 1, 2021. Available at: *https://www.nccn.org/professionals/physician_gls/pdf/antiemesis.pdf*. Accessed October 29, 2021.

7. Rizzo DJ, Brouwers M, Hurley P, et al. American Society of Clinical Oncology/American Society of Hematology clinical practice guideline update on the use of epoetin and darbepoetin in adult patients with cancer. J Clin Oncol. 2010;28:4996–5010.

8. Garon EB, Ciuleanu T, Arrieta O, et al. Ramucirumab plus docetaxel versus placebo plus docetaxel for second-line treatment of stage IV non-small-cell lung cancer after disease progression on platinum-based

therapy (REVEL): a multicentre, double-blind, randomised phase 3 trial. Lancet. 2014;384:665–673.

9. Weiss GJ, Langer C, Rosell R, et al. Elderly patients benefit from second-line cytotoxic chemotherapy: a subset analysis of a randomized phase III trial of pemetrexed compared with docetaxel in patients with previously treated advanced non-small-cell lung cancer. J Clin Oncol. 2006;24:4405–4411.

153

COLON CANCER

Drug Therapy by Design . . . . Level II

Lisa E. Davis, PharmD, FCCP, BCPS, BCOP

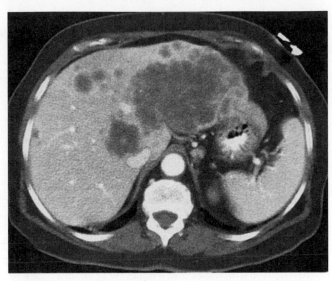

FIGURE 153-1. Abdominal/pelvic CT scan with extensive liver metastases. These multiple hypodense lesions are characteristic of metastases to the liver, the most common site for distant spread of gastrointestinal malignancies. (Reprinted with permission from Kaiser M. McGraw-Hill Manual: Colorectal Surgery. *http://www.accesssurgery.com.*)

LEARNING OBJECTIVES

After completing this case study, the reader should be able to:

- Describe the treatment goals associated with advanced stages of colon cancer.

- Design an appropriate chemotherapy regimen for colon cancer based on patient-specific data.

- Formulate a monitoring plan for a patient receiving a prescribed chemotherapy regimen for colon cancer based on patient-specific information.

- Recommend alterations in a drug therapy plan for a patient with colon cancer based on patient-specific information.

- Educate patients on the anticipated side effects of irinotecan, capecitabine, fluorouracil, oxaliplatin, bevacizumab, ziv-aflibercept, ramucirumab, regorafenib, cetuximab, panitumumab, trifluridine/tipiracil hydrochloride, nivolumab, pembrolizumab, ipilimumab, dostarlimab-gxly, and encorafenib.

PATIENT PRESENTATION

■ Chief Complaint

"I have good days and bad days, and today hasn't been a good day. I know you warned me about diarrhea, but I am still really constipated, and the pain in my back and abdomen makes me extremely uncomfortable."

■ HPI

A 47-year-old woman presents with continuing constipation and worsening back pain. She was diagnosed with stage II colon adenocarcinoma that was found in her sigmoid colon during a screening colonoscopy and resected 4 years ago. Due to the patient "feeling great" and having a change in health insurance, she did not return for routine follow-up. One year ago, she presented to her PCP for right lower extremity swelling. A duplex ultrasound demonstrated two areas of noncompressible veins, consistent with DVT, and treatment was initiated with apixaban. A CEA at that time was 14.2 ng/mL, and a chest/abdomen/pelvic CT scan (Fig. 153-1) revealed multiple hypodense lesions in the left and right hepatic lobes, likely metastatic disease.

The CT scan of the chest showed no evidence of lung metastases. A biopsy of a liver mass was positive for adenocarcinoma, and tissue was sent for molecular profiling.

The tumor was *KRAS, NRAS,* and *BRAF* gene wild-type, *ERBB2* not amplified, PDL1 negative, and classified as microsatellite stable (MSS; MMR-proficient; pMMR). *UGT1A1* genotyping showed that the patient was homozygous for the *UGT1A1* *28 allele. Three weeks later, chemotherapy was initiated with infusional fluorouracil, irinotecan (FOLFIRI), and bevacizumab.

The patient tolerated chemotherapy well overall except for persistent nausea that improved after a change in her antiemetic regimen to include granisetron transdermal system. The bevacizumab was held during two cycles for recurrent nose bleeding. The patient experienced occasional bouts of diarrhea that were managed with loperamide or diphenoxylate/atropine. Her blood pressure had increased slightly to 158/97 mm Hg after her fourth cycle of chemotherapy, and her ramipril dose was increased to 10 mg. Her blood pressure was eventually controlled with the addition of metoprolol succinate. Her tumor marker CEA dropped to 5.2 ng/mL. After her ninth cycle of FOLFIRI plus bevacizumab, she endorsed poor appetite and fatigue with abdominal pain that radiates to her back, making her feel miserable. Six days ago, she received her eleventh cycle of chemotherapy. An MRI of the abdomen and pelvis showed multiple stable and new metastatic lesions in the liver, metastatic lymphadenopathy, and upper peritoneal/omental deposits. A CT of the thorax showed multiple new, mixed-density pulmonary nodules scattered throughout all lobes.

■ PMH

Asthma × 25 years
Hypertension × 15 years
Proximal lower extremity VTE × 17 months

■ FH

The patient has a younger brother and sister; both siblings are alive and well. She has been married for 20 years and has one 16-year-old daughter. Her mother died at the age of 36 from cancer (type unknown), but her father is alive in good health. Her paternal grandfather died in his 60s from colon cancer, and her maternal grandmother died in her 70s from breast cancer.

■ SH

Employed as a school superintendent but has been unable to work since starting chemotherapy. She denies tobacco use and does not drink alcohol. She reports using THC/CBD 5 mg gummy edibles 3–4 times a week to help with sleep.

■ Meds

Albuterol 90 mcg inhalation aerosol 2 puffs, QID PRN wheezing

Apixaban 10 mg PO twice daily

Diphenoxylate/atropine, 2 tablets QID PRN for diarrhea uncontrolled with loperamide

Granisetron transdermal system 3.1 mg/24 hours, apply 24 hours before chemotherapy and remove 24 hours after completion of chemotherapy

Loperamide 2 mg, 2 tablets initially, then 1 tablet after each loose bowel movement

Metoprolol succinate 50 mg PO daily

Oxycodone extended-release (ER) 9 mg PO Q 12 H

Oxycodone immediate-release (IR) 5 mg PO Q 6 H PRN pain

Ramipril 10 mg PO daily

Triamterene/hydrochlorothiazide 25/37.5 mg PO daily

■ All

NKDA

■ ROS

The patient reports experiencing pain in her abdomen that feels like a "heavy, sharp dagger within." She reports the abdominal pain severity as 6–7 out of 10. The short-acting oxycodone "doesn't do much to reduce the pain," and she states that sometimes the pain is so uncomfortable that she becomes nauseated. She denies fever, headaches, lesions in her mouth, or difficulty swallowing. She has an occasional dry cough and experiences moderate SOB upon exertion. She has been having fewer bowel movements (about one every 3–4 days), but there is no pain or blood with passage of stool. She denies polyuria, polydipsia, and burning on urination. She has not noticed any bleeding or excessive bruising.

■ Physical Examination

Gen

Patient is a slightly underweight, uncomfortably appearing woman.

VS

BP 121/67 mm Hg, P 90 bpm, RR 20, T 36.6°C; Wt 55 kg, Ht 5'5"

Skin

Warm, dry, and pink; no rashes or lesions

HEENT

PERRLA; EOMI; pale conjunctiva; no scleral icterus; moist mucous membranes; no oral lesions

Neck/Lymph Nodes

Supple neck; no lymphadenopathy

Lungs/Thorax

Clear to A&P; no inspiratory or expiratory wheezing; non-labored respiration; port-a-cath in place

Breasts

No masses

CV

Normal heart sounds; regular rate and rhythm; no murmurs or gallops

Abd

Well-healed scar on left upper abdomen; diffuse abdominal tenderness to palpation; decreased bowel sounds

Genit/Rect

LMP 4 months ago; stool heme negative

MS/Ext

Full ROM in all four extremities

Neuro

Awake, alert, and oriented × 3; CN II–XII intact

Psych

Cooperative, appropriate mood and affect

■ Labs

Na 135 mEq/L	Hgb 9.8 g/dL	WBC 3.6 × 10³/mm³	AST 85 IU/L
K 4.0 mEq/L	Hct 28.3%	Neutros 55%	ALT 94 IU/L
Cl 103 mEq/L	Plt 185 × 10³/mm³	Bands 0.3%	Alk phos 309 IU/L
CO₂ 25 mEq/L	MCV 96 μm³	Eos 3%	LDH 311 IU/L
BUN 6 mg/dL	MCHC 32 g/dL	Lymphs 32%	T. bili 1.1 mg/dL
SCr 0.62 mg/dL		Monos 10%	CEA 6.8 ng/mL
Glu 138 mg/dL			
Ca 7 mg/dL			
Phos 2.6 mg/dL			
Mg 2.4 mg/dL			

■ Tumor Molecular Profiling

KRAS, NRAS, BRAF gene wild-type, PDL1 negative, *ERBB2* amplification not detected, MSS, MMR proficient, TMB 5 mutations/Mb

■ Urinalysis

(–) glucose, trace ketones, 2+ protein, (–) leukocyte esterase and nitrites; 1–2 RBC/hpf; 1–5 WBC/hpf

■ Abdominal CT

Marked interval progression of metastatic disease throughout the liver. Osteolytic lesion right ileac bone 5.9 cm × 2.3 cm.

■ Chest CT

Multiple metastatic nodules in both lungs, with irregular thickening of cavity walls

■ Assessment

Unresectable stage IV colon cancer, with disease progression on FOLFIRI plus bevacizumab

QUESTIONS

Collect Information

1.a. What subjective and objective information indicates the presence of colon cancer?

1.b. What additional information is needed to fully assess this patient's colon cancer?

Assess the Information

2.a. Assess the severity of colon cancer based on the subjective and objective information available.

2.b. Create a list of the patient's drug therapy problems and prioritize them. Include assessment of medication appropriateness, effectiveness, safety, and patient adherence.

Develop a Care Plan

3.a. What are the goals of pharmacotherapy for colon cancer in this case?

3.b. What nondrug therapies might be useful for this patient's colon cancer?

3.c. What feasible pharmacotherapeutic options are available for treating this patient's colon cancer?

3.d. Create an individualized, patient-centered, team-based care plan to optimize medication therapy for the colon cancer and other drug therapy problems identified in Question 2.b. Include specific drugs, dosage forms, doses, schedules, and durations of therapy.

Implement the Care Plan

4.a. What information should be provided to the patient to enhance adherence, ensure successful therapy, and minimize adverse effects?

4.b. Describe how care should be coordinated with other healthcare providers.

Follow-Up: Monitor and Evaluate

5. Explain how to monitor and evaluate the care plan for medication appropriateness, effectiveness, safety, and patient adherence by using clinical and laboratory data, patient feedback, and other information.

■ CLINICAL COURSE (PART 1)

The bevacizumab was held, and the patient's proteinuria resolved. Metoprolol was discontinued due to improved blood pressure control after following permanent discontinuation of bevacizumab. The oxycodone ER dose was increased to 18 mg PO Q 12 H, and an increase in oxycodone IR to 10 mg PO Q 4 H PRN improved her pain control. A scheduled regimen of polyethylene glycol 3350 17 grams PO twice daily maintained a regular pattern of bowel movements. Olanzapine 2.5 mg PO at bedtime was initiated to improve nausea symptoms and help with sleep. The dry cough and abdominal pain improved after two cycles of the chemotherapy regimen you recommended, and her colon cancer sites of disease remained stable during the subsequent treatment cycles. However, after the seventh cycle, she started developing numbness and painful sensations in her hands and feet, which progressively worsened. After her tenth cycle of chemotherapy, chest and abdominal CT scans showed progression of the metastases in her lungs and liver.

■ FOLLOW-UP QUESTION

1. What treatment options would be appropriate to consider at this time?

■ ADDITIONAL CASE QUESTIONS

1. What is the role of *UGT1A1* genotyping in the treatment of colon cancer?

2. What is the role of *KRAS*, *NRAS*, and *BRAF* tumor gene testing in the treatment of colon cancer?

3. What is the relevance of microsatellite instability-high (MSI-H) or mismatch repair deficient (MMR-deficient; dMMR) classification of colon cancer?

■ CLINICAL COURSE (PART 2)

The patient expressed interest in receiving further treatment for her colon cancer, and her performance status remained good (ECOG 1). A decision was made to initiate therapy with regorafenib. Her supportive therapies were further optimized, and her symptom control was acceptable. Her metastatic lesions remained stable (by clinical symptoms and CT scans) for 4 months.

■ SELF-STUDY ASSIGNMENTS

1. Develop an algorithm for management of colon cancer oxaliplatin-induced neuropathy.

2. Develop patient-specific education materials regarding management of dermatologic toxicities of anti-EGFR antibodies used in colon cancer treatment.

CLINICAL PEARL

VEGF inhibitors can be used in first- and second-line treatment regimens for metastatic colon cancer when no other targeted biologics are included. However, only bevacizumab has demonstrated benefit when added to oxaliplatin-based and irinotecan-based regimens as initial treatment and for patients receiving a different chemotherapy regimen following disease progression.

REFERENCES

1. Biller LH, Schrag D. Diagnosis and treatment of metastatic colorectal cancer. A review. JAMA. 2021;325:669–685.

2. Mocellin S, Baretta Z, Figuls MRI, et al. Second-line systemic therapy for metastatic colorectal cancer. Cochrane Database Syst Rev. 2017;1:CD006875.

3. Bennouna J, Sastre J, Arnold D, et al. Continuation of bevacizumab after first progression in metastatic colorectal cancer (ML18147): a randomised phase 3 trial. Lancet Oncol. 2013;14:29–37.

4. van Helden EJ, Menke-van der Houven van Oordt CW, Heymans MW, et al. Optimal use of anti-EGFR monoclonal antibodies for patients with advanced colorectal cancer: a meta-analysis. Cancer Metastasis Rev. 2017;36:395–406.

5. Cunningham D, Humblet Y, Siena S, et al. Cetuximab monotherapy and cetuximab plus irinotecan in irinotecan-refractory metastatic colorectal cancer. N Engl J Med. 2004;351(4):337–345.

6. Price TJ, Peeters M, Kim TW, et al. Panitumumab versus cetuximab in patients with chemotherapy-refractory wild-type KRAS exon 2 metastatic colorectal cancer (ASPECCT): a randomized, multicentre, open-label, non-inferiority phase 3 study. Lancet Oncol. 2014;15:569–579.

7. Tang W, Ren L, Liu T, et al. Bevacizumab plus mFOLFOX6 versus mFOLFOX6 alone as first-line treatment for *RAS* mutant unresectable colorectal liver-limited metastases: the BECOME randomized controlled trial. J Clin Oncol. 2020;38:3175–3184.

8. Saltz LB, Clarke S, Diaz-Rubio E, et al. Bevacizumab in combination with oxaliplatin-based chemotherapy as first-line therapy in metastatic colorectal cancer: a randomized phase III study. J Clin Oncol. 2008;26:2013–2019.

9. Berry SR, Cosby R, Asmis T, et al. Continuous versus intermittent chemotherapy strategies in metastatic colorectal cancer: a systematic review and meta-analysis. Ann Oncol. 2015;26:477–485.

10. Vogel A, Hofheinz RD, Kubicka S, et al. Treatment decisions in metastatic colorectal cancer—beyond first and second line combination therapies. Cancer Treat Rev. 2017;59:54–60.

154

PROSTATE CANCER

Missed Opportunity .... Level II

Lisa M. Holle, BS-Pharmacy, PharmD, BCOP, FHOPA, FISOPP

LEARNING OBJECTIVES

After completing this case study, the reader should be able to:

- Describe typical symptoms associated with prostate cancer at initial diagnosis and at disease progression.

- Describe the standard initial treatment options for castration-sensitive metastatic prostate cancer.

- Recommend a pharmacotherapeutic plan for patients with castrate-resistant metastatic prostate cancer.

- Counsel patients regarding the toxicities associated with the pharmacologic agents used for metastatic prostate cancer treatment.

PATIENT PRESENTATION

■ Chief Complaint

"I have blood in my urine, I'm using the bathroom all the time, and my shoulder is really hurting."

■ HPI

A 73-year-old man presents with increased urinary symptoms for the past 5 months, painless gross hematuria, shoulder pain, and a PSA level of 35.7 ng/mL. He usually has yearly physical exams and PSA checks by his local physician, and the levels have always been in the range of 4–6 ng/mL. The patient did not go in for his yearly physical last year.

■ PMH

Dyslipidemia
CHF
h/o Diverticulitis 10 years ago
h/o GERD

■ FH

Father, lung cancer diagnosed age 71, died age 73; mother, breast cancer, died at age 93. The patient has a paternal aunt and paternal grandmother who both were diagnosed with unspecified malignancies.

■ SH

Retired highway maintenance employee. Tobacco: 10 cigarettes a day for 21 years; stopped smoking at age 42. Drinks: on average one beer per day. Married with two children.

■ Meds

Valsartan 160 mg PO BID
Carvedilol 12.5 mg PO twice daily
Furosemide 40 mg PO daily
Tamsulosin 0.4 mg, two capsules PO daily
Atorvastatin 10 mg PO at bedtime
Acetaminophen 500 mg PO four times daily PRN pain
Esomeprazole 40 mg PO daily

■ All

None

■ ROS

The patient reports significant fatigue and severe pain in right shoulder. No fever, chills, or sweats. No epistaxis or dysphagia. Reports no chest pain, shortness of breath, dyspnea, or cough. No nausea, vomiting, diarrhea, or constipation. Reports dysuria × 5 months with dribbling, nocturia eight times per night, hesitancy, incomplete voiding, and recurring hematuria. He denies memory loss, diplopia, or neuropathy; no recent falls.

■ Physical Examination

Gen

This is a pleasant, elderly man who appears to be in moderate discomfort. Pain is 7 over 10 multifocally. ECOG performance status 1+.

VS

BP 136/61 mm Hg, P 80 bpm, RR 20, T 36.9°C; Wt 91.5 kg, Ht 5′6″

Skin

Warm and dry; no lesions or rashes

HEENT

Sclerae are anicteric. PERRLA; EOMI. Tympanic membranes are within normal limits bilaterally.

Neck/Lymph Nodes

No cervical or supraclavicular adenopathy

Lungs/Thorax

Lungs are clear in all fields. Respirations are even and unlabored.

CV

Normal rate and rhythm; S_1, S_2 normal; no murmurs, gallops, or rubs

Abd

A large midline abdominal hernia is present (does not appear incarcerated). No hepatosplenomegaly.

Genit/Rect

Patient is circumcised with a normal phallus; bilateral descended testicles. No inguinal hernia on examination. Prostate is markedly enlarged and is asymmetric on the right. Texture is firm, but no discrete nodule palpated. Normal rectal tone.

MS/Ext

The patient has significant pain to touch on the superior aspect of the right shoulder; there is also pain on range of motion. There is tenderness in lumbar area; 1+ ankle and pedal edema is present. Pedal pulses are 2+ bilaterally.

Neuro

CN II–XII grossly normal. Cerebellar function remains intact.

■ Labs

Na 139 mEq/L	Hgb 9.5 g/dL	WBC 7.2	Total bilirubin
K 4.0 mEq/L	Hct 27.1%	$\times 10^3/mm^3$	0.2 mg/dL
Cl 107 mEq/L	RBC $3.6 \times 10^6/mm^3$	Neutros 70.3%	ALT <12 IU/L
CO_2 24 mEq/L	Plt $215 \times 10^3/mm^3$	Baso 0.2%	AST 20 IU/L
BUN 21 mg/dL	MCV 75 μm³	Eos 2.3%	LDH 742 IU/L
SCr 0.9 mg/dL	MCHC 35.1 g/dL	Lymphs 16.6%	Alk phos 912 IU/L
Glu 114 mg/dL		Monos 10.6%	Albumin 4 g/dL
		PSA 35.7 ng/mL	Calcium 8.7 mg/dL
		Testosterone	
		276 ng/dL	

■ Bone Scan

Skeletal metastases involving the skull × 2, left femur, right shoulder, and right humerus. Lesion noted in thoracic spine (T8).

■ Cystoscopy and Bladder Neck Biopsy

High-grade carcinoma consistent with prostatic adenocarcinoma, extensively involving the bladder neck biopsy tissue

■ Transrectal Prostate Biopsy

Prostatic adenocarcinoma, Gleason score 9 (4 + 5), positive for perineural invasion

■ CT Abdomen/Pelvis

Prostate mass extending into bladder, with local extension to pelvic sidewall. Multiple small, external iliac lymph nodes are present, predominantly on the left; 2–3 cm, deep inguinal lymph nodes are also present.

■ Urinalysis

Clear; negative for glucose, ketones, leukocyte esterase, nitrites, and protein; trace hemoglobin; rare bacteria

■ Assessment

A 73-year-old man with newly diagnosed T4N1M1b prostate cancer presenting with painless gross hematuria, increased urinary symptoms, and elevated PSA of 35.7 ng/mL. Patient has high-volume, metastatic, castration-naive disease and is here for consideration of initial treatment options.

QUESTIONS

Collect Information

1.a. What subjective and objective information indicates the presence of metastatic prostate cancer?

1.b. What additional information is needed to fully assess this patient's prostate cancer?

Assess the Information

2.a. Assess the extent of this patient's metastatic prostate cancer (eg, low-volume vs high-volume) based on the subjective and objective information available.

2.b. Create a list of the patient's drug therapy problems and prioritize them. Include assessment of medication appropriateness, effectiveness, safety, and patient adherence.

Develop a Care Plan

3.a. What are the goals of pharmacotherapy for prostate cancer, given this patient's disease stage and history?

3.b. What nondrug therapies might be useful for this patient's prostate cancer?

3.c. What feasible pharmacotherapeutic alternatives are available for treating the metastatic, castration-naive prostate cancer?

3.d. Create an individualized, patient-centered, team-based care plan to optimize medication therapy for this patient's prostate cancer and other drug therapy problems. Include specific drugs, dosage forms, doses, schedules, and durations of therapy.

3.e. What alternatives would be appropriate if the initial therapy for prostate cancer cannot be used?

Implement the Care Plan

4.a. What information should be provided to the patient to enhance adherence, ensure successful therapy, and minimize adverse drug reactions?

■ CLINICAL COURSE

The testosterone level has been castrate since therapy was begun 20 months ago, and pain has been better controlled with these interventions. The patient has been adherent with his treatment plan. The PSA 3 months ago was mildly elevated at 0.6 ng/mL, whereas it had been undetectable previously. Now the PSA has increased to 38.5 ng/mL, and testosterone level is 22 ng/mL. The patient is complaining of increased pelvic pain and more bone pain in ribs and back over the past 2 months. However, he is still able to participate in church social activities and play golf on the weekends. A CT of the pelvis shows a new soft tissue mass on the posterolateral aspect of the urinary bladder on the right side and multiple new blastic lesions in the pelvis and spine. A bone scan shows numerous new intense foci in the skull, scapulae, spine, and femurs.

■ FOLLOW-UP QUESTIONS

4.b. What pharmacotherapeutic options are available to the patient for his progressive, metastatic castrate-resistant prostate cancer (CRPC)?

4.c. What therapeutic options are available for managing this patient's pain?

4.d. Describe how care should be coordinated with other healthcare providers.

Follow-Up: Monitor and Evaluate

5. Explain how to monitor and evaluate the care plan for medication appropriateness, effectiveness, safety, and patient adherence by using clinical and laboratory data, patient feedback, and other information.

■ SELF-STUDY ASSIGNMENTS

1. Locate information resources that are available to prostate cancer patients and their families.

2. Describe the clinical rationale for starting an antiandrogen 1–2 weeks before giving the first dose of an LHRH agonist.

3. Define the role of bone-modulating agents (ie, bisphosphonates, receptor activator of nuclear factor κ-B [RANK] ligand inhibitors) in men with prostate cancer.

CLINICAL PEARL

Androgen deprivation therapy is continued when a metastatic prostate cancer patient progresses from a hormone-sensitive to a castrate-resistant state (ie, has a rising PSA and/or new metastatic lesions despite a castrate level of testosterone).

REFERENCES

1. NCCN Clinical Practice Guidelines in Oncology, V1.2022 Prostate Cancer. Available at: *http://www.nccn.org/professionals/physician_gls/pdf/prostate.pdf*. Accessed November 8, 2021.

2. Virgo KS, Rumble RB, de Wit R, et al. Initial management of noncastrate advanced, recurrent, or metastatic prostate cancer: ASCO guideline update. J Clin Oncol. 2021;39(11):1274–1305.

3. Zytiga Package Insert. Horsham, PA: Janssen Biotech, Inc.; 2021.

4. Yonsa Package Insert. Cranbury, NJ: Sun Pharmaceuticals Industries, Inc.; 2021.

5. Last AR, Ference JD, Menzel ER. Hyperlipidemia: drugs for cardiovascular risk reduction in adults. Am Fam Physician 2017;15(95):78–87.

6. Wolters Kluwer Clinical Drug Information, Inc. Lexi-Drugs. Wolters Kluwer Clinical Drug Information, Inc.; November 8, 2021.

7. Nuhn P, De Bono JS, Fizazi K, et al. Update on systemic prostate cancer therapies: management of metastatic castration-resistant prostate cancer in the era of precision oncology. Eur Urol. 2019;75(1):88–99.

8. Saylor PJ, Rumble B, Tagawa S, et al. Bone health and bone-targeted therapies for prostate cancer: ASCO endorsement of a cancer care Ontario guideline. J Clin Oncol. 2020;38:1736–1743.

9. NCCN Clinical Practice Guidelines in Oncology, V2.2021. Adult cancer pain. Available at: *http://www.nccn.org/professionals/physician_gls/pdf/pain.pdf*. Accessed November 8, 2021.

155

NON-HODGKIN LYMPHOMA

Chemical Formula for Cancer .... Level II

Keith A. Hecht, PharmD, BCOP

LEARNING OBJECTIVES

After completing this case study, the reader should be able to:

- Identify and describe the components of the staging workup and the corresponding staging and classification systems for non-Hodgkin lymphoma (NHL).

- Recommend treatment for NHL with high-risk genetic features.

- Identify acute and chronic toxicities associated with the drugs used to treat NHL and the measures used to prevent or treat these toxicities.

- Identify monitoring parameters for response and toxicity in patients with NHL.

- Provide detailed patient education for the chemotherapeutic regimen selected to treat NHL.

PATIENT PRESENTATION

■ Chief Complaint

"What's the next step for my lymphoma?"

■ HPI

A 58-year-old man presents to the oncologist's office for recommendations about treatment of a newly diagnosed diffuse, large B-cell lymphoma. He had been in relatively good health other than his longstanding hypertension, hypercholesterolemia, and GERD. He initially presented to the ED 1 week ago with new-onset left lower extremity edema. He was then hospitalized for further evaluation and treatment. At that time, he stated that he had lost weight over the past few months. Vital signs on admission included elevated temperature of 100.8°F (38.2°C). Physical examination findings were significant for a round, protuberant abdomen that was soft on the right side but firm on left and 3+ pitting edema of the left lower extremity from foot to knee. Laboratory findings included serum creatinine 1.9 mg/dL, serum calcium 11.6 mg/dL, and hemoglobin 10.6 g/dL. A renal ultrasound revealed severe hydronephrosis on the left side and displacement of the bladder with compression, possibly from a mass. A CT scan without contrast of the chest, abdomen, and pelvis was performed. Results showed multiple enlarged lymph nodes, including several mediastinal nodes, paraesophageal nodes, and retrocrural nodes. A large, confluent soft tissue mass was found, extending through the retroperitoneum and involving the left pelvis. The mass encased the distal left ureter. The mass in its widest dimension was 16.3 cm. A diagnosis of lymphoma was presumed based on the extent of lymph involvement. Urologists placed a left ureteral stent and performed ultrasound-guided biopsy of the mass. Pathology showed diffuse large non-Hodgkin B-cell lymphoma. Upon confirmation of diagnosis, a bone marrow biopsy was performed. Results were not available during hospitalization. The patient was insistent on discharge to attend his daughter's wedding, so treatment was deferred after initial consultation with an oncologist in the hospital. His creatinine and calcium values were normalizing at the time of discharge.

■ PMH

HTN × 10 years
Hypercholesterolemia × 5 years
GERD × 15 years

■ FH

The patient is the oldest of seven children (four brothers and two sisters), all alive and well. He has two children, both in good health. Family history of terminal prostate cancer in his father (died at age 63). No other history of malignancy that he is aware of.

■ SH

The patient is employed by a large chemical company as a manager of the division that caters to aerospace applications. He has been with the company since graduating from college. He initially began work in the production areas and advanced to his current management position. He previously smoked 1–2 ppd for 25 years; he quit when he was diagnosed with GERD. He drinks one to two beers nightly. Diet is mostly unremarkable except that he states that he does not eat many vegetables, unless popcorn counts. He has been married for 34 years; his spouse is with him today in the clinic.

■ ROS

The patient reports continuing fever, typically ranging from 100.2 to 101°F (37.9–38.3°C). He states his lower extremity swelling is much better since hospitalization and was pleased that he was able to wear his fancy dancing shoes for his daughter's wedding. He reports an unexplained weight loss of approximately 25 lb over the past 3 months. He denies headaches, changes in vision, or fainting episodes. He reports no lesions in his mouth, difficulty swallowing, or nosebleeds. He denies orthopnea and tachycardia. He has not had any back pain. He denies any changes in urination frequency, burning on urination, urinary frequency, dribbling, or blood in the urine. He has not noticed any abnormal bleeding or bruising. He has not received any prior transfusions.

■ Meds

Lisinopril 20 mg PO once daily
Furosemide 20 mg PO once daily
Simvastatin 20 mg PO at bedtime
Famotidine 20 mg PO twice daily
Epoetin alfa 40,000 units subQ once weekly

■ All

Penicillin—rash

■ Physical Examination

Gen

Patient is a thin man in no apparent distress.

VS

BP 145/100 mm Hg, P 95 bpm, RR 14, T 37.9°C; Wt 72 kg, Ht 5'9"

Skin

No rashes or moles noted

HEENT

PERRLA; TMs clear; no masses in the tonsils, palate, or floor of the mouth; no stomatitis. Several missing teeth, but no gingival inflammation is noted.

Neck

Supple; no masses; no JVD

Chest

CTA bilaterally

CV

RRR; no MRG

Abd

Soft, nontender, appears distended. No hepatomegaly or splenomegaly noted. Bowel sounds normoactive.

Genit/Rect

Normal male genitalia

Ext

1+ pitting edema of left lower extremity

Neuro

Symmetric cranial nerve function. Symmetric facial muscle movement, and the tongue is midline. The palate is symmetric. Balance

and coordination of the upper extremities are intact, with no evidence of tremor. There is symmetric coordination of rapidly alternating movements. Motor strength in the upper and lower extremities is normal and symmetric.

Lymph Node Survey

The lymph node survey is negative for any palpable peripheral nodes in the preauricular, postauricular, submandibular, cervical, supraclavicular, infraclavicular, or axillary areas.

■ Labs

Na 132 mEq/L	Hgb 10.3 g/dL	AST 29 IU/L	Phos 4.0 mg/dL
K 4.6 mEq/L	Hct 30%	ALT 27 IU/L	Uric acid
Cl 97 mEq/L	Plt 338 × 10³/mm³	Alk phos 75 IU/L	5.6 mg/dL
CO₂ 26 mEq/L	WBC 9.9 × 10³/mm³	LDH 623 IU/L	PT 12.2 seconds
BUN 20 mg/dL	Neutros 70%	T. bili 0.6 mg/dL	aPTT
SCr 0.9 mg/dL	Bands 2%	T. prot 6.3 g/dL	21.7 seconds
Glu 112 mg/dL	Lymphs 18%	Alb 3.7 g/dL	
Ca 9.7 mg/dL	Monos 9%		
	Eos 1%		

■ Bone Marrow Biopsy

Biopsy and aspiration were negative for blasts or atypical lymphocytes.

■ Tumor Pathology

Diffuse large B-cell lymphoma, germinal center type; CD10+, CD19+, CD20+, CD23+, CD38+, CD5–. FISH indicates 75% of nuclei have MYC/IGH fusion and BCL2 rearrangement. BCL6 rearrangement was not detected.

■ Initial Assessment

Diffuse large cell lymphoma. Further staging will include PET scan, HIV test, CT of the abdomen, and a baseline cardiac assessment in light of the patient's longstanding history of HTN.

■ Clinical Course

PET scanning revealed multiple foci of increased FDG uptake, consistent with findings of CT scan. No additional areas of involvement noted. MUGA scan reveals LVEF 65%.

■ Assessment

Double-hit diffuse large B-cell lymphoma, stage III; IPI score of 2.

QUESTIONS

Collect Information

1. What subjective and objective information is consistent with the diagnosis of non-Hodgkin lymphoma (NHL)?

Assess the Information

2.a. Explain what system of staging was used and how his stage of disease was determined.

2.b. What laboratory and clinical features does this patient have that may affect his prognosis and treatment? How is the International Prognostic Index (IPI) determined?

2.c. Create a list of the patient's drug therapy problems and prioritize them. Include assessment of medication appropriateness, effectiveness, safety, and patient adherence.

Develop a Care Plan

3.a. What are the goals of pharmacotherapy in this case?

3.b. What nondrug therapies might be useful for treating this patient's drug therapy problems?

3.c. What feasible pharmacotherapeutic options are available for treating NHL in this patient?

3.d. Create an individualized, patient-centered, team-based care plan to optimize medication therapy for this patient's NHL. Include specific drugs, dosage forms, doses, schedules, and durations of therapy.

3.e. What other interventions should be made to maintain control of the patient's other concurrent diseases?

Implement the Care Plan

4.a. What information should be provided to the patient to enhance adherence, ensure successful therapy, and minimize adverse effects?

4.b. Describe how care should be coordinated with other healthcare providers.

Follow-Up: Monitor and Evaluate

5. Explain how to monitor and evaluate the care plan for medication appropriateness, effectiveness, safety, and patient adherence by using clinical and laboratory data, patient feedback, and other information.

■ CLINICAL COURSE (PART 1)

The patient tolerated the first few cycles of chemotherapy well, with only some minimal nausea and vomiting. His antihypertensive medication was modified, increasing the lisinopril to 40 mg daily and achieving average systolic BPs in the 120s and average diastolic BPs in the 70s. His left lower extremity edema resolved, and furosemide was discontinued. His fasting lipid panel was checked and was found to be within his goals. One week after completing the fourth cycle of chemotherapy, he presented to the ED with fever (101.3°F [38.5°C]), cough, dyspnea, pain on inspiration, and fatigue. Laboratory evaluation showed an ANC of $0.352 \times 10^3/mm^3$. He was admitted to the hospital for evaluation and treatment of suspected neutropenic fever with pneumonia. Blood and sputum cultures were negative. The ANC remained below $0.5 \times 10^3/mm^3$ for 3 additional days before recovering. The patient was treated with broad-spectrum antibiotics and became afebrile after 3 days. He was discharged from the hospital after the neutropenia resolved, completing a 14-day course of inpatient IV antibiotics. PET and CT scans performed while he was hospitalized to evaluate his lymphoma showed that he achieved a complete response.

■ FOLLOW-UP QUESTION

1. What measures should be taken to prevent neutropenic fever in subsequent courses of chemotherapy?

■ CLINICAL COURSE (PART 2)

The patient completed his planned course of chemotherapy without further event. Eighteen months later, he returns to the oncologist office after being diagnosed with relapsed lymphoma during a hospital admission for worsening dyspnea.

■ SELF-STUDY ASSIGNMENTS

1. What therapeutic options are available for treatment of relapsed diffuse large B-cell lymphomas?

2. What is the role of chimeric antigen receptor T-cell therapy (CAR-T) in the treatment of diffuse large B-cell lymphoma?

3. If the patient had a history of hepatitis B, what diagnostic tests would be indicated? What antiviral therapy, if any, should be considered for patients with a history of hepatitis B who are receiving chemo-immunotherapy for treatment of diffuse large B-cell lymphoma?

CLINICAL PEARL

Double-hit lymphoma is an aggressive type of B-cell NHL caused by changes in the DNA that affect the MYC gene and either the BCL2 or the BCL6 gene. It requires more aggressive chemotherapy than standard B-cell lymphomas. Some clinicians advocate for initial treatment with high-dose chemotherapy with stem cell transplantation, but evidence from clinical trials does not support this approach.

REFERENCES

1. Cheson BD, Fisher RI, Barrington SF, et al. Recommendations for initial evaluation, staging, and response assessment of Hodgkin and non-Hodgkin lymphoma: the Lugano classification. J Clin Oncol. 2014;32:3059–3067.

2. Snuderl M, Kolman OK, Chen YB, et al. B-cell lymphomas with concurrent IGH-BCL2 and MYC rearrangements are aggressive neoplasms with clinical and pathologic features distinct from Burkitt lymphoma and diffuse large B-cell lymphoma. Am J Surg Pathol. 2010;34:327–340.

3. Zhou Z, Sehn LH, Rademaker AW, et al. An enhanced International Prognostic Index (NCCN-IPI) for patients with diffuse large B-cell lymphoma treated in the rituximab era. Blood. 2014;123:837–842.

4. Coiffier B, Thieblemont C, Van Den Neste E, et al. Long-term outcome of patients in the LNH-98.5 trial, the first randomized study comparing rituximab-CHOP to standard CHOP chemotherapy in DLBCL patients: a study by the Groupe d'Etudes des Lymphomes de l'Adulte. Blood. 2010;116:2040–2045.

5. Howlett C, Snedecor SJ, Landsburg DJ, et al. Front-line, dose-escalated immunochemotherapy is associated with significant progression-free survival advantage in patients with double-hit lymphomas: a systemic review and meta-analysis. Br J Haematol. 2015;170:405–514.

6. Purroy N, Bergua J, Gallur L, et al. Long-term follow-up of dose-adjusted EPOCH plus rituximab (DA-EPOCH-R) in untreated patients with poor prognosis large B-cell lymphoma. A phase II study conducted by the Spanish PETHEMA group. Br J Haematol. 2015;169:188–198.

7. Ganz WI, Sridhar KS, Ganz SS, et al. Review of tests for monitoring doxorubicin-induced cardiomyopathy. Oncology. 1996;53:461–470.

8. Smith TJ, Bohlke K, Lyman GH, et al. Recommendations for the use of WBC growth factors: American Society of Clinical Oncology clinical practice guideline update. J Clin Oncol. 2015;33:3199–3212.

9. Hesketh PJ, Kris MG, Basch E, et al. Antiemetics: ASCO guideline update. J Clin Oncol. 2020;38:2782–2797.

10. Taplitz RA, Kennedy EB, Bow EJ, et al. Antimicrobial prophylaxis for adult patients with cancer-related immunosuppression: ASCO and IDSA clinical practice guideline update. J Clin Oncol. 2018;36(30):3043–3054.

156

HODGKIN LYMPHOMA

The Rock Climber............................Level I

Stephanie Chase, PharmD, BCOP

Cindy L. O'Bryant, PharmD, BCOP

LEARNING OBJECTIVES

After completing this case study, the reader should be able to:

- Recognize the signs and symptoms commonly associated with Hodgkin lymphoma (HL).

- Propose a pharmacotherapeutic regimen of choice among several first-line treatment options for HL.

- Identify acute and chronic toxicities associated with the medications used to treat HL and the measures used to prevent, treat, and monitor these toxicities.

- Determine monitoring parameters for treatment response and toxicity in patients with HL.

- Formulate appropriate educational information to provide to a patient receiving chemotherapy treatment for HL.

PATIENT PRESENTATION

■ Chief Complaint

"I have been having night sweats, fever, and weight loss despite healthy eating. I have also been a lot more tired lately. My neck has been swollen, my left armpit is really sensitive, and I have a growth on my neck that has gotten bigger over the past month."

■ HPI

A 27-year-old man presents to an outpatient medical oncology clinic with a 1-month history of night sweats, fever, fatigue, and a 9-kg weight loss. He noticed weight loss because he has been watching his weight while training for an upcoming 2-week climbing trip. His wife also noticed neck swelling and a neck mass that has gotten progressively larger over the past month. He initially associated the mass with a strep throat infection and went to see his primary care provider 5 weeks ago. He was started on a 10-day course of antibiotics, but the mass did not resolve. One week ago, his primary care provider scheduled an ultrasound of the neck due to persistent and worsening symptoms. At this visit, enlarged right and left supraclavicular lymph nodes and an enlarged left axillary node were palpated on physical exam. The ultrasound of the neck showed a cervical lymph node that measured approximately 11 cm in diameter. As a result, an excisional lymph node core biopsy was performed that day, which demonstrated Classic HL, nodular sclerosing (NS) subtype.

■ PMH

Epstein-Barr virus as a teenager

■ FH

The patient's mother, father, and two siblings (brother and sister) are all in good health. Paternal grandfather died of lung cancer.

■ SH

Works as structural engineer. Is a rock climber and is training for a 2-week climbing trip. Drinks socially, about three to four beers per week. He has never smoked. He does not use illicit drugs. The patient is married and wishes to start a family in the next 2 years.

■ Meds

Ibuprofen 400 mg PO Q 4–6 H PRN pain/fever

■ All

NKDA

■ ROS

(+) For fevers, night sweats, fatigue, and weight loss of approximately 9 kg over the past month.
(−) For vision changes, headaches, shortness of breath, chest pain, nausea, vomiting, diarrhea, constipation, or urinary symptoms. Denies feeling depressed or having loss of pleasure with activities. His performance status is 1 on the ECOG scale.

■ Physical Examination

Gen

The patient is a healthy-appearing man in no apparent distress.

VS

BP 118/70 mm Hg, P 64 bpm, RR 16, T 37.6°C; Wt 79.3 kg, Ht 6'1"

Skin

Soft, diffusely enlarged soft tissue swelling in the neck; no erythema or warmth; no rashes

HEENT

PERRL; EOMI; TMs intact

Lymph Nodes

Both right and left supraclavicular nodes and a left axillary node are enlarged. The left anterior cervical neck mass is palpable. No other lymph nodes are palpable bilaterally.

Chest

Respirations with normal rhythm; clear to auscultation

CV

RRR; no JVD, murmurs, or gallops

Abd

Soft and nontender with no masses; bowel sounds are normoactive

Genit/Rect

Normal male genitalia; stool is guaiac (−)

MS/Ext

Without edema

Neuro

A&O × 3; CN II–XII intact; remainder of exam is nonfocal

■ Labs

Na 137 mEq/L	Hgb 10.1 g/dL	AST 19 IU/L	PT 12.9 seconds
K 4.1 mEq/L	Hct 32.3%	ALT 22 IU/L	aPTT 27.1 seconds
Cl 103 mEq/L	Plt 310 × 10³/mm³	Alk phos 74 IU/L	Phos 3.1 mg/dL
CO₂ 24 mEq/L	WBC 10.9 × 10³/mm³	LDH 372 IU/L	Magnesium
BUN 14 mg/dL	Neutros 80.5%	T. bili 0.4 mg/dL	1.2 mEq/L
SCr 0.7 mg/dL	Lymphs 13.2%	T. prot 7.7 g/dL	Uric acid
Glu 82 mg/dL	Monos 5.4%	Alb 3.2 g/dL	7.5 mg/dL
	Eos 0.9%		ESR 63 mm/h

■ Ultrasound

There are singular, enlarged abnormal lymph nodes in the right and left supraclavicular regions. The largest node on the right measures 2.8 cm × 1.5 cm × 2.1 cm and on the left 1.8 cm × 0.9 cm × 1.3 cm. The large left anterior cervical node is 11.1 cm × 6.8 cm × 8.9 cm. The left axillary lymph node measures 5.2 cm × 4.6 cm × 4.9 cm. The nodes contain solid echogenic material and have increased vascular flow.

■ Tumor Pathology

A complete excisional lymph node biopsy identified Reed–Sternberg cells, classifying this malignancy as HL, NS subtype (Fig. 156-1). Immunohistochemistry: CD15+, CD30+, CD3–, CD20–, CD45–, CD79a–.

■ PET/Helical CT Scan

Enlarged nodes demonstrating hypermetabolic activity are noted in the bilateral supraclavicular chains, the left axillary lymph node, the mediastinum, and the superior mesenteric lymphatic chain. There is involvement of the left anterior cervical node showing bulky disease. The bilateral lungs and myocardium are negative for disease. Normal physiologic liver, GI, and urinary activity are noted. Diffuse increased uptake within the bone marrow; it is unclear whether this is lymphoma or hyperplasia.

■ Bone Marrow Biopsy

Negative for HL

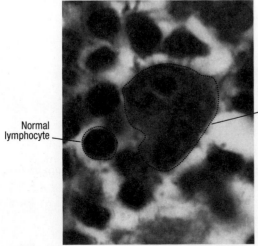

FIGURE 156-1. Reed-Sternberg cell (center) surrounded by normal lymphocytes. (Source: National Cancer Institute.)

■ Assessment

Classic HL, nodular sclerosis subtype, stage IIIB

QUESTIONS

Collect Information

1.a. What subjective and objective information is consistent with the diagnosis of Hodgkin lymphoma (HL)?

1.b. What additional information is needed to fully assess this patient's HL?

Assess the Information

2.a. Assess the severity of HL based on the subjective and objective information available.

2.b. Create a list of the patient's drug therapy problems and prioritize them. Include assessment of medication appropriateness, effectiveness, safety, and patient adherence.

Develop a Care Plan

3.a. What are the goals of pharmacotherapy for HL in this case?

3.b. What nondrug therapies might be useful for this patient's HL?

3.c. What feasible pharmacotherapeutic options are available for treating this patient's HL?

3.d. Create an individualized, patient-centered, team-based care plan to optimize medication therapy for this patient's HL and other drug therapy problems. Include specific drugs, dosage forms, doses, schedules, and durations of therapy.

Implement the Care Plan

4.a. What information should be provided to the patient to enhance adherence, ensure successful therapy, and minimize adverse effects for the treatment of HL?

4.b. Describe how care should be coordinated with other healthcare providers.

Follow-Up: Monitor and Evaluate

4.b. Explain how to monitor and evaluate the care plan for medication appropriateness, effectiveness, safety, and patient adherence by using clinical and laboratory data, patient feedback, and other information.

■ CLINICAL COURSE

The patient's treatment was administered in the outpatient setting. He received day 1 of his first cycle of chemotherapy and experienced acute nausea and vomiting. Five days after his first treatment, he experienced mild mucositis and mild constipation. He was instructed to maintain good oral hygiene, use a soft toothbrush, and avoid alcohol and spicy or acidic foods. He was started on a mouthwash (diphenhydramine, lidocaine, and aluminum/magnesium hydroxide) with instructions to swish and spit four times a day. He was educated to maintain good hydration, a high-fiber diet, and to start docusate sodium 100 mg orally once daily for constipation. He successfully received cycle 2 of chemotherapy in the outpatient clinic without incident. He was then restaged with a PET/CT scan to assess his response to chemotherapy. Restaging showed the patient had a favorable response with a Deauville score of 2, and he then received four additional cycles of chemotherapy to complete his treatment. On subsequent follow-up with an end-of-therapy (EOT) PET/CT scan, a complete response was confirmed.

■ SELF-STUDY ASSIGNMENTS

1. What are unfavorable prognostic risk factors for early-stage and advanced-stage HL, and how does this influence treatment?

2. What is the antiemetic regimen of choice to prevent acute nausea and vomiting for highly emetogenic chemotherapy?

3. What are salvage therapy options for patients with relapsing HL?

4. What is the role for hematopoietic stem cell transplantation in HL?

CLINICAL PEARL

HL can be cured with chemotherapy, even in advanced stages. To achieve a cure, it is essential that a patient receives appropriate treatment. Therapy selection is based on several key factors: (1) accurate diagnosis of the subtype of HL via immunostaining techniques; (2) appropriate staging; (3) identification of unfavorable prognostic risk factors; (4) patient age, sex, and presence of comorbid conditions; (5) baseline cardiac and pulmonary status; and (6) evaluation of all nodal and extranodal sites of involvement. A multi-agent chemotherapy regimen, with or without consolidative involved-site radiation therapy, is then initiated. The goal is to achieve a complete remission while minimizing patient exposure to acute- and long-term treatment-related toxicities.

REFERENCES

1. NCCN Clinical Practice Guidelines in Oncology: Hodgkin Lymphoma (Version 4.2021). Available at: *https://www.nccn.org/professionals/physician_gls/pdf/hodgkins.pdf*. Accessed November 1, 2021.

2. Cheson BD, Fisher RI, Barrington SF, et al. Recommendations for initial evaluation, staging, and response assessment of Hodgkin and non-Hodgkin lymphoma: the Lugano classification. J Clin Oncol. 2014;32:3059–3068.

3. Moccia AA, Donaldson J, Chhanabhai M, et al. International Prognostic Score in advanced-stage Hodgkin's lymphoma: altered utility in the modern era. J Clin Oncol. 2012;30(27):3383–3388.

4. Johnson P, Federico M, Kirkwood A, et al. Adapted treatment guided by interim PET-CT scan in advanced Hodgkin's lymphoma (RATHL Study). N Engl J Med. 2016;374(25):2419–2429.

5. Casasnovas RO, Bouabdallah R, Brice P, et al. PET-adapted treatment for newly diagnosed advanced Hodgkin lymphoma (AHL2011): a randomised, multicentre, non-inferiority, phase 3 study. Lancet Oncol. 2019;20(2):202–215.

6. Borchmann P, Goergen H, Kobe C, et al. PET-guided treatment in patients with advanced-stage Hodgkin's lymphoma (HD18): final results of an open-label, international, randomised phase 3 trial by the German Hodgkin Study Group. Lancet. 2017;390(10114):2790–2802.

7. Straus DJ, Długosz-Danecka M, Connors JM, et al. Brentuximab vedotin with chemotherapy for stage III or IV classical Hodgkin lymphoma (ECHELON-1): 5-year update of an international, open-label, randomised, phase 3 trial. Lancet Haematol. 2021;8(6):e410–e421.

8. NCCN Clinical Practice Guidelines in Oncology: Antiemesis (Version 1.2021). Available at: *https://www.nccn.org/professionals/physician_gls/pdf/antiemesis.pdf*. Accessed November 1, 2021.

9. Hodgson DC. Long-term toxicity of chemotherapy and radiotherapy in lymphoma survivors: optimizing treatment for individual patients. Clin Adv Hematol Oncol. 2015;13:103–112.

10. Schaapveld M, Aleman BM, van Eggermond A, et al. Second cancer risk up to 40 years after treatment for Hodgkin's lymphoma. N Engl J Med. 2015;373:2499–2511.

157

OVARIAN CANCER

Family Ties.................................... Level II

Amber B. Cipriani, PharmD, BCOP

Alexis Jones, PharmD, BCOP

LEARNING OBJECTIVES

After completing this case study, the reader should be able to:

- Recognize the signs and symptoms of ovarian cancer.

- Assess the need for genetic testing with ovarian cancer.

- Recommend a pharmacotherapeutic plan for the chemotherapy of newly diagnosed and relapsed ovarian cancer, as well as targeted therapy for maintenance treatment.

- Describe the dose-limiting and most common toxicities associated with the chemotherapeutic agents used to treat ovarian cancer.

PATIENT PRESENTATION

■ Chief Complaint

"I'm very anxious about getting chemotherapy. My uncles have gone through chemotherapy for colorectal cancer and became very sick. One of them was even admitted to the hospital due to the side effects. I don't want that to happen to me."

■ HPI

A 56-year-old woman presents to the gynecology oncology clinic 1 week after surgery for stage IIIB (T3b N1 M0) serous epithelial ovarian adenocarcinoma. She originally presented to her PCP 1 month ago with complaints of a 15-lb weight gain, bloating, and abdominal pain. A history and physical exam identified a left adnexal mass. CT scans of the abdomen and pelvis showed a large, soft-tissue pelvic mass. Laboratory examination revealed a CA-125 level of 490 IU/mL.

Two weeks later, the patient underwent an exploratory laparotomy, TAH-BSO, omentectomy, and bilateral pelvic and periaortic lymph node dissection with comprehensive staging by a gynecologic oncologist. On entering the abdomen, there was a relatively small amount of ascitic fluid. A large left adnexal mass measuring 15 cm × 5 cm × 10 cm and multiple small tumor nodules (≤2 cm) outside the pelvis were removed. Numerous adhesions were seen throughout the omentum and surrounding organs. At completion of the surgery, the surgeon noted that the patient was optimally debulked with an R0 resection. Ascitic fluid, peritoneal washings, left adnexal mass, left and right ovaries, multiple pelvic and periaortic lymph nodes, and omentum were sent to pathology for examination.

Gross examination of left and right ovaries revealed multiple adhesions extending from each ovary with interspersed broad regions of necrosis. Each ovary was serially sectioned for microscopic examination, which revealed numerous papillations of tumor cells destructively permeating the stroma (grade 2). Based on this information, the patient was diagnosed with stage IIIB (T3b N1 M0) serous epithelial ovarian adenocarcinoma.

PMH

Type 2 DM × 17 years
Dyslipidemia × 15 years
Peripheral neuropathy × 3 years

FH

Married × 37 years with a son age 35. Her father died of an MI at age 72, and her mother died at age 60 with ovarian cancer. Two paternal uncles (age 80 and 76 years) are alive with colorectal cancer.

SH

Consumes one glass of red wine with dinner every evening. Has a 20 pack-year history of cigarette smoking; quit 25 years ago. No recreational drug use. Poor adherence to medication as evidenced by inconsistent refill dates per pharmacy record.

Meds

Atorvastatin 40 mg PO daily
Metformin 1000 mg PO twice daily
Glyburide 10 mg PO twice daily
Lisinopril 40 mg PO daily
Gabapentin 300 mg PO twice daily

All

Penicillin (hives as a child)
Codeine ("sour stomach")

ROS

Somewhat fatigued lately, progressively worsening over the past 2 months. Reports a 15-lb weight gain over the past month. She also reports requiring more sleep than usual, about 9–10 hours per night, but cannot recall when this change occurred. Her mood is depressed because of concern about her recent cancer diagnosis. Denies any changes in sight, smell, hearing, and taste.

Physical Examination

Gen

The patient appears to be her stated age. Appears anxious in the office on exam.

VS

BP 135/85 mm Hg, P 110 bpm, RR 18, T 37.0°C; Ht 5′7″, Wt 70 kg

Skin

No erythema, rash, ecchymoses, or petechiae

LN

No cervical or axillary lymphadenopathy

HEENT

PERRLA, EOMI; TMs intact; fundus benign; OP dry

Breasts

Without masses, discharge, or adenopathy; no nipple or skin changes

Cor

RRR; no M/R/G

Pulm

CTA bilaterally

Abd

Soft, nontender; no HSM. Surgical wound healing well; no exudate or erythema; covered with 4 × 4 bandage with antibiotic ointment.

Genit/Rect

Normal female genitalia; heme (–) dark brown stool; no rectal wall tenderness or masses

Ext

No C/C/E. Residual erythema and swelling in LLE from prior DVT; no signs of ulceration.

Neuro

CN II–XII intact; sensation decreased to light touch and pinprick below the knees bilaterally; vibration sense diminished at the great toes bilaterally

Labs

Na 140 mEq/L	Hgb 12.8 g/dL	AST 25 IU/L
K 4.1 mEq/L	Hct 37%	ALT 40 IU/L
Cl 99 mEq/L	Plt 135 × 10³/mm³	T. bili 0.7 mg/dL
CO₂ 24 mEq/L	WBC 5.2 × 10³/mm³	Alb 4.0 U/L
BUN 20 mg/dL	Neutros 60%	CA-125 490 IU/mL
SCr 1.1 mg/dL	Bands 3%	
Glu 135 mg/dL	Lymphs 30%	
Ca 9.8 mg/dL	Monos 5%	
Mg 2.0 mg/dL	Eos 1%	
Phos 3.5 mg/dL	Basos 1%	

UA

WBC 1–5/hpf, RBC 0/hpf, 1+ ketones, 1+ protein, pH 5.0

Genetic Results

Patient was referred to a genetics counselor due to new diagnosis and history of ovarian cancer in her mother. Genetic testing results are pending.

Assessment/Plan

This is a 56-year-old woman with advanced stage IIIB (T2c N1 M0) serous epithelial ovarian adenocarcinoma. She underwent optimal surgical debulking (2 weeks ago) with an R0 resection by a gynecologic oncologist and presents to the clinic for follow-up care. Based on the stage of diagnosis and risk for recurrence, first-line chemotherapy is recommended.

QUESTIONS

Collect Information

1. What subjective and objective information indicates the presence of ovarian cancer?

Assess the Information

2.a. What stage of ovarian cancer does this patient have, and how does the stage of disease affect the choice of therapy?

2.b. What is the significance of the size of residual tumor after primary cytoreductive surgery?

2.c. What is the reason for performing genetic testing, and how do the results influence prognosis and treatment?

2.d. Create a list of the patient's drug therapy problems and prioritize them. Include assessment of medication appropriateness, effectiveness, safety, and patient adherence.

Develop a Care Plan

3.a. What are the goals of pharmacotherapy in this case?

3.b. What are the first-line chemotherapy options for treating ovarian cancer in this patient?

3.c. What are the specific toxicities and logistical issues related to intraperitoneal (IP) therapy?

3.d. Create an individualized, patient-centered, team-based care plan to optimize medication therapy for this patient's ovarian cancer and her other medical problems. Include specific drugs, dosage forms, doses, schedules, and durations of therapy for chemotherapy and for prevention/treatment of nausea and vomiting.

■ CLINICAL COURSE (PART 1)

The patient and oncologist agreed to begin treatment with the combination of IV docetaxel and carboplatin on day 1 every 21 days for six cycles as first-line treatment of her ovarian cancer.

Implement the Care Plan

4.a. What information should be provided to the patient to enhance adherence, ensure successful therapy, and minimize adverse effects?

4.b. Describe how care should be coordinated with other healthcare providers.

Follow-Up: Monitor and Evaluate

5. Explain how to monitor and evaluate the care plan for medication appropriateness, effectiveness, safety, and patient adherence by using clinical and laboratory data, patient feedback, and other information.

■ CLINICAL COURSE (PART 2)

The patient completed six cycles of docetaxel 75 mg/m² IV over 1 hour followed by carboplatin AUC 5 IV over 1 hour on day 1 every 21 days. She tolerated therapy very well with no dose reductions or delays. Her serum CA-125 level slowly declined over the course of treatment and was 12 IU/mL 3 weeks after her sixth cycle. Based on her CA-125 level and the negative CT scans following the fourth and sixth cycles, she was defined as a clinical complete response. Her CA-125 levels were followed monthly. Germline genetic testing results revealed a pathogenic BRCA1 mutation (deletion of exon 24). Her tumor sample was classified as HRD positive on somatic tissue-based testing.

■ FOLLOW-UP QUESTIONS

1. What are the options for first-line maintenance therapy after a patient has had a partial or complete response to platinum-based chemotherapy?

2. How would you explain "maintenance therapy" to a patient with ovarian cancer?

3. What are the implications of the genetic testing results for the patient's first-degree relatives?

■ CLINICAL COURSE (PART 3)

The patient received maintenance therapy with olaparib 300 mg PO BID. Her CA-125 levels were monitored every 3 months and remained stable. After 15 months on olaparib, her CA-125 levels began to increase monthly. Her CA-125 levels were: 10, 14, 20, 30, 43, and 88 IU/mL. A CT scan performed at 19 months after platinum

treatment discontinuation revealed a pelvic mass (6 cm × 5 cm × 4 cm) arising from the retroperitoneum and a 2-cm mass in the head of the pancreas. Laboratory data were normal except for a CA-125 level of 150 IU/mL. She was diagnosed with recurrent ovarian cancer.

■ FOLLOW-UP QUESTIONS

4. Is it preferable to treat early relapsed disease based only on a rising CA-125 level rather than delaying treatment until there are clinical signs of relapse?

5. What therapeutic options are available for this patient's relapsed disease?

6. Which of the chemotherapeutic regimens would you recommend for the patient's locally relapsed ovarian cancer? Provide the rationale for your answer.

■ CLINICAL COURSE (PART 4)

The decision was made to start IV carboplatin AUC 5 and pegylated liposomal doxorubicin 30 mg/m² on day 1 every 28 days; the patient received two cycles. Radiologic imaging just prior to the third cycle showed no evidence of disease progression. During her third cycle, she complained of having trouble putting on her shoes and pain in her feet on walking. On physical exam, the patient's feet were red, swollen, and cracked. Her CA-125 levels were 155, 158, and 160 IU/mL after each of her first three cycles of carboplatin plus pegylated liposomal doxorubicin.

■ FOLLOW-UP QUESTION

7. What are the potential adverse effects of pegylated liposomal doxorubicin therapy that require monitoring and patient education?

■ CLINICAL COURSE (PART 5)

The fourth cycle of therapy was delayed for 2 weeks and restarted when her skin lesions resolved. She completed six cycles of chemotherapy; however, upon final imaging, she still had small lesions on CT scan (none of which were >4 cm in diameter). Four months after completing six cycles of carboplatin/liposomal doxorubicin, the patient began to experience abdominal bloating and discomfort. A CT scan showed evidence of ascites and new disease within the peritoneal cavity.

■ FOLLOW-UP QUESTION

8. What options are available for salvage therapy, and which would you choose for this patient? Provide the rationale for your answer.

■ SELF-STUDY ASSIGNMENTS

1. What are the pharmacologic advantages of IV therapy versus IP therapy for ovarian cancer?

2. Why is the size of the residual tumor important with regard to IP therapy?

3. What are the probable causes of paclitaxel and docetaxel hypersensitivity?

4. What are the issues related to maintenance therapy in patients with advanced ovarian cancer after achieving complete response to consolidative chemotherapy?

5. How might cytochrome P450 3A4/5 polymorphism potentially affect docetaxel therapy of ovarian cancer?

CLINICAL PEARL

Neoadjuvant chemotherapy is an option for patients with advanced age or poor performance status who cannot undergo surgical cytoreduction followed by chemotherapy. This is given prior to the primary treatment (surgery) with the goal of reducing tumor volume and having a greater chance of cure. Neoadjuvant chemotherapy simplifies surgery by decreasing tumor volume, blood loss, and transfusions during surgery, and can reduce surgical complications and length of stays.

REFERENCES

1. The NCCN Clinical Practice Guidelines in Oncology™ Ovarian Cancer (Version 3.2021). © 2021 National Comprehensive Cancer Network Inc. Available at: *NCCN.org*. Accessed December 12, 2021.
2. Boyd J, Sonoda Y, Federici MG, et al. Clinicopathologic features of BRCA-linked and sporadic ovarian cancer. JAMA. 2000;283:2260–2265.
3. Ozols RF, Bundy BN, Greer BE, et al. Gynecologic Oncology Group. Phase III trial of carboplatin and paclitaxel compared with cisplatin and paclitaxel in patients with optimally resected stage III ovarian cancer: a gynecologic oncology group study. J Clin Oncol. 2003;21:3194–3200.
4. du Bois A, Luck HJ, Meier W, et al; Arbeitsgemeinschaft Gynakologische Onkologie Ovarian Cancer Study Group. A randomized clinical trial of cisplatin/paclitaxel versus carboplatin/paclitaxel as first-line treatment of ovarian cancer. J Natl Cancer Inst. 2003;95:1320–1329.
5. Vasey PA, Jayson GC, Gordon A, et al; Scottish Gynaecological Cancer Trials Group. Phase III randomized trial of docetaxel–carboplatin versus paclitaxel–carboplatin as first-line chemotherapy for ovarian carcinoma. J Natl Cancer Inst. 2004;96:1682–1691.
6. Armstrong DK, Bundy B, Wenzel L, et al; Gynecologic Oncology Group. Intraperitoneal cisplatin and paclitaxel in ovarian cancer. N Engl J Med. 2006;354:34–43.
7. Rustin GJ, van der Burg ME, Griffin CL, et al. Early versus delayed treatment of relapsed ovarian cancer (MRC OV05/EORTC 55955): a randomised trial. Lancet. 2010;376:1155–1163.
8. Wagner U, Marth C, Largillier R, et al. Final overall survival results of phase III GCIG CALYPSO trial of pegylated liposomal doxorubicin and carboplatin vs paclitaxel and carboplatin in platinum-sensitive ovarian cancer patients. Br J Cancer. 2010;107:588–591.
9. Pujade-Lauraine E, Hilpert F, Weber B, et al. Bevacizumab combined with chemotherapy for platinum-resistant recurrent ovarian cancer: the AURELIA Open-label Randomized Phase III Trial. J Clin Oncol. 2014;32:1302–1308.

158

ACUTE LYMPHOCYTIC LEUKEMIA

Uninvited and Unexpected Weight Loss .... Level II

Deborah A. Hass, PharmD, BCOP, BCPS

LEARNING OBJECTIVES

After completing this case study, the reader should be able to:

- Interpret the laboratory values that signify the response of acute lymphocytic leukemia (ALL) to chemotherapy.

- Describe the ancillary medications and supportive care measures that are necessary when administering chemotherapy to patients with ALL.

- Recommend the appropriate medications to treat neutropenic fever.

- Identify the backbone of therapy for treatment of adult ALL.

- State why CNS prophylaxis is routinely done in adult patients with ALL.

PATIENT PRESENTATION

■ Chief Complaint

Episodic sweating, dizziness, and progressively worsening weakness and shortness of breath on exertion × 1 month.

■ HPI

A 58-year-old man with a past medical history of diabetes, hyperlipidemia, and hypertension presents with episodic diaphoresis, dizziness, and progressively worsening weakness and dyspnea on exertion for 1 month. He has lost 40 lb in the past 9 months; despite trying to eat more recently, he is still losing 2 lb per week. Flow cytometry done 3 days ago at an outside hospital showed blastic B cells consistent with pre-B-cell lymphoblastic leukemia. The patient was found to have normocytic anemia (Hgb 9.9 g/dL). He also had a CT of the chest/abdomen/pelvis completed at the outside hospital due to weight loss and occasional abdominal pain and sensation that his stomach is "churning," although no report was sent with his records. He denies diarrhea but admits to once having an episode of dry heaving. A CXR was unremarkable. The patient was previously taking Janumet for type 2 DM, but since this workup began, he stopped it and has had blood sugars in the 100–130s.

■ PMH

DM type 2
HTN
Dyslipidemia

■ FH

Father had MI at age 60 and leukemia at age 78 and expired shortly thereafter. Mother is alive with heart disease, skin cancer, an unknown GI malignancy, and a recent diagnosis of lymphoma. He has five brothers and two sisters. One brother died at age 48 from Hodgkin lymphoma, diagnosed at age 18. Another brother has multiple sclerosis. The other three brothers and both sisters are healthy.

■ SH

Denies tobacco, EtOH, and illicit drugs. Drives a waste management truck, has three children, and lives with his wife.

■ Meds

None

■ All

NKDA

■ ROS

Constitutional: Positive for sweats, fatigue, anorexia, and weight loss. Also positive for dyspnea, nausea, abdominal pain, dizziness, and weakness.

■ **Physical Examination**

Gen

A&O × 3; NAD

VS

BP 124/58 mm Hg, P 106 bpm, RR 18, T 37.2°C; Wt 100.8 kg, Ht 5′11″, SpO$_2$: 98% (room air)

Skin

Normal, no rashes

HEENT

EOMI, no scleral icterus, no conjunctival pallor

Neck/Lymph Nodes

No cervical LAD

Lungs/Thorax

CTA bilaterally without crackles, wheezes, or rhonchi

CV

RRR; normal S$_1$, S$_2$; no murmurs, rubs, or gallops

Abd

Soft, obese, NT/ND, normoactive bowel sounds

MS/Ext

No CCE

Neuro

UE/LE strength 5/5 bilaterally

■ **Labs**

Na 137 mEq/L	Hgb 9.9 g/dL	AST 16 IU/L
K 4.1 mEq/L	Hct 27.2%	ALT 10 IU/L
Cl 100 mEq/L	MCV 93.5 μm^3	T. bili 0.5 mg/dL
CO$_2$ 28 mEq/L	RDW 17.1%	Alb 3 g/dL
BUN 19 mg/dL	Plt 95 × 10^3/mm^3	Fe 23 mcg/dL
SCr 1.2 mg/dL	WBC 7.1 × 10^3/mm^3	TIBC 252 mcg/dL
Glu 93 mg/dL	Segs 35%	T. sat 35%
	Bands 0.2%	Ferritin 159 ng/L
	Lymphs 5.2%	TSH 3.3 μIU/mL
	Monos 8.6%	PSA 0.52 ng/mL
	Myelos 1.6%	B$_{12}$ 311 ng/mL
	Blasts 49%	Folate 9.5 ng/mL

■ **Peripheral Blood Flow Cytometry**

Large population of abnormal blasts, ~49% of leukocyte population expressing CD45. Blasts have precursor B-cell phenotype and express CD19, CD22, CD34, CD38, HLA-DR, and terminal deoxynucleotidyl transferase (TdT). About 59% of blasts express CD20. Blasts are negative for surface IG, T-cell–related antigens, and myeloid antigens. The mature lymphocyte population consists of a mix of unremarkable T and B cells.

■ **Assessment and Plan**

1. Pre–B-cell lymphoblastic leukemia (Philadelphia chromosome negative):
   - Obtain LDH/uric acid
   - Bone marrow biopsy
   - MUGA scan
   - Central catheter placement
   - Will attempt to obtain CT report from outside hospital
   - Acute leukemia panel
2. Type 2 DM with controlled BS despite stopping meds recently:
   - Accu-Chek QID
   - Diabetic diet
   - Obtain UA to check for proteinuria; patient recently on ACE inhibitor but taken off. SCr ranging from 0.9 to 1.2 mg/dL at outside hospital.
3. Nausea:
   - Ondansetron PRN
4. HTN:
   - Patient recently taken off meds due to weight loss; will monitor BP and restart meds as needed
5. Thrombocytopenia:
   - Transfuse to keep platelets >10 × 10^3/mm^3
6. Anemia:
   - Transfuse to keep hemoglobin >8 g/dL
7. FEN:
   - Diabetic diet as above
   - Maintain K >4 mEq/L and Mg >2 mg/dL
8. VTE prophylaxis:
   - SCD boots

QUESTIONS

Collect Information

1.a. What subjective and objective information indicates the presence of acute lymphocytic leukemia (ALL)?

1.b. What additional information is needed to fully assess this patient's ALL?

Assess the Information

2.a. Assess the severity of ALL based on the subjective and objective information available.

2.b. Upon initial presentation, create a list of the patient's drug therapy problems and prioritize them. Include assessment of medication appropriateness, effectiveness, safety, and patient adherence.

■ CLINICAL COURSE

Within 2 days of admission, the patient receives a BM biopsy, MUGA (EF = 60%), and PICC line placement. The results of the biopsy were as follows:

The vast majority of cells in the aspirate and biopsy are large blasts with fine chromatin and many prominent cytoplasmic vacuoles. Nucleoli are not generally prominent, and flow cytometric studies indicated that this is a neoplasm of immature B cells. In addition, strong TdT expression is seen by immunohistochemistry. CD20 is expressed weakly to strongly in about half of the neoplastic cells.

WHO classification: Precursor B lymphoblastic leukemia.

The patient is started on the following medications:

- Pantoprazole delayed-release tablet 40 mg PO daily
- Ondansetron 8 mg PO Q 8 H PRN
- 0.9% normal saline by continuous IV infusion
- Allopurinol 300 mg PO daily

Following recovery from the PICC line placement, the patient was started on the R-Hyper-CVAD regimen based on Ht 180 cm, Wt 100.8 kg, and BSA = 2.2 m².

■ CHEMOTHERAPY

Regimen 1A

Cyclophosphamide 300 mg/m² (660 mg) IV over 3 hours every 12 hours for six doses on days 1–3

Mesna 600 mg/m² (1320 mg) IV over 24 hours on days 1–3, ending 12 hours after the last dose of cyclophosphamide

Vincristine 2 mg IV on days 4 and 11

Doxorubicin 50 mg/m² (110 mg) IV on day 4

Dexamethasone 40 mg PO on days 1–4 and 11–14

Rituximab 375 mg/m² (825 mg) IV on day 1. (Patient did not receive it on day 1 to prevent tumor flare.)

Regimen 1B

The patient will alternate cycles every 21 days with the following regimen, for a total of six to eight cycles depending on patient tolerability and disease progression; patient-specific doses will be based on the patient's weight at that time:

Methotrexate 200 mg/m² IV over 2 hours, followed by 800 mg/m² IV over 22 hours on day 1

Leucovorin 25 mg PO Q 6 H starting 24 hours after completion of the methotrexate infusion until methotrexate level is <0.05 µmol/mL

Cytarabine 3000 mg/m2 IV over 2 hours every 12 hours for four doses on days 2–3

Methylprednisolone 50 mg IV BID on days 1–3

CNS Prophylaxis

Methotrexate 12 mg intrathecally on day 2.

Cytarabine 100 mg intrathecally on day 8.

Repeat with each cycle of chemotherapy, depending on the risk of CNS disease. The CNS prophylaxis is given with both regimens 1 and 2.

Additional Medications with Chemotherapy

Ondansetron injection 8 mg IV push Q 12 H

Fluconazole 400 mg PO daily

Acyclovir 400 mg PO Q 12 H

Prochlorperazine 10 mg IV push Q 6 H PRN

Prochlorperazine 10 mg PO Q 6 H PRN

Lorazepam 0.5 mg PO Q 6 H PRN

■ CLINICAL COURSE

Day 2 of Induction Chemotherapy

Blood glucose remained in the 90s with one reading at 77 mg/dL early this morning. Patient denies any symptoms of hypoglycemia. He was started on a diabetic diet yesterday, which he has been tolerating. Given his recent weight loss, he may no longer have the same degree of insulin resistance as before. Continue to monitor BG levels. Hypoglycemic protocol is in place if patient's BG drops below 70 mg/dL.

Day 3 of Induction Chemotherapy

Patient c/o mild nausea but still has good appetite and is eating well; encouraged use of PRN antiemetics. Patient tolerated intrathecal chemotherapy. No acute events overnight.

Day 4 of Induction Chemotherapy

Patient spiked temp to 101°F (38.3°C). Denies any respiratory, urinary, or other symptoms. Started on cefepime 2 g IV Q 8 H.

Day 5 of Induction Chemotherapy

Patient continues to complain of nausea but has not vomited. He is able to tolerate a little solid food but reports that his appetite is not what it was. Reports two episodes of watery, nonbloody diarrhea early this morning with no further episodes since then.

Day 6 of Induction Chemotherapy

Patient reports that his appetite is improving. He still complains of nausea, which has improved only slightly, but he has had no episodes of vomiting. No further episodes of diarrhea. No acute events overnight. He will receive rituximab 375 mg/m² (825 mg) IV today.

Day 7 of Induction Chemotherapy

Patient reported chills and shaking during rituximab infusion yesterday. Acetaminophen 650 mg PO and diphenhydramine 50 mg IV were given. He felt better after that. No further symptoms during the day. Patient's only complaint is lack of bowel movement for 2 days. He is also still nauseated but is able to tolerate a regular meal without any emesis. No acute events overnight.

Day 8 of Induction Chemotherapy

Patient complains of severe hiccups throughout the day and night yesterday that prevented him from sleeping. He said that he also has epigastric discomfort associated with the hiccups. He has pain in the epigastric region that he rates as 7/10 in intensity with no radiation. It is neither sharp nor dull and feels like a "knot." He also feels very full and bloated. He says it feels better when he stands up and walks around and also subsides when the hiccups cease. No further episodes of diarrhea and no vomiting. Patient still nauseated but was able to tolerate meals. He had one small BM yesterday. No acute events overnight.

Day 15 of Induction Chemotherapy

The patient was discharged to home. He was instructed to call the hematology fellow on call at any sign of a fever or infection. He was also instructed to stay away from people who have active infections, such as an upper respiratory virus. He was told to avoid large crowds and not to do any gardening. This is all to decrease the risk of infection. He will return to the hospital in 6 days for cycle 2 of chemotherapy. He is sent home with the following prescriptions:

Fluconazole 400 mg PO daily

Acyclovir 400 mg PO Q 12 H

Prochlorperazine 10 mg PO Q 6 H PRN

2.c. Create and prioritize a new list of drug therapy problems resulting from treatment for ALL. Include assessment of medication appropriateness, effectiveness, safety, and patient adherence.

Develop a Care Plan

3.a. What are the short-term goals of pharmacotherapy in this case?

3.b. The patient will receive four cycles of R-Hyper-CVAD alternating with four cycles of high-dose methotrexate and cytarabine. What are the long-term goals of pharmacotherapy for this patient?

3.c. What nondrug therapies might be useful for this patient?

3.d. What effect will this chemotherapy regimen have on his diabetes?

3.e. What other chemotherapy regimens are available for treating this patient's ALL?

3.f. Why was the patient started on allopurinol prior to starting his chemotherapy?

3.g. Why was the patient started on fluconazole and acyclovir in the doses prescribed?

3.h. Why was the patient started on intrathecal chemotherapy with no current evidence of CNS disease?

3.i. What therapy would you recommend for a patient with relapsed or refractory ALL?

Implement the Care Plan

4.a. What information should be provided to the patient about the potential beneficial and adverse effects from the chemotherapy agents used during induction therapy?

4.b. Assume that the patient does not understand why he has to have so many courses of chemotherapy. Explain why he cannot be treated with just one cycle of chemotherapy.

4.c. Describe how care should be coordinated with other healthcare providers.

Follow-Up: Monitor and Evaluate

5. Explain how to monitor and evaluate the care plan for medication appropriateness, effectiveness, safety, and patient adherence by using clinical and laboratory data, patient feedback, and other information.

■ SELF-STUDY ASSIGNMENTS

1. Discuss the value of colony-stimulating factors in the prophylaxis or treatment of therapy-related complications in patients with ALL.

2. Discuss the response criteria used to determine if a patient with ALL has obtained a complete remission or partial remission.

3. Define the terms *stable disease* and *progressive disease* as they relate to ALL.

CLINICAL PEARL

First-line therapy for ALL must contain the backbone of an anthracycline derivative, vincristine, and a corticosteroid. Asparaginase is also a useful agent due to the leukemic cells' unique lack of endogenous asparagine. Patients with Philadelphia chromosome-positive ALL are treated with BCR-ABL tyrosine kinase inhibitors such as imatinib or dasatinib, *in addition* to the induction chemotherapy regimen, such as R-Hyper-CVAD, which this patient received.

REFERENCES

1. Thomas DA, O'Brien S, Faderl S, et al. Chemoimmunotherapy with a modified hyper-CVAD and rituximab regimen improves outcome in de novo Philadelphia chromosome-negative precursor B-lineage acute lymphoblastic leukemia. J Clin Oncol. 2010;28(24):3880–3889.

2. Weiser MA, Cabanillas ME, Konopleva M, et al. Relation between the duration of remission and hyperglycemia during induction chemotherapy for acute lymphocytic leukemia with a hyperfractionated cyclophosphamide, vincristine, doxorubicin, and dexamethasone/methotrexate-cytarabine regimen. Cancer. 2004;100:1179–1185.

3. Nam J. Dexamethasone-induced hiccups in chemotherapy may be prevented by rotating to methylprednisolone. Oncology Nurse Advisor, July 11, 2017. Available at: https://www.oncologynurseadvisor.com/home/hot-topics/side-effect-management/dexamethasone-induced-hiccups-in-chemotherapy-may-be-prevented-by-rotating-to-methylprednisolone/. Accessed December 13, 2019.

4. Wetzler M, Sanford BL, Kurtzberg J, et al. Effective asparagine depletion with pegylated asparaginase results in improved outcomes in adult acute lymphoblastic leukemia: Cancer and Leukemia Group B Study 9511. Blood. 2007;109:4164–4167.

5. Freifeld AG, Bow EJ, Sepkowitz KA, et al. Clinical practice guideline for the use of antimicrobial agents in neutropenic patients with cancer: 2010 update by the Infectious Diseases Society of America. Clin Infect Dis. 2011;52(4):e56–e93.

6. Campana D. Minimal residual disease in acute lymphoblastic leukemia. Hematology Am Soc Hematol Educ Program. 2010;2010:7–12.

7. O'Brien S, Schiller G, Lister J, et al. High-dose vincristine sulfate liposome injection for advanced, relapsed, and refractory adult Philadelphia chromosome-negative acute lymphoblastic leukemia. J Clin Oncol. 2013;31(6):676–683.

8. Kantarjian HM, DeAngelo DJ, Stelljes M, et al. Inotuzumab ozogamicin versus standard therapy for acute lymphoblastic leukemia. N Engl J Med. 2016;375(8):740–753.

9. Topp MS, Gokbuget N, Stein AS, et al. Safety and activity of blinatumomab for adult patients with relapsed or refractory B-precursor acute lymphoblastic leukaemia: a multicentre, single-arm, phase 2 study. Lancet Oncol. 2015;16(1):57–66.

10. Maude SL, Frey N, Shaw PA, et al. Chimeric antigen receptor T cells for sustained remissions in leukemia. N Engl J Med. 2014;371(16):1507–1517.

159

CHRONIC MYELOID LEUKEMIA

It's Not Always Sunny in Philadelphia. . . . . Level II

Allison L. Morse, PharmD, BCOP

Aaron Cumpston, PharmD, BCOP

LEARNING OBJECTIVES

After completing this case study, the reader should be able to:

• Identify the presenting signs and symptoms of chronic myeloid leukemia (CML).

• Determine important prognostic indicators for CML.

• Discuss available treatment options for newly diagnosed CML and refractory or relapsed CML and recommend an appropriate therapy.

• Choose appropriate parameters to monitor efficacy and potential adverse effects of treatment for CML.

• Educate patients on dosing and administration, the importance of adherence, and the most common adverse effects of the selected therapy for CML.

• Discuss potential mechanisms of resistance to first-line therapy for CML and formulate a treatment strategy for these patients.

PATIENT PRESENTATION

■ Chief Complaint

"I'm here for my routine visit for my back pain, but I have been feeling pretty tired lately and have this dull pain in my abdomen."

■ HPI

A 55-year-old man presents to his physician for an annual physical exam complaining of chronic back pain. He also complains of left-sided abdominal discomfort and fullness that has resulted in some decreased appetite and increasing fatigue and inactivity over the past 3 months. When questioned, he reports experiencing intermittent drenching night sweats for the past 2 months that seem to be more frequent now.

■ PMH

Chronic back pain secondary to injury 5 years ago
Childhood asthma, last symptoms at age 21
Appendectomy 16 years ago

■ FH

Father died at age 66 due to MI. Mother is living, 71 years old with osteoporosis, depression, and GERD. He has one sister, age 52, living in Maine with no known medical issues. Paternal grandfather had prostate cancer but passed away from unrelated causes. Patient has no natural children.

■ SH

Married and has one stepson, age 19, who attends college overseas. The patient works as a nurse in a local long-term care facility, and his wife is a tax accountant. He has no smoking history but drinks alcohol on social occasions. He denies any illicit drug use.

■ Meds

One-a-day multivitamin PO once daily
Cyclobenzaprine 10 mg PO BID as needed
Ibuprofen 800 mg PO TID as needed for mild to moderate pain
Oxycodone 10 mg PO Q 6 H as needed for severe pain

■ All

NKA

■ ROS

Positive for increased weakness and tiredness, frequent night sweats, mild shortness of breath on exertion, general musculoskeletal pain, and LUQ pain. Denies bleeding, headaches, vision changes, nausea, vomiting, chest pain, rashes, numbness or tingling in extremities, or urinary symptoms.

■ Physical Examination

Gen

Well-developed male who appears his stated age and is in no obvious distress

VS

BP 122/60 mm Hg, P 63 bpm, RR 20, T 36.3°C; Wt 77.5 kg, Ht 180 cm, pain score 0 on a 0–10 scale

Skin

Skin warm and dry, no rashes or lesions

HEENT

Head atraumatic and normocephalic; ENT without erythema or injection; mucous membranes moist; conjunctivae clear; PERRLA. No sinus discharge or tenderness. Lips, teeth, and gums without tenderness.

Neck

No JVD or thyromegaly appreciated

Lymph Nodes

No palpable cervical, supraclavicular, axillary, or inguinal adenopathy

Lungs

Diffuse expiratory wheezes bilaterally

CV

Regular rate and rhythm; S_1 and S_2 normal; 2/6 systolic murmur heard best along the upper left sternal border

Abd

Tender to palpation; tip of spleen palpable in LUQ, measuring 15 cm. Normoactive bowel sounds. No hepatomegaly.

MS/Ext

Normal gait, full range of motion in flexion and extension of the upper and lower extremities with 5/5 strength throughout. No cyanosis or edema; no synovitis or joint effusions.

Neuro

Grossly normal; CN II–XII intact; alert and oriented × 3

Psychiatric

Normal affect, behavior, memory, thought content, judgment, and speech

■ Labs

Na 139 mEq/L	Hgb 10.3 g/dL	AST 24 IU/L	Ca 8.2 mg/dL
K 3.7 mEq/L	Hct 33.8%	ALT 38 IU/L	Mg 2.2 mEq/L
Cl 105 mEq/L	Plt 470 × 10³/mm³	Alk phos 72 IU/L	Phos 3.8 mg/dL
CO₂ 27 mEq/L	WBC 123 × 10³/mm³	LDH 950 IU/L	Uric acid
BUN 28 mg/dL	PMNs 53%	T. bili 0.6 mg/dL	6.5 mg/dL
SCr 0.8 mg/dL	Bands 13%	T. prot 6.9 g/dL	LAP absent
Glu 92 mg/dL	Lymphs 7%	Alb 3.5 g/dL	
Retic 2.3%	Myelos 9%		
	Metas 10%		
	Eos 4%		
	Basos 4%		

■ Bone Marrow Biopsy

The bone marrow is markedly hypercellular (essentially 100% cellular) due to extensive proliferation of granulocytes. The granulocytic series are left-shifted; however, blasts are not increased and no Auer rods or significant dysplasia is noted. Erythroid precursors are slightly decreased and megakaryocytes are markedly increased with many small, hypolobated forms. Iron stores are decreased, and mild reticulin fibrosis is identified. Eosinophilia and basophilia are also present in the peripheral blood and bone marrow. FISH analysis is positive for BCR-ABL1 rearrangement.

Cytogenetic studies show translocation involving the long arms of chromosomes 9 and 22 [t(9q;22q)] (Philadelphia chromosome), with 95% of malignant cells analyzed found to be Ph-positive (Fig. 159-1).

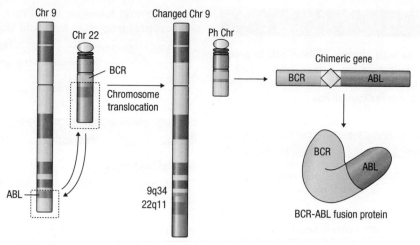

FIGURE 159-1. Specific chromosomal translocation seen in chronic myeloid leukemia (CML). The Philadelphia chromosome (Ph) is derived from a reciprocal translocation between chromosomes 9 and 22 with the breakpoint joining the sequences of the ABL oncogene with the BCR gene. The fusion of these DNA sequences allows for the generation of an entirely novel fusion protein with modified function. (Reproduced with permission from Morin PJ, Trent JM, Collins FS, Vogelstein B. Cancer genetics. In: Jameson JL, Fauci AS, Kasper DL, Hauser SL, Longo DL, Loscalzo J, eds. *Harrison's Principles of Internal Medicine*. 20th ed. New York, NY: McGraw-Hill; 2018.)

This information is consistent with the characteristics of CML, and the morphologic features are consistent with chronic phase (CML-CP).

QUESTIONS

Collect Information

1. What subjective and objective information is consistent with a diagnosis of CML-CP?

Assess the Information

2.a. Assess the severity of CML based on the subjective and objective information available.

2.b. Create a list of the patient's drug therapy problems and prioritize them. Include assessment of medication appropriateness, effectiveness, safety, and patient adherence.

Develop a Care Plan

3.a. What are the long-term therapy goals for this case?

3.b. What nondrug therapies might be useful for this newly diagnosed patient?

3.c. What feasible pharmacotherapeutic options are available for treating newly diagnosed CML-CP?

3.d. Create an individualized, patient-centered, team-based care plan to optimize medication therapy for this patient's CML and other drug therapy problems. Include specific drugs, dosage forms, doses, schedules, and durations of therapy.

Implement the Care Plan

4.a. What information should be provided to the patient prior to treatment to enhance compliance, ensure successful therapy, and minimize adverse effects?

4.b. Describe how care should be coordinated with other healthcare providers.

Follow-Up: Monitor and Evaluate

5. Explain how to monitor and evaluate the care plan for medication appropriateness, effectiveness, safety, and patient adherence by using clinical and laboratory data, patient feedback, and other information.

■ CLINICAL COURSE

The regimen you recommended was initiated. At the 2-week follow-up visit, the patient's WBC count was $34 \times 10^3/\text{mm}^3$. At the 4-week follow-up visit, his WBC count decreased to $9 \times 10^3/\text{mm}^3$. After 3 months of treatment, his WBC count was stable at $8.2 \times 10^3/\text{mm}^3$, platelet count stable at $425 \times 10^3/\text{mm}^3$, and he had a minimal cytogenetic response as evidenced by a bone marrow biopsy that revealed 70% Philadelphia chromosome-positive metaphases. After 6 months, he remained in complete hematologic response but minor cytogenetic response with 60% Ph-positive metaphases. Molecular analysis (qPCR testing for the Philadelphia chromosome) also showed less than a major response. Because he experienced a suboptimal response, mutation testing was performed and revealed the presence of a V299L mutation. Also, since beginning treatment with imatinib, the patient has noticed mild periorbital edema, moderate myalgias, and nausea. He presents to clinic today to discuss further treatment options with the healthcare team.

■ FOLLOW-UP QUESTIONS

1. What therapeutic options are available for this patient with a suboptimal response to imatinib 400 mg PO once daily?

2. Is it possible to discontinue tyrosine kinase inhibitor (TKI) therapy and maintain remission, or will the patient need lifelong therapy?

3. How would your recommendations differ if the patient had a T315I mutation instead?

■ SELF-STUDY ASSIGNMENTS

1. Describe the criteria for hematologic complete response, cytogenetic response (complete, major, partial, minor, and no response), and molecular response (early, major, deep) for therapy in patients with CML, including WBC count, splenomegaly, and percent of Ph+ marrow cells.

2. If a woman becomes pregnant while receiving TKI treatment for CML, how should the therapy be revised?

3. Discuss the progress being made to develop treatments for patients with the T315I mutation.

Mutation testing in patients with chronic phase CML is generally not performed unless the patient has a suboptimal or lack of response to first-line TKI therapy because mutations can occasionally be found in patients without resistant disease.

REFERENCES

1. Hochhaus A, Larson RA, Guilhot F, et al. Long-term outcomes of imatinib treatment for chronic myeloid leukemia. N Engl J Med. 2017;376:917–927.

2. Cortes JE, Saglio G, Kantarjian HM, et al. Final 5-year study results of DASISION: the dasatinib versus imatinib study in treatment-naïve chronic myeloid leukemia patients trial. J Clin Oncol. 2016;34(20):2333–2340.

3. Hochhaus A, Saglio G, Hughes TP, et al. Long-term benefits and risks of frontline nilotinib vs imatinib for chronic myeloid leukemia in chronic phase: 5-year update of the randomized ENESTnd trial. Leukemia. 2016;30(5):1044–1054.

4. Cortes JE, Khoury HJ, Kantarjian HM, et al. Long-term bosutinib for chronic phase chronic myeloid leukemia after failure of imatinib plus dasatinib and/or nilotinib. Am J Hematol. 2016;91(9):1206–1214.

5. Rea D. Management of adverse events associated with tyrosine kinase inhibitors in chronic myeloid leukemia. Ann Hematol. 2015;94(Suppl 2): S149–S158.

6. Baccarani M, Deininger MW, Rosti G, et al. European LeukemiaNet recommendations for the management of chronic myeloid leukemia: 2013. Blood. 2013;122(6):872–884.

7. Shah NP, Rousselot P, Schiffer C, et al. Dasatinib in imatinib-resistant or -intolerant chronic-phase, chronic myeloid leukemia patients: 7-year follow-up of study CA180-034. Am J Hematol. 2016;91(9):869–874.

8. Cortes JE, Kim DW, Pinilla-Ibarz J, et al. Ponatinib efficacy and safety in Philadelphia chromosome-positive leukemia: final 5-year results of the phase 2 PACE trial. Blood. 2018;132(4):393–404.

9. Cortes J, Lipton JH, Rea D, et al. Phase 2 study of subcutaneous omacetaxine mepesuccinate after TKI failure in patients with chronic-phase CML with T315I mutation. Blood. 2012;120:2573–2580.

10. Rea D, Mauro M, Boquimpani C, et al. A phase 3, open-label, randomized study of asciminib, a STAMP inhibitor, vs bosutinib in CML after ≥2 prior TKIs. Blood. 2021;138(21):2031–2041.

160

KIDNEY CANCER

A Time for Decision . . . . Level II

Daniel J. Crona, PharmD, PhD, CPP

LEARNING OBJECTIVES

After completing this case study, the reader should be able to:

- Evaluate first-line pharmacotherapeutic options for patients with metastatic kidney cancer.

- Formulate a monitoring plan for a patient receiving treatment for metastatic kidney cancer based on patient-specific factors and the prescribed regimen.

- Recommend subsequent treatment options for patients with relapsed or progressive metastatic kidney cancer.

- Provide appropriate and detailed educational information to patients about the targeted therapies for metastatic kidney cancer.

PATIENT PRESENTATION

■ Chief Complaint

"What treatment options do I have for my metastatic kidney cancer?"

■ HPI

A 65-year-old woman presented 3.5 years ago to her primary care physician with complaints of back pain, cough, and weight loss. She did not respond to an initial course of antibiotics for assumed pyelonephritis and developed gross hematuria a few days later. She was subsequently referred to a urologist, who detected a left kidney mass on renal ultrasound. CT scan of chest, abdomen, and pelvis revealed a 7-cm left upper-pole kidney tumor and several bilateral small, subcentimeter lung nodules. Additional imaging found no evidence of metastatic disease in her brain, bones, or liver. She was referred to a nearby cancer center for further evaluation. A core needle biopsy of the kidney mass revealed neoplastic cells, but the sample was too small and heterogeneous to definitively determine a specific histology. In order to relieve worsening symptoms and further elucidate a specific histopathology of the mass, she underwent radical nephrectomy of her left kidney. Pathologic examination revealed kidney cancer with clear-cell histology, and she recovered from surgery with resolution of back pain and hematuria. No treatment for the pulmonary nodules was undertaken because interventional radiology determined that they were not cancerous; however, the patient agreed to undergo active surveillance of the nodules over time to identify changes or progression.

Now, more than 3 years later, the patient presents to the outpatient oncology clinic for an appointment with the medical oncologist. Recently, a routine CT scan revealed lung metastases (ie, the bilateral nodules increased in number and size since the initial scans and the decision to pursue active surveillance). Imaging found no evidence of metastatic disease in her brain, bones, or liver. The patient has an estimated Karnofsky score of 90%, is interested in pursuing systemic treatment for her metastatic kidney cancer, and would like to discuss appropriate and available treatment options.

■ PMH

CKD
Hypertension
Kidney Cancer (S/P left nephrectomy)

■ FH

Mother died at age 75 due to complications related to MI, and father died at age 73 due to PE. Has one brother, age 58, who is alive and living with asthma, but who is otherwise healthy. There is no family history of cancer.

■ SH

The patient has been happily married for over 40 years, and has one grown son, age 33, who is alive and healthy. The patient reports an extensive smoking history (25 pack-years), but quit 5 years ago. She is overweight (BMI 29.3 kg/m²).

Meds

Hydrochlorothiazide 25 mg PO once daily
Enalapril 5 mg PO once daily

All

NKDA

ROS

No fever or chills; no headaches; no nausea or vomiting; feels very weak since the surgery

Physical Examination

Gen

WDWN woman in NAD

VS

BP 130/84 mm Hg, P 64 bpm, RR 18, T 37.0°C; Wt 82.4 kg, Ht 5′6″, BSA 1.96 m²

Skin

Normal turgor; no rash, lesions, or jaundice. Nephrectomy site is fully healed.

HEENT

PERRLA, EOMI; oropharynx without lesions

Neck/Lymph Nodes

Supple without adenopathy; thyroid without masses

Lung/Thorax

Slight wheezing in LUL

CV

RRR; normal S_1 and S_2; no MRG

Abd

Soft, NT/ND; (+) BS

Ext

No clubbing, cyanosis, or edema

Neuro

A&O × 3

Labs

Na 137 mEq/L	Hgb 12 g/dL	WBC 6.1 ×10³/mm³	T. bili 0.8 mg/dL
K 4.0 mEq/L	Hct 36%	Neutros 66%	AST 25 IU/L
Cl 99 mEq/L	Plt 325 ×10³/mm³	Bands 4%	ALT 27 IU/L
CO₂ 25 mEq/L		Lymphs 26%	Alk phos 125 IU/L
BUN 20 mg/dL		Monos 4%	Alb 3.8 g/dL
SCr 2.0 mg/dL			LDH 220 IU/L
Glu 75 mg/dL			Ca 8.5 mg/dL
			Mg 2.0 mg/dL

Assessment

This is a 65-year-old woman with metastatic clear-cell kidney cancer who is S/P resection of the primary tumor via radical nephrectomy. Multiple subcentimeter metastatic lung lesions persist; however, there is no evidence of additional metastatic disease. Briefly, she is not a candidate for high-dose IL-2 based on inadequate results of pulmonary function testing (both FVC and FEV₁ were <65% of predicted values) and a serum creatinine of 2.0 mg/dL. Nonpharmacologic options include surveillance and forgoing systemic treatment for now; however, she is interested in learning about possible pharmacotherapeutic options.

QUESTIONS

Collect Information

1.a. What subjective and objective information indicates the presence and severity of kidney cancer?

1.b. What additional information is needed to fully assess this patient's kidney cancer?

Assess the Information

2. Create a list of the patient's drug therapy problems and prioritize them. Include assessment of medication appropriateness, effectiveness, safety, and patient adherence.

Develop a Care Plan

3.a. What are the goals of pharmacotherapy for metastatic kidney cancer in this case?

3.b. What nondrug therapies might be useful for treating this patient's kidney cancer?

3.c. What feasible pharmacotherapeutic alternatives are available for treating metastatic kidney cancer?

3.d. Create an individualized, patient-centered, team-based care plan to optimize medications for this patient's drug therapy problems. Include specific drugs, dosage forms, doses, schedules, and durations of therapy.

3.e. Based on primary literature evidence, what are appropriate alternatives to your first-line treatment recommendations if the oncology team deems that it cannot be used?

Implement the Care Plan

4.a. What information should be provided to the patient prior to treatment to enhance adherence, ensure successful therapy, and minimize adverse effects?

4.b. Describe how care should be coordinated with other healthcare providers.

Follow-Up: Monitor and Evaluate

5. Explain how to monitor and evaluate the care plan for medication appropriateness, effectiveness, safety, and patient adherence by using clinical and laboratory data, patient feedback, and other information.

■ CLINICAL COURSE

The patient was started on the treatment you recommended and achieved partial regression of some of her metastatic pulmonary lesions. She experienced adverse effects, including hypertension (maximum BP 160/95 mm Hg), diarrhea, fatigue, mild lymphopenia, and minor elevations in liver function tests. Hypertension was controlled by increasing the enalapril dose to 10 mg once daily. Diarrhea was categorized as grade 1, attributed to the oral therapy, corticosteroids were not prescribed, and the intravenous therapy was not interrupted. Unfortunately, after 19 months of treatment, today's follow-up CT scan of the chest, abdomen, and pelvis indicates progression of the lung metastases (eg, new and larger bilateral pulmonary lesions). The patient expressed a desire to continue treatment and is here to learn about available second-line treatment options.

■ FOLLOW-UP QUESTIONS

1. Given this situation, what pharmacotherapeutic options are available? Provide the rationale for your answer.

2. How would you monitor for the potential treatment-related adverse events?

3. What education should the patient receive about the new regimen that you propose?

4. What alterations would you recommend to the patient's regimen if she were also receiving a strong inducer of hepatic CYP3A4 enzymes? What about a strong inhibitor of CYP3A4?

■ SELF-STUDY ASSIGNMENTS

1. Discuss the role of immunotherapies in metastatic kidney cancer. How has the use of immune checkpoint inhibitors, as part of combination pharmacotherapy, changed the first-line treatment landscape for metastatic kidney cancer?

2. Under what circumstances, and for which patients, is adjuvant pharmacotherapy appropriate after surgery for localized kidney cancer?

3. What role does tumor histology play in treatment selection for metastatic kidney cancer?

CLINICAL PEARL

Although the optimal management of immune-related adverse events (irAEs) for patients on combination ipilimumab plus nivolumab has been well elucidated in oncology guidelines (eg, early intervention, multidisciplinary management, corticosteroids), adverse event management for patients on an immune checkpoint inhibitor plus oral multikinase inhibitor is not as straightforward. Management of irAEs, or alternatively overlapping adverse events that can be attributed to the multikinase inhibitor (eg, diarrhea), require distinctly different management strategies.

REFERENCES

1. Heng DY, Xie W, Regan MM, et al. Prognostic factors for overall survival in patients with metastatic renal cell carcinoma treated with vascular endothelial growth factor–targeted agents: results from a large, multicenter study. J Clin Oncol. 2009;27:5794–5799.

2. Choueiri TK, Motzer RJ. Systemic therapy for metastatic renal-cell carcinoma. N Engl J Med. 2017;376:354–366.

3. Tran J, Ornstein MC. Clinical review on the management of metastatic renal cell carcinoma. JCO Oncol Pract. 2021 Sep 16;OP2100419. doi: 10.1200/OP.21.00419. Online ahead of print.

4. Rini BI, Plimack ER, Stus V, et al. Pembrolizumab plus axitinib versus sunitinib for advanced renal-cell carcinoma. N Engl J Med. 2019;380:1116–1127.

5. Motzer RJ, Alekseev B, Rha S-Y, et al. Lenvatinib plus pembrolizumab or everolimus for advanced renal cell carcinoma. N Engl J Med. 2021;384:1289–1300.

6. Choueiri TK, Powles T, Burotto M, et al. Nivolumab plus cabozantinib versus sunitinib for advanced renal-cell carcinoma. N Engl J Med. 2021;384:829–841.

7. Motzer RJ, Penkov K, Haanen J, et al. Avelumab plus axitinib versus sunitinib for advanced renal-cell carcinoma. N Engl J Med. 2019;380:1103–1115.

8. Motzer RJ, Tannir NM, McDermott DF, et al. Nivolumab plus ipilimumab versus sunitinib in advanced renal-cell carcinoma. N Engl J Med. 2018;378:1277–1290.

9. Choueiri TK, Escudier B, Powles T, et al. Cabozantinib versus everolimus in advanced renal-cell carcinoma. N Engl J Med. 2015;373:1814–1823.

10. Motzer RJ, Escudier B, McDermott DF, et al. Nivolumab versus everolimus in advanced renal-cell carcinoma. N Engl J Med. 2015;373:1803–1813.

161

MELANOMA

Overexposure . . . . Level II

Jessica Michaud Davis, PharmD, BCOP, CPP

Marina Kanos, MSN, FNP-C, RN, BSBA

LEARNING OBJECTIVES

After completing this case study, the reader should be able to:

- Identify risk factors for developing melanoma.

- Determine treatment options for metastatic melanoma.

- Prepare educational information to provide to a patient receiving treatment for metastatic melanoma.

- Discuss ways to prevent melanoma.

PATIENT PRESENTATION

■ Chief Complaint

"I have ongoing back pain for 8 weeks that has not gone away with over-the-counter treatments."

■ HPI

A 62-year-old Caucasian man presents with an 8-week history of mid-back pain. He has no history of recent injury or trauma to the area. He reports that his back pain continues to increase despite rest and applications with cold and heat. He rates his pain at its worst as 5 on 0–10 scale. The pain is present with movement and at rest. The pain does not radiate. He denies associated numbness or tingling. He has tried various medications including ibuprofen, naproxen, and acetaminophen.

■ PMH

GERD
Type 2 DM

Stage IIC melanoma of the right scapular area (T4b N0 M0; diagnosed 2 years ago in Australia; Breslow thickness 4.9 mm with ulceration. S/P wide local excision with right axillary lymph node dissection; zero out of 32 nodes showed evidence of involvement; there was no evidence of distant disease. Patient was not eligible for adjuvant treatment because it was not standard of care for stage IIC disease at the time of his diagnosis.

FH

Patient has two sisters; one with type 2 DM. Mother is 83 years old with a history of cutaneous basal cell carcinomas and stage IIA melanoma. Father died at age 71 secondary to heart disease.

SH

The patient is an advertising and commercial photographer. He is married with one daughter (age 27) who is healthy. He smoked one-half pack of cigarettes per day for 4 years while in college; has not smoked for the past 40 years. He has one to two alcoholic drinks on the weekends. He denies illicit drug use. As a child, he spent a significant amount of time outdoors in Australia. He was a summer lifeguard for 8 years. He did not routinely use sunscreen and has a history of sunburns, some blistering.

Medications

Omeprazole 20 mg orally once daily
Glipizide 10 mg orally once daily
Metformin 1000 mg orally twice daily
Ibuprofen 400 mg orally every 4–6 hours as needed for back pain

All

NKDA

ROS

Low back pain as described above. Denies fatigue, fever, chills, night sweats, recent vision changes, tinnitus, nasal congestion, sore throat, cough, dyspnea, chest pain, palpitations, nausea, vomiting, diarrhea, constipation, abdominal pain, dysuria, hematuria, bowel/bladder retention or incontinence, easy bruising, polydipsia, polyuria, rash, pruritus, new or changing skin lesions, headache, or dizziness.

Physical Examination

General

Caucasian man with mild distress due to mid-back pain

VS

BP 129/72 mm Hg, P 86 bpm, RR 16, O_2 saturation 99% on room air, T 36.8°C; Wt 90 kg, Ht 5'10"

Skin

Fair complexion with multiple (>50) nevi on trunk and bilateral upper and lower extremities. Well-healed scars on right mid-upper back and right axilla.

HEENT

Normocephalic, TMs clear with normal light reflex, PERRLA, EOMI, normal sclerae, moist oral mucosa, no pharyngeal erythema or exudate, normal nasal mucosa without drainage, no frontal or maxillary sinus tenderness

Neck

Supple, nontender, no thyromegaly, no masses

Resp

Lungs clear to auscultation bilaterally, breath sounds equal, respirations nonlabored

CV

Regular rate and rhythm, no murmurs or gallops, good pulses equal bilaterally in upper and lower extremities, no peripheral edema

Abd

Soft, nontender, nondistended, normoactive bowel sounds in all four quadrants, no organomegaly

Genitourinary

No CVA tenderness

Lymphatics

No lymphadenopathy neck, axilla, or groin; trace right upper extremity lymphedema

Musculoskeletal

Discomfort to palpation along the thoracic spine at the T7–T9 area

Neuro

Alert and oriented × 4, normal sensory and motor exam, CN II–XII intact, normal DTRs, negative Romberg, negative straight-leg raise

Psychiatric

Cooperative, appropriate mood and affect

Labs

Na 135 mEq/L, K 4.1 mEq/L, Cl 100 mEq/L, CO_2 25 mEq/L, BUN 9 mg/dL, SCr 1.0 mg/dL, Glu 75 mg/dL
Hgb 15.8 g/dL, Hct 46%, RBC 5.2 × 10⁶/mm³, Plt 322 × 10³/mm³
WBC 5.6 × 10⁶/mm³, Neutros 68%, Bands 3%, Eos 1%, Lymphs 26%, Monos 2%
T. bili 1.1 mg/dL, AST 22 IU/L, ALT 28 IU/L, Alk phos 165 IU/L, Alb 4.2 g/dL, LDH 340 IU/L, Ca 8.5 mg/dL, Mg 2.1 mg/dL, PO_4 3.6 mg/dL

CT Chest, Abdomen, and Pelvis

Two pulmonary nodules consistent with metastasis in the left upper and lower lobes. There is a lytic lesion in the vertebral body of T8.

CT-Guided Lung Biopsy

Pathology of the left lower lung nodule is consistent with metastatic melanoma. Molecular pathology confirmed BRAF V600E mutation not detected.

Assessment

A 62-year-old man with a 2-year history of melanoma with new metastases to the lungs and thoracic spine.

QUESTIONS

Collect Information

1.a. What subjective and objective information indicates the presence and severity of melanoma?

1.b. What additional information is needed to fully assess this patient's melanoma?

Assess the Information

2.a. What risk factor(s) does this patient have for developing melanoma?

2.b. Create a list of the patient's drug therapy problems and prioritize them. Include assessment of medication appropriateness, effectiveness, safety, and patient adherence.

Develop a Care Plan

3.a. What are the goals for treatment of melanoma in this case?

3.b. What nondrug therapies might be useful for this patient?

3.c. What feasible pharmacotherapeutic options are available for treating metastatic melanoma?

3.d. Create an individualized, patient-centered, team-based care plan to optimize medication therapy for this patient's metastatic melanoma and other drug therapy problems. Include specific drugs, dosage forms, doses, schedules, and durations of therapy.

Implement the Care Plan

4.a. What information should be provided to the patient to enhance adherence, ensure successful therapy, and minimize adverse effects?

4.b. Describe how care should be coordinated with other healthcare providers.

Follow-Up: Monitor and Evaluate

5. Explain how to monitor and evaluate the care plan for medication appropriateness, effectiveness, safety, and patient adherence by using clinical and laboratory data, patient feedback, and other information.

■ ADDITIONAL CASE QUESTIONS

1. The patient's daughter is concerned that she is at risk for developing melanoma. How can melanoma be prevented?

2. What is the ABCDE rule in helping to distinguish features of a normal mole from an abnormal mole?

3. How should immune-related adverse events from CTLA-4 and PD-1 checkpoint inhibitors be managed?

■ SELF-STUDY ASSIGNMENTS

1. List options for treatment if this patient had a BRAF V600E mutation.

2. Describe how the dosing of ipilimumab plus nivolumab combination therapy would differ for patients with renal cell carcinoma.

3. Infusion reactions to checkpoint inhibitors are rare but may occur. Describe how an infusion reaction may present and how it should be treated. Describe how premedications may be given before future infusions to help prevent recurrent infusion reactions.

CLINICAL PEARL

Vitiligo (the presence of hypopigmented skin lesions) is a clinically visible immune-related adverse effect of nivolumab, which is thought to occur due to the involvement of the PD-1 pathway in melanosomal proteins. The occurrence of vitiligo in melanoma patients treated with nivolumab has been associated with improved overall survival.[10]

REFERENCES

1. NCCN Clinical Practice Guidelines in Oncology. Cutaneous Melanoma. v.2.2021. Available at: www.nccn.org. Accessed November 12, 2021.

2. Larkin J, Chiarion-Sileni V, Gonzalez R, et al. Combined nivolumab and ipilimumab or monotherapy in untreated melanoma. N Engl J Med. 2015;373(1):23–34.

3. Larkin J, Chiarion-Sileni V, Gonzalez R, et al. Five-year survival with combined nivolumab and ipilimumab in advanced melanoma. N Engl J Med. 2019;381:1535–1546.

4. Robert C, Long GV, Brady B, et al. Nivolumab in previously untreated melanoma without BRAF mutation. N Engl J Med. 2015;372:320–330.

5. Robert C, Schachter J, Long GV, et al. Pembrolizumab versus ipilimumab in advanced melanoma. N Engl J Med. 2015;372:2521–2532.

6. Schachter J, Ribas A, Long GV, et al. Pembrolizumab versus ipilimumab for advanced melanoma: final overall survival results of a multicentre, randomised, open-label phase 3 study (KEYNOTE-006). Lancet. 2017;390(10105):1853–1862.

7. National Comprehensive Cancer Network. Management of Immunotherapy-Related Toxicities (Version 4.2021). Available at: https://www.nccn.org/professionals/physician_gls/pdf/immunotherapy.pdf. Accessed November 12, 2021.

8. Brahmer JR, Lacchetti C, Schneider BJ, et al. Management of immune-related adverse events in patients treated with immune checkpoint inhibitor therapy: American Society of Clinical Oncology clinical practice guideline. J Clin Oncol. 2018;36(17):1714–1768.

9. Melanoma [Internet]. New York (NY): The Skin Cancer Foundation; 2018. Available at: https://www.skincancer.org/skin-cancer-information/melanoma. Accessed December 16, 2018.

10. Freeman-Keller M, Kim Y, Cronin H, Richards A, Gibney G, Weber JS. Nivolumab in resected and unresectable metastatic melanoma: characteristics of immune-related adverse events and association with outcomes. Clin Cancer Res. 2016;22(4):886–894.

162

STEM CELL TRANSPLANTATION

Many Meds, Many Interactions . . . . Level III

Teresa C. Thakrar, PharmD, BCOP

LEARNING OBJECTIVES

After completing this case study, the reader should be able to:

- Understand the regimen-related toxicities of immunosuppression medications used for allogeneic stem cell transplantation (SCT).

- Differentiate the presenting features of immunosuppressive medication adverse events from other medications.

- Recommend optimal therapeutic plans, taking into account drug interactions, efficacy, safety, and patient adherence in post-allogeneic SCT patients.

- Design appropriate pharmacotherapeutic plans for patients who develop toxicity from immunosuppression.

PATIENT PRESENTATION

■ Chief Complaint

Bothersome headache and bilateral hand tremors with movement such as typing or holding a cup.

HPI

A 52-year-old woman presents to the BMT clinic status-post HLA-matched unrelated donor allogeneic SCT for high-risk AML. Her preparative regimen consisted of thiotepa (5 mg/kg IV Q 12 H × 3 doses) and cyclophosphamide (60 mg/kg IV Q 24 H × 2 doses). Her GVHD prophylaxis regimen consisted of tacrolimus and sirolimus, both starting on day −3. Her hospital course was complicated by febrile neutropenia, acute kidney injury, mucositis, and diarrhea. These complications had resolved at the time of discharge on day +20. Two weeks ago on day +75, she developed a skin rash and diarrhea and was diagnosed with grade 2 acute graft-versus-host disease (GVHD). She was started on methylprednisolone 80 mg (1 mg/kg) orally BID, and fluconazole was switched to posaconazole 300 mg orally once daily. She was seen recently by her PCP for dyslipidemia and hypertension, and gemfibrozil 600 mg orally twice daily was added to her existing atorvastatin 10 mg orally once daily and amlodipine 10 mg once daily.

PMH

High-risk AML treated with idarubicin and cytarabine induction, followed by high-dose cytarabine × 1 cycle. This was followed by a matched unrelated donor allogeneic SCT.

Hypertension diagnosed at age 45; previously well controlled with amlodipine prior to SCT.

Dyslipidemia diagnosed at age 39; previously well controlled with atorvastatin prior to SCT.

FH

Married with two children. Father is deceased from atherosclerotic heart disease.

Meds (at Day +120)

Posaconazole 300 mg PO daily
Esomeprazole 40 mg PO daily
Tacrolimus 2 mg PO twice daily
Methylprednisolone 80 mg PO twice daily
Valacyclovir 500 mg PO twice daily
Amlodipine 10 mg PO daily
Prochlorperazine 10 mg PO Q 8 H PRN nausea/vomiting
Sirolimus 2 mg PO once daily
Dapsone 100 mg PO daily
Atorvastatin 10 mg PO daily
Gemfibrozil 600 mg PO BID
Triamcinolone 1% cream—apply twice daily to chest and shoulders

All

Sulfa → urticaria

ROS

Worsening "annoying" motor tremors that interfere with activities of daily living such as typing and drinking. Patient also reports dull headache that started about a week ago. The rash has resolved, and she reports that the diarrhea has decreased to one to two loose stools per day.

Physical Examination

Gen

Patient is a WDWN woman.

VS

BP 158/76 mm Hg, P 92 bpm, T 37.4°C; O₂ sat 98% in room air; Wt 80 kg; Ht 5′4″

Skin

Intact, warm, dry, no rashes

HEENT

Moist mucous membranes

Neck/Lymph Nodes

Supple; no thyromegaly

Lungs

Clear without wheezes, rhonchi, or crackles

CV

RRR; normal heart sounds; no M/R/G

Abd

Slight distention, RUQ tenderness, mild hepatomegaly

MS/Ext

Grade I–II edema in LE bilaterally; postural tremors of medium amplitude in hands bilaterally

Neuro

A&O × 3

Labs

Na 135 mEq/L	Hgb 8.8 g/dL	*Fasting lipid panel*
K 3.0 mEq/L	Hct 28%	Total cholesterol 369 mg/dL
CL 112 mEq/L	Plt 110 × 10³/mm³	LDL unknown
CO₂ 19 mEq/L	WBC 4.1 × 10³/mm³	HDL 47 mg/dL
BUN 22 mg/dL	AST 55 IU/L	Trig 1,468 mg/dL
SCr 1.1 mg/dL	ALT 61 IU/L	Tacrolimus 19.6 ng/mL (target
Glu 298 mg/dL	Alk phos 222 IU/L	5–10 ng/mL)
Mg 1.2 mg/dL	LDH 70 IU/L	Sirolimus 20.5 ng/mL (target
A1C 9.5%	T. bili 0.9 mg/dL	5–10 ng/mL)
	Alb 2.9 g/dL	

Assessment

New-onset tremors, headaches, hypokalemia, hypomagnesemia, hyperglycemia, and hypertriglyceridemia

QUESTIONS

Collect Information

1.a. What subjective and objective information indicates the presence of toxicities from immunosuppressive medications?

1.b. What additional information is needed to fully assess this patient's toxicities from immunosuppressive medications?

Assess the Information

2.a. What are the likely causes for the patient's tremors and headache?

2.b. What are potential causes for development of hypertriglyceridemia and hyperglycemia?

2.c. What are the potential causes of hypokalemia and hypomagnesemia?

2.d. Create a list of the patient's drug therapy problems and prioritize them. Include assessment of medication appropriateness, effectiveness, safety, and patient adherence.

Develop a Care Plan

3.a. What are the goals of pharmacotherapy in this case?

3.b. What nondrug therapies might be useful for this patient?

3.c. What feasible pharmacotherapeutic options are available for treating the patient's dyslipidemia?

3.d. What feasible pharmacotherapeutic options are available for treating the patient's hyperglycemia?

3.e. Create an individualized, patient-centered, team-based care plan to treat all of the patient's drug therapy problems. Include specific drugs, dosage forms, doses, schedules, and durations of therapy.

Implement the Care Plan

4.a. What information should be provided to the patient and her caregivers to enhance adherence, ensure successful therapy, and minimize adverse effects?

4.b. Describe how care should be coordinated with other healthcare providers.

Follow-Up: Monitor and Evaluate

5. Explain how to monitor and evaluate the care plan for medication appropriateness, effectiveness, safety, and patient adherence by using clinical and laboratory data, patient feedback, and other information.

■ SELF-STUDY ASSIGNMENTS

1. What options are available for prevention of graft-versus-host disease after allogeneic stem cell transplantation?

2. Which vaccinations and at what schedule should patients receive after allogeneic stem cell transplantation?

CLINICAL PEARL

Allogeneic SCT is often associated with multiple medical conditions, especially metabolic syndrome and cardiovascular disease exacerbated by secondary effects from immunosuppressive medications. Patients' medication regimens also often contain drug interactions requiring careful evaluation to prevent further toxicity.

REFERENCES

1. Glotzbecker B, Duncan C, Alyea E, Campbell B, Soiffer R. Important drug interactions in hematopoietic stem cell transplantation: what every physician should know. Biol Blood Marrow Transplant. 2012;18:989–1006.

2. Cutler C, Logan BR, Nakamura R, et al. Tacrolimus/sirolimus vs tacrolimus/methotrexate as GVHD prophylaxis after matched, related donor allogeneic HCT. Blood. 2014;124(8):1372–1377.

3. Griffith ML, Savani BN, Boord JB. Dyslipidemia after allogeneic stem cell transplantation: evaluation and management. Blood. 2010;116:1197–1204.

4. Fuji S, Rovó A, Ohashi K, et al. How do I manage hyperglycemia/post-transplant diabetes mellitus after allogeneic HSCT. Bone Marrow Transplant. 2016;51(8):1041–1049.

5. Ullmann AJ, Lipton JH, Vesole DH, et al. Posaconazole or fluconazole for prophylaxis in severe graft-versus-host disease. N Engl J Med. 2007;356:335–347.

6. Tomblyn M, Chiller T, Einsele H, et al. Guidelines for preventing infectious complications among hematopoietic cell transplantation recipients: a global perspective. Biol Blood Marrow Transplant. 2009;15:1143–1238.

163

PARENTERAL NUTRITION

Getting Past the Obstruction.....................Level III

Melissa R. Pleva, PharmD, BCNSP, BCCCP

Michael D. Kraft, PharmD, BCNSP, FASPEN

LEARNING OBJECTIVES

After completing this case study, the reader should be able to:

- Describe how a bowel obstruction can lead to nutritional, fluid, and electrolyte abnormalities.

- Characterize the severity of malnutrition based on subjective and objective patient data.

- Identify potential complications related to parenteral nutrition (PN) in patients with malnutrition (eg, refeeding syndrome) and steps to avoid or manage such complications.

- Design a patient-specific PN prescription that is based on the nutritional diagnosis and other subjective and objective patient data.

- Construct and evaluate appropriate monitoring parameters for a hospitalized patient receiving PN.

PATIENT PRESENTATION

■ Chief Complaint

"My stomach hurts and I can't keep down any food or water."

■ HPI

The patient is a 49-year-old man familiar to the GI surgery service with a history of a ventral hernia, dyslipidemia, and type 2 DM. He presented to the ED earlier today with abdominal pain, nausea, vomiting, and inability to tolerate PO intake. Approximately 2 months ago, he underwent an exploratory laparotomy with small bowel resection and primary anastomosis for repair of a ventral hernia with incarcerated small bowel. His postoperative course was complicated by an anastomotic leak, peritonitis, and sepsis, and he was ultimately discharged to home after a 3-week hospital stay. For the past 4 days, he has had worsening abdominal pain and has been unable to tolerate any PO intake. His last bowel movement was 6 days ago. He has lost ~ 25 lb (~ 11 kg) from his weight prior to his surgery 2 months ago. This weight loss includes ~ 14 lb (~ 6.5 kg) since his prior discharge due to poor appetite and limited PO intake at home.

The surgical team decides to admit the patient to the hospital. On admission, they obtain an abdominal CT scan, which demonstrates dilated loops of small bowel consistent with a small bowel obstruction (SBO) and negative for anastomotic leak or abscess. The team believes this SBO is likely due to adhesions from his prior surgery.

■ PMH

Ventral hernia
Dyslipidemia
Type 2 DM

■ PSH

Exploratory laparotomy, small bowel resection with primary anastomosis for repair of ventral hernia with incarcerated small bowel 2 months ago

■ FH

Remarkable for DM in his mother, HTN and CAD in his father

■ SH

Married, lives with his wife; construction worker. Drinks two to three alcoholic beverages per week; quit smoking 2 years ago, 25 pack-year history prior to quitting.

■ ROS

Reports feeling thirsty, no appetite. Complains of moderate abdominal pain, nausea, and vomiting. Also complains his abdomen feels "crampy" and is very bloated. Complains of not passing flatus or having a bowel movement in 6 days; Denies chills, fevers, or other pain.

■ Meds Prior to Admission

Simvastatin 40 mg PO at bedtime
Glyburide/metformin 10 mg/1000 mg PO twice daily with meals

■ All

NKDA

■ Physical Examination

Gen

49-year-old man, uncomfortable because of abdominal pain, appears malnourished

VS

BP 106/70 mm Hg, P 82 bpm, RR 18, T 37.7°C; Wt 71 kg (Wt prior to surgery 2 months ago ~ 83 kg), Ht 71″ (180 cm)

Skin

Dry, flaking in some spots, poor turgor

HEENT

PERRLA, EOMI, anicteric sclerae, normal conjunctivae. Mouth is dry, pharynx is clear, some evidence of wasting on temporal lobes, eyes appear sunken in. Orbital ridge protruding somewhat, evidence of moderate–severe wasting of muscle and subcutaneous fat.

Lungs/Thorax

CTA and percussion bilaterally; bilateral protruding scapulae

CV

RRR, no murmurs

Abd

Distended; hypoactive (nearly absent) bowel sounds; diffuse tenderness throughout all four quadrants

Genit/Rect

No lesions, no internal masses

MS/Ext

(–) Cyanosis, (–) edema, 2+ dorsalis pedis and posterior tibial pulses bilaterally, moderate–severe wasting of muscle and subcutaneous fat, especially around large muscle groups (biceps, triceps, and quadriceps)

Neuro

A&O × 3; CN II–XII intact; motor 5/5 upper and lower extremity bilaterally; sensation intact and reflexes symmetric with downgoing toes

■ Labs on Admission

Na 137 mEq/L	Hgb 13.1 g/dL	AST 24 IU/L	Ca 8.2 mg/dL
K 3.6 mEq/L	Hct 38.9%	ALT 21 IU/L	Mg 1.6 mEq/dL
Cl 98 mEq/L	Plt 334 × 10³/mm³	Alk phos 41 IU/L	Phos 2.4 mg/dL
CO_2 30 mEq/L	WBC 7.5 × 10³/mm³	GGT 45 IU/L	PT 12.3 seconds
BUN 17 mg/dL		T. bili 0.9 mg/dL	INR 0.8
SCr 0.5 mg/dL		T. prot 4.9 g/dL	
Glu 142 mg/dL		Alb 2.9 g/dL	

■ Radiology

A CT scan with contrast demonstrates dilated loops of small bowel consistent with SBO; negative for anastomotic leak; negative for abscess.

■ Assessment

This is a 49-year-old man with a history of a ventral hernia, dyslipidemia, and type 2 DM, S/P exploratory laparotomy, small bowel resection with primary anastomosis, and repair of incarcerated ventral hernia 2 months ago, who is admitted with abdominal pain, nausea, vomiting, and inability to tolerate PO intake. His symptoms and CT scan are consistent with SBO. His history and physical exam also demonstrate evidence of malnutrition.

■ Clinical Course

Given that the patient has had recent abdominal surgery, as well as significant weight loss and evidence of malnutrition, the surgical team elects to manage his SBO conservatively (nonoperatively). Because of recent abdominal surgery, the team would like to avoid reentering the abdomen for surgical intervention at this time (the patient is likely to still have inflammation and adhesions from his prior operation, and additional surgical intervention can further

increase inflammation and risk of complications [eg, adhesions, fistula]). The patient is made NPO, and home PO medications are held for now. An NG tube is placed for gastric decompression, and a PICC is inserted for administration of PN and IV fluids. The team gives the patient a 1000-mL IV fluid bolus with normal saline followed by normal saline at 100 mL/hr. Once PN is initiated and the patient has been resuscitated, IV fluids will be decreased to maintain a total fluid intake of 100 mL/hr. The surgical team obtains nutrition and pharmacy consults for PN recommendations.

QUESTIONS

Collect Information

1.a. What subjective and objective information indicates the presence of malnutrition in this patient?

1.b. What additional nutrition assessment data should you obtain and why?

Assess the Information

2.a. Characterize the type and severity of malnutrition, and describe why the patient is at risk for nutritional deficiencies.

2.b. Create a list of the patient's nutrition, fluid and electrolyte, and drug therapy problems. Prioritize the problems and assess medication appropriateness, effectiveness, safety, and patient adherence.

Develop a Care Plan

3.a. What are the goals of pharmacotherapy and nutrition support therapy for this patient?

3.b. What are the options for providing nutrition support, and which form is indicated for this patient? Provide the rationale for your answer.

3.c. Create an individualized, patient-centered, team-based care plan for treating this patient's nutrition, fluid and electrolyte, and drug therapy problems.

3.d. What are the ranges of estimated daily goals for calories (kcal/kg per day), protein (g/kg per day), and hydration (mL per day or mL/kg per day) for this patient?

3.e. Design a goal PN formulation for this patient that includes the total volume (mL per day) and goal rate (mL/h), amino acids (g per day), dextrose (g per day), and IV lipid emulsion (ILE; g per day). Take into consideration the goals you developed in Question 3.a, as well as the underlying nutrition problems identified previously.

3.f. How would you initiate PN in this patient? How quickly would you advance to the goal infusion rate? Provide the rationale for your answers.

Implement the Care Plan

4.a. What information should be provided to the patient and family during his hospitalization regarding the PN?

4.b. Describe how care should be coordinated with other healthcare providers.

Follow-Up: Monitor and Evaluate

5. Explain how to monitor and evaluate the care plan for medication appropriateness, effectiveness, safety, and patient

adherence by using clinical and laboratory data, patient feedback, and other information.

■ CLINICAL COURSE

The patient was managed conservatively with bowel rest, PN, NG tube decompression, and supportive care. His symptoms improved over 4–5 days, and he began having bowel sounds and passing flatus. On hospital day 7, he had a small bowel movement, and the team began to advance his diet and taper the PN.

■ FOLLOW-UP QUESTION

1. How should PN be tapered off in this patient? Develop a plan to taper PN based on PO intake in this patient.

■ SELF-STUDY ASSIGNMENTS

1. The patient is at risk for a condition called *refeeding syndrome*. What is refeeding syndrome? What are its signs, symptoms, and potential complications? How can it be prevented? How should it be treated if signs and symptoms develop?

2. What other specific postoperative complications can develop in surgical patients with moderate to severe malnutrition? How can preoperative nutrition support impact a malnourished surgical patient's risk for postoperative complications?

3. Calculate how many milliliters per day of dextrose 70%, amino acids 10%, and ILE 20% stock solutions are needed to compound the daily PN prescription that you determined for this patient.

4. Using the calculated daily goals for amino acids, dextrose, and ILE, determine the minimum PN volume that could be compounded for this patient. Assume it will be compounded using a 10% amino acid solution, 70% dextrose solution, and 20% ILE, and use an estimate of 100 mL for all micronutrients and additives.

CLINICAL PEARLS

Refeeding syndrome is a nutritional emergency that can lead to serious complications, including death. A good rule of thumb in patients with moderate to severe malnutrition is to "start low and go slow" when initiating nutrition support and aggressively correct serum electrolyte abnormalities *before* initiating nutrition support as well as during therapy.

Achieving appropriate glycemic control while avoiding hyperglycemia and hypoglycemia can reduce morbidity and mortality. Current guidelines recommend a goal serum glucose of 140–180 mg/dL for adult hospitalized patients receiving nutrition support; hyperglycemia (>180 mg/dL), hypoglycemia (<70 mg/dL), and significant fluctuations in serum glucose should be avoided.

REFERENCES

1. White JV, Guenter P, Jenson G, et al. Consensus statement: Academy of Nutrition and Dietetics and American Society for Parenteral and Enteral Nutrition: characteristics recommended for the identification and documentation of adult malnutrition (undernutrition). JPEN J Parenter Enteral Nutr. 2012;36:275–283.

2. Kudsk KA, Tolley EA, DeWitt RC, et al. Preoperative albumin and surgical site identify surgical risk for major postoperative complications. JPEN J Parenter Enteral Nutr. 2003;27:1–9.

3. da Silva JSV, Seres DS, Sabino K, et al. ASPEN consensus recommendations for refeeding syndrome. Nutr Clin Pract. 2020;35(2):178–195.

4. Brown KA, Dickerson RN, Morgan LM, et al. A new graduated dosing regimen for phosphorus replacement in patients receiving nutrition support. JPEN J Parenter Enteral Nutr. 2006;30:209–214.

5. The American Society for Parenteral and Enteral Nutrition. Task Force for the Revision of Safe Practices for Parenteral Nutrition. Safe practices of parenteral nutrition. JPEN J Parenter Enteral Nutr. 2004;28:S39–S70.

6. Boullata JI, Gilbert K, Sacks G, et al. A.S.P.E.N. clinical guidelines: parenteral nutrition ordering, order review, compounding, labeling, and dispensing. JPEN J Parenter Enteral Nutr. 2014;38:334–377.

7. Ayers P, Adams S, Boullata J, et al. A.S.P.E.N. parenteral nutrition safety consensus recommendations. JPEN J Parenter Enteral Nutr. 2014;38:296–333.

8. Doig GS, Simpson F, Heighes PT, et al. Restricted versus continued standard caloric intake during the management of refeeding syndrome in critically ill adults: a randomised, parallel-group, multicentre, single-blind controlled trial. Lancet Respir Med. 2015;3(12):943–952.

9. McMahon MM, Nystrom E, Braunschweig C, et al. A.S.P.E.N. clinical guidelines: nutrition support of adult patients with hyperglycemia. JPEN J Parenter Enteral Nutr. 2013;37:23–36.

164

ADULT ENTERAL NUTRITION

Gut Check . . . . Level III

Carol J. Rollins, MS, RD, PharmD, BCNSP, FASPEN, FASHP

LEARNING OBJECTIVES

After completing this case study, the reader should be able to:

- List contraindications to enteral nutrition (EN) therapy.

- Calculate the protein, calorie, and fluid requirements for a patient who is to receive EN therapy.

- Recommend an appropriate enteral formula and feeding route.

- Implement an appropriate monitoring plan to achieve the desired nutritional endpoints and avoid complications.

- Design an appropriate regimen for administering medications via a feeding tube, including recommending alternate dosage forms for medications that cannot be crushed.

PATIENT PRESENTATION

A 55-year-old woman is referred to the nutrition support team for evaluation and possible initiation of parenteral nutrition. The history on the referral states: admission to the hospital 2 days ago with c/o nausea, vomiting, and abdominal pain, primarily in the epigastric and LUQ region. Continued c/o nausea and abdominal pain; no vomiting in the last 24 hours. She is NPO except for sips of water for comfort.

CLINICAL COURSE

After following appropriate procedures, you obtain the following additional information about the patient.

HPI

The patient began having symptoms of nausea and epigastric/LUQ pain about a week (per patient) prior to hospital admission. She thought this would "go away on its own by changing to a soft, low-fat diet; like in the past." She began feeling weak and dizzy the day before she asked a friend to take her to the ED. She had several episodes of vomiting before going to the ED on the day of admission. Her history indicates six episodes with symptoms of nausea and abdominal pain in the past 10 months, with two episodes in the past 6 weeks. With previous episodes, the pain was reported as less severe and lasted only a couple days; nausea occurred, but there was no vomiting; she tolerated a low-fat diet and was not weak or dizzy. She did not go to the hospital with the past episodes since the pain improved on its own.

In the ED, the patient received 5 L of 0.9% NaCl for hydration; D5%/0.45% NaCl + 20 mEq KCl/L has been infusing at 125 mL/hr since then. Imaging in the ED indicated multiple areas of cholelithiasis, potential choledocholithiasis, edema of the proximal pancreatic duct with possible stricture, and a small pancreatic pseudocyst.

Height: 66 in. Weight: no admission weight available; weight on hospital day 2 is 70 kg. Patient states, "I lost about 100 pounds over the past year; I've been 145 pounds for the past 6 months and I'm happy with that weight. When my sister died, it really scared me. I joined a virtual exercise class and started going for a walk after work; I usually attend exercise class 4–5 days a week and walk about a mile most days. My insurance pays for me to see a dietitian who helped me with a weight-loss plan that has healthy meals and snacks. My last appointment was about 3 months ago."

PMH

HTN
Pre-DM
GERD

FH

Mother died from a stroke 3 years ago; she had DM and HTN. Father is healthy; he is retired from working as a truck mechanic. Per the patient, her father's only health complaints are "aching bones" and need for glasses to read. Two brothers are healthy as far as the patient knows; however, her younger sister died from a stroke a year ago; she was obese and had complications from DM and HTN.

SH

Divorced; no contact with her ex-husband; no children. She works full time packing boxes on an assembly line. She has several breaks during the day and usually goes to the smoking area. She smokes about one pack per week, down from about two packs per day for 15 years prior to her sister's death; alcohol consumption is typically an occasional beer after work, although it was two to three beers at the end of the day before she decided to "do something to avoid ending up like my sister."

ROS

From physician's note today:

Constitutional: Moderate to severe pain and nausea
ENT: No vision changes or eye pain; no tinnitus or ear pain; no throat pain; no problem with swallowing
CV: No SOB, DOE, and chest pain
Resp: No cough or sputum production
GI: Continued persistent epigastric and LUQ abdominal pain; improved with fentanyl patch and more frequent breakthrough pain coverage; no emesis or diarrhea; complains of intermittent nausea and mild/moderate constipation

GU: No nocturia or hematuria
MS: (+) Abdominal pain; no other muscle aches or bone pain
Skin: No rashes, nodules, or itching
Neuro: No headaches, dizziness, unsteady gait, or seizures
Heme/lymph nodes: No recent blood transfusions or swollen glands

Meds

Metoprolol succinate tablet 200 mg PO daily
Morphine sulfate, immediate-release 15 mg PO Q 6 H PRN pain
Fentanyl transdermal patch 50 mcg, change every 72 hours
Lansoprazole 15 mg PO every morning
Bisacodyl tablet 5 mg PO at bedtime

All

NKDA

Physical Examination

Gen

Well-developed woman; alert and conversant

VS

BP 139/85 mm Hg, P 88 bpm, RR 20, T 37.1°C; Wt 70 kg

Skin

No nodules, masses, or rash; no ecchymoses or petechiae. Venous access device in right hand.

HEENT

PERRLA; EOMs intact. Eyes anicteric. No mouth lesions; tongue normal size.

Neck

Neck supple; no thyromegaly or masses

Lymph Nodes

No cervical, supraclavicular, axillary, or inguinal adenopathy

Heart

RRR with no gallop, rubs, or murmur

Lungs

Clear

Abd

Tender to palpation; no masses palpable; no distension

MS/Ext

No clubbing or cyanosis; 1+ bilateral ankle edema; 2+ sacral edema; no spine or CVA tenderness

Neuro

Cranial nerves intact; DTRs active and equal

Endoscopy Report

From yesterday: endoscopic ultrasound consistent with pancreatitis with swelling and edema surrounding the pancreatic duct area; suspected stricture. Fine-needle biopsy was obtained from near the pancreatic duct opening and sent to pathology. Stent placement is not possible at this time. Recommendation for repeat imaging in 2–3 weeks to determine the most appropriate plan of action; possible

TABLE 164-1	Lab Values				
Na 140 mEq/L	Hgb 8.5 g/dL	WBC 11.9 × 10³/mm³	AST 23 IU/L	Trig 105 mg/dL	
K 3.9 mEq/L	Hct 26.7%	Segs 67%	ALT 34 IU/L	Ca 7.9 mg/dL	
Cl 109 mEq/L	RBC 2.65 × 10⁶/mm³	Bands 14%	Alk phos 287 IU/L	Mg 1.9 mg/dL	
CO₂ 26 mEq/L	Plt 265 × 10³/mm³	Lymphs 17%	LDH 154 IU/L	Phos 3.5 mg/dL	
BUN 7 mg/dL	MCV 104 μm³	Monos 2%	T. bili 0.9 mg/dL	Amylase 462 mg/dL	
SCr 0.9 mg/dL			T. prot 7.1 g/dL	Lipase 591 mg/dL	
Glu 147 mg/dL			Alb 2.6 g/dL	CA 19-9 15 U/mL	
			T. chol 239 mg/dL	CEA 1.2 ng/mL	

surgery for cholecystectomy versus more extensive pancreatic resection if evidence of malignancy based on pathology report. Continue patient on NPO except sips of clear liquids.

■ Labs

See Table 164-1.

■ Other

1. Peripheral blood smear: anisocytosis 3+, poikilocytosis 2+, macrocytosis 2+, microcytosis 1+, and hypersegmented neutrophils.

2. Pancreatic biopsy results pending.

■ Assessment

Acute pancreatitis with pseudocyst, probably secondary to pancreatic duct stricture, possibly related to cholelithiasis or choledocholithiasis based on imaging completed in the ED, and/or alcohol. Serum markers for GI-related cancers are negative; pathology pending for pancreatic duct biopsy. Intolerance to diet; unable to tolerate soft, low-fat diet since hospital admission; tolerates limited volume (150–200 mL per day) of clear liquids daily. Per GI service note, patient is to remain NPO except for sips of clear liquids.

QUESTIONS

Collect Information

1. What other information is necessary to evaluate the patient and provide recommendations for a nutrition support plan of care?

Assess the Information

2.a. What is the appropriate timing for nutrition intervention?

2.b. Based on risk-versus-benefit considerations, is the consult for initiation of parenteral nutrition appropriate for this patient?

2.c. What information indicates the presence of malnutrition or increases the risk for malnutrition?

2.d. What type and degree of malnutrition does this patient exhibit? What evidence supports your assessment?

2.e. Create a list of the patient's drug therapy problems and prioritize them. Include assessment of medication appropriateness, effectiveness, safety, and patient adherence.

Develop a Care Plan

3.a. What are the goals of nutrition support in this case?

3.b. What are the potential alternatives for improving nutritional status in this patient other than initiating specialized nutrition support?

3.c. What are the potential routes for specialized nutrition support and the reason(s) why each is or is not appropriate for this patient?

3.d. By postponing invasive therapy (possible surgery for a cholecystectomy or stricture repair; awaiting pancreatic duct biopsy results to rule out pancreatic cancer) for several weeks, the potential of continuing nutrition support outside the hospital arises. What factors must be considered when evaluating home nutrition support therapy?

3.e. Estimate the protein, calorie, and fluid requirements for this patient.

3.f. What type of formula (eg, polymeric, monomeric) is most appropriate for this patient?

3.g. What administration regimen should be used for tube feedings?

3.h. Assuming that the patient is to continue her current medications during tube feedings, how should each of these be administered?

3.i. Create a care plan to manage the patient's drug therapy problems other than providing nutrition support. Include specific drugs, dosage forms, doses, schedules, and durations of therapy.

Implement the Care Plan

4.a. What information should be provided to the patient or her caregiver to enhance adherence, ensure successful therapy, and minimize adverse effects of the nutritional support therapy?

4.b. Describe how care with nutrition support should be coordinated with other healthcare providers.

Follow-Up: Monitor and Evaluate

5. Explain how to monitor and evaluate the care plan for medication appropriateness, effectiveness, safety, and patient adherence by using clinical and laboratory data, patient feedback, and other information.

■ CLINICAL COURSE

After discussing nutrition support during acute pancreatitis with the medical team, the nutrition support service discussed EN therapy with the patient. The patient consented to feeding tube placement. A 1.2-cal/mL, 55.5-g protein/L, 300-mOsm/kg polymeric formula was started using an enteral infusion pump via nasojejunal tube at 35 mL/hr for 8 hours, and then advanced to the goal rate of 65 mL/hr. Basic metabolic panel results on day 2 of EN revealed electrolyte values WNL. The WBC decreased to 10.6 × 10³/mm³ with 75% segs, 9% bands, 14% lymphs, and 2% monos. The basic metabolic panel on day 3 of EN showed stable values. The plan for discharge to home was confirmed, and arrangements for home EN were finalized. The plan is for her diet to continue as limited clear liquids (<240 mL per day) and repeat imaging in 2–3 weeks to assess the small pancreatic pseudocyst and potentially schedule her for surgery the following week for the pancreatic duct stricture. If the biopsy results indicate cancer, more extensive surgery would likely be needed.

■ SELF-STUDY ASSIGNMENTS

1. Select another case from this Casebook where the patient is receiving several medications and design an appropriate regimen for administering medications via a feeding tube, including alternative dosage forms for medications that cannot be crushed and proper dosage adjustments for different forms where necessary.

2. Educate an actual patient or do a mock education with a classmate about medication administration through a feeding tube.

3. Select another case from this Casebook where the patient is receiving several medications and determine the potential cumulative sorbitol dose if all medications were changed to oral liquid dosage forms.

4. Identify the metabolic changes associated with refeeding syndrome and the characteristics that increase the risk of this complication.

CLINICAL PEARL

Medications administered through a feeding tube frequently clog the tube and can result in adverse effects from altering the pharmaceutical characteristics (eg, crushing) of the medication; avoid administration through the tube when possible. Administer medications orally if the patient can and will take them orally. Evaluate all medications for appropriate preparation, dosing, and schedule if administered through the feeding tube.

REFERENCES

1. Evans DC, Corkins MR, Malone A, et al. The use of visceral proteins as nutrition markers: an ASPEN position paper. Nutr Clin Pract. 2021;36(1):22–28.

2. White JV, Guenter P, Jensen G, Malone A, Schofield M; Academy of Nutrition and Dietetics Malnutrition Work Group; A.S.P.E.N. Malnutrition Task Force; A.S.P.E.N. Board of Directors. Consensus statement of the Academy of Nutrition and Dietetics/American Society for Parenteral and Enteral Nutrition: characteristics recommended for the identification and documentation of adult malnutrition (undernutrition). J Acad Nutr Diet. 2012;112:730–738.

3. Mirtallo JM. Overview of parenteral nutrition. In: Mueller CM, ed. The A.S.P.E.N. Adult Nutrition Support Core Curriculum. 3rd ed. Silver Spring, MD: American Society for Parenteral and Enteral Nutrition; 2017:e-book chapter 14:25.

4. McClave SA, Taylor BE, Martindale RG, et al. Guidelines for the provision and assessment of nutrition support therapy in the adult critically ill patient: Society of Critical Care Medicine (SCCM) and American Society for Parenteral and Enteral Nutrition (A.S.P.E.N.). Section L. Acute pancreatitis. J Parenter Enteral Nutr. 2016;40(2):159–211.

5. McCleary EJ, Tajchman S. Parenteral nutrition and infection risk in the intensive care unit: a practical guide for the bedside clinician. Nutr Clin Pract. 2016;31(4):476–489.

6. Mirtallo JM, Forbes A, McClave SA, et al. International consensus guidelines for nutrition therapy in pancreatitis. J Parenter Enteral Nutr. 2012;36:284–291.

7. Kruger K, McClave SA, Martindale RG. Pancreatitis. In: Mueller CM, ed. The A.S.P.E.N. Adult Nutrition Support Core Curriculum. 3rd ed. Silver Spring, MD: American Society for Parenteral and Enteral Nutrition; 2017:e-book chapter 28:40.

8. Konrad D, Mitchell R, Hendrickson E. Home nutrition support. In: Mueller CM, ed. The A.S.P.E.N. Adult Nutrition Support Core Curriculum. 3rd ed. Silver Spring, MD: American Society for Parenteral and Enteral Nutrition; 2017:e-book chapter 38:51.

9. Boullata JI, Carrera AL, Harvey L, et al. ASPEN Safe practices for enteral nutrition therapy. J Parenter Enteral Nutr. 2017;41(1):15–103.

10. Verdell A, Rollins CJ. Drug–nutrient interactions. In: Mueller CM, ed. The A.S.P.E.N. Adult Nutrition Support Core Curriculum, 3rd ed. Silver Spring, MD, American Society for Parenteral and Enteral Nutrition; 2017:e-book chapter 18:29.

165

OBESITY

Oh, To Be 23 Again (BMI That Is) . . . . Level II

Dannielle C. O'Donnell, BS, PharmD

LEARNING OBJECTIVES

After completing this case study, the reader should be able to:

• Discuss common obesity-related comorbidities.

• Calculate body mass index (BMI), and use waist circumference to determine a patient's risk of obesity-related morbidity.

• Recommend a pharmacotherapeutic plan and treatment strategy for obese patients.

• Provide patient counseling on the expected benefits, possible adverse effects, and drug interactions with weight loss medications.

PATIENT PRESENTATION

■ Chief Complaint

"I've been through a painful divorce. I think I'm ready to try and get out and meet someone and start over, but I must've eaten my way through all of the stress of divorcing. Who's gonna even look at me when I'm this size? I may have to take up smoking again. It was easier to stay skinny when I smoked."

■ HPI

A 35-year-old woman who has struggled with body weight since her teen years presents to clinic looking for a weight loss solution. She says she feels best at 55 kg, which was how much she weighed when she was 23 years old and got married. She states that she was a "chubby" kid who worked in college to lose weight, mostly through trying to eat vegan like her roommate and going to exercise classes at the college gym. That was also when she started smoking. She and her ex-husband were smokers and stopped when she was 29 because they wanted a smoke-free home before starting a family. She remembers frustration that while she "did great going cold turkey with the cigs," she put on 10 kg in the first 6 smoke-free months. She "worked out like crazy" and dropped 7 kg before she conceived at the age of 30. She delivered a healthy baby although her pregnancy was complicated by high blood pressure and excessive weight gain (27 kg). She was happy with how quickly most of the baby weight came off while nursing, but then she plateaued 8 kg above her pre-pregnancy weight. "I don't have time to commit to exercising while juggling a job and family." She has now put on more weight over the course of the busy toddler years and then even more during the stress of the divorce and hectic new lifestyle as a single working mom. She now lives in an apartment with her 5-year-old and says she struggles financially because her ex-husband often does not pay child support on time, but she's thankful she has good medical insurance and prescription benefits through her employer. She says she has tried weight loss shakes but finds herself just "starving" and "eating her way through the fridge" in the evening after she gets her son to bed. She says she does not have time for a gym membership or money for a program that provides meals. In addition, she gets more winded with physical exertion than she used to and doesn't think she can do aerobics classes like those she found helpful in college. She doesn't think it would work with her eating one thing and cooking something else for her son. She bought some "herbal stuff" from a coworker which helped with late afternoon hunger, but thinks cigarettes would be even "less of a dent in the wallet than those supplements that I'm not sure even did very much." She also states that she lost weight when starting sertraline and titrating up to her current dose and loved it because she wasn't hungry at all, but then that seemed to wear off and she gained it all right back. To economize and accommodate her hectic single-mom schedule, they eat out a lot based on where the kids-eat-free meal nights are (ie, an all-you-can-eat buffet on Monday nights and a pancake house on Wednesday nights, drive-thru meals one or two additional nights each week). She drinks orange juice and coffee with flavored creamer in the morning and more coffee or sweet tea throughout the day. On the weekends, when she has her son, she likes to treat him with special desserts they bake together in the kitchen. When her ex-husband has the child, she doesn't have any interest in cooking for herself, so she often gets fast food or takeout. That is also a time when she feels more alone and depressed, and she snacks more when feeling lonely or stressed.

PMH

Insomnia
Adjustment disorder post-divorce

FH

Mother had an MI at age 62; father died in an MVA at age 67. Maternal grandmother died at age 63 with diabetes and "kidney problems." She states that all women in her family have struggled with their weight. No other family members have a significant medical history, although she states that her 5-year-old is "a big boy." She blames his dad, stating that when he has their son all they do is eat junk food and drink sodas, and he uses the TV and video games as a babysitter.

SH

The patient is a single working mom and a previous smoker (1 ppd × 10 years). Stopped 6 years ago. She denies IVDA. She has previously had successes, albeit short term, with weight loss by focusing on fad diets and when exercising routinely, but she is not exercising now.

Diet

Has never had formal diet instruction. Food frequency questionnaire shows a diet low in fiber, high in saturated fat, sugars, and calories. She denies regular or binge alcohol consumption.

Meds

Tylenol PM PRN sleep (one to two times per week)
Sertraline 150 mg PO once daily
Unknown "herbal" weight loss product—discontinued 3 months ago

All

Macrolides—rash

ROS

Complains of general low energy and periods of apathy that she attributes to the divorce and a preoccupation with food and her weight and feeling "undesirable," although her mood improved after sertraline was increased from 100 to 150 mg five months ago. She denies symptoms of cold or heat intolerance; changes in skin, hair, or nails; nervousness; irritability; muscle pain or weakness; palpitations; diarrhea or constipation; polyuria; polydipsia; chest pain; or shortness of breath. Despite having low energy, she relates some difficulty sleeping and reports waking up a couple of times a night to urinate or with her mind busy with all she has to do. She denies binge eating or purging.

Physical Examination

Gen

The patient is in NAD but looks tired. She is clean and dressed appropriately for the weather.

VS

BP 148/88 mm Hg (consistent with previous clinic reading), P 80 bpm, RR 16, T 36.4°C; Wt 80 kg, waist 100 cm, Ht 5′3″

Skin

Warm, with normal distribution of body hair. No significant lesions or discolorations.

Abd

Obese with multiple striae; NT; ND; (+) BS; no palpable masses

Ext

LE varicosities present. Pedal pulses 2+ bilaterally. No joint swelling or tenderness.

Labs (Fasting)

Na 138 mEq/L	A1C 5.4%
K 3.9 mEq/L	AST 24 IU/L
Cl 96 mEq/L	*Fasting lipid profile*
CO$_2$ 26 mEq/L	T. chol 208 mg/dL
BUN 13 mg/dL	LDL-C 109 mg/dL
SCr 1.0 mg/dL	HDL-C 38 mg/dL
Glu 97 mg/dL	Trig 305 mg/dL

Assessment

This is a 35-year-old woman with obesity-related comorbidities including hypertension (diagnosed today based on her 2 clinic readings) and dyslipidemia (low HDL, high triglycerides). Weight loss would decrease her risk of developing pre-diabetes or type 2 DM, osteoarthritis, and sleep apnea and can improve BP and lipids.

QUESTIONS

Collect Information

1.a. Calculate the patient's body mass index (BMI).

1.b. What subjective and objective information indicates the presence of obesity?

1.c. What additional information is needed to fully assess this patient's obesity?

Assess the Information

2.a. Assess the severity of the patient's obesity based on the subjective and objective information available.

2.b. Create a list of the patient's drug therapy problems and prioritize them. Include assessment of medication appropriateness, effectiveness, safety, and patient adherence.

2.c. What economic and psychosocial considerations are applicable to this patient?

Develop a Care Plan

3.a. What are the goals of therapy for this patient's obesity?

3.b. What nondrug therapies might be useful for this patient's obesity?

3.c. What feasible pharmacotherapeutic options are available for treating her obesity?

3.d. Create an individualized, patient-centered, team-based care plan to optimize medication therapy for this patient's obesity and other drug therapy problems. Include specific drugs, dosage forms, doses, schedules, and durations of therapy.

3.e. What alternatives would be appropriate if the initial care plan fails or cannot be used?

Implement the Care Plan

4.a. What information should be provided to the patient to enhance adherence, ensure successful therapy, and minimize adverse effects?

4.b. Describe how care should be coordinated with other healthcare providers.

Follow-Up: Monitor and Evaluate

5. Explain how to monitor and evaluate the care plan for medication appropriateness, effectiveness, safety, and patient adherence by using clinical and laboratory data, patient feedback, and other information.

■ CLINICAL COURSE

At her first return visit 3 months later, the patient had lost 4 kg (5% of her weight). By this second visit at the 6-month time point, she had lost some additional weight and weighs 73.5 kg; her waist circumference is 96 cm. She is now working out at home regularly 30 minutes each evening (typically four nights a week) with a yoga video after her son goes to bed and tries to do more on the weekends when she doesn't have her son. She uses an app on her phone and averages about 6500 steps each day. Although they still eat out frequently, she is making significantly different choices, increasing her lean meats, decreasing carbohydrates and saturated fats, monitoring portion sizes, abstaining from having seconds, and substituting a piece of fruit for dessert. She has eliminated sugary beverages (sweet tea, using Stevia in her coffee, eliminated orange juice in the morning) and is having good success sticking to her plan of not eating anything after her son goes to bed. She states that the initial nausea she had has resolved. Her appetite and evening hunger are lessened, and it is easier for her to stick to smaller portion sizes and not feel like she needs to have second helpings.

Her FBG is 92 mg/dL and A1C is 5.3%. Repeat FLP includes total cholesterol 202 mg/dL, LDL 110 mg/dL, HDL 45 mg/dL, and triglycerides 235 mg/dL. Her blood pressure has improved to 136/82 mm Hg, having also initiated lisinopril 10 mg/day at her visit 6 months ago.

At this 6 month visit, she reports adhering to the lifestyle modifications as in previous weeks and is sleeping better and is less fatigued. She has noticed a definite improvement in her clothing fit, but she is starting to become frustrated again that she has not seen any additional improvement on her home scale in the last 2 weeks and still does not like how she looks. She wants to know if there is something else she can take or if she could have the laparoscopic sleeve gastrectomy procedure since "I have good insurance and have met my deductible for the year." Although she is pleased with the improvement in her blood pressure, she is frustrated that her cholesterol didn't go down more. She is wondering if it might further help her weight loss efforts if she picked up some of "that herbal dandelion tea from Paraguay" that her coworker sells for weight loss to help move things along.

■ FOLLOW-UP QUESTIONS

1. What changes, if any, should be considered for her obesity treatment program at this 6-month visit?

2. How would you educate her regarding use of the herbal weight loss tea?

3. What changes, if any, should be made in the therapy for dyslipidemia and high blood pressure at this time?

■ SELF-STUDY ASSIGNMENTS

1. List the limitations of height–weight charts or BMI determinations. What are the most accurate methods for quantifying body fat, and why are they not routinely employed?

2. Imagine that you are a member of a pharmacy and therapeutics committee for a managed care organization. Justify whether antiobesity drugs/device should be a covered benefit, and if so, which specific agent(s) should be added to the formulary. Should there be any step-edits (a patient has to fail a trial of one agent before another is covered)? Should OTC weight loss products be covered? Justify your answer.

3. Compile a compendium of common herbal and dietary supplements that claim weight loss benefits, and make a list of the evidence for their safety and efficacy.

4. Make a list of the various prescription weight loss medications that have been introduced and subsequently withdrawn from the US and EU markets and the reasons for the withdrawal.

CLINICAL PEARL

Taking psyllium with orlistat has been reported to decrease the frequency and severity of orlistat GI adverse effects such as oily stool and leakage.

REFERENCES

1. Apovian CM, Aronne LJ, Bessesen DH, et al. Pharmacological management of obesity: an Endocrine Society clinical practice guideline. J Clin Endocrinol Metab. 2015;100(2):342–362.

2. Jensen MD, Ryan DH, Apovian CM, et al. 2013 AHA/ACC/TOS guideline for the management of overweight and obesity in adults: a report of the American College of Cardiology/American Heart Association Task Force on Practice Guidelines and The Obesity Society. Circulation. 2013;63(25 Pt B):2985–3023.

3. Garvey WT, Mechanick JI, Brett EM, et al. American Association of Clinical Endocrinologists and American College of Endocrinology

comprehensive clinical practice guidelines for medical care of patients with obesity. Endocr Pract. 2016;22(Suppl 3):1–203.

4. Toplak H, Woodward E, Yumuk V, et al. 2014 EASO position statement on the use of anti-obesity drugs. Obes Facts. 2015;8(3):166–174.

5. Khera R, Murad MH, Chandar AK, et al. Association of pharmacological treatments for obesity with weight loss and adverse events: a systematic review and meta-analysis. JAMA. 2016;315(22):2424–2434.

6. O'Neil PM, Birkenfeld AL, McGowan B, et al. Efficacy and safety of semaglutide compared with liraglutide and placebo for weight loss in patients with obesity: a randomised, double-blind, placebo and active controlled, dose-ranging phase 2 trial. Lancet. 2018;392:637–649.

SECTION 19
COMPLEMENTARY AND ALTERNATIVE THERAPIES (LEVEL III)

Kelly M. Shields, PharmD

TO THE READER

Although use of many dietary supplements has leveled off or decreased in the past few years, many patients are still interested in trying supplements, either in place of (alternative) or along with (complementary) prescription and OTC therapies. Patients have a continued desire for knowledge on the potential benefits and risks of these therapies, and often expect pharmacists and other healthcare providers to provide information they can use in determining what treatment option is preferred.

As part of providing appropriate care, clinicians have a duty to help individual patients avoid interactions with their drug therapies and prevent use of products unsafe for them because of other safety concerns. That is a fairly straightforward task when dealing with prescription and OTC therapies; there is so much information and research available that most problems and risks are well understood. If a patient is prescribed a contraindicated drug, we can ensure that they do not receive it. With dietary supplements, there is often not enough information available to make clear-cut judgments about risks. We also cannot prevent patients from taking supplements even if supplements are known to be unsafe or risky for them, because we do not control their access to those therapies. Instead, we are limited to providing as much guidance as possible to help maximize any possible benefit and minimize possible harm.

CASEBOOK QUESTIONS ABOUT DIETARY SUPPLEMENTS

The following questions regarding supplement therapy aid in the decision-making process and will be addressed in the "Clinical Course" section of the Casebook. It is assumed that necessary information about a patient's medical history and current drug regimen has already been obtained.

1. **What is the known or proposed mechanism of action?**

   - The pharmacology of FDA-approved prescription medications is generally understood, but many supplements are used with only limited knowledge about their pharmacologic activities. Botanical supplements, in particular, are extremely complex and may have multiple activities, some synergistic to the desired effect and some in opposition or unrelated. When there is little or no definitive human evidence for either efficacy or safety, we must often extrapolate based on in vitro or animal data in order to provide patients with information or instructions. For example, if a plant extract has been shown to improve glucose uptake in tissue studies, it is reasonable to expect that activity to some extent when taken by human beings. It would also be reasonable to offer cautions about use with sulfonylurea drugs or other hypoglycemic agents, even when no case studies or clinical trials have reported interactions. Depending on the risks if an interaction should happen, appropriate real-life statements to patients can range from: "If you use this supplement, you will have to do additional blood sugar checks for the first 2 weeks to make sure it's not interfering with your other medication" to "This particular supplement is not safe for you to take due to your concurrent medications."

2. **How extensive or conclusive are the clinical trial data on effectiveness?**

   - When clinical trial data conclude that a supplement has beneficial effects, it may be safer for a patient to try a supplement before a prescription drug with known adverse events. Whenever evidence of efficacy is lacking or contradictory, the severity of the patient's condition becomes more important in the risk/benefit equation. For example, a patient wishing to try a supplement for the common cold or athlete's foot is not at great risk of harm if the supplement is not effective—they will simply endure some unpleasant symptoms for a time, and then most likely use a more typical medication. On the other hand, a patient with severe hypertension who tries an ineffective supplement may be at increased risk for a cardiovascular event.

3. **What is known about safety?**

   - This question relates back to what is known about the mechanism of action: when there is a lack of information from long-term clinical trials, decisions about safety must be based on extrapolation from basic scientific studies and isolated case reports. It must be kept in mind that safety issues can be both overemphasized and underemphasized and that information (and therefore reasonable recommendations) can change. For example, ginger is often described as being associated with increased risk of bleeding. This is absolutely true at doses of 4 g per day or more but is unlikely at lower doses. However, even use at lower doses would become a major consideration in patients who have other medical conditions (eg, a clotting disorder) or if drug interactions are involved (eg, warfarin or chronic NSAID use). One safety rule of thumb for counseling patients is that *all* supplements should be stopped 10–14 days prior to scheduled surgery to minimize risks of interactions or increased risk of bleeding.

4. **Does the product have any specific quality considerations?**

   - Two questions are associated with "quality." First, is the product the "right" product—that is, the same strength or standardization as that used in the clinical trials that demonstrated any benefits? Second, is the product a "good quality product"—that is, contains what it is labeled to contain with no contaminants? The first question is answered by close attention to reliable information resources and clinical trials and to reading product labels to ensure the chosen product is the appropriate standardization or strength and doses are not subtherapeutic or toxic. The second question is best addressed by advising patients to only purchase products from manufacturers that participate in quality seal programs or that have been tested by third-party laboratories. The first choice for a quality seal program is USP's Dietary Supplement Verification Program, but UL (Underwriters' Laboratories) and NSF International also have facility cGMP audit and certification programs. Third-party laboratories with consumer-accessible information include ConsumerLab.com and Labdoor.com.

- Certain products are more likely to have specific problems with quality or carry additional risk. For example, melatonin is usually produced synthetically, but a few available products are from "natural sources," generally meaning extracted from the pituitary glands of cattle. Because the pituitary gland is in the brain, these products do carry a small but real risk of contamination with prion proteins associated with bovine spongiform encephalopathy, also known as mad cow disease. So a synthetic product would be a better quality product.

5. **Would this be an appropriate treatment choice in this particular patient?**

   - Each patient may have different motivations to try a treatment. If clinical or basic science supports potential benefit of a supplement for a given condition, the next thing to consider is the patient's own expectations of therapy and ability to self-monitor for both efficacy and safety. For example, a postmenopausal woman who suffers 10 severe hot flushes a week and wants to end them entirely will probably be disappointed with a supplement, whereas another woman who also has 10 severe hot flushes a week and would like to reduce their frequency and/or severity may be very happy with the same product. Expectations must be appropriate; only rarely will a supplement work as strongly or as quickly as a prescription drug.

6. **If the patient is going to use the product, what counseling information will allow them to maximize any possible benefit and minimize any harm?**

   - Counseling information should cover the same categories of information as prescription drugs: dose, schedule, duration of therapy, side effects, and interactions. Unfortunately, because there is usually less information available about side effects and interactions, it is impossible to warn patients about every possibility. It is best to counsel patients to contact their healthcare providers if anything "unexpected or unusual" occurs. This provides protection for the patient and allows evaluation of any possible link to the supplement, which aids in expanding the supplement knowledge base.

   - Specificity is important in counseling. For example, if a patient is going to use *Ginkgo biloba*, they need to be told to watch for easy bruising, not just that the ginkgo may increase bleeding risk. Specificity is even more important when a patient chooses to take a supplement despite being counseled against it because of safety issues.

   - In addition, there are extra categories of information to include in counseling that do not generally have to be addressed with prescription and OTC drugs: using the appropriate product and a high-quality product. For botanical supplements, it is generally necessary to specify information such as the standardization of an extract (eg, saw palmetto should be 320–960 mg of extract standardized to 85–95% fatty acids daily). For nonbotanical supplements, the salt form may need to be specified (eg, glucosamine sulfate for monotherapy has more evidence of efficacy than glucosamine hydrochloride for monotherapy and so is the preferred form).

OBTAINING CURRENT AND RELIABLE DIETARY SUPPLEMENT INFORMATION

Decisions made about using supplements are only as good as the information used in making the decisions. Unfortunately, incomplete or wrong information about dietary supplements is abundantly available, so using only reliable resources is vital. A brief list of recommended resources is provided at the end of this section, but practitioners need to know what to look for or to avoid as they come across new resources. The following suggestions should be kept in mind:

- Avoid resources published or provided by manufacturers; their primary interest is often selling the product.

- Investigate the authors or source of the information; is the resource actually created by trained professionals or by a ghost-writing group?

- Are recommendations based on careful analysis of the quality of clinical trials? Recommendations based solely on the end results of trials are often wrong; it is not possible to get good decision-making data from a badly designed or poorly conducted trial.

- Are cautions (about interactions, contraindications, or adverse effects) based on all theoretical, animal, or human data available, or only on well-documented human trials or case reports? Although it may seem counterintuitive at first, there is such a lack of high-quality reports and information in humans that theoretical data (based on in vitro experiments or theorized mechanisms of action) or animal data becomes more important in generating cautions that help keep patients safe. Often these cautions should not be as strong, of course. If a supplement has been found to affect glucose utilization in tissue cultures, a diabetic patient starting to take the supplement may be warned appropriately to monitor blood glucose more frequently, whereas a case report of loss of glycemic control in two patients using the supplement would generate a strong warning not to use the supplement.

- Does the resource include up-to-date information? Supplement information changes rapidly, so publication dates can matter tremendously.

RECOMMENDED INFORMATION RESOURCES

■ Literature Search Strategies

One of the most essential resources is a comprehensive literature search, because this can retrieve the most current information. Ideally, more than one indexing system be used (such as both Medline and EMBASE). However, healthcare professions students and professionals often do not have access to anything other than Medline. Consequently, it is essential to use very thorough search strategies, as discussed here:

- Because pertinent articles can be incompletely or wrongly indexed, search using more than just MESH (or EMTREE) terms to ensure proper retrieval. For example, to search for saw palmetto, search the MESH term (*Serenoa*), and then perform keyword searches for the common name (saw palmetto), the botanical name (*Serenoa repens*), and any alternative botanical names (*Sabul serrulata*). Consider searching misspellings; the spelling "saw palmeto" may not be common, but "gingko" instead of "ginkgo" is very common. Combining the results of these searches with "OR" will optimize retrieval of articles that may be relevant.

- Search the relevant disease state and any closely related terms. Continuing the example, search "BPH," "benign prostatic hyperplasia," "prostatic hyperplasia," "prostate hypertrophy," and "prostatic hypertrophy" as both MESH (or EMTREE) terms and keywords. It may also be useful to search symptom or outcome measure terms, such as "urinary retention" or "micturition rate."

- After combining product and disease state searches, if the retrieval set is so large as to be impossible to review, limitations can be used. For clinical decision making, the most useful types of limitations are clinical trials, evidence-based reviews, meta-analyses, and systematic reviews. Because it is not uncommon for articles about dietary supplement trials to report results of both animal and human studies, it is not recommended that a limitation of "human only" be used, because that could eliminate appropriate articles based on indexing.

■ Electronic Database Resources

- Some information about common dietary supplements can be found in major drug information compendia (eg, Micromedex, LexiComp). There are also some supplement-specific resources available. Electronic databases available for purchase include:

- Natural Medicines (*https://naturalmedicines.therapeuticresearch.com/*). It is the most comprehensive resource available and includes a wide range of individual and combination products. It contains evidence-based recommendations and summaries of clinical and basic science information that are regularly reviewed and updated. The site allows for easy checking of supplement–drug interactions. It is available for purchase by individuals as well as institutions.

- ConsumerLab.com (www.consumerlab.com). This is a third-party laboratory that tests dietary supplements for compliance with labeled content and for appropriate dissolution and contaminants. No clinical recommendations are given; the site's utility is primarily limited to aiding in the choice of a high-quality product. It is inexpensive (about $40 per year) and is also appropriate for use by consumers.

Free electronic databases include:

- The Health Information site of the National Institutes of Health Office of Dietary Supplements (*http://ods.od.nih.gov/Health-Information/*). This is a government site with links to several useful informational resources including tips for using supplements and fact sheets on a number of dietary supplements.

- Memorial Sloan-Kettering Cancer Center Integrative Medicine Service Website (*http://www.mskcc.org/mskcc/html/1979.cfm*). It includes a database of individual supplements. Information is specifically focused on use of supplements in cancer patients, a population that has a high rate of use of complementary and alternative medicine therapies. The site includes more discussion of interactions with chemotherapeutic agents than other resources.

- Computer Access to Research on Dietary Supplements (CARDS; *https://ods.od.nih.gov/Research/CARDS_Database.aspx*). This is a database of federally funded clinical trials of supplements.

- The PubMed Dietary Supplement Subset (*https://ods.od.nih.gov/Research/PubMed_Dietary_Supplement_Subset.aspx*).

This will automatically search Medline for dietary supplement-focused literature. The subset database is focused on medical use of plants, so it can be easier to search than other literature databases that contain citations for agricultural-focused studies.

- The Dietary Supplement Label Database (DSLD) became active in 2013 (*http://dsld.nlm.nih.gov/dsld/*). A project of both the National Library of Medicine and the Office of Dietary Supplements, it is a searchable database of labeling information for products both available and discontinued from the US market. It may be especially useful when gathering medication histories or when patients ask questions about brand-name products that contain multiple ingredients.

■ Print Resources

Because of limitations on the timeliness of information in print resources, it is difficult to make strong recommendations. New print resources should be evaluated according to the criteria listed above to determine their usefulness.

CASE 14: DYSLIPIDEMIA

■ Garlic and Fish Oil for Dyslipidemia

Clinical Course

The patient is already taking garlic capsules, but he is not sure about the type or dose. Because you are making changes to his current prescription regimen, you need to investigate the advisability of continuing the garlic. Because he is taking a statin drug as indicated, he should not take red yeast rice, a common supplement used for dyslipidemia, because it contains mevacolin K, a lovastatin analogue, and would be duplicative therapy. Would fish oil be a possible option for him?

■ FOLLOW-UP QUESTIONS

Garlic

1. What is the known or proposed mechanism of action?
2. How extensive or conclusive are the clinical trial data on effectiveness?
3. What is known about safety?
4. Does the product have any specific quality concerns?
5. Would this be an appropriate treatment choice in this particular patient?
6. If the patient is going to use the product, what counseling information will allow her to maximize any possible benefit and minimize any harm?

Fish Oil/Omega-3 Fatty Acids

1. What is the known or proposed mechanism of action?
2. How extensive or conclusive are the clinical trial data on effectiveness?
3. What is known about safety?
4. Does the product have any specific quality concerns?
5. Would this be an appropriate treatment choice in this particular patient?
6. If the patient is going to use the product, what counseling information will allow her to maximize any possible benefit and minimize any harm?

REFERENCES

1. Zeng T, Zhang CL, Zhao XL, Xie KQ. The role of garlic on the lipid parameters: a systematic review of the literature. Crit Rev Food Sci Nutr. 2013;53:215–230.

2. Shouk R, Abdou A, Shetty K, et al. Mechanisms underlying the antihypertensive effects of garlic bioactives. Nutr Res. 2015;34:106–115.

3. Ried K, Toben C, Fakler P. Effect of garlic on serum lipids: an updated meta-analysis. Nutr Rev. 2013;71(5):282–299.

4. Ried K. Garlic lowers blood pressure in hypertensive individuals, regulates serum cholesterol, and stimulates immunity: an updated meta-analysis and review. J Nutr. 2016;146(2):389S–396S.

5. Ried K, Travica N, Sali A. The effect of aged garlic extract on blood pressure and other cardiovascular risk factors in uncontrolled hypertensives: the AGE at Heart trial. Integr Blood Press Control. 2016;9:9–21.

6. Cho HJ, Yoon IS. Pharmacokinetic interactions of herbs with cytochrome p450 and p-glycoprotein. Evid Based Complement Alternat Med. 2015;2015:736431.

7. Innes JK, Calder PC. Marine omega-3 (N-3) fatty acids for cardiovascular health: an update for 2020. Int J Mol Sci. 2020;21(4):1362.

8. Hartweg J, Farmer AJ, Perera R, et al. Meta-analysis of the effects of n-3 polyunsaturated fatty acids on lipoproteins and other emerging lipid cardiovascular risk markers in patients with type 2 diabetes. Diabetologia. 2007;50(8):1593–1602.

9. Eslick GD, Howe PRC, Smith C, Priest R, Bensoussan A. Benefits of fish oil supplementation in hyperlipidemia: a systematic review and meta-analysis. Int J Cardiol. 2009;136:4–16.

10. Barkas F, Nomikos T, Liperopoulos E, et al. Diet and cardiovascular disease risk among individuals with familial hypercholesterolemia: systematic review and meta-analysis. Nutrients. 2020;12(8):2436.

CASE 40: NAUSEA AND VOMITING

■ Ginger for Nausea and Vomiting

Clinical Course

While discussing the patient's antiemetic regimen, he says, "I remember that my sister used to take ginger to prevent sea sickness when she went on a cruise, and my cousin used ginger when he was having chemotherapy a few years ago. Would that be good for me to try?"

■ FOLLOW-UP QUESTIONS

Ginger

1. What is the known or proposed mechanism of action?

2. How extensive or conclusive are the clinical trial data on effectiveness?

3. What is known about safety?

4. Does the product have any specific quality concerns?

5. Would this be an appropriate treatment choice in this particular patient?

6. If the patient is going to use the product, what counseling information will allow him to maximize any possible benefit and minimize any harm?

REFERENCES

1. Lete I, Allué J. The effectiveness of ginger in the prevention of nausea and vomiting during pregnancy and chemotherapy. Integrative Med Insights 2016;11:11–17.

2. Walstab J, Krüger D, Stark T, et al. Ginger and its pungent constituents non-competitively inhibit activation of human recombinant and native 5-HT$_3$ receptors of enteric neurons. Neurogastroenterol Motil. 2013;25:439–448, e302.

3. Crichton M, Marshall S, Marx W, et al. Efficacy of ginger (*Zingiber officinale*) in ameliorating chemotherapy-induced nausea and vomiting and chemotherapy-related outcomes. J Acad Nutr Diet. 2019;119(12):2055–2068.

4. Lee J, Oh H. Ginger as an antiemetic modality for chemotherapy-induced nausea and a systematic review and meta-analysis. Oncol Nurs Forum 2013;40(2):163–170.

5. Marx WM, Teleni L, McCarthy AL, et al. Ginger (*Zingiber officinale*) and chemotherapy-induced nausea and vomiting: a systematic literature review. Nutr Rev. 2013;71(4):245–254.

CASE 73: MIGRAINE HEADACHE

■ Butterbur and Feverfew for Prevention of Migraine

Clinical Course

While discussing possible alternatives to her valproic acid therapy, the patient says a friend who also has migraines had read about some herbal remedies used for migraine prevention. She asks whether any products like that could be used instead of or along with her prescription medications. The patient is very interested in a more "natural" therapy, but only if it would reduce the number of migraines she experiences.

■ FOLLOW-UP QUESTIONS

Butterbur and Feverfew

1. What are the known or proposed mechanisms of action?

2. How extensive or conclusive are the clinical trial data on effectiveness of each?

3. What is known about safety of each?

4. Does the product have any specific quality concerns?

5. Would any product be an appropriate treatment choice in this particular patient?

6. If the patient is going to use one of the products, what counseling information will allow her to maximize any possible benefit and minimize any harm?

7. Between the products, which might be a better choice for this patient?

REFERENCES

1. Sutherland A, Sweet BV. Butterbur: an alternative therapy for migraine prevention. Am J Health Syst Pharm. 2010;67:705–711.

2. Agosti R, Duke RK, Chrubasik JE, Chrubasik S. Effectiveness of *Petasites hybridus* preparations in the prophylaxis of migraine: a systematic review. Phytomedicine. 2006;13:743–746.

3. Lipton RB, Göbel H, Einhäupl KM, et al. *Petasites hybridus* root (butterbur) is an effective preventative treatment for migraine. Neurology. 2004;63:2240–2244.

4. Diener HC, Rahlfs VW, Danesch U. The first placebo-controlled trial of a special butterbur root extract for the prevention of migraine: reanalysis of efficacy criteria. Eur Neurol. 2004;51:89–97.

5. Wang YP, Yan J, Fu PP, Chou MW. Human liver microsomal reduction of pyrrolizidine alkaloid N-oxides to form the corresponding carcinogenic parent alkaloid. Toxicol Lett. 2005;155:411–420.

6. Avula B, Wang YH, Wang M, et al. Simultaneous determination of sesquiterpenes and pyrrolizidine alkaloids from the rhizomes of *Petasites hybridus* (L.) G.M. et Sch. and dietary supplements using UPLC-UV and HPLC-TOF-MS methods. J Pharm Biomed Anal. 2012;70:53–63.

7. Rajapakse T, Davenport WJ. Phytomedicine in the treatment of migraine. CNS Drugs. 2019;33(5):399–415.

8. Materazzi S, Benemei S, Fusi C, et al. Parthenolide inhibits nociception and neurogenic vasodilatation in the trigeminovascular systems by targeting the TRPA1 channel. Pain. 2013;154:2750–2758.

9. Magni P, Ruscica M, Dozio E, et al. Parthenolide inhibits the LPS-induced secretion of IL-6 and NF-κB nuclear translocation in BV-2 microglia. Phytother Res. 2012;26(9):1405–1409.

10. Pittler MH, Ernst E. Feverfew for preventing migraine. Cochrane Database Syst Rev. 2004;(1):CD002286.

CASE 80: MAJOR DEPRESSION

St. John's Wort for Depression

Clinical Course

The patient understands that she must stop the St. John's word she has been taking because of an interaction with her prescribed mirtazapine, but she wonders if it would have been helpful if she had started it when she first began feeling depressed.

■ FOLLOW-UP QUESTIONS

St. John's Wort

1. What is the known or proposed mechanism of action?
2. How extensive or conclusive are the clinical trial data on effectiveness?
3. What is known about safety?
4. Does the product have any specific quality concerns?
5. Would this be an appropriate treatment choice in this particular patient?
6. If the patient is going to use the product, what counseling information will allow her to maximize any possible benefit and minimize any harm?

REFERENCES

1. Russo E, Scicchitano F, Whalley BJ, et al. *Hypericum perforatum*: pharmacokinetic, mechanism of action, tolerability, and clinical drug-drug interactions. Phytother Res. 2014;28:643–655.
2. Butterweck V. Mechanism of action of St. John's wort in depression: what is known? CNS Drugs. 2003;17:539–562.
3. Hypericum Depression Trial Study Group. Effect of *Hypericum perforatum* (St. John's wort) in major depressive disorder. JAMA. 2002;287:1807–1814.
4. Sarris J, Fava M, Schweitzer I, Mischoulon D. St. John's wort (*Hypericum perforatum*) versus sertraline and placebo in major depressive disorder: continuation data from a 26-week RCT. Pharmacopsychiatry 2012;45:275–278.
5. Linde K, Berner MM, Kriston L. St John's wort for major depression. Cochrane Database Syst. Rev. 2008;4:CD000448.
6. Ng QX, Venkatanarayanan N, Ho CYX. Clinical use of *Hypericum perforatum* (St John's wort) in depression: a meta-analysis. J Affect Disord. 2017;210:211–221.
7. Nicolussi S, Drewe J, Butterweck V, Meyer Zu Schwabedissen HE. Clinical relevance of St. John's wort drug interactions revisited. Br J Pharmacol. 2020;177(6):1212–1226.

CASE 82: GENERALIZED ANXIETY DISORDER

■ Kava for Anxiety

Clinical Course

The patient is still worried about both the adverse effects of prescription drugs to treat his anxiety and whether he will be able to afford them. He states that he has read a lot of information about kava that "it really works for anxiety." The patient says, "Maybe I was just using a bad product last time I tried it and that's why it

didn't help much and hurt my stomach. Should I get a better product and try it again?"

■ FOLLOW-UP QUESTIONS

Kava

1. What is the known or proposed mechanism of action?
2. How extensive or conclusive are the clinical trial data on effectiveness?
3. What is known about safety?
4. Does the product have any specific quality concerns?
5. Would this be an appropriate treatment choice in this particular patient?
6. If the patient is going to use the product, what counseling information will allow him to maximize any possible benefit and minimize any harm?

REFERENCES

1. Singh YN, Singh NN. Therapeutic potential of kava in the treatment of anxiety disorders. CNS Drugs. 2002;16:731–743.
2. Sarris J, LaPorte E, Schweitzer I. Kava: a comprehensive review of efficacy, safety, and psychopharmacology. Aust NZ J Psychiatry. 2011;45:27–35.
3. Pittler M, Ernst E. Efficacy of kava extract for treating anxiety: systematic review and meta-analysis. J Clin Psychopharmacol. 2000;20:84–89.
4. Smith K, Leiras C. The effectiveness and safety of Kava Kava for treating anxiety symptoms: a systematic review and analysis of randomized clinical trials. Complement Ther Clin Pract. 2018;33:107–117.
5. Ooi SL, Henderson P, Pak SC. Kava for generalized anxiety disorder: a review of current evidence. J Altern Complement Med. 2018;24(8):770–780.
6. Sarris J, Kavanagh DJ, Byrne G, et al. The Kava Anxiety Depression Spectrum Study (KADSS): a randomized, placebo-controlled crossover trial using an aqueous extract of *Piper methysticum*. Psychopharmacology. 2009;205:399–407.
7. Sarris J, Stough C, Bouseman CA, et al. Kava in the treatment of generalized anxiety disorder. A double-blind, randomized, placebo-controlled study. J Clin Psychopharmacol. 2013;33(5):643–648.
8. Teschke R, Sarris J, Glass X, Schulze J. Kava, the anxiolytic herb: back to basics to prevent liver injury? Br J Clin Pharmacol. 2011;71(3):445–448.
9. Kuchta K, Schmidt M, Nahrstedt A. German kava ban lifted by court: the alleged hepatotoxicity of kava (*Piper methysticum*) as a case of ill-defined herbal drug identity, lacking quality control, and misguided regulatory politics. Planta Med. 2015;81(18):1647–1653.
10. Stevinson C, Huntley A, Ernst E. A systematic review of the safety of kava extract in the treatment of anxiety. Drug Safety. 2002;25:251–261.
11. Brown AC. Liver toxicity related to herbs and dietary supplements: online table of case reports. Food Chem Toxicol. 2017;107:472–501.

CASE 84: INSOMNIA

■ Melatonin for Insomnia

Clinical Course

The patient states that her neighbor had suggested that using a melatonin product to help her stay asleep. She would like to know whether that is a good option to help keep her from waking up after she has fallen asleep.

■ FOLLOW-UP QUESTIONS

Melatonin

1. What is the known or proposed mechanism of action?
2. How extensive or conclusive are the clinical trial data on effectiveness?
3. What is known about safety?

4. Does the product have any specific quality concerns?

5. Would this be an appropriate treatment choice in this particular patient?

6. If the patient is going to use the product, what counseling information will allow her to maximize any possible benefit and minimize any harm?

REFERENCES

1. Zisapel N. New perspectives on the role of melatonin in human sleep, circadian rhythms and their regulation. Br J Pharmacol. 2018;175(16):3190–3199.

2. Auld F, Maschauer EL, Morrison I, et al. Evidence for the efficacy of melatonin in the treatment of primary adult sleep disorders. Sleep Med Rev. 2017;34:10–22.

3. Luthringer R, Muzet M, Zisapel N, et al. The effect of prolonged-release melatonin on sleep measures and psychomotor performance in elderly patients with insomnia. Int Clin Psychopharmacol. 2009;24(5):239–249.

4. Sateia MJ, Buysse DJ, Krystal AD, et al. Clinical practice guideline for the pharmacologic treatment of chronic insomnia in adults: an American Academy of Sleep Medicine Clinical Practice Guideline. J Clin Sleep Med. 2017;13(2):307–349.

5. Hansen MV, Danielsen AK, Hageman I, et al. The therapeutic or prophylactic effect of exogenous melatonin against depression and depressive symptoms: a systematic review and meta-analysis. Eur Neuropsychopharmacol. 2014;24(11):1719–1728.

6. Foley HM, Steel AE. Adverse events associated with oral administration of melatonin: a critical systematic review of clinical evidence. Complement Ther Med. 2019;42:65–81.

CASE 86: TYPE 2 DIABETES MELLITUS: NEW ONSET

Fish Oil, Cinnamon, and α-Lipoic Acid for Type 2 Diabetes Mellitus

Clinical Course

While discussing the patient's diagnosis with him, he states that his neighbor with diabetes told him that she just follows her diabetic diet and takes cinnamon and something called "alip acid" and does not have to take any prescriptions for her blood sugar. He also says that he has read about fish oil being used for diabetes. The patient asks if he should start any of those to help get his blood sugar under control.

■ FOLLOW-UP QUESTIONS

Fish Oil, Cinnamon, and α-Lipoic Acid

1. What is the known or proposed mechanism of action for each?

2. How extensive or conclusive are the clinical trial data on effectiveness for each?

3. What is known about safety of each?

4. Do any of the products have any specific quality concerns?

5. Would anyone or these be an appropriate treatment choice in this particular patient?

6. If the patient is going to use any of these products, what counseling information will allow him to maximize any possible benefit and minimize any harm?

REFERENCES

1. Balk EM, Lichtenstein AH, Chung M, et al. Effects of omega-3 fatty acids on serum markers of cardiovascular disease risk: a systematic review. Atherosclerosis. 2006;189(1):19–30.

2. Gao C, Liu Y, Gan Y, et al. Effects of fish oil supplementation on glucose control and lipid levels among patients with type 2 diabetes mellitus: a meta-analysis of randomized, controlled trials. Lipids Health Dis. 2020;19(1):87.

3. Hartweg J, Perera R, Montori VM, Dinneen SF, Neil AHAWM, Farmer AJ. Omega-3 polyunsaturated fatty acids (PUFA) for type 2 diabetes mellitus. Cochrane Database Syst Rev. 2008;(1):CD003205.

4. Gao H, Geng T, Huang T, et al. Fish oil supplementation and insulin sensitivity: a systematic review and meta-analysis. Lipids Health Dis. 2017;16(1):131.

5. Lichtenstein AH, Appel LJ, Brands M, et al. Diet and lifestyle recommendations revision 2006: a scientific statement from the American Heart Association Nutrition Committee. Circulation. 2006;114:82–96.

6. Medagama AB. The glycaemic outcomes of cinnamon, a review of the experimental evidence and clinical trials. Nutr J. 2015;14:108.

7. Leach MJ, Kumar S. Cinnamon for diabetes mellitus. Cochrane Database Syst Rev. 2012;(9):CD007170.

8. Akilen R, Tsiami A, Devendra D, Robinson N. Glycated haemoglobin and blood pressure-lowering effect of cinnamon in multi-ethnic type 2 diabetic patients in the UK: a randomized, placebo-controlled, double-blind clinical trial. Diabetic Med. 2010;27:1159–1167.

9. Lu T, Sheng H, Wu J, et al. Cinnamon extract improves fasting blood glucose and glycosylated hemoglobin level in Chinese patients with type 2 diabetes. Nutr Res. 2012;32:408–412.

10. Namazi N, Khodamoradi K, Khamechi SP, et al. The impact of cinnamon on anthropometric indices and glycemic status in patients with type 2 diabetes: a systematic review and meta-analysis of clinical trials. Complement Ther Med. 2019;43:92–101.

11. Rochette L, Ghibu S, Muresan A, Vergely C. Alpha-lipoic acid: molecular mechanisms and therapeutic potential in diabetes. Can J Physiol Pharmacol. 2015;93:1021–1027.

12. Ansar H, Mazloom Z, Kazemi F, Hejazi N. Effect of alpha-lipoic acid on blood glucose, insulin resistance, and glutathione peroxidase of type 2 diabetic patients. Saudi Med J. 2011;32(6):584–588.

13. Porasuphatana S, Suddee S, Nartnampong A, et al. Glycemic and oxidative status of patients with type 2 diabetes mellitus following oral administration of alpha-lipoic acid: a randomized double-blinded placebo-controlled study. Asia Pac J Clin Nutr. 2012;21(1):12–21.

CASE 98: MANAGING MENOPAUSAL SYMPTOMS

Black Cohosh and Soy for Menopausal Symptoms

Clinical Course

This patient is considering stopping her HT because her cousin was recently diagnosed with breast cancer. She still desires relief from hot flashes and asks for additional information on other alternatives. She has heard that black cohosh should not be used in women with breast cancer, but she has a friend who also has a family history of breast cancer who has been on black cohosh for about 9 months on the recommendation of her physician. Her friend has a checkup with lab tests every 6 months. The patient asks if black cohosh or soy would be an appropriate option to help keep her hot flushes under control.

■ FOLLOW-UP QUESTIONS

Black Cohosh and Soy

1. What are the known or proposed mechanisms of action?

2. How extensive or conclusive are the clinical trial data on effectiveness for each?

3. What is known about safety of each?

4. Do the products have any specific quality concerns?

5. Would either product be an appropriate treatment choice in this particular patient?

6. If the patient is going to use either of these products, what counseling information will allow her to maximize any possible benefit and minimize any harm?

REFERENCES

1. Powell SL, Gödecke T, Nikolic D, et al. In vitro serotonergic activity of black cohosh and identification of N$_\omega$-methylserotonin as a potential active constituent. J Agric Food Chem. 2008;56:11718–11726.
2. Borrelli F, Izzo AA, Ernst E. Pharmacological effects of *Cimicifuga racemosa*. Life Sci. 2003;73:1215–1229.
3. Fritz H, Seely D, McGowan J, et al. Black cohosh and breast cancer: a systematic review. Integr Cancer Ther. 2014;13(1):12–29.
4. Castelo-Branco C, Gambacciai M, Cano A, et al. Review & meta-analysis: isopropanolic black cohosh extract iCR for menopausal symptoms—an update on the evidence. Climacteric. 2021;24(2):109–119.
5. Rebbeck TR, Troxel AB, Norman S, et al. A retrospective case-control study of the use of hormone-related supplements and association with breast cancer. Intl J Cancer. 2007;120:1523–1528.
6. Obi N, Chang-Claude J, Berger J, et al. The use of herbal preparations to alleviate climacteric disorders and risk of postmenopausal breast cancer in a German case-control study. Cancer Epidemiol Biomarkers Prev. 2009;18(8):2207–2213.
7. Naser B, Schnitker J, Minkin MJ, Garcia de Arriba S, Nolte KU, Osmers R. Suspected black cohosh hepatotoxicity: no evidence by meta-analysis of randomized controlled clinical trials for isopropanolic black cohosh extract. Menopause. 2011;18(4):366–375.
8. North American Menopause Society. The role of soy isoflavones in menopausal health: report of The North American Menopause Society/Wulf H. Utian Translational Science Symposium in Chicago, IL (October 2010). Menopause. 2011;18(7):732–753.
9. Villaseca P. Non-estrogen conventional and phytochemical treatments for vasomotor symptoms: what needs to be known for practice. Climacteric. 2012;15:115–124.
10. Schmidt M, Arjomand-Wölkart K, Birkhäuser MH, et al. Consensus: soy isoflavones as a first-line approach to the treatment of menopausal vasomotor complaints. Gyn Endocrinol. 2016;32(6):427–430.

CASE 100: BENIGN PROSTATIC HYPERPLASIA

■ *Pygeum africanum* **for BPH**

Clinical Course

As the pharmacist in the team, you perform a literature search on the use of saw palmetto for BPH. You discover that there are reports of the dietary supplement both improving and worsening symptoms of ED. In addition, your readings indicate that saw palmetto should really only be used by patients with mild to moderate BPH. Based on this information, you do not recommend use of saw palmetto for the patient's BPH symptoms. However, because the patient is requesting information on natural products, you search for alternative dietary supplements that may provide some benefit for this patient's BPH without contributing to ED. Would *Pygeum africanum* be a reasonable option to consider?

■ FOLLOW-UP QUESTIONS

1. What is the known or proposed mechanism of action?
2. How extensive or conclusive is the clinical trial data on effectiveness?
3. What is known about safety?
4. Does the product have any specific quality concerns?
5. Would this be an appropriate treatment choice in this particular patient?

6. If the patient is going to use the product, what counseling information will allow him to maximize any possible benefit and minimize any harm?

REFERENCES

1. Quiles MT, Arbós MA, Fraga A, et al. Antiproliferative and apoptotic effects of the herbal agent *Pygeum africanum* on culture prostate stromal cells from patients with benign prostatic hyperplasia (BPH). Prostate. 2010;70:1044–1053.
2. Papaioannou M, Schleich S, Roell D, et al. NBBS isolated from *Pygeum africanum* bark exhibits androgen antagonistic activity, inhibits AR nuclear translocation and prostate cancer cell growth. Invest New Drugs. 2010;28:729–743.
3. Shenouda NS, Sakla MS, Newton LG, et al. Physterol *Pygeum africanum* regulates prostate cancer in vitro and in vivo. Endocrine. 2007;31:72–81.
4. Breza J, Dzurny O, Borowka A, et al. Efficacy and acceptability of Tadenan® (*Pygeum africanum* extract) in the treatment of benign prostatic hyperplasia (BPH): a multicentre trial in central Europe. Cur Med Res Opin. 1998;14:127–139.
5. Chatelain C, Autet W, Brackman F. Comparison of once and twice daily dosage forms of *Pygeum africanum* extract in patients with benign prostatic hyperplasia: a randomized, double-blind study, with long-term open label extension. Urology. 1999;54:473–478.
6. Ishani A, MacDonald R, Nelson D, Rutks I, Wilt TJ. *Pygeum africanum* for the treatment of patients with benign prostatic hyperplasia: a systematic review and quantitative meta-analysis. Am J Med. 2000;109:654–664.
7. Wilt T, Ishani A, Mac Donald R, Rutks I, Stark G. *Pygeum africanum* for benign prostatic hyperplasia. Cochrane Data Syst Rev. 2002;(1):CD001044.

CASE 105: OSTEOARTHRITIS

■ **Glucosamine Sulfate, Glucosamine Hydrochloride, and Chondroitin for Osteoarthritis**

Clinical Course

While discussing multiple treatment options with the patient, he says, "This may seem silly, but I have a neighbor a couple years older than me who was getting some pretty bad arthritis in both knees a few years ago. He says he hardly has any pain anymore because he's taking these glucosamine and chondroitin pills. He even started back to golfing! Is there any way those could help me with my pain?"

■ FOLLOW-UP QUESTIONS

Glucosamine and Chondroitin

1. What are the known or proposed mechanisms of action?
2. How extensive or conclusive is the clinical trial data on effectiveness of each of the products or their combinations?
3. What is known about safety?
4. Do the products have any specific quality concerns?
5. Would any of these be appropriate treatment choice in this particular patient?
6. If the patient is going to use the products, what counseling information will allow him to maximize any possible benefit and minimize any harm?

REFERENCES

1. Nagaoka I, Igarashi M, Sakamoto K. Biological activities of glucosamine and its related substances. Adv Food Nutr Res. 2012;65:337–352.
2. Volpi N. Anti-inflammatory activity of chondroitin sulphate: new functions from an old natural molecule. Inflammopharmacology. 2011;19:299–306.

3. Calamia V, Mateos J, Fernández-Puente P, et al. A pharmacoproteomic study confirms the synergistic effect of chondroitin sulfate and glucosamine. Sci Rep. 2014;4:5069.

4. Kaloskinski SL, Neogi T, Hochberg MC, et al. 2019 American College of Rheumatology/Arthritis Foundation guideline for the management of osteoarthritis of the hand, hip and knee. Arthritis Rheumatol. 2020;72(2): 220–33.

5. McAlindon TE, Bannuru RR, Sullivan MC, et al. OARSI guidelines for the non-surgical management of knee osteoarthritis. Osteoarthritis Cartilage. 2014;22(3):363–388.

6. Zhu X, Sang L, Wu D, et al. Effectiveness and safety of glucosamine and chondroitin for the treatment of osteoarthritis: a meta-analysis of randomized controlled trials. J Orthop Surg Res. 2018;13:170.

7. Simental-Mendia M, Sanchez-Garcia A, Vilchez-Cavazos F, et al. Effect of glucosamine and chondroitin sulfate in symptomatic knee osteoarthritis: a systemic review and meta-analysis of randomized placebo-controlled trials. Rhematol Int. 2018;38(8):1413–1428.

CASE 110: ALLERGIC RHINITIS

■ Butterbur Extract for Allergic Rhinitis

Clinical Course

The patient reports that he has read about butterbur extract being helpful for allergy symptoms. He asks whether it would be okay to use it in addition to his prescription medications.

■ FOLLOW-UP QUESTIONS

Butterbur Extract

1. What is the known or proposed mechanism of action?

2. How extensive or conclusive are the clinical trial data on effectiveness?

3. What is known about safety?

4. Does the product have any specific quality concerns?

5. Would this be an appropriate treatment choice in this particular patient?

6. If the patient is going to use the product, what counseling information will allow him to maximize any possible benefit and minimize any harm?

REFERENCES

1. Thomet OA, Schapowal A, Heinisch IV, et al. Anti-inflammatory activity of an extract of *Petasites hybridus* in allergic rhinitis. Int Immunopharmacol. 2002;2:997–1006.

2. Dumitru AF, Shamji M, Wagenmann M, et al. Petasol butanoate complex (Ze 339) relieves allergic rhinitis-induced nasal obstruction more effectively than desloratadine. J Allergy Clin Immunol. 2011;127:1515–1521.

3. Lee DK, Haggart K, Robb FM, Lipworth BJ. Butterbur, a herbal remedy, confers complementary anti-inflammatory activity in asthmatic patients receiving inhaled corticosteroids. Clin Exp Allergy. 2004;34:110–114.

4. Guo R, Pittler MH, Ernst E. Herbal medicines for the treatment of allergic rhinitis: a systematic review. Ann Allergy Asthma Immunol. 2007;99:483–495.

5. Wu AW, Gettelfinger JD, Ting JY, et al. Alternative therapies for sinusitis and rhinitis: a systematic review utilizing a modified Delphi method. Int Forum Allergy Rhinol. 2020;10(4):496–504.

6. Anderson N, Meier T, Borlak J. Toxicogenomics applied to cultures of human hepatocytes enabled an identification of novel *Petasites hybridus* extracts for the treatment of migraine with improved hepatobiliary safety. Toxicol Sci. 2009;112:507–520.

7. Wang YP, Yan J, Fu PP, Chou MW. Human liver microsomal reduction of pyrrolizidine alkaloid N-oxides to form the corresponding carcinogenic parent alkaloid. Toxicol Lett. 2005;155:411–420.

CASE 127: INFLUENZA

■ Elderberry for Influenza

Clinical Course

As the patient is leaving, he thanks you and promises to follow your recommendations. He states that he is worried about making anyone else sick, because of his son's upcoming wedding. "My cousins keep telling me they use elderberry syrup to keep from getting sick during flu season. Could that help keep my wife from getting this flu?"

■ FOLLOW-UP QUESTIONS

Elderberry

1. What is the known or proposed mechanism of action?

2. How extensive or conclusive are the clinical trial data on effectiveness?

3. What is known about safety?

4. Does the product have any specific quality concerns?

5. Would this be an appropriate treatment choice in this particular patient or for the patient's wife?

6. If the patient is going to use the product, what counseling information will allow him to maximize any possible benefit and minimize any harm?

REFERENCES

1. Ulbricht C, Basch E, Cheung L, et al. An evidence-based systematic review of elderberry and elderflower (*Sambucus nigra*) by the Natural Standard Research Collaboration. J Diet Suppl. 2014;11(1):80–120.

2. Krawitz C, Abu Mraheil M, Stein M, et al. Inhibitory activity of a standardized elderberry liquid extract against clinically-relevant human respiratory bacterial pathogens and influenza A and B viruses. BMC Complement Altern Med. 2011;11:16.

3. Kinoshita E, Hayashi K, Katayama H, et al. Anti-influenza virus effects of elderberry juice and its fractions. Biosci Biotechnol Biochem. 2012;76(9):1633–1638.

4. Zakay-Rones Z, Varsano N, Zlotnik M, et al. Inhibition of several strains of influenza virus in vitro and reduction of symptoms by an elderberry extract (*Sambucus nigra* L.) during an outbreak of influenza B Panama. J Altern Complement Med. 1995;1:361–369.

5. Zakay-Rones Z, Thom E, Wollan T, et al. Randomized study of the efficacy and safety of oral elderberry extract in the treatment of influenza A and B virus infections. J Int Med Res. 2004;32:132–140.

6. Rauš K, Pleschka S, Klein P, et al. Effect of an echinacea-based hot drink versus oseltamivir in influenza treatment: a randomized, double-blind, double-dummy, multicenter, noninferiority clinical trial. Curr Therapeutic Res. 2015;77:66–72.

7. Hawkins J, Baker C, Cherry L, et al. Black elderberry (*Sambucus nigra*) supplementation effectively treats upper respiratory symptoms: a meta-analysis of randomized, controlled clinical trials. Complement Ther Med. 2019;42:361–365.

8. Curtis PJ, Kroom PA, Hollands WJ, et al. Cardiovascular disease risk biomarkers and liver and kidney function are not altered in postmenopausal women after ingesting and elderberry extract rich in anthocyanins for 12 weeks. J Nutr. 2009;139:2266–2271.

CONVERSION FACTORS AND ANTHROPOMETRICS*

CONVERSION FACTORS

■ SI Units

SI (*le Système International d'Unités*) units are used in many countries to express clinical laboratory and serum drug concentration data. Instead of employing units of mass (such as micrograms), the SI system uses moles (mol) to represent the amount of a substance. A molar solution contains 1 mol (the molecular weight of the substance in grams) of the solute in 1 L of solution. The following formula is used to convert units of mass to moles (mcg/mL to μmol/L or, by substitution of terms, mg/mL to mmol/L or ng/mL to nmol/L).

Micromoles per Liter (μmol/L)

$$\mu mol/L = \frac{\text{drug concentration (mcg/mL)} \times 1000}{\text{molecular weight of drug (g/mol)}}$$

Milliequivalents

An equivalent weight of a substance is that weight which will combine with or replace 1 g of hydrogen; a milliequivalent is 1/1000 of an equivalent weight.

Milliequivalents per Liter (mEq/L)

$$mEq/L = \frac{\text{weight of salt (g)} \times \text{valence of ion} \times 1000}{\text{molecular weight of salt}}$$

$$\text{weight of salt (g)} = \frac{mEq/L \times \text{molecular weight of salt}}{\text{valence of iron} \times 1000}$$

Approximate Milliequivalents

Weights of Selected Ions

Salt	mEq/g Salt	mg Salt/mEq
Calcium carbonate ($CaCO_3$)	20.0	50.0
Calcium chloride ($CaCl_2 \cdot 2H_2O$)	13.6	73.5
Calcium gluceptate ($Ca[C_7H_{13}O_8]_2$)	4.1	245.2
Calcium gluconate ($Ca[C_6H_{11}O_7]_2 \cdot H_2O$)	4.5	224.1
Calcium lactate ($Ca[C_3H_5O_3]_2 \cdot 5H_2O$)	6.5	154.1
Magnesium gluconate ($Mg[C_6H_{11}O_7]_2 \cdot H_2O$)	4.6	216.3
Magnesium oxide (MgO)	49.6	20.2
Magnesium sulfate ($MgSO_4$)	16.6	60.2
Magnesium sulfate ($MgSO_4 \cdot 7H_2O$)	8.1	123.2
Potassium acetate ($K[C_2H_3O_2]$)	10.2	98.1
Potassium chloride (KCl)	13.4	74.6
Potassium citrate ($K_3[C_6H_5O_7] \cdot H_2O$)	9.2	108.1
Potassium iodide (KI)	6.0	166.0
Sodium acetate ($Na[C_2H_3O_2]$)	12.2	82.0
Sodium acetate ($Na[C_2H_3O_2] \cdot 3H_2O$)	7.3	136.1
Sodium bicarbonate ($NaHCO_3$)	11.9	84.0
Sodium chloride (NaCl)	17.1	58.4
Sodium citrate ($Na_3[C_6H_5O_7] \cdot 2H_2O$)	10.2	98.0
Sodium iodide (NaI)	6.7	149.9
Sodium lactate ($Na[C_3H_5O_3]$)	8.9	112.1
Zinc sulfate ($ZnSO_4 \cdot 7H_2O$)	7.0	143.8

■ Valences and Atomic Weights of Selected Ions

Substance	Electrolyte	Valence	Molecular Weight
Calcium	Ca^{2+}	2	40.1
Chloride	Cl^-	1	35.5
Magnesium	Mg^{2+}	2	24.3
Phosphate (pH = 7.4)	HPO_4^- (80%) $H_2PO_4^-$ (20%)	1.8	96.0^a
Potassium	K^+	1	39.1
Sodium	Na^+	1	23.0
Sulfate	SO_4^-	2	96.0^a

^{a}The molecular weight of phosphorus only is 31; that of sulfur only is 32.1.

*Reproduced with permission from Appendices 1 and 2. In: Anderson PO, Knoben JE, Troutman WG, et al (eds). Handbook of Clinical Drug Data. 10th ed. New York: McGraw-Hill, 2002:1053-1058.

■ Anion Gap

The anion gap is the concentration of plasma anions not routinely measured by laboratory screening. It is useful in the evaluation of acid–base disorders. The anion gap is greater with increased plasma concentrations of endogenous species (eg, phosphate, sulfate, lactate, and ketoacids) or exogenous species (eg, salicylate, penicillin, ethylene glycol, ethanol, and methanol). The formulas for calculating the anion gap are as follows:

$$\text{Anion gap} = (Na^+ + K^+) - (Cl^- + HCO_3^-)$$

or

$$\text{Anion gap} = Na^+ - (Cl^- + HCO_3^-)$$

where the expected normal value for the first equation is 11–20 mmol/L, and the expected normal value for the second equation is 7–16 mmol/L. Note that there is a variation in the upper and lower limits of the normal range.

■ Temperature

Fahrenheit to Centigrade: $(°F - 32) \times 5/9 = °C$
Centigrade to Fahrenheit: $(°C \times 9/5) + 32 = °F$
Centigrade to Kelvin: $°C + 273 = K$

■ Calories

1 calorie = 1 kilocalorie = 1000 calories = 4.184 kilojoules (kJ)
1 kilojoule = 0.239 calories = 0.239 kilocalories = 239 calories

■ Weights and Measures

Metric Weight Equivalents

1 kilogram (kg) = 1000 grams
1 gram (g) = 1000 milligrams
1 milligram (mg) = 0.001 gram
1 microgram (mcg) = 0.001 milligram
1 nanogram (ng) = 0.001 microgram
1 picogram (pg) = 0.001 nanogram
1 femtogram (fg) = 0.001 picogram

Metric Volume Equivalents

1 liter (L) = 1000 milliliters
1 deciliter (dL) = 100 milliliters
1 milliliter (mL) = 0.001 liter
1 microliter (μL) = 0.001 milliliter
1 nanoliter (nL) = 0.001 microliter
1 picoliter (pL) = 0.001 nanoliter
1 femtoliter (fL) = 0.001 picoliter

Apothecary Weight Equivalents

1 scruple (Э) = 20 grains (gr)
60 grains (gr) = 1 dram (ʒ)
8 drams (ʒ) = 1 ounce (fl ʒ)
1 ounce (ʒ) = 480 grains
12 ounces (ʒ) = 1 pound (lb)

Apothecary Volume Equivalents

60 minims (♏) = 1 fluidram (fl ʒ)
8 fluidrams (fl ʒ) = 1 fluid ounce (fl ʒ)
1 fluid ounce (ft ʒ) = 480 minims
16 fluid ounces (fl ʒ) = 1 pint (pt)

Avoirdupois Equivalents

1 ounce (oz) = 437.5 grains
16 ounces (oz) = 1 pound (lb)

Weight/Volume Equivalents

1 mg/dL = 10 mcg/mL
1 mg/dL = 1 mg%
1 ppm = 1 mg/L

Conversion Equivalents

1 gram (g) = 15.43 grains
1 grain (gr) = 64.8 milligrams
1 ounce (ʒ) = 31.1 grams
1 ounce (oz) = 28.35 grams
1 pound (lb) = 453.6 grams
1 kilogram (kg) = 2.2 pounds
1 milliliter (mL) = 16.23 minims
1 minim (♏) = 0.06 milliliter
1 fluid ounce (fl oz) = 29.57 milliliter
1 pint (pt) = 473.2 milliliter
0.1 milligram = 1/600 grain
0.12 milligram = 1/500 grain
0.15 milligram = 1/400 grain
0.2 milligram = 1/300 grain
0.3 milligram = 1/200 grain
0.4 milligram = 1/150 grain
0.5 milligram = 1/120 grain
0.6 milligram = 1/100 grain
0.8 milligram = 1/80 grain
1 milligram = 1/65 grain

Metric Length Equivalents

2.54 cm = 1 inch
30.48 cm = 1 foot
1.6 km = 1 mile

ANTHROPOMETRICS

■ Creatinine Clearance Formulas

Formulas for Estimating Creatinine Clearance in Patients With Stable Renal Function

Cockcroft–Gault Formula

Adults (age ≥18 years)[1]:

$$CLcr\,(males) = \frac{(140 - age) \times weight}{Cr_s \times 72}$$

$$CLcr\,(males) = 0.85 \times above\ value^{\dagger}$$

where CLcr is creatinine clearance (in mL/min), Cr_s is serum creatinine (in mg/dL), age is in years, and weight is in kilograms.

Children (age 1–18 years)[2]:

$$CLcr = \frac{0.48 \times height \times BSA}{Cr_s \times 1.73}$$

where BSA is body surface area (in m^2), CLcr is creatinine clearance (in mL/min), Cr_s is serum creatinine (in mg/dL), and height is in centimeters.

---

†Some studies suggest that the predictive accuracy of this formula for women is better without the correction factor of 0.85.

Formula for Estimating Creatinine Clearance From a Measured Urine Collection

$$CLcr\ (mL/minute) = \frac{U \times V^{\ddagger}}{P \times T}$$

where U is the concentration of creatinine in a urine specimen (in same units as P), V is the volume of urine (in mL), P is the concentration of creatinine in serum at the midpoint of the urine collection period (in same units as U), and T is the time of the urine collection period in minutes (eg, 6 hours = 360 minutes; 24 hours = 1440 minutes).

MDRD Formula for Estimating Glomerular Filtration Rate (From the Modification of Diet in Renal Disease Study)[3]

Conventional calibration MDRD equation (used only with those creatinine methods that have not been recalibrated to be traceable to isotope dilution mass spectrometry [IDMS]).

For creatinine in mg/dL:

$$X = 186\ creatinine^{-1.154} \times age^{-0.203} \times constant$$

For creatinine in μmol/L:

$$X = 32,788 \times creatinine^{-1.154} \times age^{-0.203} \times constant$$

where X is the glomerular filtration rate (GFR), constant for white males is 1 and for females is 0.742, and constant for African Americans is 1.21. Creatinine levels in μmol/L can be converted to mg/dL by dividing by 88.4.

IDMS-Traceable MDRD Equation (Used Only With Creatinine Methods That Have Been Recalibrated to Be Traceable to IDMS)

For creatinine in mg/dL:

$$X = 175 \times creatinine^{-1.154} \times age^{-0.203} \times constant$$

For creatinine in μmol/L:

$$X = 175 \times (creatinine/88.4)^{-1.154} \times age^{-0.203} \times constant$$

where X is the glomerular filtration rate (GFR), constant for white males is 1 and for females is 0.742, and constant for African Americans is 1.21.

Ideal Body Weight (IBW)

IBW is the weight expected for a nonobese person of a given height. The following IBW formulas and various life insurance tables can be used to estimate IBW. Dosing methods described in the literature may use IBW as a method in dosing obese patients.

Adults (age ≥18 years)[4]:

IBW (males) = 50 + (2.3 × height in inches over 5 ft)
IBW (females) = 45.5 + (2.3 × height in inches over 5 ft)

where IBW is in kilograms.

Children (age 1–18 years)[2]:

Under 5 feet tall:

$$IBW = \frac{height^2 \times 1.65}{1000}$$

where IBW is in kilograms and height is in centimeters.

Five feet or taller:

IBW (males) = 39 + (2.27 × height in inches over 5 ft)
IBW (females) = 42.2 + (2.27 × height in inches over 5 ft)

where IBW is in kilograms.

REFERENCES

1. Cockcroft DW, Gault MH. Prediction of creatinine clearance from serum creatinine. Nephron. 1976;16:31–41.
2. Traub SI, Johnson CE. Comparison of methods of estimating creatinine clearance in children. Am J Hosp Pharm. 1980;37:195–201.
3. Levey AS, Bosch JP, Lewis JB, et al. A more accurate method to estimate glomerular filtration rate from serum creatinine: a new prediction equation. Modification of Diet in Renal Disease Study Group. Ann Intern Med. 1999;130:461–470.
4. Devine BJ. Gentamicin therapy. Drug Intell Clin Pharm. 1974;8:650–655.

---

‡The product of $U \times V$ equals the production of creatinine during the collection period and, at steady state, should equal 20–25 mg/kg per day for ideal body weight (IBW) in males and 15–20 mg/kg per day for IBW in females. If it is less than this, inadequate urine collection may have occurred and CLcr will be underestimated.

APPENDIX B
COMMON LABORATORY TESTS

The following table is an alphabetical listing of some common laboratory tests and their reference ranges for adults as measured in plasma or serum (unless otherwise indicated). Reference values differ among laboratories, so readers should refer to the published reference ranges used in each institution. For some tests, both SI units and conventional units are reported.

Laboratory	Conventional Units	Conversion Factor	SI Units
Acid phosphatase			
Male	2–12 units/L	16.7	33–200 nkat/L
Female	0.3–9.2 units/L	16.7	5–154 nkat/L
Activated partial thromboplastin time (aPTT)	25–40 sec		
Adrenocorticotropic hormone (ACTH)	15–80 pg/mL or ng/L	0.2202	3.3–17.6 pmol/L
Alanine aminotransferase (ALT, SGPT)	7–53 IU/L	0.01667	0.12–0.88 μkat/L
Albumin	3.5–5.0 g/dL	10	35–50 g/L
Albumin:creatinine ratio (urine)			
Normal	<30 mg/g creatinine		
Microalbuminuria	30–300 mg/g creatinine		
Proteinuria	>300 mg/g creatinine		
or	or		
Normal			
Male	<2.0 mg/mmol creatinine		
Female	<2.8 mg/mmol creatinine		
Microalbuminuria			
Male	2.0–20 mg/mmol creatinine		
Female	2.8–28 mg/mmol creatinine		
Proteinuria			
Male	>20 mg/mmol creatinine		
Female	>28 mg/mmol creatinine		
Aldosterone			
Supine	<16 ng/dL	27.7	<444 pmol/L
Upright	<31 ng/dL	27.7	<860 pmol/L
Alkaline phosphatase			
10–15 years	130–550 IU/L	0.01667	2.17–9.17 μkat/L
16–20 years	70–260 IU/L	0.01667	1.17–4.33 μkat/L
>20 years	38–126 IU/L	0.01667	0.13–2.10 μkat/L
Alpha-fetoprotein (AFP)	<15 ng/mL	1	<15 mcg/L
Alpha$_1$-antitrypsin	80–200 mg/dL	0.01	0.8–2.0 g/L
Amikacin, therapeutic	15–30 mg/L peak	1.71	25.6–51.3 μmol/L peak
	≤8 mg/L trough		≤13.7 μmol/L trough
Amitriptyline	80–200 ng/mL or mcg/L	3.4	272–680 nmol/L
Ammonia (plasma)	15.33–56.20 mcg NH$_3$/dL	0.5872	9–33 μmol NH$_3$/L
Amylase	25–115 IU/L	0.01667	0.42–1.92 kat/L
Androstenedione	50–250 ng/dL	0.0349	1.7–8.7 nmol/L
Angiotensin-converting enzyme	15–70 units/L	16.67	250–1,167 nkat/L
Anion gap	7–16 mEq/L	1	7–16 mmol/L
Anti–double-stranded DNA (anti-ds DNA)	Negative		
Anti-HAV	Negative		
Anti-HBc	Negative		
Anti-HBs	Negative		
Anti-HCV	Negative		
Anti–Sm antibody	Negative		
Antinuclear antibody (ANA)	Negative		
Apolipoprotein A-1			
Male	95–175 mg/dL	0.01	0.95–1.75 g/L
Female	100–200 mg/dL	0.01	1.0–2.0 g/L
Apolipoprotein B			
Male	50–110 mg/dL	0.01	0.5–1.10 g/L
Female	50–105 mg/dL	0.01	0.5–1.05 g/L

(continued)

Laboratory	Conventional Units	Conversion Factor	SI Units
Aspartate aminotransferase (AST, SGOT)	11–47 IU/L	0.01667	0.18–0.78 μkat/L
Beta$_2$-microglobulin	<0.2 mg/dL	10	2 mg/L
Bicarbonate	22–26 mEq/L	1	22–26 mmol/L
Bilirubin			
Total	0.3–1.1 mg/dL	17.1	5.13–18.80 μmol/L
Direct	0–0.3 mg/dL	17.1	0–5.1 μmol/L
Indirect	0.1–1.0 mg/dL	17.1	1.71–17.1 μmol/L
Bleeding time	3–7 min		
Blood gases (arterial)			
pH	7.35–7.45	1	7.35–7.45
PaO$_2$	80–105 mm Hg	0.133	10.6–14.0 kPa
PaCO$_2$	35–45 mm Hg	0.133	4.7–6.0 kPa
HCO$_3$	22–26 mEq/L	1	22–26 mmol/L
O$_2$ saturation	≥95%	0.01	0.95
Blood urea nitrogen	8–25 mg/dL	0.357	2.9–8.9 mmol/L
B-type natriuretic peptide (BNP)	0–99 pg/mL	1	0–99 ng/L
BUN-to-creatinine ratio	10:1 to 20:1		
C-peptide	0.51–2.70 ng/mL	330	170–900 pmol/L or
		0.33	0.172–0.900 nmol/L
C-reactive protein	<0.8 mg/dL	10	<8 mg/L
CA-125	<35 units/mL	1	<35 kilounits/L
CA 15-3	<30 units/mL	1	<30 kilounits/L
CA 19-9	<37 units/mL	1	<37 kilounits/L
CA 27-29	<38 units/mL	1	<38 kilounits/L
Calcium			
Total	8.6–10.3 mg/dL	0.25	2.15–2.58 mmol/L
	4.3–5.16 mEq/L	0.50	2.15–2.58 mmol/L
Ionized	4.5–5.1 mg/dL	0.25	1.13–1.28 mmol/L
	2.26–2.56 mEq/L	0.50	1.13–1.28 mmol/L
Carbamazepine, therapeutic	4–12 mg/L	4.23	17–51 μmol/L
Carboxyhemoglobin (nonsmoker)	<2%	0.01	<0.02
Carcinoembryonic antigen (CEA)			
Nonsmoker	<2.5 ng/mL	1	<2.5 mcg/L
Smoker	<5 ng/mL		<5 mcg/L
Cardiac troponin I (see troponin I)	Variable ng/mL	1	Variable mcg/L
CD4 lymphocyte count	31–61% of total lymphocytes		
CD8 lymphocyte count	18–39% of total lymphocytes		
Cerebrospinal fluid (CSF)			
Pressure	75–175 mm H$_2$O		
Glucose	40–70 mg/dL	0.0555	2.2–3.9 mmol/L
Protein	15–45 mg/dL	0.01	0.15–0.45 g/L
WBC	<10/mm^3		
Ceruloplasmin	18–45 mg/dL	10	180–450 mg/L
		0.063	1.1–2.8 μmol/L
Chloride	97–110 mEq/L	1	97–110 mmol/L
Cholesterol			
Desirable	<200 mg/dL	0.0259	<5.18 mmol/L
Borderline high	200–239 mg/dL	0.0259	5.18–6.19 mmol/L
High	≥240 mg/dL	0.0259	≥6.2 mmol/L
β-Human chorionic gonadotropin (β-hCG)	<5 milliunits/mL	1	<5 units/L
Clozapine	Minimum trough 300–350 ng/mL or mcg/L	3.06	918–1,071 nmol/L
CO$_2$ content	22–30 mEq/L	1	22–30 mmol/L
Complement component 3 (C3)	70–160 mg/dL	0.01	0.7–1.6 g/L
Complement component 4 (C4)	20–40 mg/dL	0.01	0.2–0.4 g/L
Copper	70–150 mcg/dL	0.157	11–24 μmol/L
Cortisol (fasting, morning)	5–25 mcg/dL	27.6	138–690 nmol/L
Cortisol (free, urinary)	10–100 mcg/day	2.76	28–276 nmol/day
Creatine kinase			
Male	30–200 IU/L	0.01667	0.50–3.33 μkat/L
Female	20–170 IU/L	0.01667	0.33–2.83 μkat/L
MB fraction	0–7 IU/L	0.01667	0.0–0.12 μkat/L
Creatinine clearance (CLcr) (urine)	85–135 mL/min/1.73 m^2	0.00963	0.82–1.3 mL/sec/m^2
Creatinine			
Male 4–20 years	0.2–1.0 mg/dL	88.4	18–88 μmol/L
Female 4–20 years	0.2–1.0 mg/dL	88.4	18–88 μmol/L
Male (adults)	0.7–1.3 mg/dL	88.4	62–115 μmol/L
Female (adults)	0.6–1.1 mg/dL	88.4	53–97 μmol/L

(continued)

Laboratory	Conventional Units	Conversion Factor	SI Units
Cyclosporine			
Renal transplant	100–300 ng/mL or mcg/L	0.832	83–250 nmol/L
Cardiac, liver, or pancreatic transplant	200–350 ng/mL or mcg/L	0.832	166–291 nmol/L
Cryptococcal antigen	Negative		
D-dimers	<250 ng/mL	1	<250 mcg/L
Desipramine	75–300 ng/mL or mcg/L	3.75	281–1125 mmol/L
Dexamethasone suppression test (DST) (overnight)	8:00 AM cortisol <5 mcg/dL	0.0276	<0.14 µmol/L
DHEAS			
Male	170–670 mcg/dL	0.0271	4.6–18.2 µmol/L
Female			
Premenopausal	50–540 mcg/dL	0.0271	1.4–14.7 µmol/L
Postmenopausal	30–260 mcg/dL	0.0271	0.8–7.1 µmol/L
Digoxin, therapeutic	0.5–1.0 ng/mL or mcg/L	1.28	0.6–1.3 nmol/L
Erythrocyte count (blood) See under red blood cell count			
Erythrocyte sedimentation rate (ESR)			
Westergren			
Male	0–20 mm/hr		
Female	0–30 mm/hr		
Wintrobe			
Male	0–9 mm/hr		
Female	0–15 mm/hr		
Erythropoietin	2–25 mIU/mL	1	2–25 IU/L
Estradiol			
Male	10–36 pg/mL	3.67	37–132 pmol/L
Female	34–170 pg/mL	3.67	125–624 pmol/L
Ethanol, legal intoxication	≥50–100 mg/dL	0.217	10.9–21.7 mmol/L
	≥0.05–0.1%	217	
Ethosuximide, therapeutic	40–100 mg/L or mcg/mL	7.08	283–708 µmol/L
Factor VIII or factor IX			
Severe hemophilia	<1 IU/dL	0.01	<0.01 units/mL
Moderate hemophilia	1–5 IU/dL	0.01	0.01–0.05 units/mL
Mild hemophilia	>5 IU/dL	0.01	>0.05 units/mL
Usual adult levels	60–140 IU/dL	0.01	0.60–1.40 units/mL
Ferritin			
Male	20–250 ng/mL	1	20–250 mcg/L
Female	10–150 ng/mL	1	10–150 mcg/L
Fibrin degradation products (FDP)	2–10 mg/L		
Fibrinogen	200–400 mg/dL	0.01	2.0–4.0 g/L
Folate (plasma)	3.1–12.4 ng/mL	2.266	7.0–28.1 nmol/L
Folic acid (RBC)	125–600 ng/mL	2.266	283–1360 nmol/L
Follicle-stimulating hormone (FSH)			
Male	1–7 mIU/mL	1	1–7 IU/L
Female			
Follicular phase	1–9 mIU/mL	1	1–9 IU/L
Midcycle	6–26 mIU/mL	1	6–26 IU/L
Luteal phase	1–9 mIU/mL	1	1–9 IU/L
Postmenopausal	30–118 mIU/mL	1	30–118 IU/L
Free thyroxine index (FT_4I)	6.5–12.5		
Gamma glutamyl transferase (GGT)	0–30 IU/L	0.01667	0–0.5 µkat/L
Gastrin (fasting)	0–130 pg/mL	1	0–130 ng/L
Gentamicin, therapeutic	4–10 mg/L peak	2.09	8.4–21.0 µmol/L peak
	≤2 mg/L trough		≤4.2 µmol/L trough
Globulin	2.3–3.5 g/dL	10	23–35 g/L
Glucose (fasting, plasma)	65–109 mg/dL	0.0555	3.6–6.0 mmol/L
Glucose, 2-hr postprandial blood (PPBG)	<140 mg/dL	0.0555	<7.8 mmol/L
Granulocyte count	$1.8–6.6 \times 10^3/\mu L$	10^6	$1.8–6.6 \times 10^9/L$
Growth hormone (fasting)			
Male	<5 ng/mL	1	<5 mcg/L
Female	<10 ng/mL	1	<10 mcg/L
Haptoglobin	60–270 mg/dL	0.01	0.6–2.7 g/L
HBeAg	Negative		
HBsAg	Negative		
HBV DNA	Negative		
Hematocrit			
Male	40.7–50.3%	0.01	0.407–0.503
Female	36.1–44.3%	0.01	0.361–0.443

(continued)

Laboratory	Conventional Units	Conversion Factor	SI Units
Hemoglobin (blood)			
Male	13.8–17.2 g/dL	10	138–172 g/L
		Alternative SI: 0.62	8.56–10.67 mmol/L
Female	12.1–15.1 g/dL	10	121–151 g/L
		Alternative SI: 0.62	7.5–9.36 mmol/L
Hemoglobin A$_{1c}$	4.0–6.0%	0.01	0.04–0.06
Heparin			
Via protamine titration method	0.2–0.4 mcg/mL		
Via anti–factor Xa assay	0.3–0.7 mcg/mL		
High-density lipoprotein (HDL) cholesterol	>35 mg/dL	0.0259	>0.91 mmol/L
Homocysteine	3.3–10.4 μmol/L		
Ibuprofen			
Therapeutic	10–50 mcg/mL	4.85	49–243 μmol/L
Toxic	100–700 mcg/mL or greater	4.85	485–3395 μmol/L or greater
Imipramine, therapeutic	100–300 ng/mL or mcg/L	3.57	357–1071 nmol/L
Immunoglobulin A (IgA)	85–385 mg/dL	0.01	0.85–3.85 g/L
Immunoglobulin G (IgG)	565–1765 mg/dL	0.01	5.65–17.65 g/L
Immunoglobulin M (IgM)	53–375 mg/dL	0.01	0.53–3.75 g/L
Insulin (fasting)	2–20 microunits/mL or milliunits/L	7.175	14.35–143.5 pmol/L
International normalized ratio (INR), therapeutic	2.0–3.0 (2.5–3.5 for some indications)		
Iron			
Male	45–160 mcg/dL	0.179	8.1–31.3 μmol/L
Female	30–160 mcg/dL	0.179	5.4–31.3 μmol/L
Iron-binding capacity (total)	220–420 mcg/dL	0.179	39.4–75.2 μmol/L
Iron saturation	15–50%	0.01	0.15–0.50
Lactate (plasma)	0.7–2.1 mEq/L	1	0.7–2.1 mmol/L
	6.3–18.9 mg/dL	0.111	
Lactate dehydrogenase	100–250 IU/L	0.01667	1.67–4.17 μkat/L
Lead	<25 mcg/dL	0.0483	<1.21 μmol/L
Leukocyte count	3.8–9.8 × 10³/μL	10⁶	3.8–9.8 μ10⁹/L
Lidocaine, therapeutic	1.5–6.0 mcg/mL or mg/L	4.27	6.4–25.6 μmol/L
Lipase	<100 IU/L	0.01667	1.7 μkat/L
Lithium, therapeutic	0.5–1.25 mEq/L	1	0.5–1.25 mmol/L
Low-density lipoprotein (LDL) cholesterol			
Desirable	<130 mg/dL	0.0259	<3.36 mmol/L
Borderline high risk	130–159 mg/dL	0.0259	3.36–4.11 mmol/L
High risk	≥160 mg/dL	0.0259	≥4.13 mmol/L
Luteinizing hormone (LH)			
Male	1–8 milliunits/mL	1	1–8 units/L
Female			
Follicular phase	1–12 milliunits/mL	1	1–12 units/L
Midcycle	16–104 milliunits/mL	1	16–104 units/L
Luteal phase	1–12 milliunits/mL	1	1–12 units/L
Postmenopausal	16–66 milliunits/mL	1	16–66 units/L
Lymphocyte count	1.2–3.3 × 10³/μL	10⁶	1.2–3.3 × 10⁹/L
Magnesium	1.3–2.2 mEq/L	0.5	0.65–1.10 mmol/L
	1.58–2.68 mg/dL	0.411	0.65–1.10 mmol/L
Mean corpuscular volume	80.0–97.6 μm³	1	80.0–97.6 fL
Mononuclear cell count	0.2–0.7 × 10³/μL	10⁶	0.2–0.7 × 10⁹/L
Nortriptyline, therapeutic	50–150 ng/mL or mcg/L	3.8	190–570 nmol/L
NT-ProBNP (see Pro-BNP)			
Osmolality (serum)	275–300 mOsm/kg	1	275–300 mmol/kg
Osmolality (urine)	250–900 mOsm/kg	1	250–900 mmol/kg
Parathyroid hormone (PTH), intact	10–60 pg/mL or ng/L	0.107	1.1–6.4 pmol/L
Parathyroid hormone (PTH), N-terminal	8–24 pg/mL or ng/L		
Parathyroid hormone (PTH), C-terminal	50–330 pg/mL or ng/L		
Phenobarbital, therapeutic	15–40 mcg/mL or mg/L	4.31	65–172 μmol/L
Phenytoin, therapeutic	10–20 mcg/mL or mg/L	3.96	40–79 μmol/L
Phosphate	2.5–4.5 mg/dL	0.323	0.81–1.45 mmol/L
Platelet count	140–440 × 10³/μL	10⁶	140–440 × 10⁹/L
Potassium (plasma)	3.3–4.9 mEq/L	1	3.3–4.9 μmol/L
Prealbumin (adult)	19.5–35.8 mg/dL	10	195–358 mg/L
Primidone, therapeutic	5–12 mcg/mL or mg/L	4.58	23–55 μmol/L
ProBNP	<125 pg/mL or ng/L	0.118	<14.75 pmol/L
Procainamide, therapeutic	4–10 mcg/mL or mg/L	4.23	17–42 μmol/L

(continued)

Laboratory	Conventional Units	Conversion Factor	SI Units
Progesterone			
Male	13–97 ng/dL	0.0318	0.4–3.1 nmol/L
Female			
Follicular phase	15–70 ng/dL		0.5–2.2 nmol/L
Luteal phase	200–2500 ng/dL		6.4–79.5 nmol/L
Prolactin	<20 ng/mL	1	<20 mcg/L
Prostate-specific antigen (PSA)	<4 ng/mL	1	<4 mcg/L
Protein, total	6.0–8.0 g/dL	10	60–80 g/L
Prothrombin time (PT)	10–12 sec		
Quinidine, therapeutic	2–5 mcg/mL or mg/L	3.08	6.2–15.4 µmol/L
Radioactive iodine uptake (RAIU)	<6% in 2 hr		
Red blood cell (RBC) count (blood)			
Male	$4–6.2 \times 10^6/\mu L$	10^6	$4–6.2 \times 10^{12}/L$
Female	$4–6.2 \times 10^6/\mu L$	10^6	$4–6.2 \times 10^{12}/L$
Pregnant			
Trimester 1	$4–5 \times 10^6/\mu L$	10^6	$4–5 \times 10^{12}/L$
Trimester 2	$3.2–4.5 \times 10^6/\mu L$	10^6	$3.2–4.5 \times 10^{12}/L$
Trimester 3	$3.0–4.9 \times 10^6/\mu L$	10^6	$3.0–4.9 \times 10^{12}/L$
Postpartum	$3.2–5 \times 10^6/\mu L$	10^6	$3.2–5.0 \times 10^6/L$
Red blood cell distribution width (RDW)	11.5–14.5%	0.01	0.115–0.145
Reticulocyte count			
Male	0.5–1.5% of total RBC count	0.01	0.005–0.015
Female	0.5–2.5% of total RBC count	0.01	0.005–0.025
Retinol-binding protein (RBP)	2.7–7.6 mg/dL	10	27–76 mg/L
Rheumatoid factor (RF) titer	Negative		
Salicylate, therapeutic	150–300 mcg/mL or mg/L	0.00724	1.09–2.17 mmol/L
	15–30 mg/dL	0.0724	
Sodium	135–145 mEq/L	1	135–145 mmol/L
Tacrolimus			
Renal transplant	6–12 ng/mL or mcg/L		
Liver transplant	4–10 ng/mL or mcg/L		
Pancreatic transplant	10–18 ng/mL or mcg/L		
Bone marrow transplant	10–20 ng/mL or mcg/L		
Testosterone (total)			
Men	300–950 ng/dL	0.0347	10.4–33.0 nmol/L
Women	20–80 ng/dL		0.7–2.8 nmol/L
Testosterone (free)			
Men	9–30 ng/dL	0.0347	0.31–1.04 nmol/L
Women	0.3–1.9 ng/dL		0.01–0.07 nmol/L
Theophylline			
Therapeutic	5–15 mcg/mL or mg/L	5.55	28–83 µmol/L
Toxic	20 or greater mcg/mL or mg/L	5.55	111 or greater µmol/L
Thrombin time	20–24 sec		
Thyroglobulin	<42 ng/mL	1	<42 mcg/L
Thyroglobulin antibodies	Negative		
Thyroxine-binding globulin (TBG)	1.2–2.5 mg/dL	10	12–25 mcg/L
Thyroid-stimulating hormone (TSH)	0.35–6.20 microunits/mL	1	0.35–6.20 milliunits/L
TSH receptor antibodies (TSH Rab)	0–1 unit/mL		
Thyroxine (T_4)			
Total	4.5–12.0 mcg/dL	12.87	58–155 nmol/L
Free	0.7–1.9 ng/dL	12.87	9.0–24.5 pmol/L
Thyroxine index, free (FT_4I)	6.5–12.5		
TIBC, see Iron-binding capacity (total)			
Tobramycin, therapeutic	4–10 mcg/mL or mg/L peak	2.14	8.6–21.4 µmol/L
	≤2 mcg/mL mg/L trough	2.14	≤4.28 µmol/L
Transferrin	200–430 mg/dL	0.01	2.0–4.3 g/L
Transferrin saturation	30–50%	0.01	0.30–0.50
Triglycerides (fasting)	<160 mg/dL	0.0113	<1.8 mmol/L
Triiodothyronine (T_3)	45–132 ng/dL	0.0154	0.91–2.70 nmol/L
Triiodothyronine (T_3) resin uptake	25–35%		
Troponin I	<0.6 ng/mL	1	<0.6 g/L
Uric acid	3–8 mg/dL	59.48	179–476 µmol/L
Urinalysis (urine)			
pH	4.8–8.0		
Specific gravity	1.005–1.030		
Protein	Negative		
Glucose	Negative		
Ketones	Negative		

(continued)

Laboratory	Conventional Units	Conversion Factor	SI Units
RBC	1–2 per low-power field		
WBC	3–4 per low-power field		
Valproic acid, therapeutic	50–100 mcg/mL or mg/L	6.93	346–693 µmol/L
Vancomycin, therapeutic trough for CNS infections	20–40 mcg/mL or mg/L peak	0.690	14–28 µmol/L peak
	5–20 mcg/mL or mg/L trough	0.690	3–14 µmol/L trough
	15–20 mcg/mL or mg/L trough	0.690	10–14 µmol/L trough
Vitamin A (retinol)	30–95 mcg/dL	0.0349	1.05–3.32 µmol/L
Vitamin B_{12}	180–1000 pg/mL	0.738	133–738 pmol/L
Vitamin D_3, 1,25-dihydroxy	20–76 pg/m	2.4	48–182 pmol/L
Vitamin D_3, 25-hydroxy	10–50 ng/mL	2.496	25–125 nmol/L
Vitamin E (alpha tocopherol)	0.5–2.0 mg/dL	23.22	12–46 µmol/L
WBC count	$4\text{–}10 \times 10^3/\mu L$ or $4\text{–}10 \times 10^3/mm^3$	10^6	$4\text{–}10 \times 10^9/L$
WBC differential (peripheral blood)			
Polymorphonuclear neutrophils (PMNs)	50–65%		
Bands	0–5%		
Eosinophils	0–3%		
Basophils	1–3%		
Lymphocytes	25–35%		
Monocytes	2–6%		
WBC differential (bone marrow)			
Polymorphonuclear neutrophils (PMNs)	3–11%		
Bands	9–15%		
Metamyelocytes	9–25%		
Myelocytes	8–16%		
Promyelocytes	1–8%		
Myeloblasts	0–5%		
Eosinophils	1–5%		
Basophils	0–1%		
Lymphocytes	11–23%		
Monocytes	0–1%		
Zinc	60–150 mcg/dL	0.153	9.2–23.0 µmol/L

This table was reproduced with permission from Chisholm-Burns MA, Wells BG, Schwinghammer TL, et al, eds. Pharmacotherapy Principles and Practice. New York, NY: McGraw-Hill; 2008.

Note: Many of the medical abbreviations contained in Part I of this appendix are used in the Casebook. A more extensive list of abbreviations is available on the Internet at *www.medilexicon.com* and other sites.

6MWD	Six-minute walk distance
A&O	Alert and oriented
A&P	Auscultation and percussion; anterior and posterior; assessment and plan
A&W	Alive and well
A_{1c}	Hemoglobin A_{1c}
aa	Of each (*ana*)
AA	Aplastic anemia; Alcoholics Anonymous
AAA	Abdominal aortic aneurysm
AAL	Anterior axillary line
AAO	Awake, alert, and oriented
AAP	American Academy of Pediatrics
ABC	Absolute band count; absolute basophil count; aspiration, biopsy, and cytology; artificial β-cells
Abd	Abdomen
ABG	Arterial blood gases
ABI	Ankle brachial index
ABP	Arterial blood pressure
ABPA	Allergic bronchopulmonary aspergillosis
ABW	Actual body weight
ABx	Antibiotics
AC	Before meals (*ante cibos*)
ACC	American College of Cardiology
ACE	Angiotensin-converting enzyme
ACEI	Angiotensin-converting enzyme inhibitor
ACG	American College of Gastroenterology
ACL	Anterior cruciate ligament
ACLS	Advanced cardiac life support
ACR	Albumin:creatinine ratio; American College of Rheumatology
ACS	Acute coronary syndrome
ACT	Activated clotting time
ACTH	Adrenocorticotropic hormone
AD	Alzheimer disease, right ear (*auris dextra*)
ADA	American Diabetes Association; adenosine deaminase
ADE	Adverse drug effect (or event)
ADH	Antidiuretic hormone
ADHD	Attention-deficit hyperactivity disorder
ADL	Activities of daily living
ADR	Adverse drug reaction
AED	Antiepileptic drug(s)
AERD	Aspirin-exacerbated respiratory disease
AF	Atrial fibrillation
AFB	Acid-fast bacillus; aortofemoral bypass; aspirated foreign body
Afeb	Afebrile
AFP	α-Fetoprotein
A/G	Albumin–globulin ratio
AGA	American Gastroenterological Association
AGE	Acute viral gastroenteritis
AHA	American Heart Association
AI	Aortic insufficiency
AIDS	Acquired immunodeficiency syndrome
AKA	Above-knee amputation; alcoholic ketoacidosis; all known allergies; also known as
AKI	Acute kidney injury
ALD	Alcoholic liver disease

ALFT	Abnormal liver function test
ALK	Anaplastic lymphoma kinase
ALL	Acute lymphocytic leukemia; acute lymphoblastic leukemia
ALP	Alkaline phosphatase
ALS	Amyotrophic lateral sclerosis
ALT	Alanine aminotransferase
AMA	Against medical advice; American Medical Association; antimitochondrial antibody
AMI	Acute myocardial infarction
AML	Acute myelogenous leukemia
Amp	Ampule
AMPA	α-amino-3-hydroxy-5-methyl-4-isoxazolepropionic acid
ANA	Antinuclear antibody
ANC	Absolute neutrophil count
ANLL	Acute nonlymphocytic leukemia
Anti-CCP	Anticyclic citrullinated peptide
AODM	Adult-onset diabetes mellitus
A&O × 3	Awake and oriented to person, place, and time
A&O × 4	Awake and oriented to person, place, time, and situation
AOM	Acute otitis media
AP	Anteroposterior
APACHE	Acute Physiology and Chronic Health Evaluation
APAP	Acetaminophen (*N*-acetyl-*p*-aminophenol)
aPTT	Activated partial thromboplastin time
ARB	Angiotensin receptor blocker
ARC	AIDS-related complex
ARDS	Adult respiratory distress syndrome
ARF	Acute renal failure; acute respiratory failure; acute rheumatic fever
ARNI, ARNi	Angiotensin receptor-neprilysin inhibitor
AROM	Active range of motion
AS	Left ear (*auris sinistra*)
ASA	Aspirin (acetylsalicylic acid)
ASCVD	Atherosclerotic cardiovascular disease
ASD	Atrial septal defect
ASH	Asymmetric septal hypertrophy
ASHD	Arteriosclerotic heart disease
AST	Aspartate aminotransferase
ASUC	Acute severe ulcerative colitis
ATG	Antithymocyte globulin
ATN	Acute tubular necrosis
AU	Each ear (*auris uterque*)
AUD	Alcohol use disorder
AV	Arteriovenous; atrioventricular
AVM	Arteriovenous malformation
AVR	Aortic valve replacement
AWMI	Anterior wall myocardial infarction
BAC	Blood alcohol concentration
BAL	Bronchioalveolar lavage
BBB	Bundle branch block; blood–brain barrier
BC	Blood culture
BCACP	Board Certified Ambulatory Care Pharmacist
BCG	Bacillus Calmette Guerin
BCL	B-cell lymphoma
BCNP	Board Certified Nuclear Pharmacist
BCNSP	Board Certified Nutrition Support Pharmacist
BCNU	Carmustine

BCOP	Board Certified Oncology Pharmacist		CHC	Combined hormonal contraceptives
BCP	Birth control pill		CHD	Coronary heart disease
BCPP	Board Certified Psychiatric Pharmacist		CHF	Congestive heart failure
BCPS	Board Certified Pharmacotherapy Specialist		CHO	Carbohydrate
BCR-ABL	Breakpoint cluster region-Abelson		CHOP	Cyclophosphamide, hydroxydaunorubicin (doxorubicin),
BCRP	Breast cancer resistance protein			Oncovin (vincristine), prednisone
BE	Barium enema		CI	Cardiac index
BID	Twice daily (*bis in die*)		CIS	Clinically isolated syndrome
BiPAP	Bilevel positive airway pressure		CIVI	Continuous intravenous infusion
BIS	Bispectral index		CK	Creatine kinase
BKA	Below-knee amputation		CKD	Chronic kidney disease
BM	Bone marrow; bowel movement		CKD-EPI	Chronic Kidney Disease—Epidemiology Collaboration
BMC	Bone marrow cells		CKD-MBD	Chronic kidney disease—mineral and bone disorder
BMD	Bone mineral density		CLcr	Creatinine clearance
BMR	Basal metabolic rate		CLL	Chronic lymphocytic leukemia
BMT	Bone marrow transplantation		CM	Costal margin
BNP	Brain natriuretic peptide		CMG	Cystometrogram
BOO	Bladder outlet obstruction		CML	Chronic myelogenous leukemia
BP	Blood pressure		CMRO$_2$	Cerebral metabolic rate of oxygen
BPD	Bronchopulmonary dysplasia		CMV	Cytomegalovirus
BPH	Benign prostatic hyperplasia		CN	Cranial nerve
bpm	Beats per minute		CNCP	Chronic non-cancer pain
BPRS	Brief Psychiatric Rating Scale		CNS	Central nervous system
BPS	Behavior-based pain scale		c/o	Complains of
BR	Bedrest		CO	Cardiac output; carbon monoxide
BRBPR	Bright red blood per rectum		COC	Combined oral contraceptive
BRM	Biological response modifier		COLD	Chronic obstructive lung disease
BRP	Bathroom privileges		COMT	Catechol-*O*-methyl transferase
BS	Bowel sounds; breath sounds; blood sugar		COPD	Chronic obstructive pulmonary disease
BSA	Body surface area		CP	Chest pain; cerebral palsy
BSO	Bilateral salpingo-oophorectomy		CPA	Costophrenic angle
BTFS	Breast tumor frozen section		CPAP	Continuous positive airway pressure
BUN	Blood urea nitrogen		CPK	Creatine phosphokinase
BV	Bacterial vaginosis		CPOT	Critical-Care Pain Observation Tool
Bx	Biopsy		CPP	Cerebral perfusion pressure
C&S	Culture and sensitivity		CPR	Cardiopulmonary resuscitation
CA	Cancer; calcium		CR	Complete remission; controlled release
CABG	Coronary artery bypass graft		CRF	Chronic renal failure; corticotropin-releasing factor
CAD	Coronary artery disease		CRH	Corticotropin-releasing hormone
CAH	Chronic active hepatitis		CRI	Chronic renal insufficiency; catheter-related infection
CAM	Complementary and alternative medicine		CRNA	Certified Registered Nurse Anesthetist
CAM-ICU	Confusion Assessment Method for the ICU		CRNP	Certified Registered Nurse Practitioner
CAP	Community-acquired pneumonia		CRP	C-reactive protein
CAPD	Continuous ambulatory peritoneal dialysis		CRPS	Complex regional pain syndrome
CAT	COPD Assessment Test		CRTT	Certified Respiratory Therapy Technician
CBC	Complete blood count		CS	Central Supply
CBD	Common bile duct		CSA	Cyclosporine
CBF	Cerebral blood flow		CSC	Corrected serum calcium
CBG	Capillary blood gas; corticosteroid binding globulin		CSF	Cerebrospinal fluid; colony-stimulating factor
CBT	Cognitive-behavioral therapy		CSW	Cerebral salt wasting
CC	Chief complaint		CT	Computed tomography; chest tube
CCA	Calcium channel antagonist		CTA	Clear to auscultation
CCB	Calcium channel blocker		CTB	Cease to breathe
CCE	Clubbing, cyanosis, edema		cTnI	Cardiac troponin I
CCK	Cholecystokinin		CTZ	Chemoreceptor trigger zone
CCMS	Clean catch midstream		CV	Cardiovascular
CCNU	Lomustine		CVA	Cerebrovascular accident; costovertebral angle
CCPD	Continuous cycling peritoneal dialysis		CVAT	Costovertebral angle tenderness
CCT	Central corneal thickness		CVC	Central venous catheter
CCU	Coronary care unit		CVP	Central venous pressure
CD	Crohn disease		CVVH-DF	Continuous venovenous hemodiafiltration
CDAD	*Clostridium difficile*–associated diarrhea (see CDI below)		Cx	Culture; cervix
CDC	Centers for Disease Control and Prevention		CXR	Chest X-ray
CDI	*Clostridioides* (formerly *Clostridium*) *difficile* infection; the preferred term instead of CDAD		CYP	Cytochrome P-450 enzymes
			D&C	Dilatation and curettage
CEA	Carcinoembryonic antigen		d4T	Stavudine
CF	Cystic fibrosis		D$_5$NS	5% Dextrose in normal saline
CFS	Chronic fatigue syndrome		D$_5$W5	% Dextrose in water
CFTR	Cystic fibrosis transmembrane conductance regulator		DAA	Direct acting antivirals
CFU	Colony-forming unit		DAPT	Dual antiplatelet therapy
CGM	Continuous glucose monitoring		DAS	Disease activity score
CHB	Chronic hepatitis B		DBP	Diastolic blood pressure

D/C	Discontinue; discharge
DCC	Direct current cardioversion
ddC	Zalcitabine
ddI	Didanosine
DES	Diethylstilbestrol
DEXA	Dual-energy X-ray absorptiometry
DI	Diabetes insipidus
DIC	Disseminated intravascular coagulation
Diff	Differential
DIOS	Distal intestinal obstruction syndrome
DIP	Distal interphalangeal
DIS	Dissemination in space
DIT	Dissemination in time
DJD	Degenerative joint disease
DKA	Diabetic ketoacidosis
dL	Deciliter
DM	Diabetes mellitus
DMARD	Disease-modifying antirheumatic drug
DMT	Disease-modifying therapy
DNA	Deoxyribonucleic acid
DNR	Do not resuscitate
DO	Doctor of Osteopathy
DOA	Dead on arrival; date of admission; duration of action
DOAC	Direct oral anticoagulant (see also NOAC)
DOB	Date of birth
DOE	Dyspnea on exertion
DOT	Directly observed therapy
DP	Dorsalis pedis
DPGN	Diffuse proliferative glomerulonephritis
DPI	Dry powder inhaler
DRE	Digital rectal examination
DRG	Diagnosis-related group
DRSP	Daily record of severity of problem
DS	Double strength
DSM	Diagnostic and Statistical Manual of Mental Disorders
DSMES	Diabetes self-management education and support
DSHEA	Dietary Supplement Health and Education Act (1994)
DST	Dexamethasone suppression test
DTIC	Dacarbazine
DTP	Diphtheria-tetanus-pertussis
DTR	Deep tendon reflex
DVT	Deep vein thrombosis
Dx	Diagnosis
DXA	Dual-energy X-ray absorptiometry (see also DEXA)
eAG	Estimated average glucose
EBL	Endoscopic band ligation
EBV	Epstein-Barr virus
EC	Enteric-coated, emergency contraception, emergency contraceptive
ECF	Extended care facility
ECG	Electrocardiogram
ECMO	Extracorporeal membrane oxygenator
ECOG	Eastern Cooperative Oncology Group
ECT	Electroconvulsive therapy
ED	Emergency department
EEG	Electroencephalogram
EENT	Eyes, ears, nose, throat
EF	Ejection fraction
EGD	Esophagogastroduodenoscopy
EGFR	Epidermal growth factor receptor
EIA	Enzyme immunoassay
EMG	Electromyogram
EML4-ALK	Echinoderm microtubule–associated protein-like 4–anaplastic lymphoma kinase
EMS	Emergency medical services
EMT	Emergency medical technician
Endo	Endotracheal; endoscopy
EOMI	Extraocular movements (or muscles) intact
EPO	Erythropoietin
EPS	Extrapyramidal symptoms
EPT	Early pregnancy test; expedited partner therapy
ER	Estrogen receptor; emergency room; extended release

ERCP	Endoscopic retrograde cholangiopancreatography
ERT	Estrogen replacement therapy
ESA	Erythropoiesis-stimulating agent
ESKD	End-stage kidney disease
ESLD	End-stage liver disease
ESR	Erythrocyte sedimentation rate
ESRD	End-stage renal disease
ESWL	Extracorporeal shockwave lithotripsy
ET	Endotracheal
ETOH	Ethanol
EVL	Endoscopic variceal ligation
FB	Finger-breadth; foreign body
FBDSI	Functional Bowel Disorder Severity Index
FBS	Fasting blood sugar
FDA	Food and Drug Administration
FDC	Fixed dose combinations
FDP	Fibrin degradation products
FEF	Forced expiratory flow (rate)
FEM-POP	Femoral-popliteal
FEN	Fluids, electrolytes, and nutrition
FE_{NA}	Fractional excretion of sodium
FEV_1	Forced expiratory volume in 1 second
FFP	Fresh frozen plasma
FH	Family history
FiO_2	Fraction of inspired oxygen
FISH	Fluorescence in situ hybridization
fL	Femtoliter
FLS	Fracture Liaison Service
FM	Face mask
FNA	Fine-needle aspiration
FOBT	Fecal occult blood test
FOC	Fronto-occipital circumference
FODMAPs	Fermentable oligo-, di- and monosaccharides and polyols
FOI	Flight of ideas
FPG	Fasting plasma glucose
FPIA	Fluorescence polarization immunoassay
FRAX	Fracture Risk Assessment Tool
FSH	Follicle-stimulating hormone
FTA	Fluorescent treponemal antibody
f/u	Follow-up
FUDR	Floxuridine
FUO	Fever of unknown origin
Fx	Fracture
G6PD	Glucose-6-phosphate dehydrogenase
GABA	γ-aminobutyric acid
GABHS	Group A β-hemolytic streptococcus
GAD	Generalized anxiety disorder
GB	Gallbladder
GBS	Group B *Streptococcus*; Guillain–Barré syndrome
GC	Gonococcus
G-CSF	Granulocyte colony–stimulating factor
GDH	Glutamate dehydrogenase
GDM	Gestational diabetes mellitus
GDMT	Guideline-directed medical therapy
GE	Gastroesophageal; gastroenterology
GERD	Gastroesophageal reflux disease
GFR	Glomerular filtration rate
GGT	γ-Glutamyl transferase
GGTP	γ-Glutamyl transpeptidase
GI	Gastrointestinal
GLP	Glucagon-like peptide
GM-CSF	Granulocyte-macrophage colony-stimulating factor
GN	Glomerulonephritis; graduate nurse
GnRH	Gonadotropin-releasing hormone
gr	Grain
GT	Gastrostomy tube
gtt	Drops (*guttae*)
GTT	Glucose tolerance test
GU	Gastric ulcer, genitourinary
GVHD	Graft-versus-host disease
GVL	Graft-versus-leukemia
Gyn	Gynecology

H&H	Hemoglobin and hematocrit
H&P	History and physical examination
HA or H/A	Headache
HAART	Highly active antiretroviral therapy
HAM-D	Hamilton Rating Scale for Depression
HAP	Hospital-acquired pneumonia
HAV	Hepatitis A virus
Hb, Hgb	Hemoglobin
HbA$_{1C}$	Hemoglobin A$_{1C}$
HBeAg	Hepatitis B early antigen
HBIG	Hepatitis B immune globulin
HBP	High blood pressure
HbsAg	Hepatitis B surface antigen
HBV	Hepatitis B virus
HC	Hydrocortisone; home care
HCAP	Healthcare-associated pneumonia (see new term: hospital-acquired pneumonia [HAP])
HCC	Hepatocellular carcinoma
HCG	Human chorionic gonadotropin
HCM	Hypercalcemia of malignancy
HCO$_3$	Bicarbonate
Hct	Hematocrit
HCTZ	Hydrochlorothiazide
HAV	Hepatitis A virus
HBV	Hepatitis B virus
HCV	Hepatitis C virus
Hcy	Homocysteine
HD	Hodgkin disease; hemodialysis
HDL	High-density lipoprotein
HE	Hepatic encephalopathy
HEC	High-emetic-risk chemotherapy
HEENT	Head, eyes, ears, nose, and throat
HeFH	Heterozygous familial hypercholesterolemia
HEMT	Highly effective modulator therapy
HEPA	High-efficiency particulate air
HF	Heart failure
HFA	Hydrofluoroalkane
H. flu	*Haemophilus influenza*
HF*p*EF	Heart failure with preserved ejection fraction
HF*r*EF	Heart failure with reduced ejection fraction
HFSA	Heart Failure Society of America
HGH	Human growth hormone
HH	Hiatal hernia
HHS	Hyperosmolar hyperglycemic state
Hib	*Haemophilus influenzae* type b
HIV	Human immunodeficiency virus
HJR	Hepatojugular reflux
HL	Hodgkin lymphoma
HLA	Human leukocyte antigen; human lymphocyte antigen
HMG-CoA	Hydroxy-methylglutaryl coenzyme A
H/O	History of
HOB	Head of bed
HPA	Hypothalamic–pituitary axis
HPF	High-power field
HPI	History of present illness
HPV	Human papilloma virus
HR	Heart rate
HRQOL	Health-related quality of life
HRT	Hormone replacement therapy (see new term: hormone therapy, HT)
HS	At bedtime (*hora somni*)
HSCT	Hematopoietic stem cell transplantation
HSM	Hepatosplenomegaly
HSV	Herpes simplex virus
HT	Hormone therapy
HTN	Hypertension
HVPG	Hepatic venous pressure gradient
Hx	History
I&D	Incision and drainage
I&O	Intake and output
IABP	Intra-arterial balloon pump
IADL	Instrumental activities of daily living

IBD	Inflammatory bowel disease
IBS	Irritable bowel syndrome
IBS-C	Irritable bowel syndrome with constipation
IBS-D	Irritable bowel syndrome with diarrhea
IBS-SSS	Irritable Bowel Syndrome Symptom Severity Score
IBW	Ideal body weight
ICD	Implantable cardioverter defibrillator, impulse control disorder
ICDSC	Intensive Care Delirium Screening Checklist
ICP	Intracranial pressure
ICS	Intercostal space
ICU	Intensive care unit
ID	Identification; infectious disease
IDDM	Insulin-dependent diabetes mellitus
IFN	Interferon
Ig	Immunoglobulin
IgA	Immunoglobulin A
IgD	Immunoglobulin D
IHC	Immunohistochemistry
IHD	Ischemic heart disease
IJ	Internal jugular
ILE	Intravenous lipid emulsion
IM	Intramuscular; infectious mononucleosis
IMV	Intermittent mandatory ventilation
INH	Isoniazid
INR	International normalized ratio
IOP	Intraocular pressure
IOR	Ideas of reference
IP	Intraperitoneal
IPG	Impedance plethysmography
IPI	International prognostic index
IPN	Interstitial pneumonia
IPPB	Intermittent positive pressure breathing
IPS	Idiopathic pneumonia syndrome
IPV	Inactivated polio vaccine
IRB	Institutional Review Board
ISA	Intrinsic sympathomimetic activity
ISDN	Isosorbide dinitrate
ISH	Isolated systolic hypertension
ISMN	Isosorbide mononitrate
IT	Intrathecal
ITP	Idiopathic thrombocytopenic purpura
IU	International unit
IUD	Intrauterine device
IV	Intravenous; Roman numeral IV; symbol for Class 4 controlled substances
IVC	Inferior vena cava; intravenous cholangiogram
IVDA	Intravenous drug abuse (*Note*: Usage inappropriate; see IVDU)
IVDU	Intravenous drug use®
IVF	Intravenous fluids
IVIG	Intravenous immunoglobulin
IVP	Intravenous pyelogram; intravenous push
IVPB	Intravenous piggyback
IVSS	Intravenous Soluset
IWMI	Inferior wall myocardial infarction
JODM	Juvenile-onset diabetes mellitus
JRA	Juvenile rheumatoid arthritis
JVD	Jugular venous distention
JVP	Jugular venous pressure
K	Potassium
kcal	Kilocalorie
KCL	Potassium chloride
KDIGO	Kidney Disease: Improving Global Outcomes
KOH	Potassium hydroxide
KRAS	Kirsten rat sarcoma viral oncogene homolog
KUB	Kidney, ureters, bladder
KVO	Keep vein open
L	Liter
LAD	Left anterior descending; left axis deviation
LADA	Latent autoimmune diabetes in adulthood
LAO	Left anterior oblique

LAP	Leukocyte alkaline phosphatase	MRI	Magnetic resonance imaging
LBBB	Left bundle branch block	MRSA	Methicillin-resistant *Staphylococcus aureus*
LBP	Low back pain	MRSE	Methicillin-resistant *Staphylococcus epidermidis*
LCM	Left costal margin	MS	Mental status; mitral stenosis; musculoskeletal; multiple sclerosis; morphine sulfate
LDH	Lactate dehydrogenase		
LDL	Low-density lipoprotein	MSE	Mental status exam
LE	Lower extremity	MSM	Men who have sex with men
LES	Lower esophageal sphincter	MSW	Master of social work
LFT	Liver function test	MTD	Maximum tolerated dose
LHRH	Luteinizing hormone-releasing hormone	MTP	Metatarsophalangeal
LIMA	Left internal mammary artery	MTX	Methotrexate
LLE	Left lower extremity	MUD	Matched unrelated donor
LLL	Left lower lobe	MUGA	Multiple gated acquisition
LLQ	Left lower quadrant (abdomen)	MVA	Motor vehicle accident
LLSB	Left lower sternal border	MVI	Multivitamin
LMD	Local medical doctor	MVR	Mitral valve replacement; mitral valve regurgitation
LMP	Last menstrual period	MVS	Mitral valve stenosis; motor, vascular, and sensory
LMWH	Low molecular weight heparin		
LOA	Looseness of association	NAAT	Nucleic acid amplification test
LOC	Loss of consciousness; laxative of choice	NAD	No acute (or apparent) distress
LOS	Length of stay	NAFLD	Nonalcoholic fatty liver disease
LP	Lumbar puncture	NASH	Nonalcoholic steatohepatitis
LPF	Low-power field	N/C	Noncontributory; nasal cannula
LPN	Licensed practical nurse	NC/AT	Normocephalic/atraumatic
LPO	Left posterior oblique	NDDI-E	Neurological Disorders Depression Inventory for Epilepsy
LPT	Licensed physical therapist		
LR	Lactated Ringer	NG	Nasogastric
LS	Lumbosacral	NGT	Nasogastric tube
LTCF	Long-term care facility	NGTD	No growth to date (on culture)
LUE	Left upper extremity	NHL	Non-Hodgkin lymphoma
LUL	Left upper lobe	NIDDM	Non–insulin-dependent diabetes mellitus
LUQ	Left upper quadrant	NIH	National Institutes of Health
LUTS	Lower urinary tract symptoms	NKA	No known allergies
LVEF	Left ventricular ejection fraction	NKDA	No known drug allergies
LVH	Left ventricular hypertrophy	NL	Normal
MAOI	Monoamine oxidase inhibitor	NMDA	*N*-methyl-D-aspartate
MAP	Mean arterial pressure	NMOSD	Neuromyelitis optica spectrum disorder
MAR	Medication administration record	NNRTI	Nonnucleoside reverse transcriptase inhibitor
MART	Maintenance and reliever therapy	NOAC	Nonwarfarin (also new, novel, or non–vitamin K) oral anticoagulant
mcg	Microgram		
MCH	Mean corpuscular hemoglobin	NOS	Not otherwise specified
MCHC	Mean corpuscular hemoglobin concentration	NP	Nurse practitioner
MCL	Midclavicular line	NPH	Neutral protamine Hagedorn; normal pressure hydrocephalus
MCP	Metacarpophalangeal		
MCV	Mean corpuscular volume	NPI	Neuropsychiatric Inventory
MD	Medical doctor	NPN	Nonprotein nitrogen
MDD	Major depressive disorder	NPO	Nothing by mouth (*nil per os*)
MDI	Metered-dose inhaler	NRAS	Neuroblastoma RAS viral (v-ras) oncogene homolog
MDRD	Modified Diet in Renal Disease	NRS	Numeric rating scale
MED	Morphine-equivalent dose	NRTI	Nucleoside reverse transcriptase inhibitor
MEFR	Maximum expiratory flow rate	NS	Neurosurgery; normal saline
mEq	Milliequivalent	NSAID	Nonsteroidal anti-inflammatory drug
mg	Milligram	NSCLC	Nonsmall cell lung cancer
MHC	Major histocompatibility complex	NSR	Normal sinus rhythm
MI	Myocardial infarction; mitral insufficiency	NSS	Normal saline solution
MIC	Minimum inhibitory concentration	NSTEMI	Non-ST-elevation myocardial infarction
MICU	Medical intensive care unit	NSVD	Normal spontaneous vaginal delivery
MIDAS	Migraine Disability Assessment	NTG	Nitroglycerin
mL	Milliliter	NT/ND	Nontender/nondistended
MM	Multiple myeloma	N/V	Nausea and vomiting
MMA	Methylmalonic acid	NVD	Nausea/vomiting/diarrhea; neck vein distention; nonvalvular disease; neovascularization of the disk
MMEFR	Maximal midexpiratory flow rate		
MMR	Measles-mumps-rubella	NYHA	New York Heart Association
MMSE	Mini mental state examination	O&P	Ova and parasites
MOG	Myelin oligodendrocyte glycoprotein	OA	Osteoarthritis
MOM	Milk of magnesia	OB	Obstetrics
MoCA	Montreal Cognitive Assessment	OBS	Organic brain syndrome
MOUD	Medication for Opioid Use Disorder	OCB	Oligoclonal band
MPV	Mean platelet volume	OCD	Obsessive–compulsive disorder
MRD	Minimal residual disease	OCG	Oral cholecystogram
MRAB	Medication-related aberrant behavior	OCT	Optical coherence tomography
MRG	Murmur/rub/gallop	OD	Right eye (*oculus dexter*); overdose; Doctor of Optometry
		ODT	Orally disintegrating tablet
		OFC	Occipitofrontal circumference

OGT	Oral glucose tolerance test	PNH	Paroxysmal nocturnal hemoglobinuria
OHTx	Orthotopic heart transplantation	PO	By mouth (*per os*)
OIH	Opioid-induced hyperalgesia	POAG	Primary open-angle glaucoma
OLTx	Orthotopic liver transplantation	POD	Postoperative day
OME	Otitis media with effusion	POS	Polycystic ovarian syndrome
ONJ	Osteonecrosis of the jaw	PP	Patient profile
OOB	Out of bed	PPBG	Postprandial blood glucose
OPD	Outpatient department	ppd	Packs per day
OPG	Ocular plethysmography	PPD	Purified protein derivative
OPV	Oral poliovirus vaccine	PPE	Personal protective equipment
OR	Operating room	PPH	Past psychiatric history
ORS	Oral rehydration solution	PPI	Proton pump inhibitor
ORT	Oral rehydration therapy	PPMS	Primary progressive multiple sclerosis
OS	Left eye (*oculus sinister*)	PPN	Peripheral parenteral nutrition
OSA	Obstructive sleep apnea	pr	Per rectum
OT	Occupational therapy	PR	Progesterone receptor; partial remission
OTC	Over-the-counter	PRA	Panel-reactive antibody; plasma renin activity
OU	Each eye (*oculus uterque*)	PRBC	Packed red blood cells
OUD	Opioid use disorder	PRN	When necessary; as needed (*pro re nata*)
P	Pulse, plan, percussion, pressure	PSA	Prostate-specific antigen
P&A	Percussion and auscultation	PSCT	Peripheral stem cell transplant
P&T	Peak and trough	PSE	Portal systemic encephalopathy
PA	Physician assistant; posterior–anterior; pulmonary artery	PSH	Past surgical history
PAC	Premature atrial contraction	PSVT	Paroxysmal supraventricular tachycardia
$PaCO_2$	Arterial carbon dioxide tension	PT	Prothrombin time; physical therapy; patient; posterior tibial
PAH	Pulmonary arterial hypertension	PTA	Prior to admission
PaO_2	Arterial oxygen tension	PTCA	Percutaneous transluminal coronary angioplasty
PAOP	Pulmonary artery occlusion pressure	PTE	Pulmonary thromboembolism
PAP smear	Papanicolaou smear	PTH	Parathyroid hormone
PARP	Poly ADP ribose polymerase	PTHrP	Parathyroid hormone-related peptide
PAT	Paroxysmal atrial tachycardia	PTSD	Posttraumatic stress disorder
PBI	Protein-bound iodine	PTT	Partial thromboplastin time
PBSCT	Peripheral blood stem cell transplantation	PTU	Propylthiouracil
PC	After meals (*post cibum*)	PUD	Peptic ulcer disease
PCA	Patient-controlled analgesia	PVC	Premature ventricular contraction
PCI	Percutaneous coronary intervention	PVD	Peripheral vascular disease
PCKD	Polycystic kidney disease	Q	Every (*quaque*)
PCN	Penicillin	QA	Quality assurance
PCOS	Polycystic ovarian syndrome	QD	Every day (*quaque die*)
PCP	Primary care physician; phencyclidine; *Pneumocystis* (*carinii*) *jirovecii* pneumonia	QI	Quality improvement
		QID	Four times daily (*quater in die*)
PCR	Polymerase chain reaction	QNS	Quantity not sufficient
PCV	Pneumococcal conjugate vaccine	QOD	Every other day
PCWP	Pulmonary capillary wedge pressure	QOL	Quality of life
PDA	Patent ductus arteriosus	QOLIE	Quality of Life in Epilepsy
PDE	Phosphodiesterase	QS	Quantity sufficient
PE	Physical examination; pulmonary embolism	R&M	Routine and microscopic
PEEP	Positive end-expiratory pressure	RA	Rheumatoid arthritis; right atrium
PEFR	Peak expiratory flow rate	RADT	Rapid antigen detection test
PEG	Percutaneous endoscopic gastrostomy; polyethylene glycol	RAIU	Radioactive iodine uptake
PERLA	Pupils equal, react to light and accommodation	RANKL	Receptor activator of nuclear factor-κβ ligand
PERRLA	Pupils equal, round, and reactive to light and accommodation	RAO	Right anterior oblique
		RASS	Richmond Agitation Sedation Scale
PET	Positron emission tomography	RBBB	Right bundle branch block
PFT	Pulmonary function test	RBC	Red blood cell
pH	Hydrogen ion concentration	RCA	Right coronary artery
PharmD	Doctor of Pharmacy	RCM	Right costal margin
PHQ	Patient health questionnaire	RCT	Randomized controlled trial
PI	Principal investigator; protease inhibitor	RDA	Recommended daily allowance
PICC	Peripherally inserted central catheter	RDP	Random donor platelets
PID	Pelvic inflammatory disease	RDS	Respiratory distress syndrome
PIP	Proximal interphalangeal	RDW	Red cell distribution width
PKU	Phenylketonuria	REM	Rapid eye movement
PLMS	Periodic limb movement of sleep	RES	Reticuloendothelial system
PMD	Private medical doctor	RF	Rheumatoid factor; renal failure; rheumatic fever
PMH	Past medical history	Rh	Rhesus factor in blood
PMI	Point of maximal impulse	RHD	Rheumatic heart disease
PMN	Polymorphonuclear leukocyte	RLE	Right lower extremity
PMP	Prescription monitoring program	RLL	Right lower lobe
PMS	Premenstrual syndrome	RLQ	Right lower quadrant (abdomen)
PNC-E	Postnecrotic cirrhosis-ethanol	RLS	Restless legs syndrome
PND	Paroxysmal nocturnal dyspnea	RML	Right middle lobe

RN	Registered nurse		SRMD	Stress-related mucosal damage
RNA	Ribonucleic acid		SSKI	Saturated solution of potassium iodide
R/O	Rule out		SSRI	Selective serotonin reuptake inhibitor
ROM	Range of motion		STAT	Immediately; at once
ROS	Review of systems		STD	Sexually transmitted disease
RPGN	Rapidly progressive glomerulonephritis		STEMI	ST-elevation myocardial infarction
RPh	Registered pharmacist		STI	Sexually transmitted infection
RPR	Rapid plasma reagin		SUA	Serum uric acid
RR	Respiratory rate; recovery room		SUP	Stress ulcer prophylaxis
RRMS	Relapsing-remitting multiple sclerosis		SV	Stroke volume
RRR	Regular rate and rhythm		SVC	Superior vena cava
RRT	Registered respiratory therapist		SVR	Supraventricular rhythm; systemic vascular resistance, sustained virologic response
RSE	Refractory status epilepticus		SVRI	Systemic vascular resistance index
RSV	Respiratory syncytial virus		SVT	Supraventricular tachycardia
RT	Radiation therapy		SW	Social worker
RTA	Renal tubular acidosis		SWI	Surgical wound infection
RTC	Return to clinic		Sx	Symptoms
RT-PCR	Reverse transcriptase-polymerase chain reaction		T	Temperature
RUE	Right upper extremity		T&A	Tonsillectomy and adenoidectomy
RUL	Right upper lobe		T&C	Type and crossmatch
RUQ	Right upper quadrant (abdomen)		TAH	Total abdominal hysterectomy
RVH	Right ventricular hypertrophy		TB	Tuberculosis
S_1	First heart sound		TBG	Thyroid-binding globulin
S_2	Second heart sound		TBI	Total body irradiation; traumatic brain injury
S_3	Third heart sound (ventricular gallop)		T. bili	Total bilirubin
S_4	Fourth heart sound (atrial gallop)		T/C	To consider
SA	Sinoatrial		TCA	Tricyclic antidepressant
SAAG	Serum ascites–albumin gradient		TCN	Tetracycline
SAD	Seasonal affective disorder		TED	Thromboembolic disease; thyroid eye disease
SAH	Subarachnoid hemorrhage		TEE	Transesophageal echocardiogram
SaO_2	Arterial oxygen percent saturation		TEN	Toxic epidermal necrolysis
SAS	Sedation-Agitation Scale		TENS	Transcutaneous electrical nerve stimulation
SBE	Subacute bacterial endocarditis		TFT	Thyroid function test
SBFT	Small bowel follow-through		TG	Triglyceride
SBGM	Self blood glucose monitoring		THA	Total hip arthroplasty
SBO	Small bowel obstruction		THC	Tetrahydrocannabinol
SBP	Systolic blood pressure; spontaneous bacterial peritonitis		TIA	Transient ischemic attack
SC	Subcutaneous; subclavian		TIBC	Total iron-binding capacity
SCD	Sequential compression device		TID	Three times daily (*ter in die*)
SCID	Severe combined immunodeficiency		TIH	Tumor-induced hypercalcemia
SCLC	Small cell lung cancer		TIPS	Transjugular intrahepatic portosystemic shunt
SCr	Serum creatinine		TKA	Total knee arthroplasty
SDP	Single donor platelets		TKI	Tyrosine kinase inhibitor
SEM	Systolic ejection murmur		TLC	Therapeutic lifestyle changes
SG	Specific gravity		TLI	Total lymphoid irradiation
SGOT	Serum glutamic oxaloacetic transaminase		TLS	Tumor lysis syndrome
SCT	Stem cell transplantation		TM	Tympanic membrane
SGLT	Sodium-glucose linked transporter		TMJ	Temporomandibular joint
SGPT	Serum glutamic pyruvic transaminase		TMP/SMX	Trimethoprim-sulfamethoxazole
SH	Social history		TMs	Tympanic membranes
SI/HI	Suicide ideation/homicide ideation		TNF	Tumor necrosis factor
SIADH	Syndrome of inappropriate antidiuretic hormone secretion		TnI	Troponin I (cardiac)
SIDS	Sudden infant death syndrome		TnT	Troponin T
SIMV	Synchronized intermittent mandatory ventilation		TNTC	Too numerous to count
SIRS	Systemic inflammatory response syndrome		TOD	Target organ damage
SJS	Stevens–Johnson syndrome		TPI	Trigger-point injection
SL	Sublingual		TPN	Total parenteral nutrition
SLE	Systemic lupus erythematosus		TPR	Temperature, pulse, respiration
SMART	Single maintenance and reliever therapy		T. prot	Total protein
SMBG	Self-monitoring of blood glucose		TRAb	Thyrotropin receptor antibodies
SNF	Skilled nursing facility		TSH	Thyroid-stimulating hormone
SNRI	Serotonin–norepinephrine reuptake inhibitor		TSS	Toxic shock syndrome
SNS	Sympathetic nervous system		TTP	Thrombotic thrombocytopenic purpura
SOB	Shortness of breath; side of bed		TUIP	Transurethral incision of the prostate
SOS	Sinusoidal obstruction syndrome		TURP	Transurethral resection of the prostate
S/P	Status post		TWD	Total weekly dose
SPEP	Serum protein electrophoresis		Tx	Treat; treatment
SPF	Sun protection factor		UA	Urinalysis; uric acid; unstable angina
SPMS	Secondary progressive multiple sclerosis		UC	Ulcerative colitis
SPS	Sodium polystyrene sulfonate		UCD	Usual childhood diseases
SR	Sustained release		UDS	Urine drug screen
SRI	Serotonin reuptake inhibitor			

UE	Upper extremity
UFC	Urinary-free cortisol
UFH	Unfractionated heparin
UGI	Upper gastrointestinal
UOQ	Upper outer quadrant
UPDRS	Unified Parkinson's Disease Rating Scale
UPT	Urine pregnancy test
URI	Upper respiratory infection
USP	United States Pharmacopeia
UTI	Urinary tract infection
UV	Ultraviolet
VA	Veterans' Affairs
VAMC	Veterans' Affairs Medical Center
VAP	Ventilator-associated pneumonia
VBL	Variceal band ligation
VDRL	Venereal Disease Research Laboratory
VEP	Visual evoked potential
VF	Ventricular fibrillation
VL	Viral load
VLDL	Very low-density lipoprotein
VNA	Visiting Nurses' Association

VO	Verbal order
VOD	Veno-occlusive disease
VP-16	Etoposide
V_A/Q	Ventilation/perfusion
VRE	Vancomycin-resistant *Enterococcus*
VS	Vital signs
VSS	Vital signs stable
VT	Ventricular tachycardia
VTE	Venous thromboembolism
WA	While awake
WBC	White blood cell
W/C	Wheelchair
WDWN	Well-developed, well-nourished
Wes ESR	Westergren erythrocyte sedimentation rate
WHO	World Health Organization
WNL	Within normal limits
W/U	Workup
Y-BOCS	Yale-Brown Obsessive–Compulsive Scale
yo	Year-old
yr	Year
ZDV	Zidovudine

PART II: PREVENT MEDICATION ERRORS BY AVOIDING DANGEROUS ABBREVIATIONS, SYMBOLS, AND DOSE DESIGNATIONS

Institute for Safe Medication Practices (ISMP)

The ISMP's list of error-prone abbreviations, symbols, and dose designations can be found here: *https://www.ismp.org/recommendations/error-prone-abbreviations-list*. These items have been reported to be frequently misinterpreted and involved in harmful medication errors. They should **NEVER** be used when communicating medical information. This includes internal communications, telephone/verbal prescriptions, computer-generated labels, labels for drug storage bins, medication administration records, as well as pharmacy and prescriber computer order entry screens.

116

VITAMIN B$_{12}$ DEFICIENCY

Seriously Lacking Motivation.................... Level II

Jon P. Wietholter, PharmD, BCPS, FCCP

CASE SUMMARY

A 55-year-old woman presents to an outpatient clinic with complaints of tongue pain, fatigue, paresthesias, anorexia, and early satiety. These complaints have bothered her for months to years, but she has recently noticed increased tongue swelling and pain. The physical exam and laboratory tests reveal findings consistent with vitamin B$_{12}$ deficiency including low hemoglobin, hematocrit, and vitamin B$_{12}$ level; elevated MCV and MCH; a low-grade fever; mild tachycardia; mild splenomegaly; and decreased pinprick, vibratory, and temperature sensations in the lower extremities. The peripheral blood smear showed abnormalities commonly seen in vitamin B$_{12}$ deficiency. Additionally, she is taking both metformin and omeprazole, which are potential causes of vitamin B$_{12}$ deficiency. Several options for replacement of vitamin B$_{12}$ are available, and intramuscular (IM), deep subcutaneous (SC), and oral replacement are all potential options for this patient.

QUESTIONS

Collect Information

1.a. **What subjective and objective information indicates the presence of vitamin B$_{12}$ deficiency?**

- Complaints of fatigue and lethargy[1,2]
- (+) red, smooth, swollen, sore tongue with loss of papillae (atrophic glossitis)[2,3]
- (+) paresthesias, and decreased pinprick, vibratory, and temperature sensations in both lower extremities[2,3]
- Decreased hemoglobin, hematocrit, and red blood cell (RBC) count[2,4]
- Decreased serum vitamin B$_{12}$ level
- Elevated MCV and MCH levels[1,4]
- Mild splenomegaly
- Persistent low-grade fever
- Mild tachycardia[1]
- Anorexia and early satiety (feels fuller more quickly when eating)
- Mild thrombocytopenia[1–3]

- Peripheral blood smear containing macro-ovalocytosis, hypersegmented granulocytes, large platelets, and macrocytic RBCs with megaloblastic changes[1,3]

1.b. **What additional information is needed to fully assess this patient's vitamin B$_{12}$ deficiency?**

- The main causes of cobalamin deficiency are pernicious anemia, insufficient nutritional vitamin B$_{12}$ intake, ileal disease and/or resection, medications, and food-cobalamin malabsorption usually caused by atrophic gastritis (typically caused by *Helicobacter pylori* infection or long-term antacid use).[1–3]
- Information about the patient's diet would be valuable. Humans are not able to synthesize vitamin B$_{12}$, so it must be provided in the diet.[1,3,4] Vitamin B$_{12}$ deficiency is more common in vegetarians and vegans due to lack of intake of meat, fish, and dairy products.[1,2]
- Knowing the length of time she has been taking her chronic medications would be helpful to determine whether metformin and/or omeprazole could be playing a role in her vitamin B$_{12}$ deficiency.[2,4]
- Currently, any vitamin B$_{12}$ level <150 pmol/L or <200 pg/mL is considered deficient.[2,4] Elevated homocysteine (>12 mmol/L) and methylmalonic acid (MMA) (>0.37 mmol/L) levels can also be used due to their increased sensitivity for cobalamin deficiency (95.9% and 98.4%, respectively); normal homocysteine and MMA levels exclude vitamin B$_{12}$ deficiency.[3–5] An MMA level has increased specificity for vitamin B$_{12}$ deficiency and is recommended in patients with borderline vitamin B$_{12}$ levels (<350 pg/mL).[1–3,6] A low serum holotranscobalamin (holoTC) level (<35 pmol/L) is the earliest marker of vitamin B$_{12}$ deficiency and more closely correlates with the biologically active fraction of vitamin B$_{12}$.[1,4,6]

Assess the Information

2.a. **Assess the severity of vitamin B$_{12}$ deficiency based on the subjective and objective information available.**

- The patient has clinically relevant vitamin B$_{12}$ deficiency of at least moderate severity due to atrophic glossitis and paresthesias.

2.b. **Create a list of the patient's drug therapy problems and prioritize them. Include assessment of medication appropriateness, effectiveness, safety, and patient adherence.**

- *Problem #1:* Vitamin B$_{12}$ deficiency that requires treatment with pharmacotherapy.
- *Problem #2:* Potential adverse drug reaction of vitamin B$_{12}$ deficiency possibly caused by metformin and/or omeprazole.[3,4]
- *Problem #3:* Controlled diabetes mellitus type 2 treated with metformin (A1C <7%).
- *Problem #4:* GERD treated with omeprazole with uncertain control based on available information.

Develop a Care Plan

3.a. What are the goals of pharmacotherapy for vitamin B$_{12}$ deficiency in this case?

- Reverse symptoms related to vitamin B$_{12}$ deficiency, if possible.
- Replenish vitamin B$_{12}$ stores.
- Correct abnormal laboratory values associated with vitamin B$_{12}$ deficiency anemia.
- Prevent further complications of vitamin B$_{12}$ deficiency via dietary changes and/or pharmacotherapy.

3.b. What nondrug therapies might be useful for this patient's vitamin B$_{12}$ deficiency?

- Increasing nutritional intake of vitamin B$_{12}$ is indicated if diet is deemed to be the source of her deficiency. It may take several years to develop a deficiency due to poor dietary intake or malabsorption.[1] Metabolic vitamin B$_{12}$ requirements are 2–5 mcg/day, and the recommended daily allowance for adults in the United States is 2.4–2.8 mcg/day.[1,2] Foods rich in vitamin B$_{12}$ include meat, fish, eggs, cheese, milk, and yogurt so increased consumption of these products should be recommended.
- Physical therapy and occupational therapy are valuable options in patients with problems related to balance, gait, or arm function. Assistance with ambulation might be needed in later stages of vitamin B$_{12}$ deficiency via a cane or walker.

3.c. What feasible pharmacotherapeutic options are available for treating vitamin B$_{12}$ deficiency?

- *Cyanocobalamin* and *hydroxocobalamin* are pharmacologic agents used to replete vitamin B$_{12}$. Cyanocobalamin is the preferred option and is available in parenteral and oral formulations.
- Traditional treatment for severe deficiency involves parenteral administration of vitamin B$_{12}$ via IM or deep SC injection as cyanocobalamin.[2] Various dosing regimens are used; one common schedule is to administer 1000 mcg IM daily for 1–2 weeks, then 1000 mcg IM weekly for 4–8 weeks, followed by 1000 mcg IM monthly thereafter. Some clinicians skip the daily portion and begin with 1000 mcg IM weekly for 1–2 months followed by 1000 mcg IM monthly thereafter; this facilitates adherence with therapy. Additionally, symptoms associated with longstanding vitamin B$_{12}$ deficiency may take several months to resolve, so daily injections are often seen as unnecessary.
- Oral cyanocobalamin administration is as effective as parenteral administration for replacing vitamin B$_{12}$ stores if given in adequate doses; it avoids the discomfort of chronic injections and is more economical.[5,7] The current dosing recommendation is 1000–2000 mcg orally daily for 1–2 weeks, followed by 1000 mcg daily thereafter.
- Sublingual, intranasal, and lozenge cyanocobalamin preparations are also available and can be used in vitamin B$_{12}$ deficiency. The recommended dose is 350–2000 mcg sublingually daily, 500 mcg inhaled in one nostril weekly, or 1000 mcg of lozenges daily.
- Hydroxocobalamin is only available parenterally, and the usual dose is 1000 mcg IM either every other day or weekly until vitamin B$_{12}$ deficiency is corrected, followed by 1000 mcg IM every 1–2 months thereafter.

3.d. Create an individualized, patient-centered, team-based care plan to optimize medication therapy for vitamin B$_{12}$ deficiency and other drug therapy problems. Include specific drugs, dosage forms, doses, schedules, and durations of therapy.

Problem #1: Vitamin B$_{12}$ deficiency that requires treatment with pharmacotherapy

- Based on the patient's presentation, it is appropriate to initiate cyanocobalamin therapy. Because she has numerous signs and symptoms of vitamin B$_{12}$ deficiency, an appropriate regimen would be cyanocobalamin 1000 mcg IM daily for 1 week, followed by 1000 mcg IM weekly for 4 weeks, followed by 1000 mcg IM monthly for the rest of her life. If the patient or her husband can administer the injections appropriately, therapy can be given at home.
- If the patient responds well to injectable therapy, it would be reasonable to switch to oral cyanocobalamin with a dose of 1000 mcg daily. If oral cyanocobalamin is chosen initially and she does not respond adequately, a switch to parenteral therapy is warranted.

Problem #2: Potential adverse drug reaction of vitamin B$_{12}$ deficiency possibly caused by metformin and/or omeprazole[3,4]

- Metformin is thought to cause vitamin B$_{12}$ deficiency through malabsorption in the ileum.[4] A systematic review also concluded that metformin reduced vitamin B$_{12}$ levels in a dose-dependent manner.[8]
- Prolonged use of acid suppression therapy with proton-pump inhibitors and H$_2$-receptor antagonists appears to be associated with vitamin B$_{12}$ deficiency due to impaired cobalamin release from dietary protein sources.[3–4]
- Because both metformin and omeprazole can contribute to vitamin B$_{12}$ deficiency, their continued use for her diabetes and GERD should be reassessed, as described further.

Problem #3: Controlled diabetes mellitus type 2 treated with metformin (A1C <7%)

- This patient's A1C is 6.8%, meeting the American Diabetes Association (ADA) target of <7%. However, use of metformin should be reassessed to determine if its benefit outweighs its risk for potential vitamin B$_{12}$ deficiency. Because her diabetes is controlled on the current regimen, it may be appropriate to continue metformin while replacing vitamin B$_{12}$; alternatively, one could discontinue the metformin and attempt to control her diabetes with a different oral agent not linked to vitamin B$_{12}$ deficiency.

Problem #4: GERD treated with omeprazole with uncertain control based on available information

- Because omeprazole may contribute to vitamin B$_{12}$ deficiency, the provider should assess how well controlled her GERD has been and, if possible, discontinue omeprazole. H$_2$-receptor antagonists are also associated with this problem, making chronic acid suppressive therapy problematic in this patient. If feasible, low-dose on-demand acid suppressive therapy may be more appropriate than chronic daily therapy. Simply replacing vitamin B$_{12}$ orally while continuing omeprazole would be another possible option; since oral cyanocobalamin is not protein-bound, its absorption should not be impaired by acid suppressive therapy.[4]

Implement the Care Plan

4.a. What information should be provided to the patient to enhance adherence, ensure successful therapy, and minimize adverse effects?

General instructions

- This medication is called vitamin B$_{12}$ or *cyanocobalamin*. Vitamin B$_{12}$ deficiency may occur because of inadequate dietary intake, pernicious anemia (an inability to absorb vitamin B$_{12}$ after dietary intake), stomach disorders, medications, infections, or prior surgery.

- It is important to continue using vitamin B$_{12}$ for as long as your provider indicates (which may be lifelong) to correct the deficiency and prevent its recurrence.

- Inform your provider of any prescription and/or nonprescription medications you have used to manage your symptoms. Also inform your provider if symptoms worsen significantly at any point during treatment.

- Store the medication away from heat, direct light, moisture, and children.

- During treatment with vitamin B$_{12}$, it may be necessary to have periodic laboratory testing performed to monitor how well you are responding.

Injectable cyanocobalamin

- If you are taking an injectable form of cyanocobalamin, you may need to receive your shots in your provider's office; alternatively, they may be given to you by a home care nurse or someone who has been trained to give the injections.

- If you are self-administering the injections, you will need appropriate-size needles and syringes and a container for proper disposal of needles after use. Injections should be given into a muscle (intramuscularly) with common locations being the gluteal (buttocks) or deltoid (upper arm) muscles.

- Vitamin B$_{12}$ injections should be protected from light.

- If a dose is missed, take the dose as soon as you remember and return to your normal schedule. If a provider is responsible for administering your shot, reschedule your appointment immediately. Do not take two doses of the medication at the same time.

Oral cyanocobalamin

- If you are using the lozenge or sublingual form of cyanocobalamin, place it under your tongue and allow it to melt. Some lozenges can be swallowed but should be held in your mouth for at least 30 seconds prior to swallowing.

Intranasal cyanocobalamin

- If you are using the intranasal form of cyanocobalamin, separate your weekly dose by at least 1 hour from any hot liquids. Before the initial intranasal dose, prime the device by pumping the unit until a spray appears. At that point, prime the device two more times before instilling the weekly dose into your nostril.

- Intranasal cyanocobalamin should be protected from light.

Adverse effects of cyanocobalamin

- Common adverse effects while using this medication include pain or irritation at the injection site (with the injectable form), headache, rhinitis, and GI upset. Serious adverse effects include hives, vision changes, chest tightness, or trouble breathing; contact your provider immediately if these occur,

4.b. Describe how care should be coordinated with other healthcare providers.

- The medical provider can educate the patient about vitamin B$_{12}$ deficiency and its prognosis. Follow-up visits should happen regularly, particularly early in the treatment course.

- A pharmacist can help with counseling on the cyanocobalamin product prescribed, including appropriate administration technique and common or serious adverse effects.

- Referral to a dietician may be beneficial if it is determined that the vitamin B$_{12}$ deficiency is due to a dietary cause.

- Referral to a physical or occupational therapist may be beneficial if the patient begins to have issues with balance, gait, or arm function.

- If symptoms continue or worsen despite appropriate pharmacotherapy, referral to a hematologist may be appropriate.[1]

Follow-Up: Monitor and Evaluate

5.   **Explain how to monitor and evaluate the care plan for medication appropriateness, effectiveness, safety, and patient adherence by using clinical and laboratory data, patient feedback, and other information.**

Medication appropriateness and effectiveness

- Reticulocytosis typically begins in 2–5 days and peaks at 1 week. Hemoglobin and hematocrit concentrations usually rise within 7–10 days, and hypersegmented neutrophils characteristically disappear in 1–2 weeks. Hematologic abnormalities should normalize within 2 months if vitamin B$_{12}$ deficiency is solely responsible (hemoglobin 12–16 g/dL for females and 13–18 g/dL for males).[2,3] If laboratory values do not normalize, patient adherence to the prescribed cyanocobalamin should be assessed and confirmed.

- Patients may subjectively improve within hours after cyanocobalamin therapy initiation. Complaints of weakness and fatigue should improve dramatically over the course of treatment. It is likely that the neurologic symptoms will also resolve over months, although this does not always occur.[2,3]

Medication safety

- Monitor the patient for the most common adverse effects of cyanocobalamin, which include headache, asthenia, GI upset, and rhinitis.

- Instruct the patient to contact her provider immediately if vision changes, wheezing, chest tightness, blue skin color, seizures, or swelling of the face, lips, tongue, or throat occur after administration.

- Monitor the patient for adverse effects associated with reticulocytosis, including hypokalemia due to increased potassium utilization in hematopoiesis. Rebound thrombocytosis may precipitate thrombotic events.

- Monitor complete blood counts and vitamin B$_{12}$ levels periodically. One strategy is to monitor the vitamin B$_{12}$ level 1 month after beginning replacement therapy and every 3–6 months thereafter. Annual follow-up evaluations have also been recommended.[5]

- It would be reasonable to monitor MMA and homocysteine levels in addition to the patient's serum vitamin B$_{12}$ level.[3,6]

Patient adherence

- Ask the patient if she has any difficulty getting medication refills on time or affording her medication.

- Ask how often she misses a dose and what action she takes when she does.

- Encourage the patient to keep all follow-up appointments with her healthcare providers.

REFERENCES

1. Green R. Vitamin B$_{12}$ deficiency from the perspective of a practicing hematologist. Blood. 2017;129(19):2603–2611.

2. Langan RC, Goodbred AJ. Vitamin B$_{12}$ deficiency: recognition and management. Am Fam Physician. 2017 Sep 15;96(6):384–389.

3. Briani C, Dalla Torre C, Citton V, et al. Cobalamin deficiency: clinical picture and radiological findings. Nutrients. 2013;5:4521–4539.

4. Miller JW. Proton pump inhibitors, H$_2$-receptor antagonists, metformin, and vitamin B-12 deficiency: clinical implications. Adv Nutr. 2018 Jul 1; 9(4):511S–518S.

5. Chan CQ, Low LL, Lee KH. Oral vitamin B$_{12}$ replacement for the treatment of pernicious anemia. Front Med. (Lausanne) 2016;3(38):1–6.

6. Oberley MJ, Yang DT. Laboratory testing for cobalamin deficiency in megaloblastic anemia. Am J Hematol. 2013;88:522–526.

7. Wang H, Li L, Qin LL, Song Y, Vidal-Alaball J, Liu TH. Oral vitamin B$_{12}$ versus intramuscular vitamin B$_{12}$ for vitamin B$_{12}$ deficiency. Cochrane Database Syst Rev. 2018 Mar 15;3(3):CD004655.

8. Liu Q, Li S, Quan H, Li J. Vitamin B$_{12}$ status in metformin treated patients: systematic review. PLoS One 2014;9(6):e100379. doi: 10.1371/journal.pone.0100379.

130

DIABETIC FOOT INFECTION

Let's Nail That Infection . . . . Level II

Renee-Claude Mercier, PharmD, BCPS-AQ ID, PhC, FCCP

Paulina Deming, PharmD, PhC

CASE SUMMARY

In this 67-year-old man with poorly controlled type 2 diabetes mellitus and several comorbid conditions, an ingrown toenail has become infected, causing significant erythema and swelling of the right foot with purulent discharge from the wound. Physical and laboratory findings, including an elevated white blood cell (WBC) count, erythrocyte sedimentation rate (ESR), and fever, suggest a potential systemic infection secondary to cellulitis. The patient undergoes incision and drainage of the lesion, and tissue is submitted to the laboratory for culture. Due to the presence of systemic signs of infection, empiric antimicrobial treatment must be initiated before results of wound culture and sensitivity testing are known. Because of the patient's comorbidities and the size and severity of the wound infection, parenteral antibiotic therapy should be initiated. In addition, acutely infected wounds are most commonly infected with virulent pathogens such as aerobic Gram-positive bacteria (especially *Staphylococcus aureus*). However, broad-spectrum coverage for Gram-negative and anaerobic bacteria should also be instituted due to the location of the wound (bottom of foot), its size and severity, foul-smelling drainage, and the patient's history of poorly controlled diabetes. This patient has risk factors for antibiotic-resistant organisms such as methicillin-resistant *Staphylococcus aureus* (MRSA) infection (ie, recent hospitalization and existing chronic illnesses), and empiric coverage of this organism should be considered. When tissue cultures are reported as positive for MRSA and *Bacteroides fragilis*, the reader is asked to narrow to more

specific therapy, which traditionally includes parenteral vancomycin or either oral or parenteral linezolid or tedizolid with anaerobic coverage (metronidazole or clindamycin). Second-line agents include daptomycin, telavancin, ceftaroline, oritavancin, or dalbavancin all in combination with a drug with anaerobic coverage (metronidazole or clindamycin). This infection will require 5–14 days of therapy, so the patient will most likely be discharged on outpatient antibiotic therapy. Once there are signs of clinical improvement with no evidence of systemic toxicity, antibiotics may be transitioned from parenteral to oral therapy. Although antimicrobial therapy may be completed as an outpatient, attention must be given to the patient's social and economic situation. Better glycemic control and education regarding techniques for proper foot care are important components of a comprehensive treatment plan for this patient.

QUESTIONS

Collect Information

1.a. **What subjective and objective information indicates the presence of a diabetic foot infection?**

- Swollen, sore, and red foot. Induration extending from first metatarsal to midfoot (4 × 5 cm)
- Purulent foul-smelling drainage with cellulitis
- 2+ edema of the foot increasing in amplitude
- Elevated WBC count ($17.3 \times 10^3/mm^3$)
- X-ray showing tissue swelling from first metatarsal to midfoot consistent with cellulitis

1.b. **What additional information is needed to fully assess this patient's diabetic foot infection?**

- Risk factors for infection in this patient include:
  ✓ Ingrown toenail; attempted self-treatment
  ✓ Poorly controlled diabetes
  ✓ Vascular calcifications in the foot per X-ray indicate a decreased blood supply
  ✓ Decreased sensation of bilateral lower extremities
  ✓ Poor foot care (presence of fungus and overgrown toenails)
  ✓ Recent hospitalization
- Deep culture of the wound for both anaerobes and aerobes:
  ✓ Common aerobic isolates: *S. aureus*, *Streptococcus* spp., *Enterococcus* spp., *Proteus mirabilis*, *Escherichia coli*, *Klebsiella* spp., and *Pseudomonas aeruginosa*.
  ✓ Common anaerobic isolates: *Peptostreptococcus* and *B. fragilis*.[1]

Assess the Information

2.a. **Assess the severity of the diabetic foot infection based on the subjective and objective information available.**

- **Mild:** Local infection involving only the skin and subcutaneous tissues without systemic signs. Erythema >0.5 cm and ≤2 cm.
- **Moderate:** Local infection with erythema >2 cm, or involving structures deeper than skin and subcutaneous tissues, and *no* systemic inflammatory response signs (SIRS).
- **Severe (this patient):** Local infection with SIRS, which includes at least two of the following:
  ✓ Temperature >38°C or <36°C
  ✓ Heart rate >90 bpm

✓ Respiratory rate >20 breaths/min or PaCO$_2$ <32 mm Hg

✓ WBC count >12,000 or <4000 cells/mcL or ≥10% immature forms

2.b. Create a list of the patient's drug therapy problems and prioritize them. Include assessment of medication appropriateness, effectiveness, safety, and patient adherence.

- *Problem #1:* Cellulitis and infection of the right foot in a patient with diabetes, requiring treatment.

- *Problem #2:* Poorly controlled type 2 diabetes mellitus despite therapy with three medications.

- *Problem #3:* Renal insufficiency secondary to diabetic nephropathy, treated appropriately with lisinopril but without available information on progression of renal disease.

- *Problem #4:* Dyslipidemia treated with atorvastatin but with no available information on the efficacy of therapy.

- *Problem #5:* Hypertension treated with lisinopril and currently controlled (blood pressure [BP] 126/79 mm Hg), but without information about long-term BP control.

2.c. What economic and psychosocial considerations are applicable to this patient?

- Poor adherence to current treatment for diabetes likely contributed to this situation. Lack of access to medical care, and challenges with health literacy may have contributed to nonadherence. Diabetic foot infections are complications of poorly controlled diabetes and hyperglycemia that can lead to neuropathy, decreased blood supply to extremities, and impaired immune status.

- A simplified drug regimen (monotherapy and less frequent dosing, whenever possible) should be selected because of his history of poor medication adherence. Addressing barriers to adherence will also be an important component of this patient's success with current treatment and prevention of future recurrence.

- The patient receives his healthcare primarily at First Choice Clinic, a Federally Qualified Health Center. This may become an important consideration in selecting his future therapeutic plan.

- For this patient to receive appropriate wound care and home IV therapy if judged necessary, the healthcare team must establish that his family or a home healthcare nurse will be able to provide assistance.

Develop a Care Plan

3.a. What are the goals of pharmacotherapy for diabetic foot infection in this case?

- Eradicate the bacteria.

- Prevent the development of osteomyelitis and the need for amputation.

- Preserve as much normal limb function as possible.

- Improve control of diabetes mellitus.

- Prevent infectious complications.

- Avoid adverse medication reactions.

3.b. What nondrug therapies might be useful for this patient's diabetic foot infection?

- Appropriate wound care by experienced podiatrists (incision and drainage, debridement of the wound, and toenail clipping), nurses (wound care, dressing changes of wound, and foot care teaching), and physical therapists (whirlpool treatments, wound debridement, and teaching about minimal weight bearing with a walker or crutches).

- Bed rest, minimal weight bearing, leg elevation, and control of edema.

- Proper education about wound care and the importance of good diabetes control, diet, glucometer use, adherence to the medication regimens, and foot care in this patient with diabetes.

3.c. What feasible pharmacotherapeutic options are available for the treatment of diabetic foot infection?

- Based on the most recent 2012 clinical practice guideline for the diagnosis and treatment of diabetic foot infections, treatment differs based on infection severity (mild vs moderate vs severe)[1]:

Mild

- Oral antimicrobial therapy may be used in mild, uncomplicated diabetic foot infections *only*.[1,2] The following agents could be considered preferred oral options because they target *S. aureus* and *Streptococcus* spp.:

  ✓ *Amoxicillin/clavulanate*

  ✓ *Dicloxacillin*

  ✓ *Clindamycin*

  ✓ *Cephalexin*

  ✓ *Levofloxacin*

- If MRSA coverage is needed, then use either *doxycycline, minocycline,* or *trimethoprim/sulfamethoxazole* (activity against streptococci is uncertain).

- Although these regimens cover the most likely causative organisms, it is important to note that except for levofloxacin none of the antibiotics given above cover *P. aeruginosa*.

Moderate/severe

- Treatment of *moderate* infection may be with oral agents or initial parenteral therapy while *severe* infections should be treated with parenteral agents at least until infection is controlled and signs of systemic infection have subsided.[1] Consider coverage for MSSA, streptococci, *Enterobacteriaceae*, and obligate anaerobes. Options for IV monotherapy include:

  ✓ *Piperacillin/tazobactam*

  ✓ *Imipenem/cilastatin*

  ✓ *Meropenem*

  ✓ *Cefepime* or *levofloxacin* could be used; however, additional coverage against obligate anaerobes should be considered with either *metronidazole* or *clindamycin*. *Levofloxacin* is also not optimal for *S. aureus* coverage.

- These agents cover all of the most likely causative organisms, including anaerobes and *P. aeruginosa*. However, imipenem/cilastatin is a potent β-lactamase inducer, so therapy with the other agents may be preferable initially.

- The following agents could also be used as IV therapy, but they do not cover *P. aeruginosa*:

  ✓ *Ampicillin/sulbactam*

  ✓ *Ertapenem*

  ✓ *Cefoxitin or cefotetan*

  ✓ Third-generation cephalosporin (*ceftriaxone/cefotaxime*) plus IV *clindamycin combination*

- A combination of *clindamycin IV* or *oral metronidazole* plus either *aztreonam* or *an oral* or *IV fluoroquinolone (ciprofloxacin* or *levofloxacin)* could be used in patients with moderate-to-severe infections who are allergic to penicillin and cephalosporins. *Moxifloxacin* is also now recommended for treatment of moderate infections and offers the advantage of once-daily dosing, no need of renal adjustments, and being relatively broad spectrum including most obligate anaerobic organisms. The use of clindamycin provides added coverage for MSSA as compared to metronidazole.

- MRSA may be a suspected causative organism in some cases. There are two genetically distinct types of MRSA that can be of concern in diabetic foot infections: community-associated MRSA (CA-MRSA) and healthcare-associated MRSA (HA-MRSA). While acquisition of HA-MRSA is associated with well-defined risk factors (history of prolonged hospital or nursing home stay, past antimicrobial use, indwelling catheters, pressure sores, surgery, or dialysis), risk factors for acquisition of CA-MRSA are not as well established. CA-MRSA is susceptible to more antibiotics than is HA-MRSA.[3]

- *Vancomycin IV, daptomycin IV, linezolid or tedizolid oral or IV, ceftaroline IV,[4] dalbavancin IV, or oritavancin IV* may be used if HA-MRSA is a suspected causative organism. Persons who are at high risk for HA-MRSA wound infection include those who: (a) have a previous history of HA-MRSA infection/colonization; (b) have positive nasal cultures for HA-MRSA; (c) have a recent history (within the past year) of prolonged hospitalization or intensive care unit stay; or (d) receive frequent and/or prolonged courses of broad-spectrum antibiotics.[5,6] Should the above-stated agents be used empirically, Gram-negative and anaerobic coverage will need to be added to provide adequate empiric coverage.

- Should CA-MRSA be more of a concern (eg, in a patient with no HA-MRSA risk factors who is admitted from an area where the CA-MRSA rate is relatively high), the antibiotic regimen should include any of those agents active against HA-MRSA or *clindamycin, sulfamethoxazole/trimethoprim, doxycycline or minocycline*.[3]

- Aminoglycosides should generally be avoided in diabetic patients because they are at increased risk for developing diabetic nephropathy and renal failure.

- *Becaplermin 0.01% gel (Regranex)* is FDA approved for treatment of diabetic ulcers on the lower limbs and feet. Becaplermin is a genetically engineered form of platelet-derived growth factor, a naturally occurring protein in the body that stimulates diabetic ulcer healing. It is to be used as adjunctive therapy, *in addition to* infection control and wound care. In one clinical trial, becaplermin applied once daily in combination with good wound care significantly increased the incidence of complete healing when compared with placebo gel (50% vs 35%, respectively). Becaplermin gel also significantly decreased the time to complete healing of diabetic ulcers by 32% (about 6 weeks faster). The incidence of adverse events, including infection and cellulitis, was similar in patients treated with becaplermin gel, placebo gel, or good diabetic wound care alone.[7] Further studies are needed to assess which patients might best benefit from becaplermin use, particularly considering its cost (average wholesale price $1200 per 15-gram tube).

3.d. **Create an individualized, patient-centered, team-based care plan to optimize medication therapy for diabetic foot infection and this patient's other drug therapy problems. Include specific drugs, dosage forms, doses, schedules, and durations of therapy.**

Problem #1: Cellulitis and infection of the right foot in a patient with diabetes, requiring treatment

- This diabetic foot infection has significant involvement of the skin and skin structures with deep tissue involvement.

Moreover, the area of cellulitis and induration exceeds 2 cm (4 × 5 cm). Because this is an acutely infected wound, aerobic Gram-positive bacteria (especially *S. aureus*) are the most likely causative organisms.[1] However, broad-spectrum coverage for Gram-negative and anaerobic bacteria should also be instituted due to the location of the wound (bottom of foot), foul-smelling discharge, its size and severity, and the patient's diabetes. This patient does have risk factors for HA-MRSA infection (ic, recent hospitalizations and existing chronic illnesses), and empiric coverage of this organism should be considered as well. Initial empiric IV therapy is recommended in severe diabetic foot infections such as this one.

- A number of treatment options are appropriate for empiric therapy of this patient's diabetic foot infection. Drug selection may be based on institutional cost and drug availability through the formulary system. Dosage should be adjusted for the patient's renal function, as appropriate. This patient's calculated creatinine clearance, based on total body weight (patient's weight is below ideal body weight), is 25 mL/min. Antimicrobial resistance within the area and based on patient's prior culture and susceptibility should also be taken into consideration when selecting an empiric regimen.[8]

- All antibiotic regimens appropriate for this patient include two or more antibiotics (one to cover HA-MRSA and other Gram-positive bacteria, and one or two to cover gram-negative and anaerobic bacteria). It would be best to limit it to no more than two antibiotics to optimize nursing ease and patient adherence and to minimize drug costs and toxicity. In most institutions, the patient would be started on vancomycin in addition to piperacillin/tazobactam as a first-line regimen. This is a dual therapy regimen that covers MRSA, gram-negative aerobic as well as anaerobic bacteria while reserving the carbapenems for use when necessary. There are concerns about increased renal toxicity associated with combined vancomycin and piperacillin/tazobactam use that warrant at least weekly to biweekly renal function monitoring.

- To cover MRSA, the preferred regimen due to experience and cost will often be:

  ✓ Vancomycin 1 g IV Q 48 H (or other dosing regimen to achieve vancomycin trough of 10–15 mg/L)

- To cover Gram-negative bacteria and anaerobes, the following agent is often preferred due to its spectrum and safety profile (dosed for renal dysfunction when indicated):

  ✓ Piperacillin/tazobactam 2.25 g IV Q 6 H

- Start tolnaftate 1% topical cream BID as a treatment for his athlete's foot fungal infection that may have served as a portal of entry for bacteria.

Problem #2: Poorly controlled type 2 diabetes mellitus despite therapy with three medications

- As evidenced by an A1C of 11.8% (goal <7%) and recent episode of hyperglycemic hyperosmolar state (HHS). Metformin is contraindicated in this patient due to his SCr of 2.4 mg/dL and eGFR <30 mL/min/1.73 m². However, his renal function may improve with hydration, and this should be monitored.

- Nonadherence with medication administration and home glucose monitoring.

- The patient's eGFR is <30 mL/min/1.73 m², which is a contraindication to metformin use; it should be discontinued. The insulin regimen with both short- and long-acting insulins should be optimized to make sure patient has access to both forms and knows how to use them appropriately with regular blood sugar monitoring. Daily journaling would help the medical provider make appropriate adjustment at future appointments.

Problem #3: Renal insufficiency, treated appropriately with lisinopril but without available information on progression of renal disease

- In light of the chronic kidney disease associated with diabetes, the patient is appropriately prescribed an angiotensin-converting inhibitor, lisinopril. He may also have a component of acute kidney injury due to current illness and would benefit from hydration. As renal function improves, vancomycin dosing should be adjusted based on blood concentration and piperacillin/tazobactam dose will need to increase accordingly as well.

- The patient's history of renal insufficiency should be assessed to determine the rate at which his renal function is declining.

Problem #4: Dyslipidemia treated with atorvastatin but with no available information on the efficacy of therapy

- At a future visit with his primary care provider, the most recent fasting lipid panel should be reviewed to assess the efficacy of the current regimen of atorvastatin 40 mg daily. If appropriate, another fasting lipid panel should be obtained. The patient should also be asked about his adherence with therapy and whether he is experiencing any potential adverse medication reactions.

Problem #5: Hypertension treated with lisinopril but without information about long-term BP control

- Although the current BP indicates control (BP 126/79 mm Hg), the history of long-term control is unavailable. At a future visit with the healthcare provider, the medical record should be reviewed to assess long-term control. The patient should also be asked about adherence to the current regimen of lisinopril 20 mg daily and whether he is experiencing any potential adverse medication reactions.

3.e. **What alternatives would be appropriate if the initial care plan for the infection fails or cannot be used?**

- To cover MRSA, if vancomycin cannot be used as first-line agent, then any one of the following agents is considered part of the preferred regimen:
  - ✓ Linezolid 600 mg PO Q 12 H; or
  - ✓ Tedizolid 200 mg PO Q 24 H; or
  - ✓ Daptomycin 240 mg IV Q 48 H is a second-line option.
  - ✓ Ceftaroline 300 mg IV Q 12 hours is also a second-line option (covers some common Gram-negative organisms).
  - ✓ Dalbavancin 1125 mg IV infused over 30 minutes as a single dose is a second-line option.
  - ✓ Oritavancin 1200 mg IV infused over 3 hours as a single dose is a second-line option (although dosing adjustment in severe renal impairment CrCl <30 mL/min has not been studied).
  - ✓ Telavancin (10 mg/kg [600 mg] Q 48 H) should be considered as a third-line option.

- To cover Gram-negative bacteria and anaerobes, piperacillin/tazobactam is often considered as first-line agent although any one of the following agents could be considered (dosed for renal dysfunction when indicated):
  - ✓ Ampicillin/sulbactam 3 g IV Q 8 H
  - ✓ Ertapenem 500 mg IV Q 24 H
  - ✓ Imipenem/cilastatin 250 mg IV Q 6 H
  - ✓ Meropenem 1 g IV Q 12 H

- Other acceptable IV alternatives for Gram-negative and anaerobic coverage, with dose adjustments appropriate for the patient's renal function, include the combination of either clindamycin or metronidazole plus either a third- or fourth-generation cephalosporin (ceftazidime or cefepime), aztreonam, or a fluoroquinolone. However, this would cause the patient to be on a three-drug empiric regimen (including the antibiotic active against HA-MRSA), which may be costlier, inconvenient, and associated with more adverse drug reactions than monotherapy or dual therapy options (eg, clindamycin, fluoroquinolones, and cephalosporins are more highly associated with *Clostridioides difficile* colitis than other antibiotics).

Implement the Care Plan

4.a. **What information should be provided to the patient to enhance adherence, ensure successful therapy, and minimize adverse effects?**

- A home health nurse will come to your home to show you and your family how the infusion set works.

- We will need to see you in the clinic each week to make sure the antibiotic is working. At these visits, we will draw some blood so that we can check for adverse medication reactions.

- Vancomycin should be infused slowly, over 1–2 hours, to prevent flushing and BP decreases that are associated with rapid infusion.

- Contact your physician or me if any adverse medication reactions, such as rash, shortness of breath, diminished hearing or ringing in the ears, or decreased urine production, occur while taking this medicine.

- Contact your home healthcare provider if pain, redness, or swelling is observed at the IV site.

- Avoid alcohol intake as you may experience a significant drug interaction with metronidazole that could be characterized by intense flushing, breathlessness, headache, increased or irregular heart rate, low BP, nausea, and vomiting.

- *Note:* The patient needs to be made aware that osteomyelitis and limb amputation are possible consequences of these infections in diabetic patients. He also needs to be provided with personnel resources (telephone numbers and addresses) to contact if unusual reactions occur while on therapy, if infection worsens, or if he has questions or concerns. Adherence to outpatient clinic follow-up visits is of prime importance for success in this case.

4.b. **Describe how care should be coordinated with other healthcare providers.**

- The patient's primary care provider will need to follow up for management of diabetes, hypertension, and dyslipidemia as well as medication adherence. An appointment with the provider should occur within the next 2–3 weeks after release from the hospital to adjust the patient's medication as necessary and address any barriers to adherence.

- Pharmacists are often available within several days from hospital discharge in primary care clinics to help with medication reconciliation and medication therapy management, which can decrease the burden on other primary care providers who have limited appointment availability. Pharmacists may also be able to assist with applicable patient assistance programs to facilitate drug acquisition and adherence. The primary care provider and pharmacist should emphasize education and the importance of adherence at every visit.

- Scheduling a meeting with a diabetes educator while in the hospital may facilitate adherence postdischarge.
- An infectious disease consult in the hospital will be beneficial to help coordinate with the outpatient parenteral antimicrobial clinic to complete IV antibiotic in the outpatient setting if selected to complete the course. The patient should be seen in the outpatient parenteral antimicrobial therapy (OPAT) clinic within 1 week after discharge.
- Referral to a wound care specialist will be required upon discharge from the hospital for appropriate debridement of the wound and dressing changes.

Follow-Up: Monitor and Evaluate

5. **Explain how to monitor and evaluate the care plan for medication appropriateness, effectiveness, safety, and patient adherence by using clinical and laboratory data, patient feedback, and other information.**

Medication appropriateness and effectiveness

- Regardless of the drug chosen, improvement in the signs and symptoms of infection and healing of the wound with prevention of limb amputation are the primary endpoints.
- Observe for decreased swelling, induration, and erythema. Improvement should be observed after 72–96 hours of appropriate antimicrobial therapy and surgical debridement.
- A decrease in cloudy drainage and formation of new scar tissue are signs of positive response to therapy that may take as long as 7–14 days to be seen.
- Obtain a WBC count and differential every 48–72 hours for the first week or until normalization if <1 week, and weekly thereafter until the end of therapy. Continue monitoring until therapy is completed because neutropenia is associated with many antibiotics (eg, ampicillin/sulbactam, vancomycin).
- ESR and CRP are excellent makers of inflammation to follow while on therapy. Baseline levels then weekly levels should be drawn; normalization of the levels is anticipated by the end of therapy and are predictors of positive outcomes.
- Assess the patient's infection daily for changes in swelling, induration, and erythema. Measure temperature at least twice daily and obtain a WBC count daily if it was initially increased. Improvements in these physical signs and laboratory parameters should be observed after 72–96 hours of appropriate antimicrobial therapy and surgical debridement. If the area of swelling and erythema increases, or if response to therapy appears inadequate, it may be necessary to broaden therapy so that Gram-negative bacteria are covered as well. Response to therapy is often patient-dependent, and in some cases, improvement may not be seen until after 7–10 days of treatment.
- The duration of therapy is controversial. The latest guidelines recommend continuing antibiotic therapy until, but not beyond, resolution of all signs and symptoms of infection, but not through complete healing of the wound. Treatment as short as 5 days have been recommended although wound healing in diabetic patients is often very slow. Therapy should be continued for at least 2 weeks total in severe infection.
- The patient should remain hospitalized until he is afebrile for 24–48 hours, has signs of improvement and positive response to therapy (decreased swelling, redness, purulent drainage; normalization of the WBC, ESR, or CRP), and outpatient wound care has been established, either by proper teaching to the patient (and his family) or through home healthcare services.

- The patient should be seen in clinic at least once weekly while on therapy to assess therapeutic efficacy and safety. At each visit, a CBC should be obtained to evaluate for vancomycin-associated neutropenia or thrombocytopenia. An SCr should be obtained as well, and if any significant changes in renal function are observed, the vancomycin dose should be adjusted or the drug stopped and changed to a nonnephrotoxic agent. An ESR or CRP should be monitored weekly as a marker of inflammation and response to therapy.

Medication safety

- Vancomycin used at high dose (trough goal of 15–20 mg/L) has been associated with higher incidence of renal dysfunction, and patient already has an impaired renal function that increases the risk. Routine weekly SCr levels may be recommended to prevent vancomycin-associated nephrotoxicity and ototoxicity that can develop with accumulation of the drug should the patient's renal function worsen. It would be reasonable to order a weekly vancomycin trough level also to ensure that an adequate trough level (~10–15 mg/L) is being achieved. Several healthcare systems have now adopted area under the curve (AUC) as the preferred monitoring parameter to optimize vancomycin efficacy and safety and levels should be obtained according to hospital protocols adjusting for AUC of 400–600 mg*hr/L for MRSA infections.
- Question the patient to detect any adverse medication reactions related to the drug or infusion (eg, rash, nausea, vomiting, and diarrhea) daily for the first 3–5 days and then weekly thereafter.

Patient adherence

- A thorough review of medication adherence using patient self-report, pill count, or refill history, medication tolerability, and associated adverse medication reactions should be performed at each patient visit.

■ FOLLOW-UP CASE QUESTIONS

1. **What therapeutic alternatives are available for treating this patient after results of cultures are known to contain MRSA and *B. fragilis*?**
   - Once the culture results are available and the involved organism(s) is (are) considered pathogenic and responsible for the infectious process, therapy should be targeted at the specific organism(s).
     - ✓ Vancomycin given IV is often considered the drug of choice for skin and soft tissue infections caused by MRSA, as it has established efficacy, is generally well tolerated, and is inexpensive.
     - ✓ Linezolid is an effective treatment for MRSA skin and soft tissue infections and has the advantage of oral administration, but it is expensive. A weekly CBC must be obtained from patients receiving linezolid because it carries a significant risk of thrombocytopenia that may require treatment discontinuation (0.3–10.0%).
     - ✓ Daptomycin is a lipopeptide antibiotic approved for treatment of complicated skin and soft tissue infections due to susceptible organisms including MRSA. It is expensive and is generally restricted to prevent the development of resistance.
     - ✓ Telavancin has been approved for treatment of complicated skin and soft tissue infections due to susceptible organisms including MRSA. It is fairly expensive, has been associated with renal dysfunction, and should be reserved for resistant bacteria or failure of first- and second-line therapy.

✓ Ceftaroline has been approved for the treatment of complicated skin and soft tissue infections due to susceptible organisms including MRSA. It covers *Enterobacteriaceae* but lacks coverage against anaerobes, extended-spectrum β-lactamase (ESBL), AmpC β-lactamase or *Klebsiella pneumoniae* carbapenemase (KPC) producing strains, and *P. aeruginosa*. It is administered at least twice daily, but it lacks data in diabetic foot infection and should be reserved for patients failing first-line agents.

✓ Dalbavancin and oritavancin are approved as single-dose IV agents for treatment of acute bacterial skin and soft tissue infection caused by Gram-positive bacteria. Neither agent has activity against Gram-negative organisms. Oritavancin must be infused over 3 hours compared to 30 minutes for dalbavancin. Both agents are well tolerated, although oritavancin has more drug and laboratory interactions than dalbavancin and it has not yet been studied in patients who have a CrCl of approximately 25 mL/min. Both agents are also very expensive.

- None of the above agents has anaerobic coverage, and therefore metronidazole or clindamycin will need to be added. Either agent could be used orally or parentrally. Metronidazole may be associated with a disulfiram reaction if the patient consumes alcohol again. Liver enzymes should be monitored at baseline and then weekly while on metronidazole and with clindamycin in patients with severe hepatic disease. Clindamycin has an increased risk of *C. difficile* colitis.

- Evidence for oral therapy as an acceptable alternative has been growing over the last few years with reports such as the OVIVA trial which supported oral treatment in bone and joint infections.[9] Treatment with trimethoprim/sulfamethoxazole, doxycycline or minocycline combined with either metronidazole or clindamycin would also be considered appropriate after resolution of all systemic signs of infections as described above.

2. Design an optimal drug treatment plan for treating the mixed infection while he remains hospitalized.

- The patient's therapy should be streamlined to vancomycin 1 g IV Q 48 H (per renal function). After the third dose, a vancomycin trough level should be recommended and therapy adjusted to maintain a trough ≥10 mg/L. Metronidazole 500 mg PO Q 8 H should be initiated to cover the *B. fragilis*.

3. Design an optimal pharmacotherapeutic plan for completion of treatment after he is discharged from the hospital.

- The decision about completion of therapy with IV versus oral therapy is often based on clinical experience because few clinical trials have been performed on long-term treatment of diabetic foot infections.[9,10]

- In this patient, determination of IV vs oral therapy will depend on patient's ability to receive IV therapy at home based on resources available for the patient. If possible, due to decreased blood supply and uncontrolled diabetes, continued use of IV vancomycin would probably be the best choice. Either the drug could be infused at home, most likely with the wife's or daughter's assistance and frequent nursing care visits, or the patient may be required to visit a home infusion clinic to receive therapy, depending on what is economically feasible. Discharge planning should be involved in this case to ensure a smooth transition to outpatient therapy.

REFERENCES

1. Lipsky BA, Berendt AR, Cornia PB, et al. 2012 Infectious Diseases Society of America clinical practice guideline for the diagnosis and treatment of diabetic foot infections. Clin Infect Dis. 2012;54:132–173.
2. Levin ME. Management of the diabetic foot: preventing amputation. South Med J. 2002;95:10–20.
3. Echániz-Aviles G, Velazquez-Meza ME, Vazquez-Larios Mdel R, Soto-Noguerón A, Hernández-Dueñas AM. Diabetic foot infection caused by community-associated methicillin-resistant *Staphylococcus aureus* (USA300). J Diabetes. 2015;7(6):891–892.
4. Lipsky BA, Cannon CM, Ramani A, et al. Ceftaroline fosamil for treatment of diabetic foot infections: the CAPTURE study experience. Diabetes Metab Res Rev. 2015;31(4):395–401.
5. Lipsky BA, Tabak YP, Johannes RS, Vo L, Hyde L, Weigelt JA. Skin and soft tissue infections in hospitalised patients with diabetes: culture isolates and risk factors associated with mortality, length of stay and cost. Diabetologia. 2010;53:914–923.
6. Liu C, Bayer A, Cosgrove SE, et al. Clinical practice guidelines by the Infectious Diseases Society of America for the treatment of methicillin-resistant *Staphylococcus aureus* infections in adults and children. Clin Infect Dis. 2011;52:1–38.
7. Martí-Carvajal AJ, Gluud C, Nicola S, et al. Growth factors for treating diabetic foot ulcers. Cochrane Database Syst Rev. 2015;10: CD008548.
8. Guillamet CV, Kollef MH. How to stratify patients at risk for resistant bugs in skin and soft tissue infections? Curr Opin Infect Dis. 2016;29(2): 116–123.
9. Li HK, Rombach I, Zambellas R, et al. Oral versus intravenous antibiotics for bone and joint infection. N Engl J Med. 2019;380:425–436.
10. Nicolau DP, Stein GE. Therapeutic options for diabetic foot infections: a review with an emphasis on tissue penetration characteristics. J Am Podiatr Med Assoc. 2010;100:52–63.